Cone Beam Computed Tomography in Orthodontics: Indications, Insights, and Innovations

Cone Beam Computed Tomography in Orthodontics: Indications, Insights, and Innovations

Sunil D. Kapila, BDS, MS, PhD

Robert W. Browne Endowed Professor and Chair
Department of Orthodontics and Pediatric Dentistry
The University of Michigan School of Dentistry
Ann Arbor, Michigan

WILEY Blackwell

Wiley-Blackwell is an imprint of John Wiley & Sons, formed by the merger of Wiley's global Scientific, Technical and Medical business with Blackwell Publishing.

Editorial offices: 2121 State Avenue, Ames, Iowa 50014-8300, USA
The Atrium, Southern Gate, Chichester, West Sussex, PO19 8SQ, UK
9600 Garsington Road, Oxford, OX4 2DQ, UK

For details of our global editorial offices, for customer services and for information about how to apply for permission to reuse the copyright material in this book please see our website at www.wiley.com/wiley-blackwell.

Library of Congress Cataloging-in-Publication Data
Cone beam computed tomography in orthodontics : indications, insights, and innovations / [edited by] Sunil Kapila.
p. ; cm.
Includes bibliographical references and index.
ISBN 978-1-118-44848-9 (hardback)
I. Kapila, Sunil (Sunil D.), 1958– , editor.
[DNLM: 1. Cone-Beam Computed Tomography–methods. 2. Orthodontics–methods. 3. Malocclusion–radiography. 4. Radiography, Dental–methods. WU 400]
RK523
617.6'43075722–dc23
2014032720

A catalogue record for this book is available from the British Library.

Wiley also publishes its books in a variety of electronic formats. Some content that appears in print may not be available in electronic books.

Cover images supplied by Sebastian Baumgaertel, Sunil D. Kapila, Birte Melsen, and Michel Dalstra
Cover design by Andy Meaden

Set in 9.5/11.5 pt PalatinoLTStd-Roman by Toppan Best-set Premedia Limited
Printed and bound in Singapore by Markono Print Media Pte Ltd

1 2014

To my wife, Yvonne, and our children Anjuli, Sahil, and
Simran for their unconditional love and support.
To my father, Dharam Inder, and late mother, Ved Kumari,
for their nurturing guidance and numerous sacrifices.

Contents

List of Contributors

Abeer AlHadidi, DDS, MS, Dipl ABOMR
Assistant Professor
Faculty of Dentistry
University of Jordan
Amman, Jordan

Christos Angelopoulos, DDS, MS
Adjunct Professor
Oral and Maxillofacial Imaging
Columbia University
College of Dental Medicine
New York City, New York

Rajiv Balachandran, BDS, MDS
Senior Resident
Division of Orthodontics and Dentofacial Deformities
Centre for Dental Education and Research
All India Institute of Medical Sciences
New Delhi, India

Sebastian Baumgaertel, DMD, MSD, FRDC(C)
Clinical Associate Professor
Department of Orthodontics
School of Dental Medicine
Case Western Reserve University
Cleveland, Ohio

Erika Benavides, DDS, PhD
Clinical Assistant Professor
Department of Periodontics and Oral Medicine
Division of Pathology, Medicine and Radiology
School of Dentistry
The University of Michigan
Ann Arbor, Michigan

Sharon L. Brooks, DDS, MS
Professor Emerita
School of Dentistry
The University of Michigan
Ann Arbor, Michigan

Paolo M. Cattaneo, MSc, PhD
Associate Professor
Orthodontics
Department of Dentistry
Aarhus University
Denmark

Lucia H.S. Cevidanes, DDS, MS, PhD
Assistant Professor
Department of Orthodontics and Pediatric Dentistry
School of Dentistry
The University of Michigan
Ann Arbor, Michigan

R. Scott Conley, DMD
Robert W. Browne Endowed Professor of Dentistry
Clinical Associate Professor & Graduate Clinic Director
Department of Orthodontics and Pediatric Dentistry
School of Dentistry
The University of Michigan
Ann Arbor, Michigan

Michel Dalstra, MSc, PhD
Associate Professor
Orthodontics
Department of Dentistry
Aarhus University
Aarhus, Denmark

Paul C. Edwards, MSc, DDS, FRCD(C)
Professor
Department of Oral Pathology, Medicine and Radiology
School of Dentistry
Indiana University
Indianapolis, Indiana

Sean P. Edwards, DDS, MD, FRCD(C)
Clinical Associate Professor of Dentistry
Chief, Pediatric Oral and Maxillofacial Surgery
CS Mott Children's Hospital
Residency Program Director
Section of Oral and Maxillofacial Surgery
Department of Surgery
The University of Michigan Medical Center
Ann Arbor, Michigan

Carla A. Evans, DDS, DMSc
Professor and Department Head
Department of Orthodontics
College of Dentistry
University of Illinois at Chicago
Chicago, Illinois

Carlos Flores-Mir, DDS, MSc, DSc, FRCD(C)
Associate Professor and Head
Division of Orthodontics
University of Alberta
Alberta, Canada

Bernard Friedland, BChD, MSc, JD
Director, Predoctoral Program in Oral Radiology
Assistant Professor of Oral Medicine, Infection, and Immunity
Harvard School of Dental Medicine
Boston, Massachusetts

Anna-Kari Hajati, DDS, PhD
Private Practitioner
Stockholm, Sweden

Mark G. Hans, DDS, MSD
Chair, Department of Orthodontics
School of Dental Medicine
Case Western Reserve University
Cleveland, Ohio

Bruce S. Haskell, DMD, MA, PhD
Clinical Professor of Orthodontics
University of Louisville
Louisville, Kentucky

Laura Iwasaki, DDS, MSc, PhD
Associate Professor and Leo A. Rogers Chair
Department of Orthodontics and Dentofacial Orthopedics
University of Missouri—Kansas City
Kansas City, Missouri

Bin Jiang, MD
Associate Professor
Department of Radiology
Beijing Tongren Hospital
Capital Medical University
Beijing, China

Devasenathipathy Kandasamy, MD, DNB, FRCR
Assistant Professor
Department of Radiodiagnosis
All India Institute of Medical Sciences
New Delhi, India

Sunil D. Kapila, BDS, MS, PhD
Robert W. Browne Endowed Professor and Chair
Department of Orthodontics and Pediatric Dentistry
Graduate Orthodontics Program Director
School of Dentistry
The University of Michigan
Ann Arbor, Michigan

Om P. Kharbanda, BDS, MDS, M Orth RCS, M MEd, FDS RCS Hon
Professor and Head
Division of Orthodontics and Dentofacial Deformities
Centre for Dental Education and Research
All India Institute of Medical Sciences
New Delhi, India

Yoon-Ji R. Kim, DDS, MSD, PhD
Clinical Instructor
Department of Orthodontics
Kangdong Sacred Heart Hospital
Hallym University Medical Center
Seoul, Korea

Leonardo Koerich de Paula, MS, DDS
Department of Orthodontics
Federal University of Rio de Janeiro
Rio de Janeiro, Brazil

John B. Ludlow, DDS, MS
Professor of Oral and Maxillofacial Radiology
North Carolina Oral Health Institute
University of North Carolina
Chapel Hill, North Carolina

Birte Melsen, DDS, Certified Specialist in Orthodontics, Dr. Ordont.
Emeritus Professor
Department of Orthodontics
Aarhus University
Aarhus, Denmark

Aaron D. Molen, DDS, MS
Lecturer
Section of Orthodontics
Division of Associated Clinical Specialties
University of California, Los Angeles
School of Dentistry
Los Angeles, California
Private Practice
Auburn, Washington

Jeanne M. Nervina, DMD, PhD
Adjunct Assistant Professor
Department of Orthodontics and Pediatric Dentistry
School of Dentistry
The University of Michigan
Ann Arbor, Michigan

Tung Nguyen, DMD, MS
Assistant Professor
Department of Orthodontics
University of North Carolina
Chapel Hill, North Carolina

Jeffrey C. Nickel, DMD, MSc, PhD, MRCD (C), Dipl ABO
Associate Professor and Director
Advanced Education Program in Orthodontics and Dentofacial Orthopedics
Department of Orthodontics and Dentofacial Orthopedics
Department of Oral Biology
School of Dentistry
University of Missouri—Kansas City
Kansas City, Missouri

Snehlata Oberoi, DDS, MDS
Associate Professor of Clinical Orofacial Sciences
Center for Craniofacial Anomalies
University of California, San Francisco
San Francisco, California

Juan Martin Palomo, DDS, MSD
Associate Professor and Program Director
Department of Orthodontics
Director, Craniofacial Imaging Center
School of Dental Medicine
Case Western Reserve University
Cleveland, Ohio

Beatriz Paniagua, PhD
Research Assistant Professor
Psychiatry
University of North Carolina at Chapel Hill
Chapel Hill, North Carolina

Yang-Ho Park, DDS, MSD, PhD
Professor
Department of Orthodontics
Kangdong Sacred Heart Hospital
Hallym University Medical Center
Seoul, Korea

William C. Scarfe, BDS, FRACDS, MS
Professor
Oral and Maxillofacial Radiology
University of Louisville School of Dentistry
Louisville, Kentucky

Kirt E. Simmons, DDS, PhD
Director, Craniofacial and Special Needs Orthodontics
Arkansas Children's Hospital
University of Arkansas for Medical Sciences
Little Rock, Arkansas

Manish Valiathan, DDS, MSD
Associate Professor,
Department of Orthodontics
Director, Surgical and Craniofacial Fellowship Program
School of Dental Medicine
Case Western Reserve University
Cleveland, Ohio

Michael W. Vannier, MD
Professor
Department of Radiology
University of Chicago
Chicago, Illinois

Karin Vargervik, DDS
Larry L. Hillblom Distinguished Professor in Craniofacial Anomalies
Director, UCSF Center for Craniofacial Anomalies
University of California, San Francisco
San Francisco, California

Neeraj Wadhawan, BDS, MDS
Senior Research Officer
Department of Orthodontics and Dentofacial Deformities
Centre for Dental Education and Research
All India Institute of Medical Sciences
New Delhi, India

Preface

Since its introduction to dentistry slightly over a decade ago, cone beam computed tomography (CBCT) has undergone a rapid evolution and considerable integration into orthodontics. However, despite the rapidly increasing popularity of CBCT and progress in applying it to clinical orthodontics, the profession has lacked a cohesive, comprehensive, and objective reference that provides clinicians with the background needed to utilize this technology optimally for treating their patients. Also, the specific indications and protocols for acquiring CBCT images and extracting appropriate clinical information have not been resolved fully. This textbook provides timely, impartial, and state-of-the-art information on the indications and protocols for CBCT imaging in orthodontics, clinical insights gained from these images, and innovations driven by these insights. As such, it is the most current and authoritative textbook on CBCT in orthodontics.

The book is organized to progress sequentially through specific topics so as to build the knowledgebase logically in this important and rapidly evolving field.

- **Part 1** on *Technology Assessment and Enhancements* provides the foundational information on CBCT technology, radiation exposure and risks, the transition from 2D to 3D imaging, and emerging technologies and future evolutions in computed tomography.
- **Part 2** contains chapters describing the *Protocols and Principles for CBCT Imaging in Orthodontics* that focus on developing evidence-based criteria for CBCT imaging, the medico-legal implications of CBCT to the professional, and the protocols and integration of this technology in orthodontic practice.
- **Part 3** provides critical information on CBCT-based *Diagnosis and Treatment Planning* that includes how to interpret CBCT scans and identify incidental pathologies, and the evolving discoveries and possible uses of CBCT to assess the temporomandibular joint, airway, and dentoalveolar boundary conditions.
- **Part 4** covers practical aspects of CBCT's *Clinical Applications and Treatment Outcomes* and encompasses a range of topics including root morphology and position, impacted and transposed teeth, rapid palatal expansion, outcomes with bone anchored maxillary protraction, temporary anchorage devices, virtual surgical treatment planning and outcomes, facial asymmetries, and craniofacial anomalies.

In reading the book, it will become evident that the insights gained from CBCT are contributing to novel or refined approaches to diagnosis, treatment, and biomechanics planning; assessment of treatment outcomes; and identifying opportunities for novel areas of research. Indeed, future evolutions in CBCT technology and improvements in the clinician's ability to extract and utilize clinically important information contained within the image dataset likely will lead to enhanced treatment outcomes and efficiencies in a broader spectrum of cases than currently possible.

The many authors who contributed to this book include recognized authorities in CBCT and 3D imaging, several of whom also have expertise in specific aspects of orthodontic treatment. They comprise oral maxillofacial radiologists, orthodontists, medical radiologists, engineers, oral and maxillofacial surgeons, and an oral pathologist. In addition to invited manuscripts from these experts, this volume includes chapters and videos of presentations given by well-known authorities in this field at the 39th Annual Moyers Symposium and the 38th Annual International Conference on Craniofacial Research (Presymposium). I believe that readers will find this book and accompanying DVDs a valuable resource for the appropriate and optimized application of CBCT to patient care and research.

Sunil D. Kapila, BDS, MS, PhD
Robert W. Browne Endowed Professor and Chair
Department of Orthodontics
and Pediatric Dentistry
Graduate Orthodontics Program Director
School of Dentistry
The University of Michigan
Ann Arbor, Michigan

Acknowledgments

This book and videos are a culmination of the efforts of a group of individuals without whose support this project would not have been brought to fruition. Among these individuals are Ms. Kris De Koster, who was instrumental in editing the chapters, tables, and figures, and assuring their quality for publication; Dr. Michael Rudolph, who videographed, edited, and formatted the presentations for the DVDs; all the manuscript authors and presenters at the Moyers Symposium and the Presymposium whose knowledge and contributions in the field of cone beam computed tomography (CBCT) make this an invaluable book to orthodontists and other clinicians who utilize this technology in patient care and research; the moderators at the Moyers Symposium and Presymposium—Drs. Lucia Cevidanes, Scott Conley, Nan Hatch, James McNamara Jr., Jeanne Nervina, William Scarfe, and Kirt Simmons—whose active participation made for a highly stimulating meeting; and Dr. Allan Farman, for his dedicated efforts in helping organize the 39th Annual Moyers Symposium. I am very grateful for their varied contributions and support in helping to bring this worthwhile endeavor to completion.

S.D.K.

Cone Beam Computed Tomography in Orthodontics: Indications, Insights, and Innovations

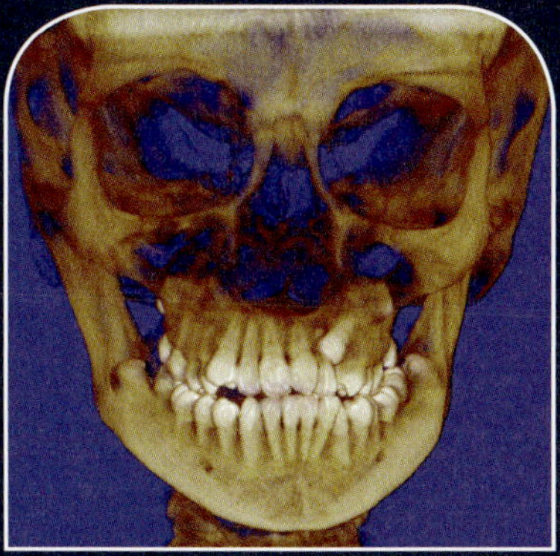
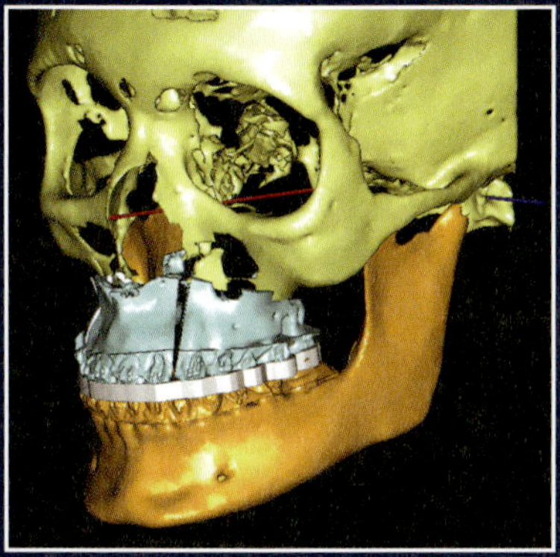

PART 1
Technology Assessment and Enhancements

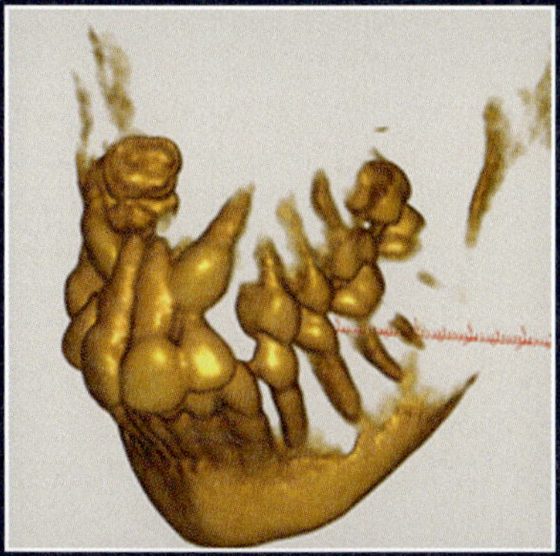
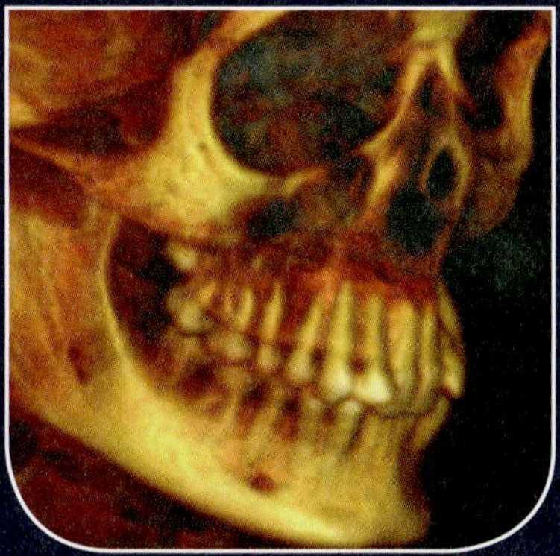

1 Contemporary Concepts of Cone Beam Computed Tomography in Orthodontics

Sunil D. Kapila, BDS, MS, PhD

INTRODUCTION

Truly transformative innovations are rare in most fields, but their emergence can generate a buzz that reverberates across disciplines. This is true especially in medicine and dentistry, which would stagnate without groundbreaking technologies that improve diagnosis, treatment planning, and prevention of disease. Among the advances in healthcare, radiological innovations are uniquely important as they have propelled advances in virtually most medical and dental specialties directly or indirectly. In this book, we examine how this technological cross-pollination works by detailing the broad impact of three-dimensional (3D) radiographic imaging on orthodontic diagnosis and treatment planning.

Several different technologies, including structured light, laser surface imaging, magnetic resonance imaging (MRI), computed tomography (CT), and cone beam computed tomography (CBCT), are currently available for 3D imaging. While these technologies differ in their operational details, all of them generate 3D images using the same general principles. In each of these imaging modalities, an emitted energy beam passing through or reflected from the body is modified by the structures that it encounters. A specialized sensor captures the modified energy beam, which then is converted into a 3D image by sophisticated software. Surface models, such as dental casts or slices through the 3D volume, which clearly display internal structures, can then be generated to improve diagnosis and treatment planning. Factors such as the desired image resolution, radiation exposure, soft tissue versus hard tissue visualization, and region of interest are used to determine which imaging modality is suited best for any given patient. Because of the need for orthodontists to image the craniofacial skeleton optimally and derive volumetric information, X-ray–based imaging is the best choice among these imaging technologies.

Cone Beam Computed Tomography in Orthodontics: Indications, Insights, and Innovations, First Edition. Sunil D. Kapila.

Within the volumetric 3D imaging subset, CBCT, as opposed to the more expensive CT or MRI or higher radiation CT technologies, currently is the most preferred approach for such imaging.

Since the introduction of CBCT to dentistry, which first was discussed comprehensively at the 2002 symposium "Craniofacial Imaging in the 21st Century" and documented in the proceedings of the meeting (Kapila & Farman, 2003), this technology has undergone a rapid evolution and considerable integration into orthodontics (Kapila *et al.*, 2011). Typically the pattern of integration of a new technology into a discipline, such as CBCT's utilization in dentistry, starts with early enthusiastic adopters who hope to extend the technology's boundaries beyond its capabilities or utility, while others wait for evidence to justify the use of such technology and still others remain skeptical that the new technology will have any impact on their modality of practice, patient care, or treatment outcomes. Given the exponentially increasing research and clinical information on CBCT, it is likely that the latter group is dwindling as more clinicians begin to recognize the usefulness of CBCT, at least for patients presenting with specific clinical challenges. On the other end of the spectrum, the routine use of CBCT on every orthodontic patient remains a controversial issue since it is not clear that the information derived from CBCT enhances diagnosis or helps in modifying treatments in several case types, which is important particularly when weighed against the risks of radiation exposure.

This varied utilization of CBCT among clinicians exists within the context of research evidence, published case reports, or anecdotal observations on topics ranging from impacted teeth to temporomandibular joint (TMJ) morphology, many of which suggest that important information indeed can be obtained through CBCT imaging. Nevertheless, scientific evidence that the utilization of CBCT alters diagnosis and improves treatment plans or outcomes has only recently begun to emerge for some of its suggested applications. Also, for several of these recommendations in which the use of CBCT is logical and/or supported by scientific evidence, the specific indications for acquisition of CBCT images and protocols for imaging and extracting appropriate information have not been resolved fully. Finally, the information obtained from CBCT imaging requires a substantial level of expertise for interpretation that orthodontists currently may not have achieved (Ahmed *et al.*, 2012), which has attendant medico-legal implications. Thus, despite the rapidly increasing popularity of CBCT and progress in understanding and applying it to clinical orthodontics, and possibly because of the large quantities of often disparate information on this imaging technology, a cohesive, comprehensive, and objective approach to its uses and advantages in orthodontic applications currently is lacking.

This textbook provides detailed, impartial, and state-of-the-art insights, indications, protocols, procedures, innovations, and medico-legal implications of CBCT. The insights gained from CBCT are contributing to novel or refined approaches to diagnosis, treatment, and biomechanic planning (Chapters 9–23), assessment of treatment outcomes (Chapters 12–15, 17, 19–23), and providing opportunities for novel areas of research (Chapters 4, 5, 12–23). These insights have been facilitated largely by the relative advantages of CBCT imaging over radiographic two-dimensional (2D) imaging.

This chapter provides an essential overview of the topics presented in this book with the goal of highlighting the current knowledge on CBCT technology, its applications in defining 3D craniofacial anatomy and treatment outcomes, incidental findings and their medico-legal implications, and evidence-based indications and protocols for clinical applications of CBCT. In reading this chapter and book, it will become apparent that while some applications and areas have advanced sufficiently with demonstrated scientific evidence for the efficacy of CBCT in enhancing diagnosis and treatment planning, the use of CBCT in other clinical situations still is evolving. Thus, depending on where this field is in specific types of cases, the topics may range from current science to implied clinical applications to actual utility in patients who present with specific clinical findings. It is likely that as the field advances and more evidence of the efficacy of CBCT emerges, its applications in orthodontics will increase or be modified. This will enable clinicians to realize the ultimate goal of increased treatment efficiency or outcomes or both in many more clinical scenarios.

EVOLUTION IN AND BASICS OF CBCT TECHNOLOGY

CBCT technology owes its inception to the discovery of X-rays by the physicist Wilhelm Conrad Röntgen in 1895, which enabled the first ever non-invasive visualization inside the human body. The discovery of X-rays was a landmark achievement in the medical field and contributed to innovative changes in how medicine and surgery are practiced. Since its initial discovery, radiographic imaging has found widespread applications in many healthcare fields. Although the images derived from the original planar X-ray technology have proven to be valuable diagnostically, they are 2D images of 3D objects, which have inherent caveats and considerable loss of information that could be of value in clinical practice or in research discoveries. Other limitations of 2D radiographic imaging include magnification, geometric distortion, superimposition of structures, projective displacements (which may elongate or foreshorten an object's perceived dimensions), rotational errors, and linear projective transformation (Tsao *et al.*, 1983; Quintero *et al.*, 1999; Adams *et al.*, 2004).

The subsequent exponential advances in computer hardware and software technologies and electrical engineering resulted in the next significant breakthrough in radiography, namely, the development of CT independently by Hounsfield and Cormack in the early 1970s (Raju, 1999; Oransky, 2004). This technological advancement enabled the generation of 3D images and the ability to view an object in its entirety from all possible viewpoints. The advantages of CT relative to 2D radiography resulted in its rapid adoption in many medical and dental fields. Successive enhancements in CT technology attributable to improvements in hardware have resulted in units with faster scanning times and relatively high image quality. In the two decades following the introduction of CT, the spiral or helical CT in effect became the standard instrument for medical imaging, which was supplanted by the multislice CT (MSCT) or multirow detector CT (MDCT) in 1998. Although medical CT has been used for craniofacial imaging from its earliest days, its utilization for this purpose increased only when high-resolution scanners with slice thicknesses of 2 mm were developed in the 1980s (Mozzo *et al.*, 1998). However, due to the high levels of radiation, cost of the imaging units, and inaccessibility, use of medical CT for craniofacial imaging generally has been limited to patients for whom the risk-benefit ratio was considered favorable, such as for those with craniofacial anomalies, trauma, or cancer.

CBCT scanners were developed for craniofacial imaging in the late 1990s, in part to overcome several of the limitations of MSCT. In 2001, the Food and Drug Administration (FDA) approved CBCT scanners for sale in the United States, which led to their introduction into dentistry that year. CBCT differs from MSCT in the shape of the beam, the configuration of the detectors, and the software algorithms used to reconstruct the images (Figure 1.1; see also Chapter 2). These hardware and software modifications enable CBCT to capture images of the desired region of interest (ROI) with only one or two rotations, thereby decreasing the radiation exposure and time required to scan the patient compared with MSCT scans. Another advantage of CBCT scanners is their availability as compact and relatively inexpensive units that can be installed in private clinics, including those of general dentists, oral surgeons, and orthodontists (Vannier, 2003). The growing popularity and use of CBCT is evident by the more than 40 different CBCT units that now are available from more than 20 manufacturers (Molen, 2011; see also Chapters 2, 4, and 6). It is apparent that the development and availability of these specialized low-radiation-dose CBCT scanners for imaging craniofacial structures has driven the adoption and integration of 3D digital imaging into dentistry and increasingly is becoming an important source of 3D volumetric data supplemented with 2D multiplanar reconstructions (MPR; Figure 1.2) in clinical orthodontics.

Historically, 2D imaging, including traditional radiographs and photographs, combined with 3D data obtained from models and clinic examination, has been a mainstay of orthodontic diagnosis and treatment planning. In contrast, in cases where indicated, the acquisition of clinical information entirely from 3D imaging, including CBCT, would allow for the evaluation and analysis of the true anatomy providing clinically accurate 3D representations of craniofacial structures, teeth, and

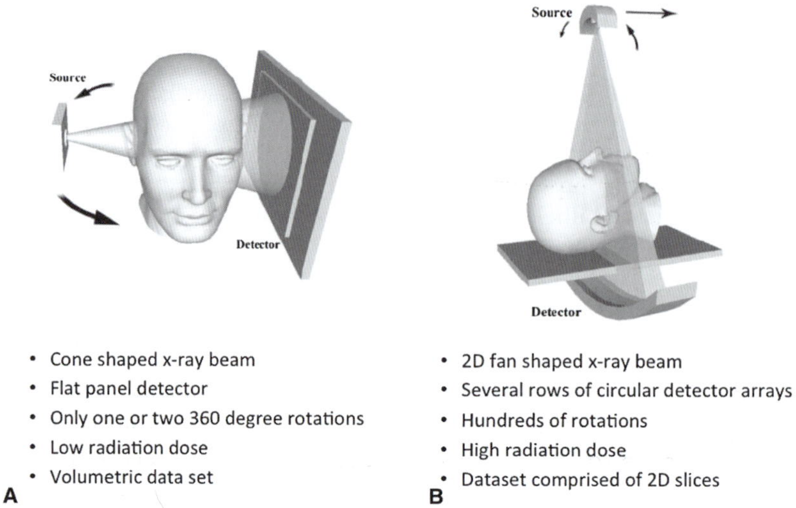

Figure 1.1 Diagrammatic representation of CBCT (*A*) and MSCT (*B*) units and summary of key differences between these two types of CT imaging modalities. (Modified and reprinted with permission from Miracle & Mukherji, 2009.)

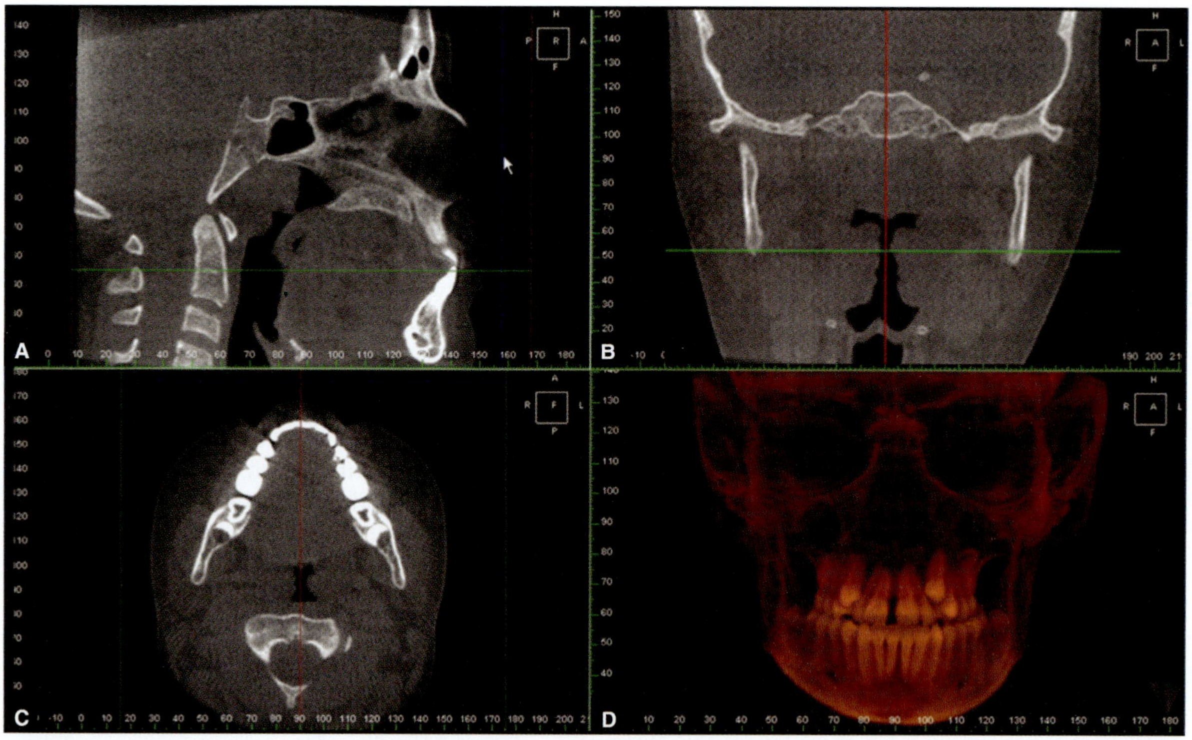

Figure 1.2 CBCTs provide multidimensional perspectives, including 2D cross-sections in the sagittal (*A*), coronal (*B*), and axial (*C*) planes. The image can be scanned through slice planes to reveal details of the anatomy in any of the three planes of space. The 3D volumetric-rendered view (*D*) can be rotated in all three planes of space to reveal the anatomic structures, their relationships, and the volumes of the dental, skeletal, and airway anatomy. In this case, the sagittal, axial, and coronal views reveal enlarged adenoids and tonsils. A narrow and asymmetric maxilla that is rotated to the patient's right and impacted maxillary canines is noticeable in the rendered view.

roots with no superimposition of structures. Unlike several other 3D imaging methods (e.g., structured light or surface laser scanning), CBCT imaging, in addition to providing acceptable representation of soft tissue surface anatomy, has the advantage over most other 3D imaging modalities of incorporating details of underlying skeletal and dental structures, albeit with the caveat that the patient is exposed to radiation.

The pace of CBCT innovations and applications to orthodontics is reflected by the rapidly expanding numbers and quality of publications on this topic. A PubMed search using the key words CBCT or cone beam computed tomography and orthodontics generated 558 references published in English up to the end of 2013. These include three published in 2003, none in 2004, five each in 2005 and 2006, 14 in 2007, 18 in 2008, 55 in 2009, 71 in 2010, 98 in 2011, 132 in 2012, and 157 in 2013. Of these publications, a substantial subset are original or research studies that can be classified broadly into the following categories: (1) technology assessment and enhancements, (2) craniofacial and airway morphometric analyses in health and disease, (3) CBCT use in analyzing treatment outcomes, (4) incidental findings and medico-legal implications, and (5) evidence-based indications, uses, and efficacy of CBCT in diagnosis and treatment planning, all of which are discussed in greater depth in the remainder of this chapter.

TECHNOLOGY ASSESSMENT AND ENHANCEMENTS

Technology assessment studies that include radiation exposure, accuracy of measurements and images, comparison of 3D with 2D images, and advances in software and hardware technologies provide important information needed for the effective and safe utilization of CBCT.

Radiation exposure

Radiation exposure is determined by several variables, including the type of unit used, field of exposure, pulsed versus continuous exposure, milliamperage seconds (mAs), peak kilovoltage (kVp), beam filtration, and number basis of images, several of which can be controlled by the technician or clinician. A wide variation in radiation exposure has been reported for different CBCT units (Brooks, 2009; see also Chapters 2 and 3). The field of view (FOV)-dependent effective dose of CBCT varies: 68–1074 μSv for large (>15 cm), 69–560 μSv for medium (10–15 cm), and 189–652 μSv for small (8–10 cm) FOV (Silva *et al.*, 2008; Ludlow, 2009a, 2009b; also see Chapter 3). The effective dose for a craniofacial (large or extended) FOV CBCT scan ranges from 114 to 282 μSv when using a 10-year-old phantom and from approximately 81 to 216 μSv effective dose when using an adolescent phantom (Theodorakou *et al.*, 2012). In contrast, although MSCT provides better soft tissue visualization than CBCT, it has a higher radiation dose of 280–1410 μSv for a maxilla-mandibular image (Loubele *et al.*, 2005; Garcia Silva *et al.*, 2008a; Okano *et al.*, 2009; Suomalainen *et al.*, 2009) and generates greater scatter from metal restorations than CBCT, which impacts the quality of the image (Farman & Scarfe, 2006; see also Chapters 2 and 3). Thus, relative to MSCT, CBCT provides appropriate levels of detail at a substantially reduced radiation exposure.

Radiation exposure is an important factor when considering whether to take a CBCT or conventional 2D radiographs. Compared with conventional 2D orthodontic radiographic series of a panoramic radiograph (2.7–24.3 μSv), a lateral cephalogram (<6 μSv) and a full-mouth series (<1.5 μSv per radiograph, or approximately 27 μSv for 18 radiographs; Garcia Silva *et al.*, 2008a, 2008b; Ludlow *et al.*, 2008; Ludlow & Ivanovic, 2008; Palomo *et al.*, 2008; Okano *et al.*, 2009), CBCT radiation exposure can be equivalent to or greater than traditional imaging depending on the FOV and age of the patient (Silva *et al.*, 2008; SEDENTEXCT, 2011; also see Chapter 3). More specifically, when comparing radiation exposure for the large or extended FOV CBCT preferred by those clinicians who undertake CBCT in lieu of the standard orthodontic imaging, the CBCT radiation exposure derived using an adolescent or child phantom is approximately two- to tenfold greater than the combined effective radiation dose of approximately 30 μSv from a cephalogram and panoramic radiograph (Table 1.1). The use of

Table 1.1 Comparison of effective radiation doses from conventional 2D radiography, CBCTs using pediatric phantoms for dentoalveolar (small and medium) and craniofacial (large) FOVs, MSCT, and background radiation. Most of the radiation data are provided in ranges and medians (in parentheses).

Type of radiography	Specific radiograph or methods	Effective dose (μSv)
2D radiography	Intraoral (PAs and bitewings)	27
	Panoramic	2.7–24.3
	Cephalometric	<6
Dentoalveolar FOV CBCT	10-year-old phantom	16–214 (43)
	Adolescent phantom	18–70 (32)
Craniofacial FOV CBCT	10-year-old phantom	114–282 (186)
	Adolescent phantom	81–216 (135)
Conventional CT	MSCT	280–1410
Background radiation		8

Sources of data include Loubele *et al.*, 2005; Garcia Silva *et al.*, 2008a, 2008b; Ludlow *et al.*, 2008; Okano *et al.*, 2009; Palomo *et al.*, 2008; Theodorakou *et al.*, 2012.

Table 1.2 Radiation risk in relation to age. This approach assumes a multiplicative risk projection model averaged for the two sexes. In fact, the risk for females always is higher relatively than for males.

Age group (years)	Multiplication factor for risk
<10	×3
10–20	×2
20–30	×1.5
30–50	×0.5
50–80	×0.3
80+	Negligible risk

Data are derived from ICRP (1991) and represent relative attributable lifetime risk standardized to the relative risk of 1 at age 30, which is considered the population average risk. (Reprinted with permission from SEDENTEXCT, 2009.)

a dentoalveolar FOV CBCT where indicated combined with a cephalometric radiograph also has a lower effective radiation exposure than a craniofacial FOV, although this difference in radiation exposure is much less marked than when comparing the traditional 2D radiographic series with a large or extended FOV CBCT. Another approach for understanding the potential effects of radiation exposure from radiographic imaging is to compare this exposure with that from background radiation. Given that the background radiation in the United States is approximately 8μSv per day, a large FOV would expose the patient to an equivalent of 10 to 35 days of background radiation.

A final consideration for radiation risks, particularly for orthodontic patients, most of whom are children or adolescents, is *attributable lifetime radiation risk* (ICRP, 1991, 2008). This determination is based on the assumption that younger subjects are at a higher risk to the adverse effects of radiation exposure over their lifetimes than are older patients because of their length of remaining life, greater proportion of mitotic cells, and lower radiation resistance of tissues. Table 1.2 summarizes the age-related lifetime radiation risk multiplication factor based on a relative risk of one at age 30 years, which is used as the population average risk. These data show that relative to the risk of radiation exposure to a 30-year-old, children less than 10 years old have a three-fold greater radiation risk and those between 10 and 20 years have a two-fold greater attributable radiation risk; this suggests that extra caution should be exercised prior to exposing children and young adults to radiographic examination.

Overall, irrespective of the patient's age, it is important to weigh the risks of radiation exposure against the expected clinical benefits of imaging, given the possible sequelae of exposure to radiation (see also Chapters 3 and 6). The latter determination is based on an objective assessment of whether any additional information obtained from these scans is likely to enhance diagnosis and/or treatment planning prior to taking CBCT imaging. Conversely, it should be emphasized that radiation risks alone are not an adequate reason for not taking a CBCT scan when indicated. Instead, knowledge of radiation exposure and risks should be used to make informed decisions on when CBCT could prove to be beneficial for extracting additional diagnostic information and/or providing optimal treatment to the patient. Finally, when deciding on undertaking radiographic imaging it is important to exercise the "As Low As Reasonably Achievable" (ALARA) principle (Farman & Scarfe, 2006).

Accuracy of CBCT-derived cephalograms and measurements versus gold standard

Studies have also been performed to determine the translatability and utility of CBCT relative to the most commonly used current methods of morphologic assessment, namely, cephalometrics and panoramic radiographs. Techniques for reconstructing cephalograms from CBCT have been developed (Farman & Scarfe, 2006) and measurements from these reconstructions can be compared directly with measurements from traditional cephalograms to assess their accuracy (Kumar *et al.*, 2008). Such studies have revealed no significant differences in linear and angular measurements from cephalograms reconstructed from the NewTom 3G CBCT (NewTom Germany AG, Marburg, Germany) relative to conventional 2D cephalograms (Kumar *et al.*, 2008). While these comparisons provide important information, it probably is more important to determine the accuracy of measurements from CBCT surface-rendered volumetric images to direct "gold standard" anatomical measurements made on the object of interest. Findings from studies on this subject have shown that the mean percentage measurement error for 3D CBCT is higher significantly (2.3%) than replicate skull measurements (0.6%; Periago *et al.*, 2008). Additionally, most of the midsagittal 3D CBCT measurements were smaller systematically and significantly when using Dolphin 3D (Dolphin Imaging and Management Systems, Chatsworth, CA) software than those made directly from the skull, reflecting some potential need for image correction algorithms in the software. Similar but smaller systematic differences in 3D CBCT measurements made using NewTom HQR DVT 9000 and Hitachi MercuRay (Hitachi Medical Corp, Tokyo, Japan) versus true measurements on the skull have been reported by others (Stratemann *et al.*, 2008). Fortunately, the majority of measurements from 3D CBCT were within 2 mm of those made directly from the skull, indicating that while the differences may be significant statistically for research purposes, they may not be relevant clinically.

As pointed out in several chapters, the direct comparison of cephalograpms with CBCT imaging may be a transitional step in the adoption of this new technology into the field. Novel approaches currently are being devised for 3D analyses and superimpositions for assessment of treatment outcomes (Chapters 19 and 21), monitoring disease progression and responses to therapy (Chapter 12), and research purposes (Chapter 4) that likely will result in the traditional 2D analyses methods becoming less relevant in specific case types and in research in orthodontics.

Comparison of CBCT versus panoramic radiograph

Qualitative assessments also have been made to determine whether CBCT images provide more detailed information than routine orthopantomograms or panoramic radiographs in various orthodontically relevant situations. A subjective comparison of reconstructed panoramic images from two CBCT units (NewTom 9000 and Arcadis Orbic 3D; Siemens Medical Solutions, Erlangen, Germany) with routine panoramic projection demonstrated a gain in information over conventional radiography for localizing impacted and retained teeth, the presence or absence of root resorption, cleft lip and palate (CL/P), and third molar evaluation, but not for changes in the TMJ (Korbmacher *et al.*, 2007). Other studies have shown that CBCT provides a more accurate assessment of root parallelism, root resorption, and localization of impacted teeth than do panoramic or other 2D radiographs (Peck *et al.*, 2007; Alqerban *et al.*, 2009a, 2009b, 2011a, 2011b; Van Elslande *et al.*, 2010; Bouwens *et al.*, 2011; Durack *et al.*, 2011; Ponder *et al.*, 2012; Ren *et al.*, 2012; see also later and Chapters 15 and 16).

Technology enhancements

As described in Chapters 2, 4, 5, 20, and 21, CBCT hardware and software technologies continue to undergo rapid evolution and enhancement. Indeed, CBCT units now are available with varied configurations that include adjustable or even customizable FOVs. Other discoveries and improvements in X-ray source technologies, detectors, and post-processing of images will offer further opportunities for reduction in radiation and customization of imaging protocols. Additional developments in software include introduction of user-friendly treatment planning software and the increasing automation in 3D superimposition that will be of utility in both clinical and research applications. Progress also is being made in applying new methodologies that facilitate the merging of 3D datasets from different sources and in verifying the efficacy of these enhancements in clinical decision-making. A key extension in the utility of 3D imaging involves rapid progress in technologies such as 3D printing that increasingly are becoming available for fabrication of surgical splints and specialized orthodontic appliances that also have substantial yet untapped practical applications (see also Chapter 20).

CBCT MORPHOMETRIC ANALYSES IN HEALTH AND DISEASE

CBCT-based 3D craniofacial and dental morphometrics is important for defining normal and abnormal 3D anatomy of structures with a potential for longer-term utility in diagnosis and treatment planning. Much work to date on this topic has focused on quantitative and qualitative determinations of the morphology of craniofacial structures, airway, TMJ, roots, and dentoalveolar boundary conditions.

Qualitative and quantitative assessments of craniofacial morphometrics

3D imaging allows for analysis of normal size, shape, and volume of various craniofacial structures and facilitates the determination of differences in these variables between bilateral structures (Stratemann *et al.*, 2010). Although CBCT has the potential for defining craniofacial growth changes in 3D, its sole use for this purpose is highly unlikely due to radiation concerns. To date, three main methods have been utilized for analyzing 3D anatomy and changes due to treatment in craniofacial structures. The first method extends approaches that are utilized in 2D cephalometry to derive linear and angular measurements from 3D images (Jung *et al.*, 2009; Kim *et al.*, 2010, 2011). This approach has the caveat of reducing 3D dimensions into 2D measurements. The second method, called Closest Point analysis (Figure 12.8 and Figure 12.9B) determines the smallest displacements between two structures but does not account for changes in shape (Cevidanes *et al.*, 2007; Almeida *et al.*, 2011; Motta *et al.*, 2011). Shape correspondence (Figure 12.9B) is the third method that determines the displacement of a given landmark between two time points and represents these as either vectors or color-coded maps to depict the directionality and amount of movements, respectively (Paniagua *et al.*, 2010; see also Chapters 12, 19, and 22). In the future, it is likely that the latter and similar approaches will replace or complement linear and angular measurements made from 3D or planar reconstructions for determining treatment changes from CBCT images.

Root morphology, resorption, and angulations

Root length, form, and resorption traditionally have been assessed via periapical radiographs, while post-orthodontic root parallelism and relationships customarily are determined using panoramic radiographs. Recent studies show that CBCT provides enhanced visualization of roots, making it a valuable tool for assessing pre- or post-orthodontic root resorption and parallelism. Using true anatomic root and tooth length as a gold standard, it has been shown that CBCT is at least as good as periapical radiography for assessing root and tooth length (Lund *et al.*, 2010; Sherrard *et al.*, 2010). Because of its ability to generate precise images of small root defects,

CBCT provides more accurate insights into root resorption as well as greater sensitivity and specificity in detecting these lesions than do panoramic or other 2D radiographs (Alqerban *et al.*, 2009a, 2009b, 2011; Durack *et al.*, 2011; Ponder *et al.*, 2012; Ren *et al.*, 2012). Also relative to CBCT, panoramic radiographs underestimate external apical root resorption (EARR; Segal *et al.*, 2004; Dudic *et al.*, 2009) such that *in vivo* root resorption is diagnosed on 43% of all teeth on panoramic radiographs compared with 69% of all teeth on the CBCT images (Dudic *et al.*, 2009). For maxillary incisors, root resorption is not diagnosed 20% of the time with panoramic radiographs and 14% of the time with CBCT images. Finally, while 2D radiographs provide visualization of only the apex and the mesial and distal root surfaces, CBCT imaging adds insights into the effects of treatment on buccal and lingual root surfaces. This has led to the novel discovery that root loss not only is present at the root apex or is symmetrical around the root surface, but also shows a slanting pattern on surfaces adjacent to the direction of tooth movement. This finding highlights the efficacy of CBCT's 3D rendering capacity for accurate diagnosis of both EARR and other types of root resorption.

Since root parallelism is an important goal of orthodontic treatment, its accurate determination could add valuable information in assessing the quality of treatment outcomes and, possibly, of post-treatment stability. Several studies show that panoramic radiographs generate numerous errors in the assessment of root angulation. Specifically relative to true angulations, the roots of maxillary anterior teeth often appear tipped mesially, while posterior teeth appear inclined distally, and roots of all mandibular teeth appear tipped more mesially on panoramic radiographs (McKee *et al.*, 2002; Garcia-Figueroa *et al.*, 2008; Owens & Johal, 2008). Recent studies comparing gold standard direct measurements on typodonts or skulls demonstrate that CBCT images, though not perfect, provide improved angular measurements relative to those derived from 2D radiographs (Peck *et al.*, 2007; Van Elslande *et al.*, 2010; Bouwens *et al.*, 2011). Despite these findings, the assessment of root parallelism currently does not qualify as an indication for CBCT imaging.

Bone quality and quantity assessments

Evaluating the status of the alveolar housing or boundary conditions is gaining increasing importance as a component of orthodontic patient evaluation (see also Chapter 14). For example, changes in bone height and width measurements increasingly are being utilized for assessing orthodontic treatment outcomes (Garrett *et al.*, 2008; Kartalian *et al.*, 2010; Tai *et al.*, 2010a; Cattaneo *et al.*, 2011; Corbridge *et al.*, 2011; see also Chapter 14). Although dentoalveolar bone morphology and its relationship to underlying roots is an important component of orthodontic diagnosis and treatment, some controversy remains on the accuracy, reliability, and reproducibility of CBCT in assessing bone morphology, quantity, and quality. The accuracy of bone width dimensions depends on CBCT machine-specific settings including mAs, kVp, exposure time, and sensor size, and patient-specific variables including age, bone density, and periodontal biotype (Molen, 2010). Studies have shown that bone width particularly above a specific bone thickness threshold can be determined from CBCT with a relatively high level of reliability and reproducibility and, therefore, accuracy (Leung *et al.*, 2010; Patcas *et al.*, 2012). Although CBCT provides accurate assessment of alveolar bone height, caution must be exercised in evaluating fenestrations due to the high number of false positives in the determination of these defects (Leung *et al.*, 2010; Patcas *et al.*, 2012).

Both the quantity and quality of the cortical bone and the quality of underlying trabecular bone may be important in determining primary stability of temporary anchorage devices (TADs), which, in turn, is relevant to secondary TAD stability over the longer term (Dalstra *et al.*, 2004; Wilmes *et al.*, 2006; Marquezan *et al.*, 2012; see also Chapter 18). Bone density often serves as a surrogate for bone quality and typically is measured using Hounsfield Units (HU)—a method previously devised for MSCT. HU measurements allow clinicians to assess the health of tissues. For example, alveolar bone density at a proposed dental implant site can be measured with MSCT prior to surgery to determine whether the density is sufficient to support the implant or whether a bone graft should be performed first. The HU scale assigns unit values to air, soft tissues, water, and hard tissues based on their ability to attenuate an X-ray beam. On the HU scale, air has an HU value of −1000, water is 0, and dense bone is ≥+1000. Soft tissues, which have high water content, have HU values that fall between water and dense bone. Because all conventional CT machines are calibrated to ensure that the grayscale measurements on each scan are accurate, all HU measurements taken on conventional CT-generated images can be compared directly with each other. In contrast to MSCT, because the grayscale on CBCT images is not calibrated, this technology cannot be used to measure bone density accurately; in fact, it is arbitrary, which means that tissue densities on two CBCT scans, even if taken on the same patient, cannot be measured or compared directly (Katsumata *et al.*, 2006, 2007; Swennen & Schutyser, 2006). Thus, while a CBCT image can be used to determine if an edentulous site has sufficient alveolar bone thickness to support a dental implant, it cannot be used to determine if the bone density is sufficient to withstand the surgical placement and long-term functional stresses of implant treatment. Efforts are ongoing to develop algorithms that convert specific parameters, such as a voxel volume (VV) grayscale, derived from CBCT to quantify bone density.

TMJ anatomy and morphology

Although little information currently is available on the efficacy of CBCT in enhancing the diagnosis of TMJ disorders over routine radiography, CBCT has been shown to be more efficacious than conventional tomography and MRI in detecting osseous changes (Honey *et al.*, 2007; Alkhader *et al.*, 2010). Comparison of asymptomatic control and osteoarthritic TMJs by shape correspondence also has shown significant differences between the morphologies of healthy and degenerative condyles (Cevidanes *et al.*, 2010a). This study also revealed a significant correlation of both pain intensity and pain duration with the variations in 3D morphology of the osteoarthritic condyles. While these findings suggest the potential utility of CBCT as a diagnostic aid in TMJ osteoarthritis (OA), it is important to understand that structural bony changes of the TMJ alone do not reveal whether or not the disease is active, and no direct correlation between TMJ morphological changes and clinical findings in OA or other arthritides exists.

Airway morphology and relationship to obstructive sleep apnea (OSA)

As reported later in this book (see Chapter 13) and in a recent publication (Schendel & Hatcher, 2010), CBCT can be used to image the airway accurately to provide cross-sectional area, minimum cross-section, and total airway volume (Figure 1.3). Initial investigations on airway patency, function, and disorders utilizing CBCT have provided preliminary answers including dimensions of normal airway anatomy in adults (Smith, 2009),

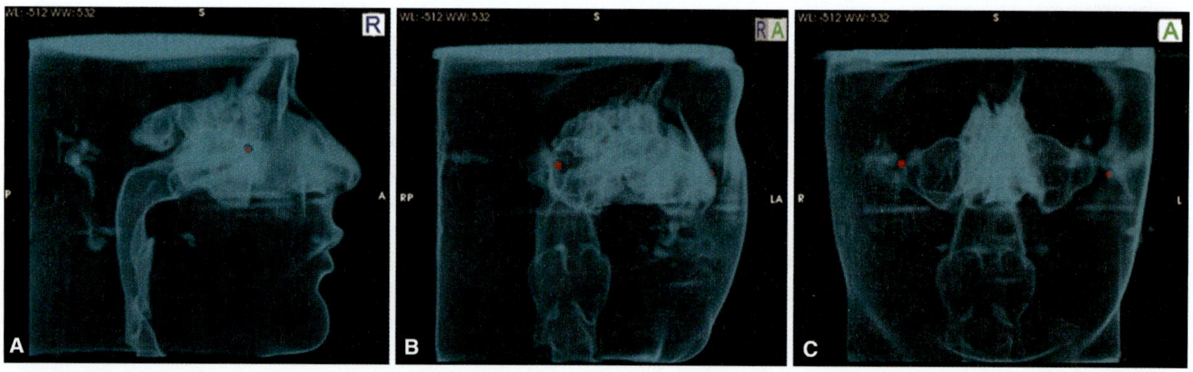

Figure 1.3 3D airway visualization in the lateral (*A*), three-quarter (*B*), and frontal (*C*) views. Both qualitative and quantitative assessments of the airway can be made by thresholding specific tissue density either through features built into the software program, as performed here, or by customized selection of a window of density to obtain refined and accurate 3D volumetric, cross-sectional area, and linear measurements of the airway.

relationship of 2D to 3D measurements (Lenza *et al.*, 2010), differences in airway morphology in obstructive sleep apnea (OSA) and non-OSA subjects (Haponik *et al.*, 1983; Galvin *et al.*, 1989; Avrahami & Englender, 1995; Caballero *et al.*, 1998; Schwab *et al.*, 2003; Yucel *et al.*, 2005), and the effects of rapid palatal expansion (RPE) and orthognathic surgery on airway dimensions (Samman *et al.*, 1992; Chen *et al.*, 2007; Degerliyurt *et al.*, 2008; Oliviera de Felippe *et al.*, 2008; Hong *et al.*, 2011; see also Chapters 13, 17, and 22). Several of these studies show no relationship between 2D linear and 3D cross-sectional areas of airway, which suggests that the use of 2D data may not be valid for assessing airway patency. Also up to this time, no studies have demonstrated that qualitative or quantitative assessments of CBCT are capable of predicting OSA accurately.

UTILITY OF CBCT IN ASSESSING TREATMENT OUTCOMES

Because CBCT is 3D and not subject to the error and overlap found in lateral or posterior-anterior cephalometry, it provides the capability of assessing treatment outcomes in all three planes of space as well as volumetrically. As a result of these advantages over routine radiography, CBCT is becoming an important tool in assessing outcomes of orthodontic and surgical therapies. These include the determination of the effects of treatments on orthopedic versus orthodontic changes, root resorption, bone boundary conditions, airway, alveolar grafting in CL/P, and orthognathic surgery as discussed later and in Chapters 12, 14, 15, and 17–23.

Maxillary expansion

CBCT has enabled more in-depth dissection of responses of bone and teeth to maxillary expansion than was possible through 2D radiography or study models. For example, studies on four-banded maxillary expanders have revealed that although the first premolar, second premolar, and first molar all have similar magnitudes of total overall expansion (which includes skeletal expansion, dental tipping, and alveolar bone bending), the skeletal expansion is greater in the anterior than posterior maxilla (Rungcharassaeng *et al.*, 2007; Garrett *et al.*, 2008; Kartalian *et al.*, 2010). These differences in findings between skeletal and overall expansion result from increasingly greater alveolar bone bending and the buccal crown tip going back from the first premolar to the first molar. Of the total expansion obtained in one of these studies with an adolescent sample (mean age 13.8 ± 1.7 years), 38% was orthopedic, 13% was due to alveolar bending, and 49% resulted from dental tipping (Garrett *et al.*, 2008). These studies confirm that besides sutural expansion, RPE produces both dental and alveolar tipping, and suggest that much of post-expansion relapse probably occurs from "rebound" from the alveolar bending and dental tipping, since these two modalities of expansion are hard to retain. Additionally, the sample showed an increase in nasal width and decrease in maxillary sinus width (Garrett *et al.*, 2008). In contrast to expansion using the fixed RPE appliance, a removable Schwarz appliance achieves expansion in both arches through alveolar buccal tipping (Tai *et al.*, 2010a, 2010b).

Treatment effects on alveolar boundary conditions

Alveolar boundary conditions are the depth, height, and morphology of alveolar bone relative to tooth root dimensions, angulation, and spatial position (Kapila *et al.*, 2011; see also Chapter 14). Boundary conditions are determined not only by dentoalveolar anatomy prior to treatment, but also by the bone's adaptability during tooth movement and its morphology following the final positioning of teeth. Thus, in the context of orthodontic tooth movement, boundary conditions can be considered to be dynamic and dependent on the patient's pre-treatment bone and gingival biotype as well as bone physiology. This implies that pre-treatment status of alveolar boundary conditions and their potential adaptation may dictate the limits of both the planned tooth movement and the final desired spatial position and angulation of the tooth.

The effect of orthodontic treatment and various appliances on bone morphology and boundary conditions in three planes of space can be assessed relatively well with CBCT, though not perfectly due to some of its technological limitations (see earlier and Chapter 14). This approach has been used to discern the potential effects of treatment- or patient-specific variables on the integrity and morphology of bone around tooth roots in full-fixed appliance therapy and with both rapid and slow expansion (Rungcharassaeng *et al.*, 2007; Garrett *et al.*, 2008; Kartalian *et al.*, 2010; Tai *et al.*, 2010a; Cattaneo *et al.*, 2011; Corbridge *et al.*, 2011; Johnson, 2011; Welmerink, 2012). Thus, it has been shown that routine orthodontic therapy using full-fixed appliances is accompanied by significant changes in bone width even with small amounts of buccal movement of posterior teeth (Johnson, 2011; Welmerink, 2012). This finding raises the question of whether biologically compatible expansion is possible using specific combinations of fixed appliances and wires as claimed by some manufacturers. A recent study tested such claims by evaluating the effects of active (In-Ovation R; Dentsply GAC, Islandia, NY) and passive (Damon 3 MX; Ormco Corp, Orange, CA) self-ligating brackets on alveolar boundary conditions (Cattaneo *et al.*, 2011). Buccal cortical bone thickness on the second premolars decreased significantly with both types of appliances, even though the change in buccolingual tip of the teeth was the same with both systems. Thus these findings do not support the claims that specific appliances generate biologically compatible forces in which the bone remodels to maintain its integrity despite substantial arch expansion during treatment. Similarly, it also is known that buccal crown tipping during RPE is accompanied by a concomitant decrease in both buccal bone thickness and buccal marginal bone height (Rungcharassaeng *et al.*, 2007). Finally, slow palatal expansion using quadhelix or Schwarz appliances decreases and increases, respectively, buccal and lingual bone thicknesses (Tai *et al.*, 2010a, 2010b; Corbridge *et al.*, 2011).

Bimaxillary protrusion in which orthodontic treatment aims to reduce the dentoalveolar prominence is an example of a patient- plus treatment-specific variable that can contribute to compromised alveolar boundary resulting in dehiscences following incisor retraction (Sarikaya *et al.*, 2002). Similarly, post-orthodontic increase in incisal proclination is known to be a risk factor for dehiscences (Fuhrmann, 1996). Such incisor proclination-related recession may be worse in patients with thin initial symphysis bone width (Wehrbein *et al.*, 1996; Artun & Grobety, 2001). In general, it appears that both patient- and treatment-specific variables such as pre-treatment boundary conditions, the magnitude of expected dental movements, and the potential adaptability of the bone to remodel adequately with these movements may be important to the quality and quantity of bone retained following orthodontic treatment.

Quantifying CL/P defects and outcomes of alveolar bone grafts

Several studies have been performed using CBCT to determine its diagnostic efficacy in CL/P and to evaluate the success of alveolar bone grafts and paths of eruption of canines through grafted bone sites in these patients (Hamada *et al.*, 2005; Oberoi *et al.*, 2009, 2010; Quereshy *et al.*, 2011; Garib *et al.*, 2012; Zhang *et al.*, 2012). In comparing CBCT with panoramic radiographs, it has been shown that while the panoramic radiograph enables the approximation of vertical bone height of the bone bridge, it does not permit determination of the buccal-palatal width of the bone, both of which can be discerned with CBCT (Hamada *et al.*, 2005). Additionally, the CBCT images enable the visualization of the 3D morphology of the bone bridge, the relationship between the bone bridge and roots of neighboring teeth, and their periodontal condition. A subsequent study that compared patients before and after cleft grafting demonstrated an 84% bone fill of the cleft defect 1 year following the graft (Oberoi *et al.*, 2009). This information is important in the decision process for implant placement. Additional studies have reported a large range for graft volume of between 6.1 mm^3 (Oberoi *et al.*, 2009) and 489 mm^3 (Quereshy *et al.*, 2011) at cleft sites for unilateral CL/P. Such determinations from CBCT are valuable in pre-surgical planning of graft site reconstruction and bone harvesting. In addition, studies on canine eruption following grafting demonstrate no significant differences in absolute incisal, facial, and mesial distances traveled between cleft-side and non-cleft-side canines. However, the movement of the cleft-side canines does not mimic that of the non-cleft-side canines and more of the cleft-side canines tend to be impacted. It remains to be determined whether the alveolar boundary conditions and bone quality of the bone graft contribute to these differences in canine eruption. These findings and their clinical implications are discussed in greater detail in Chapter 23.

Orthognathic surgery

CBCT continues to provide useful information for diagnosis, treatment planning and assessment of treatment outcomes for orthognathic surgery cases, which are discussed in greater detail in Chapters 20–22. These studies include the determination of changes in 3D hard and soft tissue facial anatomy (McCance *et al.*, 1992; Soncul & Bamber, 2004; Honrado *et al.*, 2006; Jung *et al.*, 2009; Baik & Kim, 2010; Lim *et al.*, 2010; Ryckman *et al.*, 2010; Park *et al.*, 2012; Kim *et al.*, 2013), maxilla-mandibular relationships and positional changes in the condyle (Magalhaes *et al.*, 1995; Lee & Park, 2002; Baek *et al.*, 2006, 2009; Cevidanes *et al.*, 2007; Mucedero *et al.*, 2008; Draenert *et al.*, 2010; Kim *et al.*, 2010, 2011, 2012; Jakobsone *et al.*, 2011), post-surgical relapse (Busby *et al.*, 2002; Cevidanes *et al.*, 2007; Proffit *et al.*, 2007), and airway dimensions (Cevidanes *et al.*, 2007; Chen *et al.*, 2007; Degerliyurt *et al.*, 2008; Carvalho Fde *et al.*, 2010; Almeida *et al.*, 2011; Hong *et al.*, 2011; Motta *et al.*, 2011). As discussed in Chapter 21, the changes resulting from orthognathic surgery can be determined in 3D by performing a superimposition of the pre- and post-treatment scans on the anterior cranial base, enabling depiction of the magnitude and direction of treatment changes via color maps or vectors (Cevidanes *et al.*, 2005, 2010b).

The effects of surgery on airway patency also have begun to be elucidated and generally show that post-surgical changes in the cross-sectional area of the airway vary depending on the type of surgery and the site at which the airway is being assessed (see also Chapter 22). Thus, for example, mandibular setback surgery decreases the airway sagittal cross-section at the soft palate but not at the posterior nasal spine. In contrast, while both a single-jaw mandibular setback and two-jaw maxillary advancement/mandibular setback procedure are accompanied by narrowing of the airway, the two-jaw surgery tends to demonstrate comparatively fewer negative effects on the airway (Samman *et al.*, 1992; Chen *et al.*, 2007; Degerliyurt *et al.*, 2008; Hong *et al.*, 2011). These findings have implications for selecting optimal surgical approaches for OSA patients and are presented in greater detail in Chapter 22.

INCIDENTAL FINDINGS, DIAGNOSTICIAN SKILLS, AND MEDICO-LEGAL IMPLICATIONS

Identifying incidental findings and determining their frequency is important for insights into medico-legal implications and the capability of the diagnostician to interpret the images optimally. Incidental findings represent clinically relevant abnormal findings in radiographic images for which the image was not prescribed initially. The frequency of incidental findings varies between studies depending on the sample age, FOV studied, and methods for lesion characterization (Miles, 2005, 2009; Cha *et al.*, 2007; Rogers *et al.*, 2011). Given that CBCT has substantially more data than 2D radiographs and, therefore, captures more lesions both within and outside the dento-maxillofacial area, the rate of incidental findings is considerably higher in CBCT scans than in traditional radiographs. Indeed, whereas incidental findings are detected in approximately 3.5–8% of panoramic radiographs (Tetradis & Kantor, 1999; Kuhlberg & Norton, 2003; Bondemark *et al.*, 2006; Asaumi *et al.*, 2008), the frequency of detecting incidental findings in CBCTs is as high as 25–54% (Miles, 2005; Cha *et al.*, 2007). The use of larger FOV images typically preferred by orthodontists as opposed to those favored by most other dental providers increases the likelihood of incidental findings in the imaged volume and its attendant consequences. Furthermore, the utilization of CBCT as a screening test with the expectation of discovering incidental findings when there are no relevant signs or symptoms or other appropriate justification for undertaking this type of imaging is not justified due to the risks of radiation (see also Chapter 6).

The most common incidental findings in CBCT include those associated with airways, the TMJ, endodontic lesions, developmental dental conditions, impacted teeth, soft tissue calcifications, and lesions of bone (Caglayan & Tozoglu, 2012; Price *et al.*, 2012). Of the incidental findings reported by Price and colleagues (2012), 16.1% required intervention or referral, 15.6% required monitoring, while the remainder (68.3%) required no further treatment. This finding and others suggest that while most incidental lesions do not carry serious consequences for the patient, more serious unsuspected lesions, including those of the cranial base and cervical spine (Kau *et al.*, 2005; Nair *et al.*, 2007; Popat *et al.*, 2008; Miles, 2009) that require follow-up or treatment, may be present in CBCTs (see also Chapter 10). Up to 60–86% of incidental findings have been reported to be in extragnathic sites (Cha *et al.*, 2007; Abdul-Kader, 2008), which typically are less familiar to a radiologically untrained diagnostician (Ahmed *et al.*, 2012). It also currently is not known what proportion of incidental findings in CBCT scans are relevant orthodontically and would lead to modifications in treatment approaches. Such knowledge would be critical in determining whether the prevalence of treatment-modifying findings is adequately high to justify the more universal use of CBCT in orthodontics.

It is important to recognize that the diagnostician, whether the radiology specialist or an appropriate healthcare provider who chooses to interpret a radiographic image, bears legal and ethical responsibilities for identifying all anomalies in the entire prescribed FOV that may potentially affect the patient's health and, when needed, for referring the patient for follow-up (Turpin, 2007; Friedland, 2009; Miles, 2009; AAO Insurance Company, 2010; see also Chapter 7). The current guidelines also state that all CBCT scans should be read in their entirety, with all regions covered by the scan being the responsibility of the diagnostician (Turpin, 2007). Because no laws exist yet as to who should read the CBCT scans, the diagnostician can be either the orthodontist or the radiologist. If an orthodontist elects to interpret the information from CBCT scans, he or she has accepted a greater duty to the patient than that to which he or she otherwise would be obligated (AAO Insurance Company, 2010). Because of these reasons and the higher propensity for incidental findings in CBCT scans than in 2D radiographs, it is important that diagnosticians have the necessary knowledge and ability to identify pathologies within the entire scan.

The above considerations lead to an important question, namely, "What is the capability of the orthodontist to identify non-orthodontically relevant findings and to make appropriate referrals when necessary?" Lack of recognition of incidental lesions can have substantial medico-legal ramifications (Zinman *et al.*, 2010; see also Chapter 7), while the inadvertent diagnosis of false-positive findings by the untrained eye has the potential to add unnecessary healthcare costs due to secondary tests and treatments, as well as to contribute needless anxiety to the patient and family. In the study by Ahmed and associates (2012), orthodontists and orthodontic residents were found to miss approximately 67% of lesions and had a 50% false-positive detection rate in CBCT images. Following a 3-hour training by an oral and maxillofacial radiologist, the error rate in these two measures dropped to 43% and 35%, respectively. Although no data currently are available for error rates with CBCT or CT for oral and maxillofacial radiologists, historical norms of missed lesion error rates in medical radiology range from 4 to 13.5% (Renfrew *et al.*, 1992; Wechsler *et al.*, 1996; Berlin, 2005) versus about 43% post-training error rate for orthodontists obtained in this study. These studies show for the first time that orthodontists and orthodontic residents currently do not have the necessary background to read and interpret CBCT scans optimally and that an appropriately trained diagnostician such as an oral and maxillofacial radiologist should be consulted for the interpretation of CBCT scans, as recommended by others (Turpin, 2007; AAO Insurance Company, 2010). These findings also suggest that increased training of orthodontists in viewing normal and abnormal anatomy in CBCT images would provide additional valuable skills for them to further identify important components further relevant to orthodontic diagnosis and treatment planning.

INDICATIONS: EFFICACIOUS USE OF CBCT IN ORTHODONTIC DIAGNOSIS AND TREATMENT PLANNING

CBCT and 3D imaging in orthodontic diagnosis and treatment planning

Accurate imaging is an essential requirement in orthodontics for deriving an appropriate diagnosis, formulating an optimal treatment plan, and monitoring and documenting treatment progress and outcome. Until recently, the information needed to arrive at a diagnosis and treatment plan has relied on a combination of 2D data obtained from photographs and conventional radiographs and 3D visualization derived through clinical examination of the patient and analysis of plaster casts. Recent advances in digital technology have provided the means to evaluate study models, as well as facial, skeletal, and dental morphology and relationships using CBCT, in 3D.

Despite the increasing popularity of CBCT, there is a range of opinions among clinicians on the overall utility of CBCT in orthodontics. This spans from those who advocate for its routine use for all orthodontic patients to those who recommend its use in specific cases in which conventional radiography cannot supply satisfactory diagnostic information and where the CBCT-derived information may enhance diagnosis and/or lead to refinements or alterations in treatment plans (Isaacson *et al.*, 2008; SEDENTEXCT, 2009, 2011). The latter approach to CBCT imaging has been endorsed by the American Association of Orthodontists (AAO), which adopted a resolution stating that while the organization recognizes that "there may be clinical situations where a cone beam computed tomography (CBCT) radiograph may be of value, the use of such technology is not *routinely* required for orthodontic radiography" (AAO, 2010). This implies that the justification for using CBCT in orthodontics is linked intricately to its diagnostic and therapeutic efficacies, for which research has been performed in a relatively small subset of clinical problems that include impacted teeth, CL/P, and orthognathic surgery. Thus, determining the efficacy of CBCT in enhancing orthodontic diagnosis and therapeutic decisions is a key area in need of substantial future research focus, not only to validate the utility of the technology in specific situations, but also to define clinical protocols that will generate optimal information with minimal radiation exposure, as discussed later.

Hierarchy of evidence in the use of CBCT

Although CBCT clearly enhances the visualization of normal and abnormal anatomy and pathologies, scientific evidence on the impact of the additional information obtained in refining or changing orthodontic treatment plans in several clinical situations remains to be determined. Nevertheless, with increasing clinical utilization and research studies, a hierarchy of indicators for CBCT imaging is emerging. Ideally, the utilization of any new technology should be supported by the highest level of evidence generated from rigorous scientific studies that demonstrate that its use enhances diagnosis in a significant number of cases when compared with currently available technology and, in the longer term, is shown to improve treatment results, efficacy, and efficiency (Figure 1.4; SEDENTEXCT, 2009, 2011; see also Chapter 6). In the absence of such proof, the next level of evidence that can be used to justify use of the technology is provided by published case reports showing its contribution to improved diagnosis, treatment plan or outcome, or any combination of these for a specific type of case, which could be applicable to other similar cases. If these two levels of evidence are not available, a clinician still may choose to utilize the technology if he or she believes that it likely would enhance the diagnosis and/or alter the treatment plan. Any one of these three tiers of evidence is important particularly in justifying the use of a technology such as CBCT, which has associated risks of radiation exposure and increased costs of imaging and interpretation as compared with the technologies it is intended to replace. When used for any of these three scenarios, it should be anticipated that the CBCT likely will provide information that could result in one or more of the following outcomes: (1) enhance diagnosis by localizing the site of aberration as for impacted and transposed teeth, (2) quantify the magnitude of defect or deformity as for CL/P,

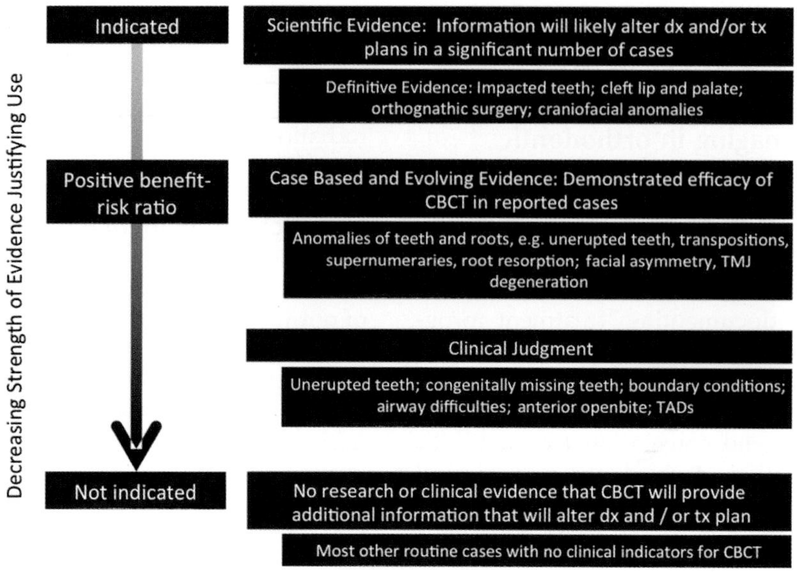

Figure 1.4 Clinical scenarios in which the use of CBCT may be indicated on the basis of research evidence or case- or clinical judgment–based determination of the need for imaging. All three levels of indicators require a careful consideration of the benefit-to-risk analyses prior to undertaking CBCT.

(3) help to provide a differential diagnosis on whether the defect is skeletal, dental, or both, (4) identify the jaw(s) involved and determine whether the aberration is bilateral or unilateral (e.g., as in orthognathic surgery, asymmetry, craniofacial anomaly, and openbite cases), and (5) help point to possible cause(s) of these findings such as for openbites or asymmetries resulting from TMJ degeneration. The expected benefit of the enhanced 3D information derived from CBCT relative to that obtained from traditional 2D radiographs ultimately may span from a refinement of treatment to a total modification in the treatment rendered.

Whether supported by research evidence or a potential positive benefit-to-risk outcome, the decision to undertake a CBCT examination should be made only after the clinician has carefully evaluated the patient history and chief complaint, performed a clinical examination, and, where indicated, taken traditional 2D radiographs (Figure 1.5). Such a careful selection of patients for CBCT imaging will ensure maximum benefit while avoiding unnecessary risks to patients who do not need this diagnostic imaging. Based on a synthesis of current scientific evidence, case reports, and other available information, the section below summarizes clinical scenarios where CBCT may be beneficial and ways to use this imaging modality under specific circumstances. The examples provided are by no means all-inclusive, and the proposed benefits of CBCT in some instances may be conjectural at this point. These and additional possible applications of CBCT in specific case types are discussed in greater detail in several chapters in Sections III and IV of this book.

Research evidence-based use of CBCT

Impacted and transposed teeth

Impacted and transposed teeth possibly are the most common indications for CBCT imaging in orthodontics. Of the many clinical situations presented to the orthodontist, impacted teeth are one in which CBCT has been shown to improve diagnosis and contribute to modifications in treatment planning in a significant number of subjects (Walker *et al.*, 2005; Haney *et al.*, 2010; Katheria *et al.*, 2010; Botticelli *et al.*, 2011; see also Chapter 16). CBCT

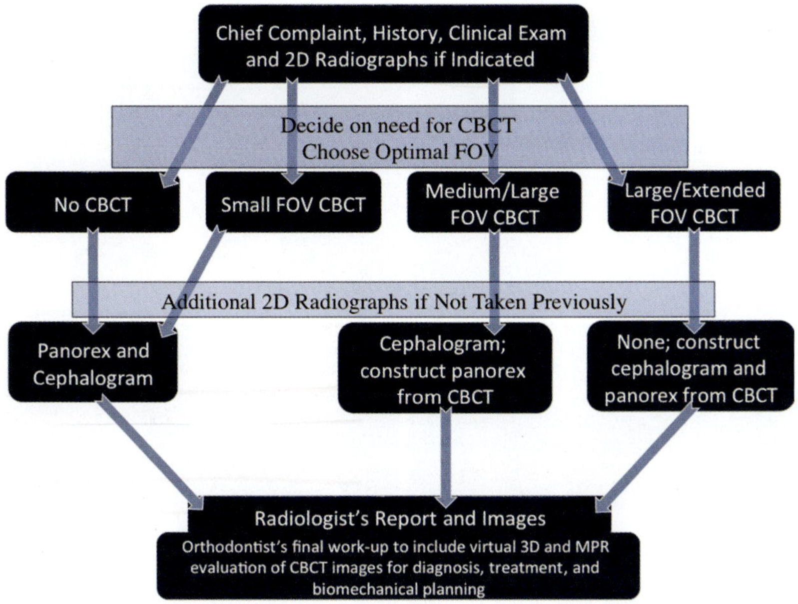

Figure 1.5 Decision tree for CBCT and 2D radiographic imaging of the orthodontic patient. Decisions on whether or not to take a CBCT and the choice of FOV should be made on the basis of a thorough knowledge of the chief complaint, history, clinical examination, and, if needed, 2D radiographs. The selection of any further 2D radiographs required should be based on the CBCT FOV and whether the patient has had any 2D radiographs taken during the initial work-up. The orthodontist then should utilize all the information collected, including that from the radiologist's report and virtual evaluation of the CBCT, to refine the diagnosis and derive an optimal treatment and biomechanical plan.

enhances the ability to localize impacted canines accurately, evaluate their proximity to other teeth, determine the follicle size and presence of pathology, estimate space conditions, and assess resorption of adjacent teeth (Walker *et al.*, 2005; Haney *et al.*, 2010; Botticelli *et al.*, 2011; Alqerban *et al.*, 2011b; Figure 1.6 and Figure 1.7). Additionally, CBCT imaging not only aids in tooth localization and choice of site for surgical access for a significant number impacted teeth, but also contributes to a significantly higher confidence in diagnosis and treatment planning relative to the combination of panoramic, periapical, and occlusal radiographs that traditionally have been used for this purpose (Haney *et al.*, 2010). More important, the findings also demonstrate that the original treatment plans derived from 2D radiographs are changed for more than 25% of the impacted teeth when orthodontists viewed these teeth in CBCT images. These findings are in concordance with those reported by others (Katheria *et al.*, 2010; Botticelli *et al.*, 2011). The scientific evidence for the utility of CBCT in both refining diagnosis and modifying treatment plans for significant numbers of impacted teeth validates its use for impacted teeth. Some of this scientific evidence on the superiority of CBCT to 2D radiography could be applicable to supernumerary and transposed teeth.

From a clinical standpoint, besides providing detailed information on impacted and transposed tooth location and associated root resorption and pathologies, CBCT facilitates the accurate definition of the relationship of these teeth to neighboring structures and teeth, assists in planning surgical access and bond placement, and helps in defining the optimal direction for extrusion into the oral cavity. The latter information is useful for two reasons. First, it can help minimize or prevent damage to adjacent tooth roots by defining a safe tractional path or, where this is not possible, it can help in the determination of proactive movement of any interfering tooth and root out of the

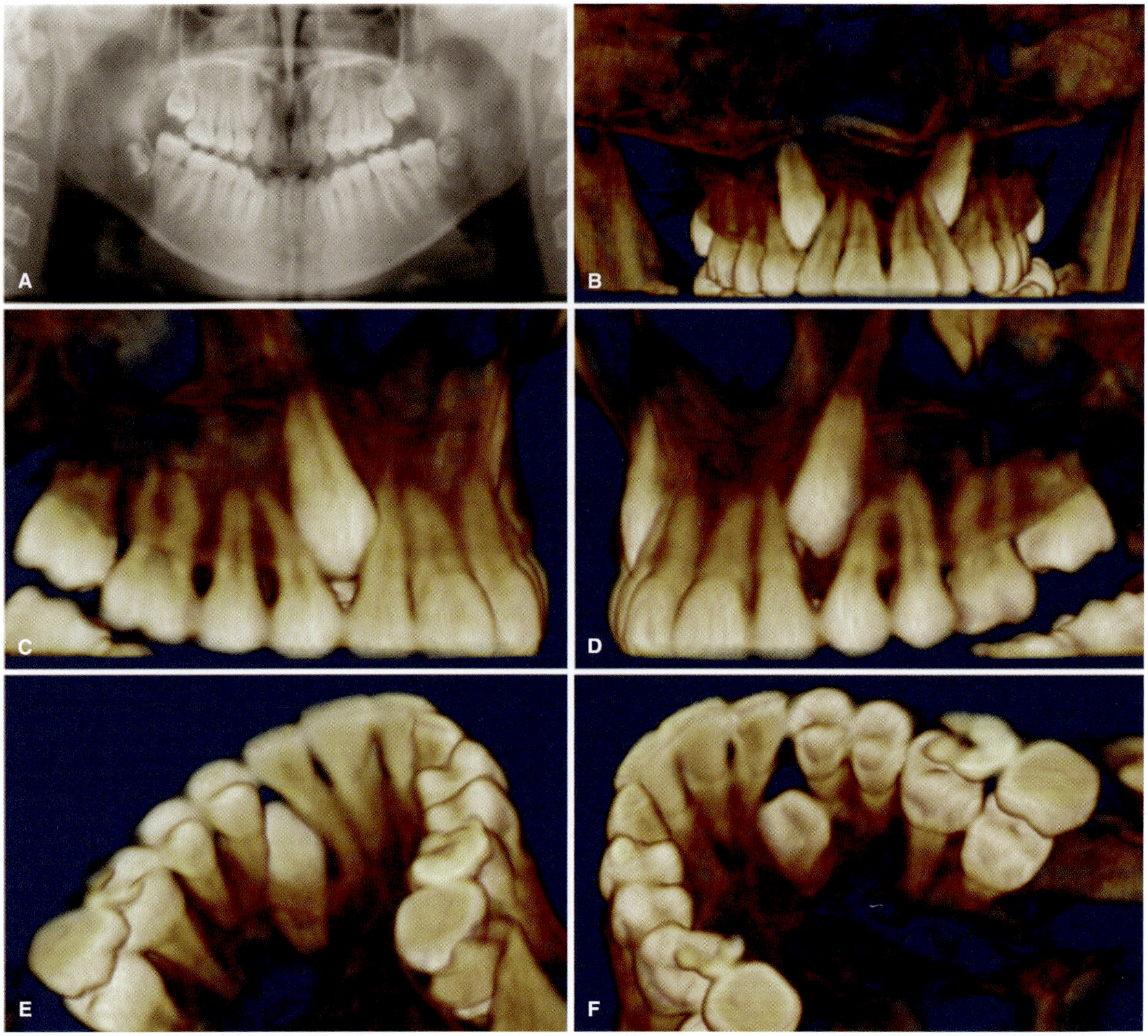

Figure 1.6 Depiction of impacted maxillary canines using a conventional 2D panorex (*A*) and 3D volumetric renderings (*B–F*). The 3D images permit clear visualization of the location and relationships of the impacted canines to adjacent structures, as well as the presence of any root resorption. The detailed information obtained facilitates treatment decisions, including determination of teeth to be extracted in extraction cases such as the one in this figure, optimal surgical approach, appropriate placement of attachments, and biomechanics planning.

tractional path so as to avoid damage. Second, the determination of the direction and path(s) for traction from CBCT aids in designing the appliance or spring optimally to move the tooth most efficiently into the dental arch and occlusion (see also Chapter 16). Increased accuracy of tooth size measurement with CBCT compared with 2D radiographs can aid in determining and developing proactively the space needed to fit the tooth into the arch. Overall, it can be expected that the optimal and accurate utilization of information derived from CBCT to customize treatment for impacted and transposed teeth should result in increased efficiency and enhanced success rates for tooth retrieval.

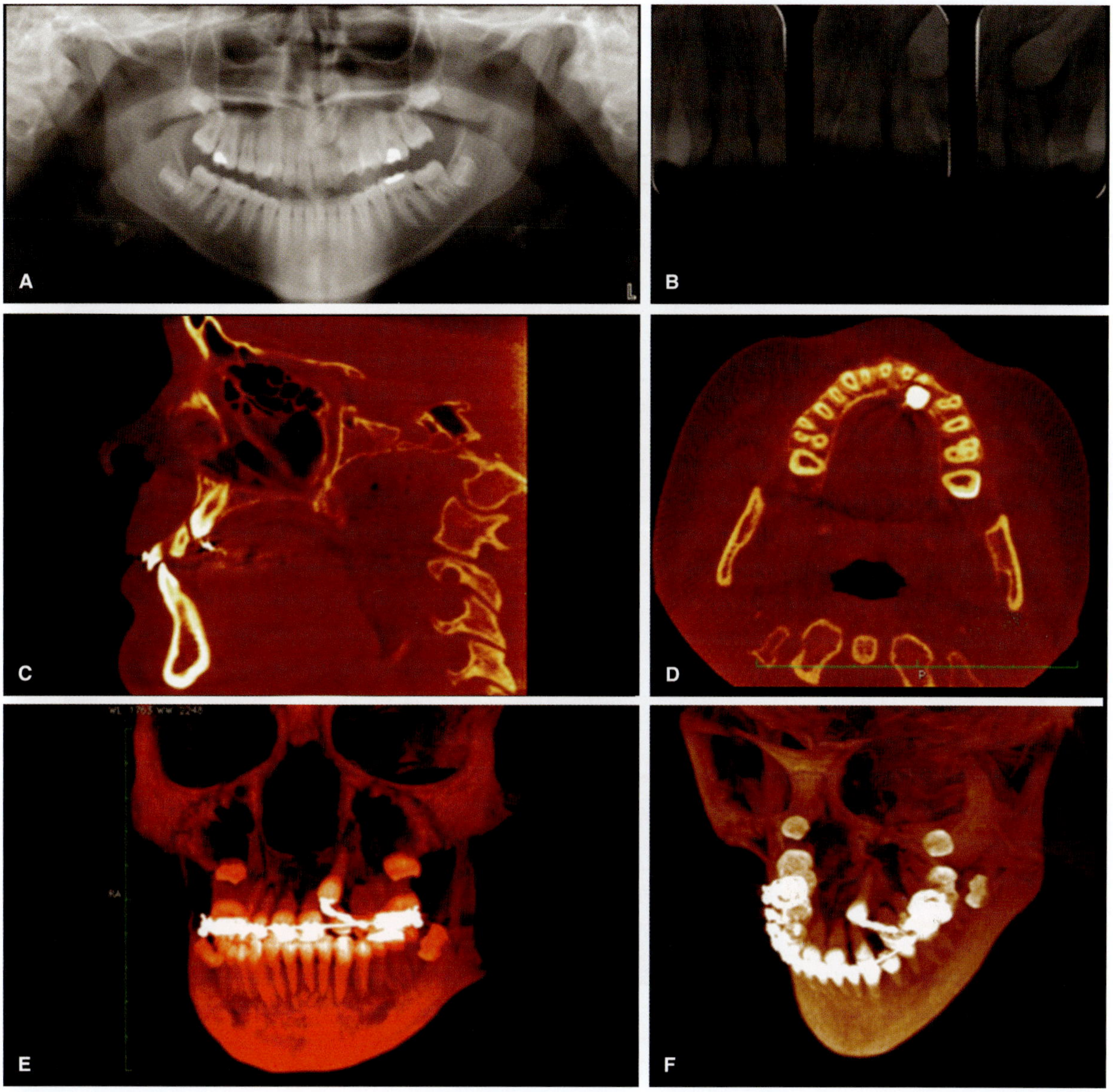

Figure 1.7 Utility of CBCT in diagnosis of localization of impacted teeth and identification of associated root resorption. 2D images are prone to superimposition and other limitations for this purpose that can be overcome with use of 3D radiography that can be useful in identifying precise location of the impacted tooth, its relationship with other structures, and any associated root resorption. In this case, pre-treatment panoramic (*A*) and periapical (*B*) radiographs are not adequate for precise location of the impacted tooth or discerning if root resorption truly is present. Approximately a year into treatment during which time the tooth failed to erupt, a CBCT scan was taken to reveal lateral and central incisor root resorption, as seen here in sagittal (*C*) and axial (*D*) sections and 3D volumetric renderings (*E* and *F*).

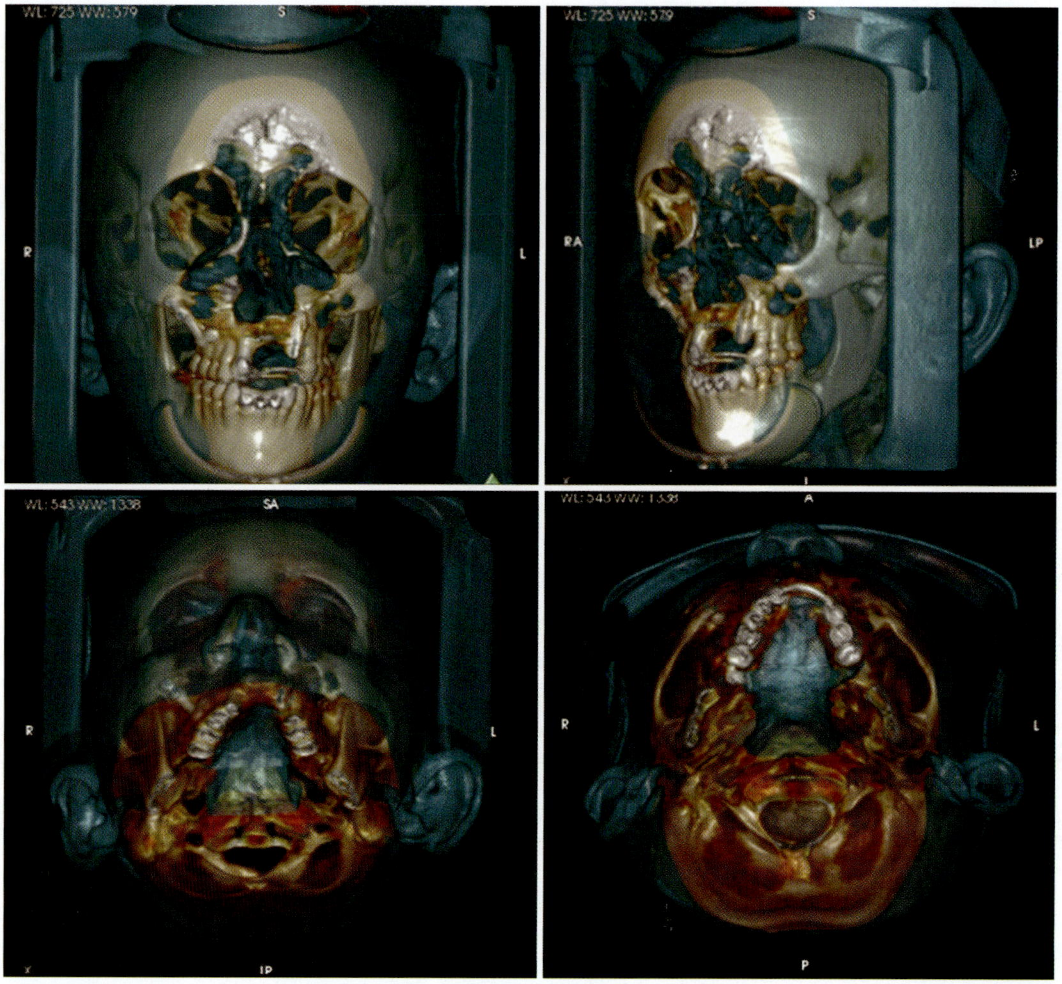

Figure 1.8 3D volumetric reconstructions of a patient with bilateral CL/P are useful in obtaining detailed information on the magnitude of the defect and the status and position of teeth at the defect site. This information can be valuable for diagnosis and treatment planning.

Cleft lip and palate (CL/P)

3D information has been shown to be valuable in determining the volume of the alveolar defect and, therefore, the amount of bone needed for grafting in CL/P patients and for determining the success of bone fill following surgery (Oberoi *et al.*, 2009; Shirota *et al.*, 2010; Figure 1.8). Other valuable information obtained from CBCT in CL/P patients includes the numbers, quality, and location of teeth in proximity to the cleft site (Zhou *et al.*, 2013), the eruption status and path of canines in grafted cleft sites (Oberoi *et al.*, 2010), and diagnosing for implant placement (see also Chapter 23).

Orthognathic and craniofacial anomalies surgical planning and implementation

CBCT combined with computer-aided surgical simulation (CASS) or computer-aided orthognathic surgery (CAOS) offers many novel enhancements including refining diagnosis and optimizing treatment objectives in 3D and virtual treatment

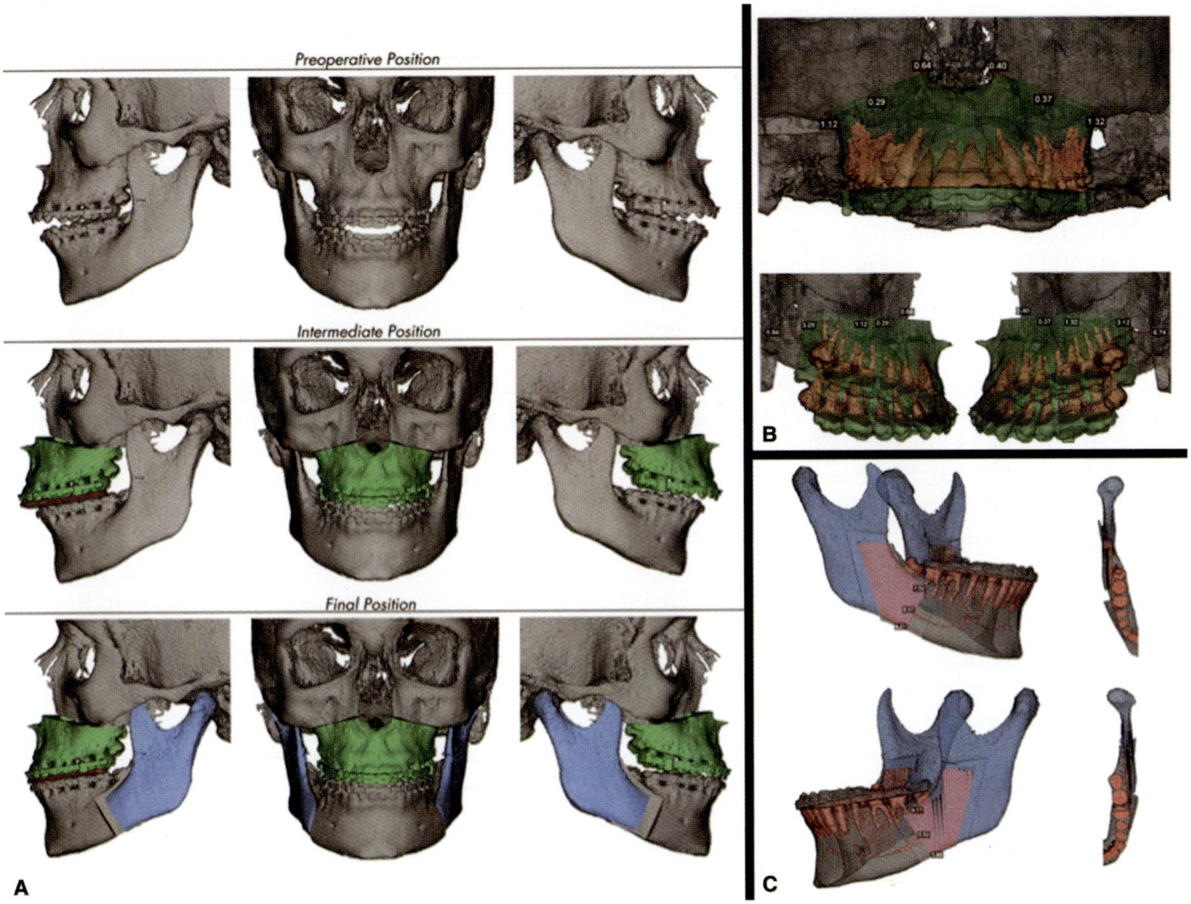

Figure 1.9 Virtual surgical treatment planning for a patient to visualize and determine the magnitude of maxillary and mandibular movements, as well as any complication such as proximal segment interferences that may arise during surgery. The patient's treatment objectives include maxillary impaction to address the openbite and bimaxillary advancement to mitigate obstructive sleep apnea. *A*: An intermediate step involving maxillary advancement and impaction is planned followed by determination of the corresponding mandibular advancement. *B*: Depiction of the magnitude of maxillary movements. *C*: Depiction of mandibular movements and potential proximal segment interferences. The virtual treatment plan then is used to generate an intermediate occlusal wafer and a surgical splint using stereolithography (SLA) or selective laser sintering (SLS).

planning to improve surgical procedures and outcomes (Xia *et al.*, 2000a, 2000b; Hassfeld & Muhling, 2001; Troulis *et al.*, 2002; Gateno *et al.*, 2003, 2007; see also Chapters 20–22). In particular, virtual surgical procedures facilitate the planning of osteotomies, minimizing damage to structures such as nerves, visualizing and planning for interferences such as those of proximal segments, and fabrication of customized fixation devices for orthognathic surgery (Figure 1.9). CBCT with or without co-registered 3D images from other sources such as those from dental casts also can be used to construct physical anatomic models that typically are fabricated in a 1:1 ratio by 3D printing such as stereolithography (SLA) or selective laser sintering (SLS). These physical models can be used to simulate or test treatment options and construct anatomically correct replacement grafts, although they now are used less commonly for this purpose than virtual models. The importance of these approaches as a tool during surgical procedures has been validated by several investigations showing that computer-aided surgery facilitates the prediction of potential surgical complications, decreases the length of surgery, and results in outcomes similar to or better than those of traditional approaches (Xia *et al.*, 2000a, 2000b; Hassfeld & Muhling, 2001; Troulis *et al.*, 2002; Gateno *et al.*, 2003, 2007). Thus, CBCT should be considered an important diagnostic and treatment planning adjunct for cases that will be treated with orthognathic or craniofacial surgery.

3D CBCT imaging is useful particularly in the diagnosis and treatment planning of asymmetries, where discrepancies often manifest in all three planes of space. Facial asymmetries may involve perturbations in the size and shape of the maxilla and/or the mandible in which any number of anatomic structures, including the condyle, condylar neck, ramus, and body of the mandible can be affected. Combined asymmetry in pitch, roll, and yaw produce deformities in the skeletal bases and dental arches. The differences in the bilateral anatomy determined through CBCT facilitates a refined and quantifiable diagnosis of asymmetries that, if clinically significant, may alter a given treatment plan in both growing individuals and adults. When large differences exist between bilateral structures, CBCT scans enable the use of a technique called "mirroring," in which the normal side is mirrored onto the discrepant side so as to simulate and visualize the desired end result, as well as to plan the surgery to facilitate correction (Metzger *et al.*, 2007; see also Chapter 21). Other surgical cases in which 3D CBCT imaging is likely to offer advantages over 2D radiography in diagnosis and treatment planning include those with CL/P (as discussed earlier) and craniofacial anomalies such as hemifacial microsomia, cleidocranial dysplasia, and ectodermal dysplasia.

Case-based and clinical judgment-based use of CBCT

Other than the above clinical entities, the utility of CBCT in other orthodontic situations has been demonstrated through case reports or may be justified based on the provider's clinical judgment of a positive benefit-to-risk analysis. These clinical scenarios encompass anomalies of teeth and roots, including supernumerary teeth, transpositions, and root resorption; TMJ degeneration; suspect boundary conditions; airway concerns; and the determination of possible contributors to or causes of open bites.

Supernumerary teeth

The presence of supernumerary teeth can pose a challenge in the ability to distinguish which tooth is actually the "supernumerary" and which is the "normal tooth" (Katheria *et al.*, 2010). Accurate measurements and the determination of the precise location of the tooth from CBCT images may allow the clinician to make an informed decision on which tooth or teeth to extract on the basis of size, shape, and retrievability of the teeth; the most optimal surgical approach; as well as help to minimize damage to the normal tooth. These points are illustrated well in a case (Figure 1.10) showing the advantages of CBCT over routine radiography in deriving optimal diagnostic information and refined treatment approaches.

Root resorption

For generalized root resorption or that associated with impacted teeth, CBCT scans provide more sensitive and accurate information than do periapical or panoramic radiographs (Alqerban *et al.*, 2009b, 2011b; Durack *et al.*, 2011; Ponder *et al.*, 2012; Ren *et al.*, 2012; see also Chapter 15; Figure 1.7). Thus, detection of mild to moderate pretreatment root resorption by CBCT that may go undetected by 2D radiographs could lead to modifications in treatment plans, such as avoiding extractions in borderline cases to reduce the duration of treatment and magnitude of tooth movement to mitigate additional root resorption. However, there currently is no information that there are differences in the detection of substantial EARR between 2D and CBCT radiography or that its discovery by CBCT during treatment would lead to a treatment decision different from that made if the resorption was detected in 2D radiographs, which typically would entail stopping the treatment at least temporarily. In contrast, it is

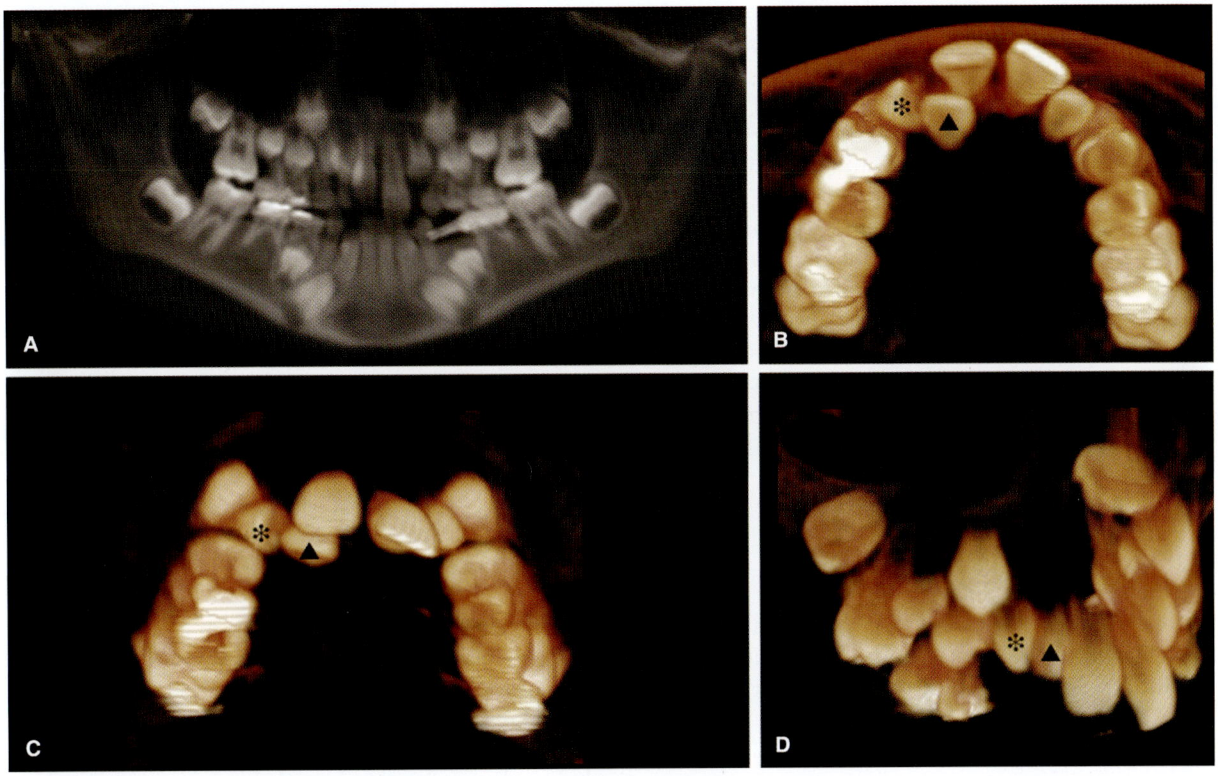

Figure 1.10 CBCT images offer important information and finer details in treatment planning of supernumerary teeth. *A*: A panoramic view extracted from the CBCT scan shows the presence of a supernumary tooth in the upper right lateral incisor area with delayed eruption of the maxillary right central incisor. It is difficult to discern from the panoramic view (or even from periapical radiographs, not shown) which of the two teeth, marked * and ▲ would be optimal morphologically to serve as the lateral incisor. Since the contralateral lateral incisor has not erupted yet, it cannot be examined clinically for size and form for comparison. *B–D*: Various 3D views from CBCT scans allow the comparison of the two teeth on the right lateral incisor area with the unerupted left lateral incisor. An analysis of the mesiodistal measurements of these unerupted teeth revealed that the tooth marked * most closely matches the contralateral lateral incisor morphologically and dimensionally, with tooth marked ▲ being almost 1 mm larger mesiodistally than the contralateral lateral incisor. (Reprinted with permission from Kapila *et al.*, 2011.)

plausible that detection of buccal or lingual root resorption by CBCT that is not visualized by 2D radiographs could differentiate pre- or in-treatment decisions made with the two imaging modalities. The question that remains to be answered in this scenario is how and when a clinician would decide that a patient has undergone such buccal and/or lingual root resorption to justify taking CBCT scan. Because of these considerations, additional work remains to be performed to validate the diagnostic utility and protocols for the use of CBCT for generalized root resorption.

For root resorption associated with impacted teeth, CBCT scans provide substantially superior visualization of roots than routine radiographs by eliminating artifacts resulting from superimposition of structures and depicting the 3D root structure from all possible directions (Alqerban *et al.*, 2009b, 2011b; Figure 1.7). This enhanced information derived from CBCT scans relative to that from

2D images may be critical in changing treatment plans, including the option to extract a resorbed lateral incisor rather than a premolar in an extraction case. Although such treatment decisions appear to be a logical clinical outcome with the use of CBCT, the effects of the superior information derived from CBCT images in modifying treatment decisions as well as determining the threshold of root resorption at which a clinician opts to extract a tooth with a resorbed root rather than a healthy premolar remain to be seen. Finally, the detection by CBCT of abnormal anatomy of the root, such as dilacerated roots—particularly in the bucco-lingual direction not seen in 2D radiographs—also may help determine the amount and direction that a dilacerated tooth can be moved or may aid in the decision to extract it.

Miscellaneous dental anomalies

Other dental anomalies that may benefit from CBCT imaging over traditional radiographs include delayed or unerupted teeth and congenitally missing teeth.

Alveolar boundary conditions

CBCT imaging can help verify alveolar boundary conditions that typically are not observable by 2D radiographs that either may be inadequate prior to treatment or may become compromised during tooth movement. Compromised or limited pretreatment alveolar boundary conditions may limit or interfere with the planned or potential tooth movement, as well as the final desired spatial position and angulation of the teeth. Failure to diagnose compromised alveolar bone prior to treatment and to factor this into the treatment plan likely will lead to worsening of the problem during orthodontic treatment. The visualization and characterization of boundary conditions is performed best by carefully analyzing MPR and volumetric CBCT information during the initial workup (Figure 1.11), which may aid in implementing alternative treatment strategies when indicated.

As with other types of cases, it is best to be selective about which cases may benefit from CBCT scans for assessing alveolar boundary conditions. These include those presenting with alveolar bone phenotypes that clinically appear too narrow to accommodate significant labio- or bucco-lingual displacements or changes in angulations of teeth (Figure 1.11), those with compromised periodontium and/or gingival anatomy, those where the planned orthodontic movements are substantial enough such that the bone anatomy is not likely to adapt to these movements, and those where the movement of the tooth may entail translocating it past another tooth or obstruction (Figure 14.3). As discussed in Chapter 14, specific clinical situations that may pose challenges related to boundary conditions include those with existing thin or compromised labial and/or buccal anatomy of the alveolar bone, transposed or ectopic teeth, bimaxillary protrusion involving an extraction treatment plan, camouflage treatment of compensated dentoalveolar structures where round-trip orthodontic mechanics is used, dilacerated roots, and where bone is deficient or missing (i.e., CL/P). Precise information on alveolar boundary conditions also may be helpful in treatment planning decisions for situations that require moving teeth close to the alveolar boundaries such as in borderline nonextraction cases or in situations where teeth are being decompensated, such as commonly is performed in orthognathic surgery cases. CBCT-aided diagnosis of fenestrations may be useful in planning treatment to torque roots back into bone using sophisticated biomechanics combined with TADs.

TMJ degeneration, progressive bite changes, functional shifts, and responses to therapy

A radiographic examination of the TMJ is an important component in the diagnosis and monitoring of responses to therapy in TMJ diseases in which the articulating osseous tissues or joint spatial relationships are compromised (Okeson, 1996). However, conventional 2D radiography of the TMJ including panoramic radiographs and cephalograms do not provide an accurate characterization of the joint because of distorted images with superimposed structures. Although TMJ tomograms are superior to other 2D radiographs of the TMJ, they provide only information limited to a few sections of the joint. In contrast, CBCT images the entire joint with visualization of minor to overt osseous hard tissue morphologic changes

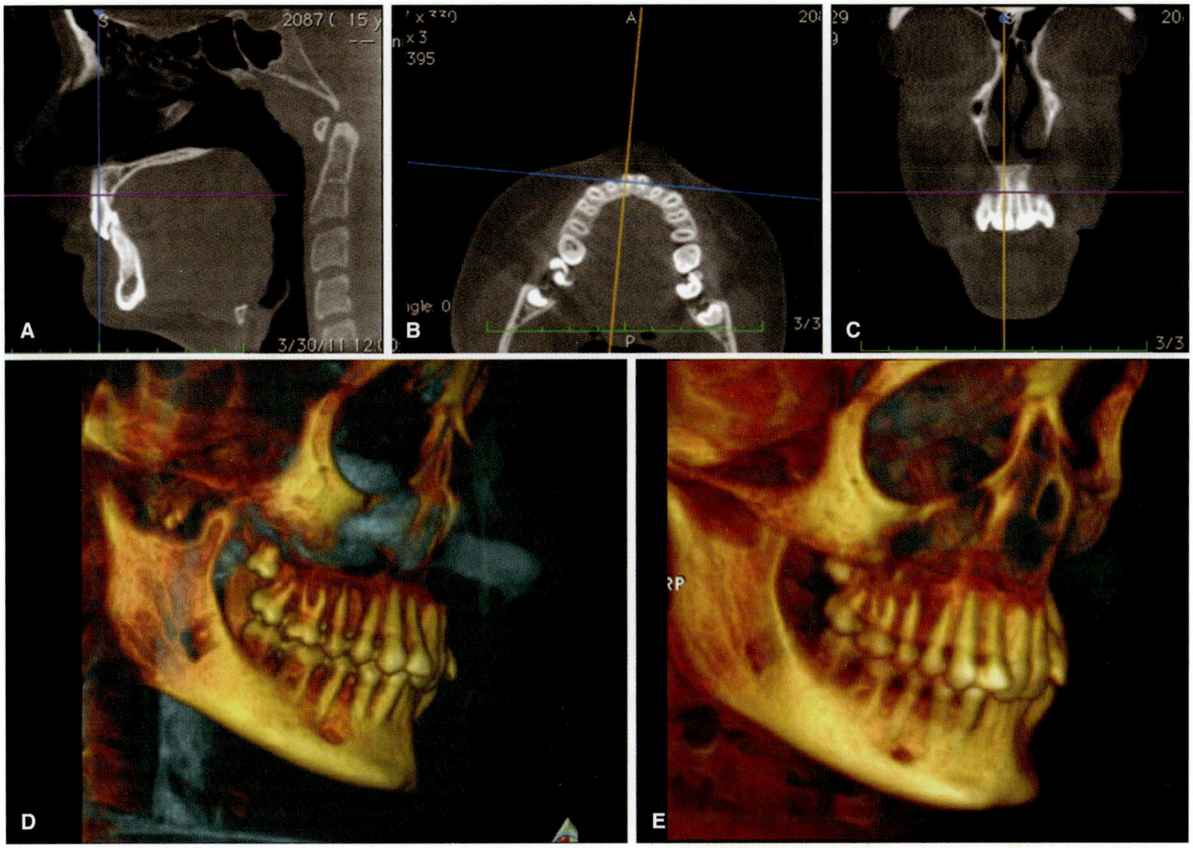

Figure 1.11 Determination of anterior boundary conditions in a case with severely retroclined maxillary and mandibular incisors using sagittal (*A*), axial (*B*) and coronal (*C*) multiplanar, and 3D volumetric (*D* and *E*) reconstructions. This patient with a severe Class II division 2 malocclusion presents with upper incisor roots that have limited buccal bone support that could be placed into a better relationship with the bone through lingual root torque. In contrast, the lower incisors are retroclined severely and the boundary conditions may not adapt adequately during orthodontic flaring of these teeth. Information such as this could be helpful in planning treatment and defining the optimal methods to move teeth.

and congruency of bone surfaces that define the joint space resulting from pathology and adaptive processes and allows for accurate detection and evaluation of pathological changes (Honda *et al.*, 2006; Honey *et al.*, 2007; Figure 1.12). Radiographic signs of bony changes associated with TMJ arthritides include irregular and possibly thickened cortical outlines (sclerosis), erosions, osteophyte formation, subchondral cysts, and flattening and narrowing of the joint space (Gynther *et al.*, 1996; Ahmad *et al.*, 2009; Alexiou *et al.*, 2009). Since these changes occur in a spectrum of TMJ diseases including OA, rheumatoid arthritis (RA), idiopathic condylar resorption, and other less common diseases, CBCT alone without history and clinical findings cannot distinguish between these disorders but can be useful for refining their diagnosis or responses to therapies. For example, early diagnosis and treatment of destructive inflammatory conditions, if determined clinically and/or by imaging, could prove advantageous since it has been shown that early intervention is important for controlling further bone destruction successfully (Allaart *et al.*, 2006), which, in turn, can be monitored by CBCT (Finzel *et al.*, 2011).

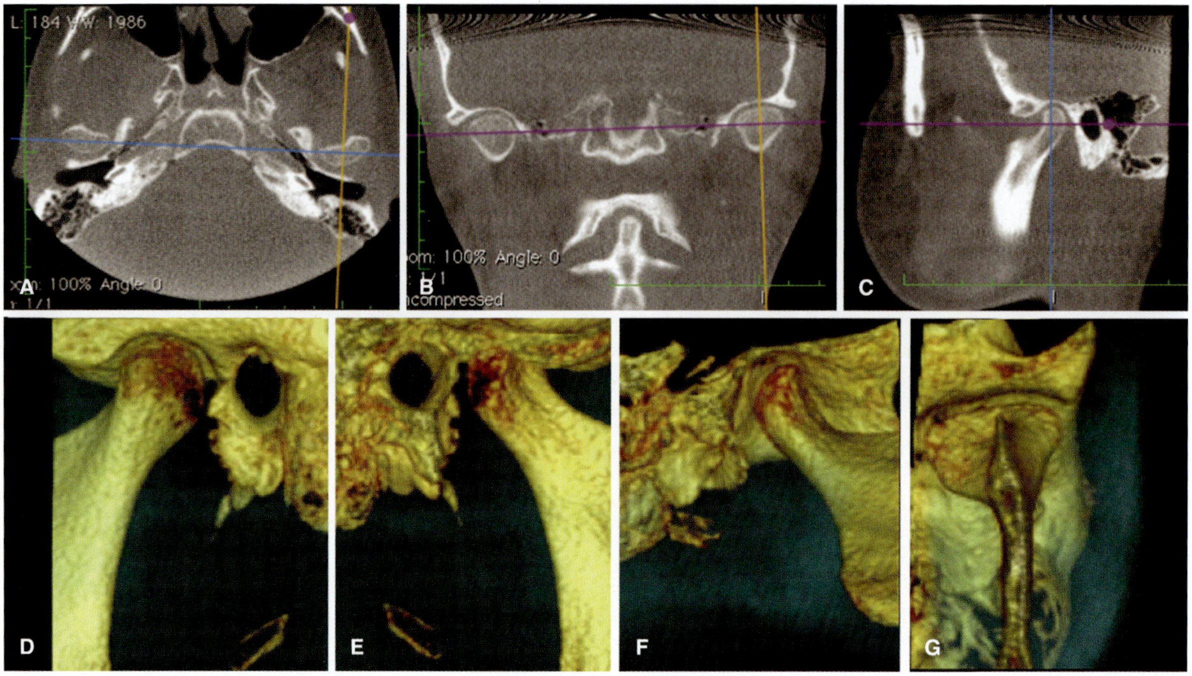

Figure 1.12 Visualization of the TMJ in the axial (*A*), coronal (*B*), and sagittal (*C*) planes, as well as 3D volumetric reconstructions here visualized from the buccal (*D*), medial (*E*), medio-inferior (*F*), and antero-inferior (*G*). Such detailed visualization without any superimposition of structures and in 3D can help in the identification of pathologic changes, including sclerosis, flattening, erosions, osteophytes, abnormalities in joint spaces, and responses of the joint tissues to therapy. Although these changes are visualized more clearly by CBCT than 2D radiography, there is little current evidence that the findings lead to changes in treatment plans.

While relatively infrequent, some patients who have TMJ pathologies such as temporomandibular joint disorders (TMJDs) or developmental disorders, including condylar hyperplasia, hypoplasia, or aplasia, undergo adverse morphologic and functional changes that include progressive bite changes, dental and skeletal compensations, and limitation or deviation of jaw movements (Helenius *et al.*, 2005; Koyama *et al.*, 2007; Alexiou *et al.*, 2009; Yura *et al.*, 2010) that contribute to unpredictable orthodontic outcomes. When these conditions occur during development, they can result in perturbed growth of the condyle on the affected joint, a decrease in ipsilateral mandibular growth, and accompanying compensations in the maxilla, tooth position, occlusion, and cranial base (Guyuron, 1988). Bilateral degenerative changes in the TMJ also may alter the facial growth pattern, resulting in adverse skeletal and dental changes in the vertical, horizontal, and transverse directions and contributing to mandibular retrusion, anterior open bite, and Class II malocclusion (Yura *et al.*, 2010). Because of the large numbers of structures involved and the inherent limitations of 2D radiography, changes resulting from these disorders are difficult to characterize accurately with conventional 2D radiography. In contrast, by allowing the concurrent visualization of the TMJs and assessment of the maxillo-mandibular-spatial relationships and occlusion, CBCT images provide the opportunity to visualize and quantify the local and regional effects associated with the TMJ abnormalities. With further advances in the field, CBCT may provide the ability to monitor the effects of therapy on condylar morphology and repair and aid in assessing both the efficacy and potential prognosis of the treatment (see also Chapter 12). Although not yet studied or validated, CBCT may also offer some advantages in diagnosing the initial skeletal and dental relationships in patients with large centric relation/centric occlusion (CR/CO) shifts such that images taken in CR would provide a frame of reference of the pre-treatment findings in three planes to aid in treatment decisions.

Temporary anchorage devices (TADs)

While there is not a high level of indication for CBCT scans in the placement of TADs, these images can prove helpful for macro-anatomical analyses through visualization of neighboring structures such as tooth roots, sinuses, and nerves that can be valuable for avoiding damage or complications (see also Chapter 18), as well as for micro-anatomical evaluation of the quantity and quality of cortical bone that may determine primary and secondary TAD stability. These determinations can aid in identifying optimal sites for TAD placement, thereby enhancing the chances of success. For example, it has been shown that a location 4 mm palatal to the incisive foramen provides excellent bone volume for palatal bone screws (King *et al.*, 2007; Gracco *et al.*, 2008). A technique involving a high-resolution 0.1 mm slice thickness CBCT and rapid prototyping to fabricate surgical guides also has been described for placing TADs on the buccal aspect of the jaws. Although the use of CBCT for TAD placement may not be justified in routine cases and locations at this point, it could have applications where a TAD needs to be placed in sites with complex anatomical structures or relationships (Jung *et al.*, 2012). In such situations, unless the CBCT is needed for other reasons as well, a limited FOV CBCT scan typically may be adequate.

Case types not indicated for CBCT utilization

Cases in which clinical examination with or without 2D radiographs indicates that CBCT will not provide valuable new information typically do not justify the utilization of CBCT. Although CBCT is used to a limited extent for constructing custom fixed appliances and/or fabricating custom wires, the utilization of CBCT for this purpose also remains questionable. This is because other non-radiologic digital imaging technologies are available that serve as adequate alternatives and the radiation exposure with CBCT makes the benefit-to-risk ratio for the utilization of this technology for this purpose extremely low. Even though CBCT provides information on roots that would not be available with other scanning modalities, no data presently are available to suggest that this enhanced information results in better or more efficient treatments. Finally, CBCT images taken primarily to enhance patient and parent education are not a justified use of this technology.

PROTOCOLS FOR UTILIZING AND INTERPRETING CBCT IN ORTHODONTICS

Imaging goals and protocols

CBCT imaging goals in orthodontics should include evaluation and, where indicated, measurement of anatomic features, size, and relationships. Anatomic features include orthodontic landmarks and anatomic descriptors that help to differentiate between normal and abnormal anatomy. An imaging protocol for orthodontic purposes should take several factors into consideration. First, the image should incorporate the desired FOV that, in turn, is determined by the ROI. The provider first must decide what the CBCT image needs to accomplish for a specific patient. This determination is made on the basis of a thorough clinical exam supplemented by 2D radiography when necessary (Figure 1.5). Depending on the needs of the patient determined by this evaluation, the orthodontist may prescribe a small, medium, large, or extended FOV. The small FOV is used for assessing individual teeth (impacted teeth, root morphology, supernumeraries), quadrants, or sites for TAD placement (Figure 1.13). The medium or large FOV includes the mandible, the maxilla, or parts of both and typically would be used when requiring information on occlusal relationships, localized asymmetries, or bilateral TMJ evaluations or when the condition(s) of interest (i.e., potentially adverse boundary conditions) are present in both arches or jaws. The large or extended FOV includes the

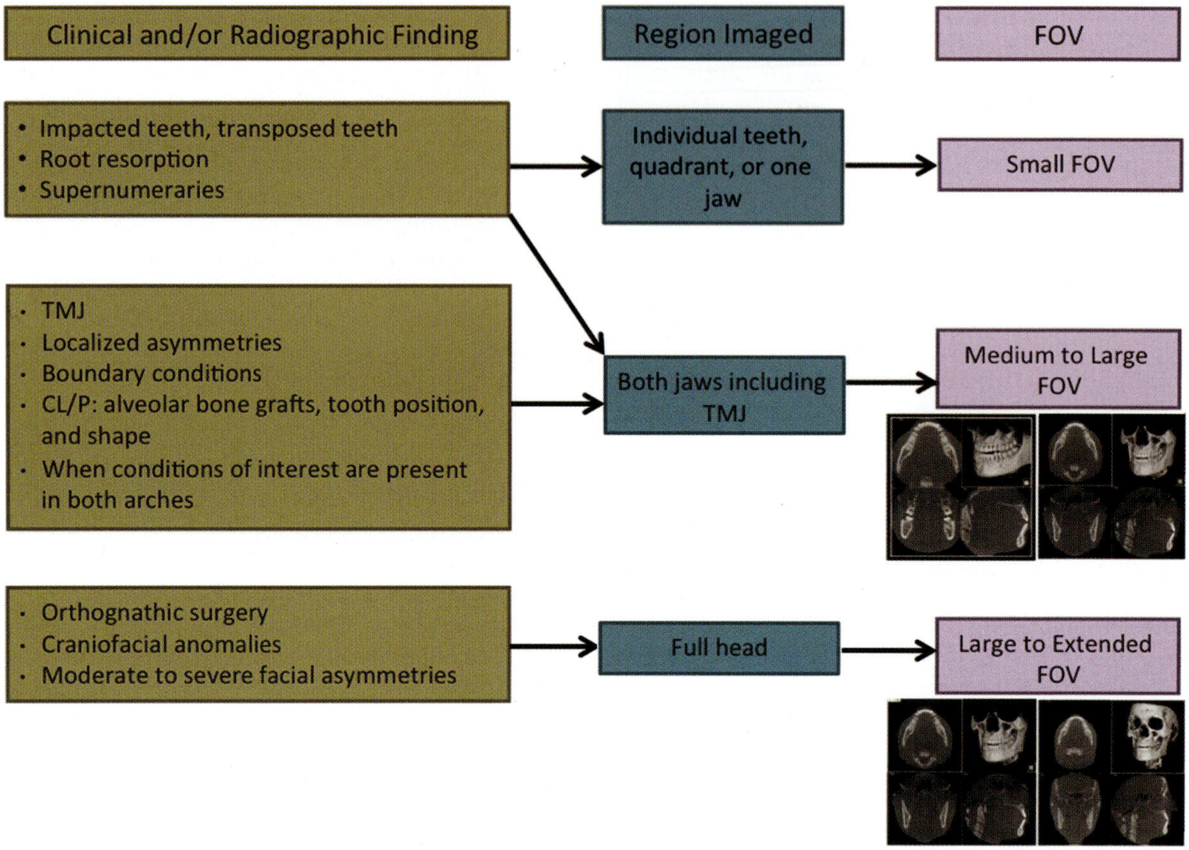

Figure 1.13 Protocol for the selection of appropriate CBCT FOV to obtain additional information following the discovery of specific findings from history and clinical examination. The choice of the FOV is based on the diagnostic objectives for the imaging as determined through a careful clinical assessment of the patient. The recommended FOV for specific needs also is dependent on the size of the individual. Thus, if the image of the entire craniofacial region is needed, it might entail using a large FOV for a child and an extended FOV for an adult. The FOV should default to the larger FOV indicated in each category when findings at distinct sites are being investigated so as to incorporate these ROIs in the FOV.

whole head and helps to visualize relationships between skeletal bases and between teeth and skeletal bases, as well as significant anomalies in patients requiring orthognathic surgery or having craniofacial anomalies. Obviously, the FOV also will be determined by the physical size of the subject; thus, a large FOV that primarily captures the maxilla and mandible of a large adult may be adequate to image the whole head of a child. It also is important to keep in mind that a smaller FOV not only decreases the radiation exposure to the patient but also has the added benefit of increasing the image quality, since the flat panel detector picks up less scattered radiation.

As discussed earlier, the initial interpretation of a CBCT scan should be performed by a diagnostician who has the necessary expertise for this purpose (Figure 1.14). Given the current status of the orthodontist's skills in interpreting CBCTs (Ahmed *et al.*, 2012), the scans ideally should be read by a radiologist. Once the CBCT report including relevant images is derived and communicated by the diagnostician, the orthodontist should extract additional details on the clinical entity

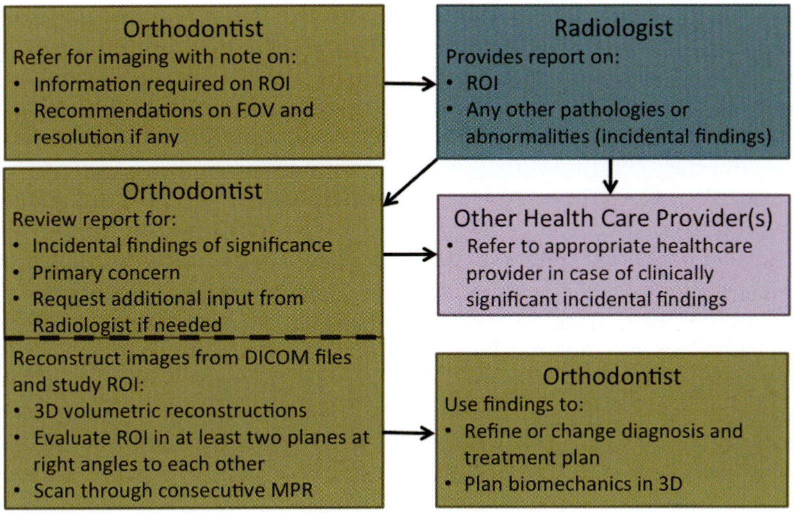

Figure 1.14 Protocol on image prescription and CBCT information extraction and management followed by appropriate patient referral and derivation of diagnostic information.

being imaged and any clinically relevant incidental findings from a review of the report and images provided. When clinically significant incidental findings are observed, the orthodontist and/or the radiologist should refer the patient to the appropriate healthcare provider. The orthodontist also should examine the entire volume virtually, particularly the ROI, to maximize the retrieval of clinically relevant information that may not be obvious in the radiologist's report. Therefore, it is important for the orthodontist to learn to use and manipulate 3D imaging software. Toward this goal, several user-friendly software programs now are available commercially and are relatively easy to utilize and master.

Following appropriate orientation of the images on the computer, the orthodontist should view the entire ROI from at least two planes at right angles to each other that will offer a multidimensional perspective, as well as the volumetric rendering in a 3D format (Figure 1.2; see also Chapters 2 and 8). In all, this protocol will enable the clinician to view an entire scan through 2D images in the axial, coronal, and sagittal planes, in addition to a 3D-rendered view, which can be rotated 360° or translated in three planes of space, offering up to six degrees of freedom. The information thus obtained should be used to refine diagnosis, modify the treatment plan, and optimize the biomechanics when indicated.

AREAS REQUIRING FURTHER STUDY

Despite promising studies and anecdotal support for the use of CBCT scans for specific clinical applications, the ultimate question to be answered is what true measurable quantitative and/or qualitative impact the observations from the scans have in modifying or enhancing diagnosis and altering or refining treatment plans. It is likely that future studies not only will address these questions, but also will help in modifying imaging protocols and image outputs, and possibly changing the overall strategies in which we approach the treatment of specific types of cases. For example, while CBCT scans are proving to be valuable in localizing impacted teeth, it is expected that the information gained increasingly will dictate the biomechanics by which we tract teeth, the direction of traction through the shortest possible path while minimizing damage to adjacent teeth, the optimal proactive placement of roots of neighboring teeth so that they are not damaged, and optimization of the placement of the tooth as it appears in the oral cavity (see also Chapter 16). Several additional examples are outlined later that offer rich opportunities for inquiry that may help better to define, delineate, and justify the utilization of CBCT in specific types of cases.

CBCT imaging is beginning to provide critical information on bone boundary conditions that previously was not available. Current orthodontic treatment entails moving teeth as best as possible within the constraints of the bone encasing the roots. Often, little consideration is given to the limits that the bone is capable of adapting around the roots and many clinicians practice mechanics in which teeth often are subjected to round-tripping. Thus, for example, in crowded cases treated with extraction therapy and continuous archwires, it is likely that the incisors will be flared before being retracted to their final position following space consolidation. It is not known yet if this compromises the quantity or quality of bone support, leads to increased incidence of fenestrations, or perhaps even increases root resorption. Such negative consequences could apply to other types of round-tripping tooth movements or to expansion beyond the permissible boundary conditions in all three planes. Further complicating the potential for these adverse responses are the possible effects that the pre-treatment bone biotype and alveolar anatomy may have on the likelihood for orthodontically mediated tissue damage. If supported by future research evidence, information from CBCT increasingly may become important in identifying patients whose bone anatomy and biotype will not be able to accommodate dental expansion to manage crowded arches, thus aiding in treatment decisions (see also Chapter 14). Such studies then could help provide guidelines that could be added to our diagnostic armamentarium when planning orthodontic treatments and also aid in identifying patients whose diagnosis and treatment would need to be modified on the basis of this CBCT data. As further scientific information on the limitations imposed by alveolar boundary conditions on orthodontic treatment become available, prior to commencing treatment the clinicians may be able to address additional questions such as: (1) Can the desired tooth movement be accomplished within the existing boundary conditions? (2) Will the boundary conditions be affected positively or negatively by skeletal or dento-alveolar expansion or tooth retraction? (3) What are the effects of compromised bone as in periodontal disease on the ability to move teeth in the sagittal or transverse planes? (4) What are the limits of bone adaptability and how is this affected by age, periodontal health, and the pre-treatment bone and anatomic phenotype of the patient?

While root resorption has been associated with various factors such as root morphology and use of heavy forces, many of these links remain tenuous (Weltman *et al.*, 2010). 3D images derived from CBCT scans may offer better insights into key causative factors for apical root resorption, particularly if performed at high resolution on a limited FOV. This information would enable clinicians to take necessary measures to minimize damage to roots during orthodontic treatment. Similar studies could help to distinguish the systemic and/or local basis for the mild localized versus moderate to severe generalized root resorption phenotypes that likely have different underlying biologic reasons and, thus, possibly contribute to more refined methods to manage or prevent these adverse responses. Also, a careful assessment of the correlations between 3D changes in root morphology during orthodontic treatment and biomarkers may offer novel non-invasive diagnostic assays that could be used to identify subjects predisposed to or undergoing orthodontic root resorption. This would enable the clinician to make appropriate and timely decisions on treatment options. Additionally, it is possible that high-resolution CBCT scans might offer definitive diagnostic information on tooth ankylosis in the future, which is an important question in need of investigation. Finally, CBCT imaging could help answer numerous questions within the broad thematic areas of orthognathic surgery, CL/P, craniofacial anomalies, developing asymmetries, as well as airway morphology, OSA, and TMJ disorders.

CONCLUSIONS

Since its introduction into dentistry in 1998, CBCT has become an increasingly important source of 3D volumetric information in clinical orthodontics. Over this period, valuable CBCT data have been accumulated on technology assessment, craniofacial morphology in health and disease, treatment outcomes, and efficacy of CBCT images in diagnosis and treatment planning. This chapter provides a summary of the current understanding of and evidence for the clinical utility of CBCT in orthodontics, reviews the findings that use this technology in answering clinically relevant questions, describes the current indications and protocols for the use of CBCT in specific cases, and poses key questions that need to be addressed through additional studies that would help to validate or determine other future uses of this technology in orthodontics. Although CBCT continues to gain substantial popularity, its use currently is recommended in cases in which conventional radiography cannot supply satisfactory diagnostic information including impacted teeth, CL/P, and planning of orthognathic or craniofacial surgery patients. CBCT on other types of cases also can be performed where there is likely to be a positive benefit-to-risk outcome such as supernumerary teeth, identification of root resorption caused by unerupted teeth, evaluating boundary conditions, TMJ degeneration, and progressive bite changes and for placement of TADs in complex situations.

References

Abdul-Kader, H. (2008) Medicolegal perspective: interpretation of pretreatment orthodontic radiographs. *World Journal of Orthodontics*, 9, 14–20.

Adams, G.L., Gansky, S.A., Miller, A.J., *et al.* (2004) Comparison between traditional 2-dimensional cephalometry and a 3-dimensional approach on human dry skulls. *American Journal of Orthodontics and Dentofacial Orthopedics*, 126 (4), 397–409.

Ahmad, M., Hollender, L., Anderson, Q., *et al.* (2009) Research diagnostic criteria for temporomandibular disorders (RDC/TMD): development of image analysis criteria and examiner reliability for image analysis. *Oral Surgery, Oral Medicine, Oral Pathology, Oral Radiology and Endodontology*, 107 (6), 844–860.

Ahmed, F., Brooks, S.L., & Kapila, S. (2012) The efficacy of identifying maxillofacial lesions in cone beam computed tomographs by orthodontists and orthodontic residents. *American Journal of Orthodontics and Dentofacial Orthopedics*, 141, 451–459. http://dx.doi.org/10.1016/j.ajodo.2011.10.025.

Alexiou, K., Stamatakis, H., & Tsiklakis, K. (2009) Evaluation of the severity of temporomandibular joint osteoarthritic changes related to age using cone beam computed tomography. *Dentomaxillofacial Radiology*, 38 (3), 141–147.

Alkhader, M., Ohbayashi, N., Tetsumura, A., *et al.* (2010) Diagnostic performance of magnetic resonance imaging for detecting osseous abnormalities of the temporomandibular joint and its correlation with cone beam computed tomography. *Dentomaxillofacial Radiology*, 39 (5), 270–276.

Allaart, C.F., Goekoop-Ruiterman, Y.P., de Vries-Bouwstra, J.K., *et al.* (2006) Aiming at low disease activity in rheumatoid arthritis with initial combination therapy or initial monotherapy strategies: the BeSt study. *Clinical and Experimental Rheumatology*, 24 (6 Suppl 43), S77–S82.

Almeida, R.C., Cevidanes, L.H., & Carvalho, F.A. (2011) Soft tissue response to mandibular advancement using 3D CBCT scanning. *International Journal of Oral and Maxillofacial Surgery*, 40 (4), 353–359.

Alqerban, A., Jacobs, R., Lambrechts, P., *et al.* (2009a) Root resorption of the maxillary lateral incisor caused by impacted canine: a literature review. *Clinical Oral Investigations*, 13 (3), 247–255.

Alqerban, A., Jacobs, R., Souza, P.C., *et al.* (2009b) *In-vitro* comparison of two cone-beam computed tomography systems and panoramic imaging for detecting simulated canine impaction-induced external root resorption in maxillary lateral incisors. *American Journal of Orthodontics and Dentofacial Orthopedics*, 136 (6), 764, e1–e11.

Alqerban, A., Jacobs, R., & Fieuws, S. (2011a) Comparison of six cone-beam computed tomography systems for image quality and detection of simulated canine impaction-induced external root resorption in maxillary lateral incisors. *American Journal of Orthodontics and Dentofacial Orthopedics*, 140 (3), e129–e139.

Alqerban, A., Jacobs, R., & Fieuws, S. (2011b) Comparison of two cone beam computed tomographic systems versus panoramic imaging for localization of impacted maxillary canines and detection of root resorption. *European Journal of Orthodontics*, 33 (1), 93–102.

American Association of Orthodontists. Statement on the Role of CBCT in Orthodontics (26-10 H). eBulletin May 7, 2010. Available at: http://www.aaomembers.org/Resources/Publications/ebulletin-05-06-10.cfm, accessed March 18, 2011.

American Association of Orthodontists Insurance Company. (2010) Cone beam technology: legal caveats. *The Bulletin*, 28, 24–25.

Artun, J. & Grobety, D. (2001) Periodontal status of mandibular incisors after pronounced orthodontic advancement during adolescence: a follow-up evaluation. *American Journal of Orthodontics and Dentofacial Orthopedics*, 119 (1), 2–10.

Asaumi, J.I., Hisatomi, M., Yanagi, Y., *et al.* (2008) Evaluation of panoramic radiographs taken at the initial visit at a department of paediatric dentistry. *Dentomaxillofacial Radiology*, 37 (6), 340–343.

Avrahami, E. & Englender, M. (1995) Relation between CT axial cross-sectional area of the oropharynx and obstructive sleep apnea syndrome in adults. *American Journal of Neuroradiology*, 16 (1), 135–140.

Baek, S.H., Kim, T.K., & Kim, M.J. (2006) Is there any difference in the condylar position and angulation after asymmetric mandibular setback? *Oral Surgery, Oral Medicine, Oral Pathology, Oral Radiology and Endodontology*, 101 (2), 155–163.

Baek, S.H., Kim, K., & Choi, J.Y. (2009) Evaluation of treatment modality for skeletal class III malocclusion with labioversed upper incisors and/or protrusive maxilla: surgical movement and stability of rotational maxillary setback procedure. *Journal of Craniofacial Surgery*, 20 (6), 2049–2054.

Baik, H.S. & Kim, S.Y. (2010) Facial soft-tissue changes in skeletal Class III orthognathic surgery patients analyzed with 3-dimensional laser scanning. *American Journal of Orthodontics and Dentofacial Orthopedics*, 138 (2), 167–178.

Berlin, L. (2005) Errors of omission. *American Journal of Roentgenology*, 185 (6), 1416–1421.

Bondemark, L., Jeppsson, M., Lindh-Ingildsen, L., *et al.* (2006) Incidental findings of pathology and abnormality in pretreatment orthodontic panoramic radiographs. *Angle Orthodontist*, 76 (1), 98–102.

Botticelli, S., Verna, C., Cattaneo, P.M., *et al.* (2011) Two-versus three-dimensional imaging in subjects with unerupted maxillary canines. *European Journal of Orthodontics*, 33 (4), 344–349.

Bouwens, D.G., Cevidanes, L., Ludlow, J.B., *et al.* (2011) Comparison of mesiodistal root angulation with post-treatment panoramic radiographs and cone-beam computed tomography. *American Journal of Orthodontics and Dentofacial Orthopedics*, 139 (1), 126–132.

Brooks, S.L. (2009) CBCT dosimetry: orthodontic considerations. *Seminars in Orthodontics*, 15 (1), 14–18.

Busby, B.R., Bailey, L.J., Proffit, W.R., *et al.* (2002) Long-term stability of surgical class III treatment: a study of 5-year postsurgical results. *The International Journal of Adult Orthodontics and Orthognathic Surgery*, 17 (3), 159–170.

Caballero, P., Alvarez-Sala, R., Garcia-Rio, F., *et al.* (1998) CT in the evaluation of the upper airway in healthy subjects and in patients with obstructive sleep apnea syndrome. *Chest*, 113 (1), 111–116.

Caglayan, F. & Tozoglu, U. (2012) Incidental findings in the maxillofacial region detected by cone beam CT. *Diagnostic and Interventional Radiology*, 18 (2), 159–163.

Carvalho Fde, A., Almeida, R.C., Almeida, M.A., *et al.* (2010) Efficiency of light-emitting diode and halogen units in reducing residual monomers. *American Journal of Orthodontics and Dentofacial Orthopedics*, 138 (5), 617–622.

Cattaneo, P.M., Treccani, M., Carlsson, K., *et al.* (2011) Transversal maxillary dento-alveolar changes in patients treated with active and passive self-ligating brackets: a randomized clinical trial using CBCT-scans and digital models. *Orthodontics & Craniofacial Research*, 14 (4), 222–233.

Cevidanes, L.H., Bailey, L.J., Tucker, G.R., Jr., *et al.* (2005) Superimposition of 3D cone-beam CT models of orthognathic surgery patients. *Dentomaxillofacial Radiology*, 34 (6), 369–375.

Cevidanes, L.H., Bailey, L.J., Tucker, S.F., *et al.* (2007) Three-dimensional cone-beam computed tomography for assessment of mandibular changes after orthognathic surgery. *American Journal of Orthodontics and Dentofacial Orthopedics*, 131 (1), 44–50.

Cevidanes, L.H., Hajati, A.K., Paniagua, B., *et al.* (2010a) Quantification of condylar resorption in temporomandibular joint osteoarthritis. *Oral Surgery, Oral Medicine, Oral Patholology, Oral Radiolology and Endodontology*, 110 (1), 110–117.

Cevidanes, L.H., Motta, A., Proffit, W.R., *et al.* (2010b) Cranial base superimposition for 3-dimensional evaluation of soft-tissue changes. *American Journal of Orthodontics and Dentofacial Orthopedics*, 137 (4 Suppl), S120–S129.

Cha, J.Y., Mah, J., & Sinclair, P. (2007) Incidental findings in the maxillofacial area with 3-dimensional cone-beam imaging. *American Journal of Orthodotics and Dentofacial Orthopedics*, 132 (1), 7–14.

Chen, F., Terada, K., Hua, Y., *et al.* (2007) Effects of bimaxillary surgery and mandibular setback surgery on pharyngeal airway measurements in patients with Class III skeletal deformities. *American Journal of Orthodontics and Dentofacial Orthopedics*, 131 (3), 372–377.

Corbridge, J.K., Campbell, P.M., Taylor, R., *et al.* (2011) Transverse dentoalveolar changes after slow maxillary expansion. *American Journal of Orthodontics and Dentofacial Orthopedics*, 140 (3), 317–325.

Dalstra, M., Cattaneo, P.M., & Melsen, B. (2004) Load transfer of miniscrews for orthodontic anchorage. *Orthodontics*, 1, 53–62.

Degerliyurt, K., Ueki, K., Hashiba, Y., *et al.* (2008) A comparative CT evaluation of pharyngeal airway changes in class III patients receiving bimaxillary surgery or mandibular setback surgery. *Oral Surgery, Oral Medicine, Oral Pathology, Oral Radiology and Endodontology*, 105 (4), 495–502.

Draenert, F.G., Erbe, C., Zenglein, V., *et al.* (2010) 3D analysis of condylar position after sagittal split osteotomy of the mandible in mono- and bimaxillary orthognathic surgery: a methodology study in 18 patients. *Journal of Orofacial Orthopedics*, 71 (6), 421–429.

Dudic, A., Giannopoulou, C., Leuzinger, M., *et al.* (2009) Detection of apical root resorption after orthodontic treatment by using panoramic radiography and cone-beam computed tomography of super-high resolution. *American Journal of Orthodontics and Dentofacial Orthopedics*, 135 (4), 434–437.

Durack, C., Patel, S., Davies, J., *et al.* (2011) Diagnostic accuracy of small volume cone beam computed tomography and intraoral periapical radiography for the detection of simulated external inflammatory root resorption. *International Endodontic Journal*, 44 (2), 136–147.

Farman, A.G. & Scarfe, W.C. (2006) Development of imaging selection criteria and procedures should precede cephalometric assessment with cone-beam computed tomography. *American Journal of Orthodontics and Dentofacial Orthopedics*, 130 (2), 257–265.

Finzel, S., Rech, J., Schmidt, S., *et al.* (2011) Repair of bone erosions in rheumatoid arthritis treated with tumour necrosis factor inhibitors is based on bone apposition at the base of the erosion. *Annals of the Rheumatic Diseases*, 70 (9), 1587–1593.

Friedland, B. (2009) Medicolegal issues related to cone-beam CT. *Semininars in Orthodontics*, 15 (1), 77–84.

Fuhrmann, R. (1996) Three-dimensional interpretation of periodontal lesions and remodeling during orthodontic treatment: part III. *Journal of Orofacial Orthopedics*, 57 (4), 224–237.

Galvin, J.R., Rooholamini, S.A., & Stanford, W. (1989) Obstructive sleep apnea: diagnosis with ultrafast CT. *Radiology*, 171 (3), 775–778.

Garcia Silva, M.A., Wolf, U., Heinicke, F., *et al.* (2008a) Cone-beam computed tomography for routine orthodontic treatment planning: a radiation dose evaluation. *American Journal of Orthodontics and Dentofacial Orthopedics*, 133 (640), e1–e5.

Garcia Silva, M.A., Wolf, U., Heinicke, F., *et al.* (2008b) Effective dosages for recording Veraviewepocs dental panoramic images: analog film, digital, and panoramic scout for CBCT. *Oral Surgery Oral Medicine, Oral Pathology, Oral Radiology and Endodontology*, 106 (4), 571–577.

Garcia-Figueroa, M.A., Raboud, D.W., Lam, E.W., *et al.* (2008) Effect of buccolingual root angulation on the mesiodistal angulation shown on panoramic radiographs. *American Journal of Orthodontics and Dentofacial Orthopedics*, 134 (1), 93–99.

Garib, D.G., Yatabe, M.S., Ozawa, T.O., *et al.* (2012) Alveolar bone morphology in patients with bilateral complete cleft lip and palate in the mixed dentition: cone beam computed tomography evaluation. *The Cleft Palate-Craniofacial Journal*, 49 (2), 208–214.

Garrett, B.J., Caruso, J.M., Rungcharassaeng, K., *et al.* (2008) Skeletal effects to the maxilla after rapid maxillary expansion assessed with cone-beam computed tomography. *American Journal of Orthodontics and Dentofacial Orthopedics*, 134 (1), 8–9.

Gateno, J., Teichgraeber, J.F., & Xia, J.J. (2003) Three-dimensional surgical planning for maxillary and midface distraction ostogenesis. *The Journal of Craniofacial Surgery*, 14 (6), 833–839.

Gateno, J., Xia, J.J., & Teichgraeber, J.F. (2007) Clinical feasibility of computer-aided surgical simulation (CASS) in the treatment of complex cranio-maxillofacial deformities. *Journal of Oral and Maxillofacial Surgery*, 65 (4), 728–734.

Gracco, A., Lombardo, L., Cozzani, M., *et al.* (2008) Quantitative cone-beam computed tomography evaluation of palatal bone thickness for orthodontic miniscrew placement. *American Journal of Orthodontics and Dentofacial Orthopedics*, 134 (3), 361–369.

Guyuron, B. (1988) Facial deformity with juvenile rheumatoid arthritis. *Plastic and Reconstructive Surgery*, 81 (6), 948–951.

Gynther, G.W., Tronje, G., & Holmlund, A.B. (1996) Radiographic changes in the temporomandibular joint in patients with generalized osteoarthritis and rheumatoid arthritis. *Oral Surgery, Oral Medicine, Oral Pathology, Oral Radiology and Endodontology*, 81 (5), 613–618.

Hamada, Y., Kondoh, T., Noguchi, K., *et al.* (2005) Application of limited cone beam computed tomography to clinical assessment of alveolar bone grafting: a preliminary report. *Cleft Palate and Craniofacial Journal*, 42 (2), 128–137.

Haney, E., Gansky, S.A., Lee, J.S., *et al.* (2010) Comparative analysis of traditional radiographs and cone-beam computed tomography volumetric images in the diagnosis and treatment planning of maxillary impacted canines. *American Journal of Orthodontics and Dentofacial Orthopedics*, 137 (5), 590–597.

Haponik, E.F., Smith, P.L., Bohlman, M.E., *et al.* (1983) Computerized tomography in obstructive sleep apnea: correlation of airway size with physiology during sleep and wakefulness. *American Review of Respiratory Disease*, 127 (2), 221–226.

Hassfeld, S. & Muhling, J. (2001) Computer assisted oral and maxillofacial surgery: a review and an assessment of technology. *International Journal of Oral and Maxillofacial Surgery*, 30 (1), 2–13.

Helenius, L.M., Hallikainen, D., Helenius, I., *et al.* (2005) Clinical and radiographic findings of the temporomandibular joint in patients with various rheumatic diseases: a case control study. *Oral Surgery, Oral Medicine, Oral Pathology, Oral Radiology and Endodontology*, 99 (4), 455–463.

Honda, K., Larheim, T.A., Maruhashi, K., *et al.* (2006) Osseous abnormalities of the mandibular condyle: diagnostic reliability of cone beam computed tomography compared with helical computed tomography based on an autopsy material. *Dentomaxillofacial Radiology*, 35 (3), 152–157.

Honey, O.B., Scarfe, W.C., Hilgers, M.J., *et al.* (2007) Accuracy of cone-beam computed tomography imaging of the temporomandibular joint: comparisons with panoramic radiology and linear tomography. *American Journal of Orthodontics and Dentofacial Orthopedics*, 132 (4), 429–438.

Hong, J.S., Park, Y.H., Kim, Y.J., *et al.* (2011) Three-dimensional changes in pharyngeal airway in skeletal Class III patients undergoing orthognathic surgery. *Journal of Oral and Maxillofacial Surgery*, 69 (11), e401–e408.

Honrado, C.P., Lee, S., Bloomquist, D.S., *et al.* (2006) Quantitative assessment of nasal changes after maxillomandibular surgery using a 3-dimensional digital imaging system. *Archives of Facial Plastic Surgery*, 8 (1), 26–35.

ICRP, International Commission on Radiological Protection. (1991) The 1990 recommendations of the International Commission on Radiological Protection, publication 60. *Annals of ICRP*, 21, 1–201.

ICRP, International Commission on Radiological Protection. (2008) The 2007 recommendations of the International Commission on Radiological Protection, publication 103. *Annals of ICRP*, 37, 1–332.

Isaacson, K.G., Thom, A.R., Horner, K., *et al.* (2008) *Orthodontic Radiographs: Guidelines*, 3rd ed. British Orthodontic Society, London.

Jakobsone, G., Stenvik, A., Sandvik, L., *et al.* (2011) Three-year follow-up of bimaxillary surgery to correct skeletal Class III malocclusion: stability and risk factors for relapse. *American Journal of Orthodontics and Dentofacial Orthopedics*, 139 (1), 80–89.

Johnson, D.P. (2011) Effects of curve of Wilson correction and pre-treatment boundary conditions on quantitative changes in alveolar bone morphology. Master of Science thesis, The University of Michigan.

Jung, B.A., Wehrbein, H., Wagner, W., *et al.* (2012) Preoperative diagnostic for palatal implants: is CT or CBCT necessary? *Clinical Implant Dentistry and Related Research*, 14 (3), 400–405.

Jung, Y.J., Kim, M.J., & Baek, S.H. (2009) Hard and soft tissue changes after correction of mandibular prognathism and facial asymmetry by mandibular setback surgery: three-dimensional analysis using computerized tomography. *Oral Surgery, Oral Medicine, Oral Pathology, Oral Radiology and Endodontology*, 107 (6), 763–771, e8.

Kapila, S. & Farman, A.G. (2003) Craniofacial imaging in the 21st century. Proceedings of the 2002 COAST conference, Asilomar Conference Center, Pacific Grove, California. *Orthodontics and Craniofacial Research*, 6 (Suppl 1).

Kapila, S., Conley, R.S., & Harrel, W. (2011) Current status of cone beam computed tomography imaging in orthodontics. *Journal of Dentomaxillofacial Radiology*, 40 (1), 24–34. http://dx.doi.org/10.1259/dmfr/12615645.

Kartalian, A., Gohl, E., Adamian, M., *et al.* (2010) Cone-beam computerized tomography evaluation of the maxillary dentoskeletal complex after rapid palatal expansion. *American Journal of Orthodontics and Dentofacial Orthopedics*, 138 (4), 486–492.

Katheria, B.C., Kau, C.H., Tate, R., *et al.* (2010) Effectiveness of impacted and supernumerary tooth diagnosis from traditional radiography versus cone beam computed tomography. *Pediatric Dentistry*, 32 (4), 304–309.

Katsumata, A., Hirukawa, A., Noujeim, M., *et al.* (2006) Image artifact in dental cone-beam CT. *Oral Surgery, Oral Medicine, Oral Patholology, Oral Radiology and Endodontology*, 101 (5), 652–657.

Katsumata, A., Hirukawa, A., Okumura, S., *et al.* (2007) Effects of image artifacts on gray-value density in limited-volume cone-beam computerized tomography. *Oral Surgery, Oral Medicine, Oral Patholology, Oral Radiology and Endodontology*, 104 (6), 829–836.

Kau, C.S., Richmond, J., Palomo, M., *et al.* (2005) Current products and practice: three dimensional cone beam computerized tomography in orthodontics. *Journal of Orthodontics*, 32 (4), 282–293.

Kim, B.R., Oh, K.M., Cevidanes, L.H., *et al.* (2013) Analysis of 3D soft tissue changes after 1- and 2-jaw orthognathic surgery in mandibular prognathism patients. *Journal of Oral and Maxillofacial Surgery*, 71 (1), 151–161.

Kim, Y.I., Jung, Y.H., Cho, B.H., *et al.* (2010) The assessment of the short and long-term changes in the condylar position following sagittal split ramus osteotomy (SSRO) with rigid fixation. *Journal of Oral Rehabilitation*, 37 (4), 262–270.

Kim, Y.I., Cho, B.H., Jung, Y.H., *et al.* (2011) Cone-beam computerized tomography evaluation of condylar changes and stability following two-jaw surgery: Le Fort I osteotomy and mandibular setback surgery with rigid fixation. *Oral Surgery, Oral Medicine, Oral Pathology, Oral Radiology and Endodontology*, 111 (6), 681–687.

Kim, Y.J., Oh, K.M., Hong, J.S., *et al.* (2012) Do patients treated with bimaxillary surgery have more stable condylar positions than those who have undergone single-jaw surgery? *Journal of Oral and Maxillofacial Surgery*, 70 (9), 2143–2152.

King, K.S., Lam, E.W., Faulkner, M.G., *et al.* (2007) Vertical bone volume in the paramedian palate of adolescents: a computed tomography study. *American Journal of Orthodontics and Dentofacial Orthopedics*, 132 (6), 783–788.

Korbmacher, H., Kahl-Nieke, B., Schollchen, M., *et al.* (2007) Value of two cone-beam computed tomography systems from an orthodontic point of view. *Journal of Orofacial Orthopedics*, 68 (4), 278–289.

Koyama, J., Nishiyama, H., & Hayashi, T. (2007) Follow-up study of condylar bony changes using helical computed tomography in patients with temporomandibular disorder. *Dentomaxillofacial Radiology*, 36 (8), 472–477.

Kuhlberg, A.J. & Norton, L.A. (2003) Pathologic findings in orthodontic radiographic images. *American Journal of Orthodontics and Dentofacial Orthopedics*, 123 (2), 182–184.

Kumar, V., Ludlow, J., Cevidanes, L.H., *et al.* (2008) *In vivo* comparison of conventional and cone beam CT synthesized cephalograms. *The Angle Orthodontist*, 78 (5), 873–879.

Lee, W. & Park, J.U. (2002) Three-dimensional evaluation of positional change of the condyle after mandibular setback by means of bilateral sagittal split ramus osteotomy. *Oral Surgery, Oral Medicine, Oral Pathology, Oral Radiology and Endodontology*, 94 (3), 305–309.

Lenza, M.G., Lenza, M.M., Dalstra, M., *et al.* (2010) An analysis of different approaches to the assessment of upper airway morphology: a CBCT study. *Orthodontics & Craniofacial Research*, 13 (2), 96–105.

Leung, C.C., Palomo, L., Griffith, R., *et al.* (2010) Accuracy and reliability of cone-beam computed tomography for measuring alveolar bone height and detecting bony dehiscences and fenestrations. *American Journal of Orthodontics and Dentofacial Orthopedics*, 137 (Suppl 4), S109–S119.

Lim, Y.K., Chu, E.H., Lee, D.Y., *et al.* (2010) Three-dimensional evaluation of soft tissue change gradients after mandibular setback surgery in skeletal Class III malocclusion. *The Angle Orthodontist*, 80 (5), 896–903.

Loubele, M., Jacobs, R., Maes, F., *et al.* (2005) Radiation dose vs. image quality for low-dose CT protocols of the head for maxillofacial surgery and oral implant planning. *Radiation Protection Dosimetry*, 117 (1–3), 211–216.

Ludlow, J.B. (2009a) Dosimetry of small FOV tomography using OP 200 VT & Scanora 3D. 60th annual session of the American Academy of Oral and Maxillofacial Radiology (AAOMR), Louisville, KY, October 22.

Ludlow, J.B. (2009b) Dose and risk in dental diagnostic imaging with emphasis on dosimetry of CBCT. *Korean Journal of Oral and Maxillofacial Radiology*, 39 (4), 175–184.

Ludlow, J.B. & Ivanovic, M. (2008) Comparative dosimetry of dental CBCT devices and 64 row CT for oral and maxillofacial radiology. *Oral Surgery, Oral Medicine, Oral Pathology, Oral Radiology and Endodontology*, 106 (1), 930–938.

Ludlow, J.B., Davies-Ludlow, L.E., & White, S.C. (2008) Patient risk to common dental radiographic examinations: the impact of 2007 ICRP recommendations regarding dose calculation. *Journal of the American Dental Association*, 139 (9), 1237–1243.

Lund, H., Gröndahl, K., & Gröndahl, H.G. (2010) Cone beam computed tomography for assessment of root length and marginal bone level during orthodontic treatment. *The Angle Orthodontist*, 80 (3), 466–473.

Magalhaes, A.E., Stella, J.P., & Tahasuri, T.H. (1995) Changes in condylar position following bilateral sagittal split ramus osteotomy with setback. *International Journal of Adult Orthodontics and Orthognathic Surgery*, 10 (2), 137–145.

Marquezan, M., Lau, T.C., Mattos, C.T., *et al.* (2012) Bone mineral density. *The Angle Orthodontist*, 82 (1), 62–66.

McCance, A.M., Moss, J.P., Fright, W.R., *et al.* (1992) A three dimensional analysis of soft and hard tissue changes following bimaxillary orthognathic surgery in skeletal III patients. *British Journal of Oral and Maxillofacial Surgery*, 30 (5), 305–312.

McKee, I.W., Williamson, P.C., Lam, E.W., *et al.* (2002) The accuracy of four panoramic units in the projection of mesiodistal tooth angulations. *American Journal of Orthodontics and Dentofacial Orthopedics*, 121 (2), 166–175.

Metzger, M.C., Hohlweg-Majert, B., Schon, R., *et al.* (2007) Verification of clinical precision after computer-aided reconstruction in craniomaxillofacial surgery. *Oral Surgery, Oral Medicine, Oral Pathology, Oral Radiology and Endodontology*, 104 (4), e1–e10.

Miles, D.A. (2005) Clinical experience with cone-beam volumetic imaging: report of findings in 381 cases. *Computed Tomography*, 20, 416–424.

Miles, D.A. (2009) Interpreting the cone beam data volume for occult pathology. *Seminars in Orthodontics*, 15, 70–76.

Miracle, A.C. & Mukherji, S.K. (2009) Conebeam CT of the head and neck. Part 1: physical principles. *American Journal of Neuroradiolology*, 30 (6), 1088–1095.

Molen, A.D. (2010) Considerations in the use of cone-beam computed tomography for buccal bone measurements. *American Journal of Orthodontics and Dentofacial Orthopedics*, 137 (4), S130–S135.

Molen, A.D. (2011) Comparing cone-beam computed tomography systems from an orthodontic perspective. *Seminars in Orthodontics*, 17 (1), 34–38.

Motta, A.T., Cevidanes, L.H., Carvalho, L.H., *et al.* (2011) Three-dimensional regional displacements after mandibular advancement surgery: one year of follow-up. *Journal of Oral and Maxillofacial Surgery*, 69 (5), 1447–1457.

Mozzo, P., Poracci, C., Tacconi, A., *et al.* (1998) A new volumetric CT machine for dental imaging based on the cone-beam technique: preliminary results. *European Radiology*, 8 (9), 1558–1564.

Mucedero, M., Coviello, A., Baccetti, T., *et al.* (2008) Stability factors after double-jaw surgery in Class III malocclusion: a systematic review. *The Angle Orthodontist*, 78 (6), 1141–1152.

Nair, M.K., Pettigrew, J.C., Jr., & Mancuso, A.A. (2007) Intracranial aneurysm as an incidental finding. *Dentomaxillofacial Radiolology*, 36 (2), 107–112.

Oberoi, S., Chigurupati, R., Gill, P., *et al.* (2009) Volumetric assessment of secondary alveolar bone grafting using cone beam computed tomography. *The Cleft Palate–Craniofacial Journal*, 46 (5), 503–511.

Oberoi, S., Gill, P., Chigurupati, R., *et al.* (2010) Three-dimensional assessment of the eruption path of the canine in individuals with bone-grafted alveolar clefts using cone beam computed tomography. *The Cleft Palate–Craniofacial Journal*, 47 (5), 507–512.

Okano, T., Harata, Y., Sugihara, Y., *et al.* (2009) Absorbed and effective doses from cone beam volumetric imaging for implant planning. *Dentomaxillofacial Radiolology*, 38, 79–85.

Okeson, J.P. (1996) *Orofacial Pain: Guidelines for Assessment, Diagnosis and Management. American Academy of Orofacial Pain*. Quintessence, Chicago, IL.

Oliviera de Felippe, N.L., Da Silveira, A.C., Viana, G., *et al.* (2008) Relationship between rapid maxillary expansion and nasal cavity size and airway resistance: short- and long-term effects. *American Journal of Orthodontics and Dentofacial Orthopedics*, 134 (3), 370–382.

Oransky, I. (2004) Sir Godfrey N. Hounsfield. *Lancet*, 364 (9439), 1032.

Owens, A.M. & Johal, A. (2008) Near-end of treatment panoramic radiograph in the assessment of mesiodistal root angulation. *The Angle Orthodontist*, 78 (3), 475–481.

Palomo, J.M., Rao, P.S., & Hans, M.G. (2008) Influence of CBCT exposure conditions on radiation dose. *Oral Surgery, Oral Medicine, Oral Pathology, Oral Radiology and Endodontology*, 105 (6), 773–782.

Paniagua, B., Cevidanes, L., Zhu, H., *et al.* (2010) Outcome quantification using SPHARM-PDM toolbox in orthognathic surgery. *International Journal of Computer Assisted Radiology and Surgery*, 6 (5), 617–626.

Park, S.B., Yoon, J.K., Kim, Y.I., *et al.* (2012) The evaluation of the nasal morphologic changes after bimaxillary surgery in skeletal Class III maloccusion by using the superimposition of cone-beam computed tomography (CBCT) volumes. *Journal of Craniomaxillofacial Surgery*, 40 (4), e87–e92.

Patcas, R., Muller, L., Ullrich, O., *et al.* (2012) Accuracy of cone-beam computed tomography at different resolutions assessed on the bony covering of the mandibular anterior teeth. *American Journal of Orthodontics and Dentofacial Orthopedics*, 141 (1), 41–50.

Peck, J.L., Sameshima, G.T., Miller, A., *et al.* (2007) Mesiodistal root angulation using panoramic and cone beam CT. *The Angle Orthodontist*, 77 (2), 206–213.

Periago, D.R., Scarfe, W.C., Moshiri, M., *et al.* (2008) Linear accuracy and reliability of cone beam CT derived 3-dimensional images constructed using an orthodontic volumetric rendering program. *The Angle Orthodontist*, 78 (3), 387–395.

Ponder, S., Benavides, E., Kapila, S., *et al.* (2012) Quantification of external root resorption by low- vs. high-resolution cone beam computed tomography and periapical radiography: a volumetric and linear analysis. *American Journal of Orthodontics and Dentofacial Orthopedics*, 143 (6), 77–91.

Popat, H., Drage, N., & Durning, P. (2008) Mid-line clefts of the cervical vertebrae: an incidental finding arising from cone beam computed tomography of the dental patient. *British Dental Journal*, 204 (6), 303–306.

Price, J.B., Thaw, K.L., Tyndall, D.A., *et al.* (2012) Incidental findings from cone beam computed tomography of the maxillofacial region: a descriptive retrospective study. *Clinical Oral Implants Research*, 23 (11), 1261–1268.

Proffit, W.R., Turvey, T.A., & Phillips, C. (2007) The hierarchy of stability and predictability in orthognathic surgery with rigid fixation: an update and extension. *Head & Face Medicine*, 3, 21.

Quereshy, F.A., Barnum, G., Demko, C., *et al.* (2011) Use of cone beam computed tomography to volumetrically assess alveolar cleft defects: preliminary results.

Journal of Oral and Maxillofacial Surgery, 70 (1), 188–191.

Quintero, J., Trosien, A., Hatcher, D., *et al.* (1999) Craniofacial imaging in orthodontics: historical perspective, current status, and future developments. *The Angle Orthodontist*, 69 (6), 491–506.

Raju, T.N. (1999) The Nobel chronicles. 1979: Allan MacLeod Cormack (b 1924) and Sir Godfrey Newbold Hounsfield (b 1919). *Lancet*, 354 (9190), 1653.

Ren, H., Chen, J., Deng, F., *et al.* (2012) Comparison of cone-beam computed tomography and periapical radiography for detecting simulated apical root resorption. *The Angle Orthodontist*, 83 (2), 189–195.

Renfrew, D., Franken, E.A., Jr., Berbaum, K.S., *et al.* (1992) Error in radiology: classification and lessons in 182 cases presented at a problem conference. *Radiology*, 183 (1), 145–150.

Rogers, S.A., Drage, N., & Durning, P. (2011) Incidental findings arising with cone beam computed tomography imaging of the orthodontic patient. *The Angle Orthodontist*, 81 (2), 350–355.

Rungcharassaeng, K., Caruso, J.M., Kan, J.Y., *et al.* (2007) Factors affecting buccal bone changes of maxillary posterior teeth after rapid maxillary expansion. *American Journal of Orthodontics and Dentofacial Orthopedics*, 132 (4), 428, e1-e8.

Ryckman, M.S., Harrison, S., Oliver, D., *et al.* (2010) Soft-tissue changes after maxillomandibular advancement surgery assessed with cone-beam computed tomography. *American Journal of Orthodontics and Dentofacial Orthopedics*, 137 (4), S86–S93.

Samman, N., Tong, A.C., Cheung, D.L., *et al.* (1992) Analysis of 300 dentofacial deformities in Hong Kong. *International Journal of Adult Orthodontics and Orthognathic Surgery*, 7 (3), 181–185.

Sarikaya, S., Haydar, B., Ciger, S., *et al.* (2002) Changes in alveolar bone thickness due to retraction of anterior teeth. *American Journal of Orthodontics and Dentofacial Orthopedics*, 122 (1), 15–26.

Schendel, S.A. & Hatcher, D. (2010) Automated 3-dimensional airway analysis from cone-beam computed tomography data. *Journal of Oral and Maxillofacial Surgery*, 68 (3), 696–701.

Schwab, R.J., Pasirstein, M., Pierson, R., *et al.* (2003) Identification of upper airway anatomic risk factors for obstructive sleep apnea with volumetric magnetic resonance imaging. *American Journal of Respiratory and Critical Care Medicine*, 168 (5), 522–530.

Segal, G.R., Schiffman, P.H., & Tuncay, O.C. (2004) Meta-analysis of the treatment-related factors of external apical root resorption. *Orthodontics and Craniofacial Research*, 7 (2), 71–78.

SEDENTEXCT Guideline Development Panel. (May 2009) Radiation Protection: Cone Beam CT for Dental and Maxillofacial Radiology Provisional Guidelines 2009 (v. 1.1 May 2009). Available at: http://www.sedentexct.eu, accessed June 10, 2013.

SEDENTEXCT Guideline Development Panel. (2011) Radiation Protection: Cone Beam CT for Dental and Maxillofacial Radiology: Evidence Based Guidelines 2011 (v. 2.0 Final). Available at: http://www.sedentexct.eu, accessed June 10, 2013.

Sherrard, J.F., Rossouw, P.E., Benson, B.W., *et al.* (2010) Accuracy and reliability of tooth and root lengths measured on cone-beam computed tomographs. *American Journal of Orthodontics and Dentofacial Orthopedics*, 137 (4), S100–S108.

Shirota, T., Kurabayashi, H., Ogura, H., *et al.* (2010) Analysis of bone volume using computer simulation system for secondary bone graft in alveolar cleft. *International Journal of Oral and Maxillofacial Surgery*, 39 (9), 904–908.

Silva, M.A., Wolf, U., Heinicke, F., *et al.* (2008) Cone-beam computed tomography for routine orthodontic treatment planning: a radiation dose evaluation. *American Journal of Orthodontics and Dentofacial Orthopedics*, 133 (5), 640, e1-e5.

Smith, J.M. (2009) The normal adult airway in 3-dimensions: a cone-beam computed tomography evaluation establishing normative values. MS thesis, University of Michigan.

Soncul, M. & Bamber, M.A. (2004) Evaluation of facial soft tissue changes with optical surface scan after surgical correction of Class III deformities. *Journal of Oral and Maxillofacial Surgery*, 62 (11), 1331–1340.

Stratemann, S.A., Huang, J.C., Maki, K., *et al.* (2008) Comparison of cone beam computed tomography imaging with physical measures. *Dentomaxillofacial Radiology*, 37 (2), 80–93.

Stratemann, S.A., Huang, J.C., Maki, K., *et al.* (2010) Evaluating the mandible with cone-beam computed tomography. *American Journal of Orthodontics and Dentofacial Orthopedics*, 137 (4), S58–S70.

Suomalainen, A., Kiljunen, T., Käser, Y., *et al.* (2009) Dosimetry and image quality of four dental cone beam computed tomography scanners compared with multislice computed tomography scanners. *Dentomaxillofacial Radiology*, 38 (6), 367–378.

Swennen, G.R. & Schutyser, F. (2006) Three-dimensional cephalometry: spiral multislice vs. cone-beam computed tomography. *American Journal of Orthodontics and Dentofacial Orthopedics*, 130 (3), 410–416.

Tai, K., Hotokezaka, H., Park, J.H., *et al.* (2010a) Preliminary cone-beam computed tomography study evaluating dental and skeletal changes after treatment with a mandibular Schwarz appliance. *American Journal of Orthodontics and Dentofacial Orthopedics*, 138 (3), 262, e1–e11.

Tai, K., Park, J.H., Mishima, K., *et al.* (2010b) Using superimposition of 3-dimensional cone-beam computed tomography images with surface-based registration in growing patients. *Journal of Clinical Pediatric Dentistry*, 34 (4), 361–367.

Tetradis, S. & Kantor, M.L. (1999) Prevalence of skeletal and dental anomalies and normal variants seen in cephalometric and other radiographs of orthodontic patients. *American Journal of Orthodontics and Dentofacial Orthopedics*, 116 (5), 572–577.

Theodorakou, C., Walker, A., Horner, K., *et al.* (2012) Estimation of paediatric organ and effective doses from dental cone beam CT using anthropomorphic phantoms. *British Journal of Radiology*, 85 (1010), 153–160.

Troulis, M.J., Everett, P., Seldin, E.B., *et al.* (2002) Development of a three-dimensional treatment planning system based on computer tomographic data. *International Journal of Oral and Maxillofacial Surgery*, 31 (4), 349–357.

Tsao, D.H., Kazanoglu, A., & McCasland, J.P. (1983) Measurability of radiographic images. *American Journal of Orthodontics and Dentofacial Orthopedics*, 84 (3), 212–216.

Turpin, D. (2007) Befriend your oral and maxillofacial radiologist. *American Journal of Orthodontics and Dentofacial Orthopedics*, 131 (6), 697.

Van Elslande, D., Heo, G., Flores-Mir, C., *et al.* (2010) Accuracy of mesiodistal root angulation projected by cone-beam computed tomographic panoramic-like images. *American Journal of Orthodontics and Dentofacial Orthopedics*, 137 (4), S94–S99.

Vannier, M.W. (2003) Craniofacial computed tomography scanning: technology, applications and future trends. *Orthodontics and Craniofacial Research*, 6 (Suppl 1), 23–30.

Walker, L., Enciso, R., & Mah, J. (2005) Three-dimensional localization of maxillary canines with cone-beam computed tomography. *American Journal of Orthodontics and Dentofacial Orthopedics*, 128 (4), 418–423.

Wechsler, R.J., Spettell, C.M., Kurtz, A.B., *et al.* (1996) Effects of training and experience in interpretation of emergency body CT scans. *Radiology*, 199 (3), 717–720.

Wehrbein, H., Bauer, W., & Diedrich, P. (1996) Mandibular incisors, alveolar bone, and symphysis after orthodontic treatment: a retrospective study. *American Journal of Orthodontics and Dentofacial Orthopedics*, 110 (3), 239–246.

Welmerink, A.D. (2012) Effects of non-extraction orthodontic therapy and boundary conditions on quantitative changes in alveolar bone morphology. Master of Science thesis, University of Michigan.

Weltman, B., Vig, K.W., Fields, H.W., *et al.* (2010) Root resorption associated with orthodontic tooth movement: a systematic review. *American Journal of Orthodontics and Dentofacial Orthopedics*, 137 (4), 462–476.

Wilmes, B., Rademacher, C., Olthoff, G., *et al.* (2006) Parameters affecting primary stability of orthodontic mini-implants. *Journal of Orofacial Orthopedics*, 67 (3), 162–174.

Xia, J., Ip, H.H., Samman, N., *et al.* (2000a) Computer-assisted three-dimensional surgical planning and simulation: 3D virtual osteotomy. *International Journal of Oral and Maxillofacial Surgery*, 29 (1), 11–17.

Xia, J., Samman, N., Yeung, R.W., *et al.* (2000b) Three-dimensional virtual reality surgical planning and simulation workbench for orthognathic surgery. *International Journal of Oral and Maxillofacial Surgery*, 15 (4), 265–282.

Yucel, A., Unlu, M., Haktanir, A., *et al.* (2005) Evaluation of the upper airway cross-sectional area changes in different degrees of severity of obstructive sleep apnea syndrome: cephalometric and dynamic CT study. *American Journal of Neuroradiology*, 26 (10), 2624–2629.

Yura, S., Ooi, K., Kadowaki, S., *et al.* (2010) Magnetic resonance imaging of the temporomandibular joint in patients with skeletal open bite and subjects with no dentofacial abnormalities. *British Journal of Oral and Maxillofacial Surgery*, 48 (6), 459–461.

Zhang, W., Shen, G., Wang, X., *et al.* (2012) Evaluation of alveolar bone grafting using limited cone beam computed tomography. *Oral Surgery, Oral Medicine, Oral Pathology and Oral Radiology*, 113 (4), 542–548.

Zhou, W., Li, W., Lin, J., *et al.* (2013) Tooth lengths of the permanent upper incisors in patients with cleft lip and palate determined with cone beam computed tomography. *Cleft Palate–Craniofacial Journal*, 50 (1), 88–95.

Zinman, E.J., White, S.C., & Tetradis, S. (2010) Legal considerations in the use of cone beam computer tomography imaging. *Journal of the California Dental Association*, 38 (1), 49–56.

2 Functional and Technical Characteristics of Different Cone Beam Computed Tomography Units

Om P. Kharbanda, BDS, MDS, M Orth RCS, M MEd, FDS RCS Hon, Neeraj Wadhawan, BDS, MDS, Rajiv Balachandran, BDS, MDS, Devasenathipathy Kandasamy, MD, DNB, FRCR, and Sunil D. Kapila, BDS, MS, PhD

INTRODUCTION

By providing three-dimensionally (3D) accurate representation of craniofacial structures, cone beam computed tomography (CBCT) has opened up new paradigms in diagnosis, treatment planning, and assessment of treatment outcomes in orthodontics and orthognathic surgery. This technology also has found applications in many other fields of dentistry, particularly in implant dentistry, imaging of craniofacial trauma, and facial reconstruction; additional applications are being envisaged in endodontics and periodontics. Useful medical applications of CBCT technology include imaging for otorhinolaryngology (ear, nose and throat [ENT]), skull base, radiotherapy planning, intra-operative imaging, angiography, and even mammography (Broderick *et al.*, 2007; Miracle & Mukherji, 2009a,b; Angelopoulos *et al.*, 2012).

CBCT, an X-ray–based imaging modality, is similar to multi-slice computed tomography (MSCT), also referred to as multi-detector computed tomography (MDCT), but with far less radiation exposure, reduced cost, and high spatial resolution (Miracle & Mukherji, 2009a). The increasing popularity of CBCT has been facilitated mainly by reductions in radiation and costs resulting from advances in flat panel detector (FPD) technology and processing power of computer hardware supported with advanced software applications.

Most CBCT scanners are intended for use in the imaging of the head and neck region. In 1998, the first CBCT machine for imaging of the maxillofacial region (Mozzo *et al.*, 1998) was marketed for commercial use (Miracle & Mukherji, 2009a). By 2005, there were five manufacturers supplying CBCT machines. Currently, there are over 20 manufacturers providing over 40 different CBCT units (Molen, 2011; also see Chapter 6). These units vary in their configuration, hardware, and image reconstruction capabilities, which continue to evolve rapidly. The overall goal of this chapter is to provide the reader with a working knowledge of the capabilities and specifications of the broad

Cone Beam Computed Tomography in Orthodontics: Indications, Insights, and Innovations, First Edition. Sunil D. Kapila.

array of CBCT scanners that currently are available. More specifically, this chapter compares and contrasts several of the commonly used CBCT units and discusses their relative merits for use in orthodontics. The review of CBCT scanners is preceded by some of the essential information on CT imaging, including a discussion of concepts such as resolution, noise, artifacts, and determinants of radiation exposure.

CHARACTERISTICS OF A CT IMAGE

The principle of CBCT is the same as that of conventional CT except for differences in the type of beam used, configuration of the detectors, and reconstruction algorithms used (Figure 2.1). The use of two-dimensional (2D) FPDs in CBCT enables the scanner to obtain the required information of the region of interest (ROI) in a single rotation or, in some cases, in two rotations, which decreases the exposure time drastically relative to MSCTs. Depending on the equipment and reconstruction algorithm used, the scan arc can be 360° or less. In essence, the machine acquires multiple images of the structure at various angles during a rotation. The total number of images acquired depends on frame rate, speed of rotation, and scan arc. The greater the number of images acquired, the greater the radiation dose and the better the image quality. In contrast to MSCT, X-rays in CBCT are used more efficiently, which decreases the load on the X-ray tubes.

An image from a MSCT or CBCT has three fundamental characteristics or components that are common to all medical imaging techniques: (1) resolution, (2) image noise, and (3) artifacts. These, in turn, are controlled by machine parameters such as peak tube voltage (kVp), milliamperage seconds (mAs), scanning time, field of view (FOV), frame rate, speed of rotation, arc of the trajectory, type of detector, reconstruction algorithm, and radiation scatter. The effects of some of these machine parameters on resolution, image noise, and artifacts are summarized below and in Table 2.1.

Resolution

In medical imaging, resolution typifies the ability of an imaging modality to resolve closely placed objects. Resolution can be classified further into

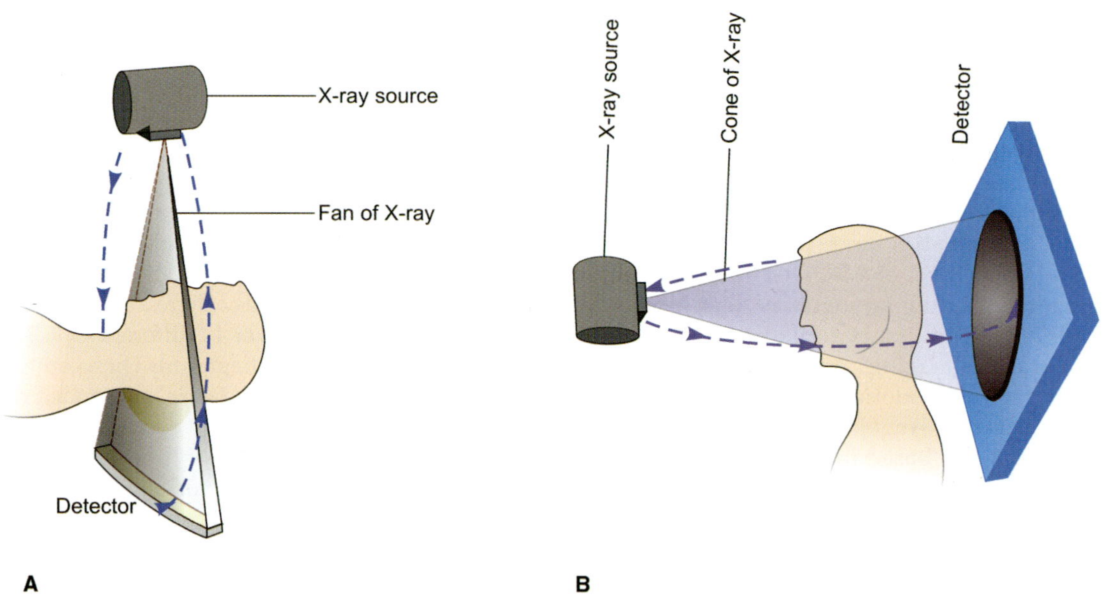

Figure 2.1 Key hardware configuration differences between MSCT (*A*) and CBCT (*B*). (Adapted from Ghosh *et al.*, 2013.)

Table 2.1 Scan parameters influencing image quality.

Tube voltage (kVp)	High	Increased energy of the X-ray beam, increased tissue penetration, good signal to noise ratio
	Low	Better contrast resolution, lower signal to noise ratio and lower dose for a given tube current
Tube current (mA)	High	Good signal to noise ratio, thereby increasing the contrast resolution
	Low	Lower patient dose, poor signal to noise ratio
Scan time	Long	Prone to motion related artifacts
	Short	Superior temporal resolution, fewer artifacts
Field of view (FOV)	Large	Larger area is covered, lower spatial resolution
	Small	Better spatial resolution
Slice thickness	Large	Good signal to noise ratio, lower *z*-axis resolution
	Small	Partial volume effect is reduced, poor signal to noise ratio
Reconstruction algorithm	Smooth	Image appears smother and less noisy, spatial resolution suffers
	High frequency	Better spatial resolution but noisier image

spatial resolution, contrast resolution, and temporal resolution (Mahesh, 2009).

Spatial resolution

Spatial resolution is the ability of a scanner to distinguish closely placed objects. The better the resolution, the better the image quality. Spatial resolution is measured in two planes: axial plane (x–y plane) and longitudinal plane (z-axis). The key factors controlling spatial resolution in a CT scan are related mainly to receptor characteristics, focal spot size, detector size, scanner geometry, type of reconstruction filter used, and patient motion.

A major advantage of CBCT is the excellent spatial resolution obtained by the use of FPDs (0.4 mm or lower), which can provide isotropic voxels of high resolution up to 80 μm (0.08 mm) compared with 500–1000 μm voxels in MSCT. The current generation of CBCT scanners have the ability to acquire data at voxel size 0.08–0.4 mm (Angelopoulos *et al.*, 2012). However, a machine with a smaller voxel size does not translate necessarily into higher clinical resolution. As the voxel size reduces, fewer photons reach each voxel, thus reducing the data acquired by each voxel. Due to tissue- and beam-related differences, adjacent voxels are affected by a different number of photons, resulting in an inhomogeneous image, which leads to loss of contrast and increased image noise.

The resolution power of a scanner is measured clinically by its ability to distinguish closely spaced bars in a CT phantom and is specified as line pairs per centimeter (lp/cm) or per millimeter (lp/mm; Mahesh, 2009; see also Chapter 8). Current CBCT scanners offer a resolution of as low as 5 lp/mm compared with 2–3 lp/mm for CT scanners (Angelopoulos *et al.*, 2012).

Modulation transfer function (MTF) is a more objective and quantitative way of determining spatial resolution. It is defined as the ratio of output modulation to input modulation and relates the percentage of actual contrast conferred to a spatial frequency of inserts in a phantom. MTF values range between 0 and 1 and usually are depicted graphically (Figure 2.2). Manufacturers often use 50, 10, 20, and 0% MTF to indicate the frequencies (lp/cm) corresponding to the points on the MTF curves (Mahesh, 2009). High MTF values in the low frequency range are needed to outline coarse details, while high MTF values in the high frequency range are necessary to portray fine details and sharp edges (Suomalainen *et al.*, 2009). The data reported by most manufacturers on the MTF values are derived under experimental conditions using phantom heads. However, due to the many

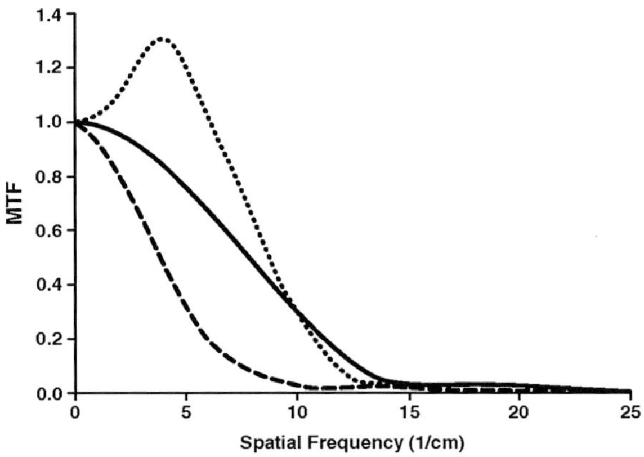

Figure 2.2 Modulation transfer function (MTF) of sinus protocols with CBCT (solid line) and MSCT (bone reconstruction with H70, dotted line; soft-tissue reconstruction with H41, dashed line). (Reprinted from Yu *et al.*, 2010, with permission from the American Roentgen Ray Society.)

variables including the presence of soft tissues, artifacts, and patient motion, the resolving power of scanners under clinical conditions may be lower than that reported by manufacturers.

Temporal resolution

Temporal resolution is the ability of an imaging system to discriminate several sequentially acquired projection data in time (Miracle & Mukherji, 2009a). A system with higher temporal resolution would have more contrast resolution. Solid state FPDs of CBCT systems have limited temporal resolution ability compared with ceramic detectors of MSCT systems (Orth *et al.*, 2008), which limits the frame rate and contributes to streak artifacts, thus reducing low contrast detectability (Akpek *et al.*, 2005).

Contrast resolution

Contrast resolution, or low contrast detectability (LCD), is the ability of an imaging device to distinguish differences in tissue attenuation or the capability of an imaging system to distinguish objects from the background (Goldman, 2007; Mahesh, 2009). A system with high LCD has an increased capability to resolve objects from the background and, therefore, is considered to have high sensitivity. Contrast resolution is an important determinant of image quality. When the contrast resolution decreases, the visualization of tissue differences in the low contrast areas such as soft tissues becomes poor. CT contrast is measured on a scale of −1000 to 1000 Hounsfield units (HU). The major factors influencing contrast resolution include tube current, slice thickness, thickness of the region being imaged, detector sensitivity, reconstruction algorithm, and image display (Mahesh, 2009).

CBCT inherently has poor LCD, which results in suboptimal soft tissue imaging. CBCT systems typically have an LCD of 10 HU (Dörfler *et al.*, 2008) compared with 1 HU resolution of modern MSCT (Miracle & Mukherji, 2009a,b). Despite this caveat, the visualization of high contrast structures such as bones is not affected in CBCT imaging. The prime cause of lower contrast resolution in CBCT is the scatter radiation, which is inherent to the geometry of the CBCT system due to the cone beam's large *z*-axis coverage. Older generation scanners employed image intensifier CCD detectors (Kau *et al.*, 2009) and had limited resolution of grayscale. However, current CBCT systems offer contrast range anywhere between 12- and 16-bit grayscale (Molen, 2011).

Image noise

Image noise is the CT equivalent of radiographic mottling and occurs due to a reduced number of photons reaching the receptor plates, a phenomenon called photon starvation (Hounsfield, 1976; Goldman & Fowlkes, 2000). This difference of photon density reaching the receptor causes differential contrast in adjacent voxels and graininess of the image, causing loss of image quality. Due to this phenomenon, even radiographically uniform density structures appear to have a slightly different value of Hounsfield units on CT images.

Image noise is affected by the following factors: tube current (mA), scan (rotation) time, slice thickness, peak voltage (kVp), and choice of filter (Goldman, 2007). For example, smooth filters blur image, which reduces its visual impact, whereas sharp filters enhance noise. For imaging of soft tissues, smooth filters are preferred because noise generally interferes more than image blur. For hard tissue imaging or for imaging structures with edges, sharp filters are preferred because blur interferes more than noise. The quality of output of a scanner at typical noise levels for soft tissue imaging usually is a good test of the scanner's overall performance.

Artifacts

Artifacts are details seen on an image that do not represent the actual anatomic structures that have been imaged (Goldman, 2007; Miracle & Mukherji, 2009a,b). Many types of CT image artifacts exist and can be divided broadly as: (1) physics-based; (2) patient-based; and (3) scanner-based (Barrett & Keat, 2004). The resulting types of artifacts include streaking, shading, rings, and cupping (Scarfe & Farman, 2008). Artifacts lead to reduction in image quality, reducing its diagnostic value and causing misinterpretation of detail.

CLASSIFICATION OF SCANNERS

From a practical standpoint, the types of scanners currently available can be categorized by the positioning of the patient within the unit and by the FOV of the scanner.

Classification based on patient positioning

The various CBCT scanners grouped on the basis of patient positioning in the scanner are listed below. Examples are shown in Figure 2.3.

- Supine imaging position: Newtom 3G and Newtom 5G (Quantitative Radiology, Verona, Italy) and SkyView (MyRay, Cefla Dental Group, Imola, Italy)
- Sitting imaging position: i-CAT Next Generation (Imaging Sciences International, Hatfield, PA), KaVo 3D eXam (KaVo Dental GmbH, Bismarckring, Germany), 3DE Accuitomo (J. Morita, Kyoto, Japan), Scanora (Soredex, Orion Corporation, Helsinki, Finland), and Galileos® (Sirona Dental Systems, Bensheim, Germany)
- Standing imaging position: Newtom VGi (Quantitative Radiology), ProMax (Planmeca OY, Helsinki, Finland), Galileos® (Sirona Dental Systems), and AugeZIO series (Asahi Roentgen, Kyoto, Japan).

Some CBCT units offer the option to scan with the patient in either standing or sitting position; however, none offers the option of both supine and standing positions. A unit with supine imaging position is more useful in hospital settings (e.g., trauma centers) in which patients with maxillofacial trauma or multiple injuries including head injuries are tended. Scanners with supine position also are necessary for planning radiation guidance in oncology and intraoperative planning. For the purposes of orthodontic imaging and other dental applications, CBCT units with sitting or standing features are preferred for ease of accessibility. These units require less space and their configuration decreases the likelihood of claustrophobia to the patient. In addition, due to scan time of several seconds to more than half a minute, the units offering a sitting option may be less prone to movement artifacts than those in which patients have to stand.

Classification based on field of view (FOV)

FOV is widely used to classify CBCT machines (Table 2.2, Table 2.3, Table 2.4 and Table 2.5). As presented by Scarfe & Farman (2008), FOVs for craniofical imaging can be classified as follows:

- *Localized imaging* utilizes a small FOV of 5 cm or less for scanning anatomy such as of dento-alvelaor structures and the TMJ.
- *Single arch imaging* is performed with a FOV of 5–7 cm.
- *Interarch imaging* requires a FOV of approximately 7–10 cm.
- *Maxillofacial imaging* requires a large FOV of 10–15 cm (mandible to nasion).
- *Craniofacial imaging* is used for capturing the entire craniofacial structures and requires an extended FOV of 15 cm or more.

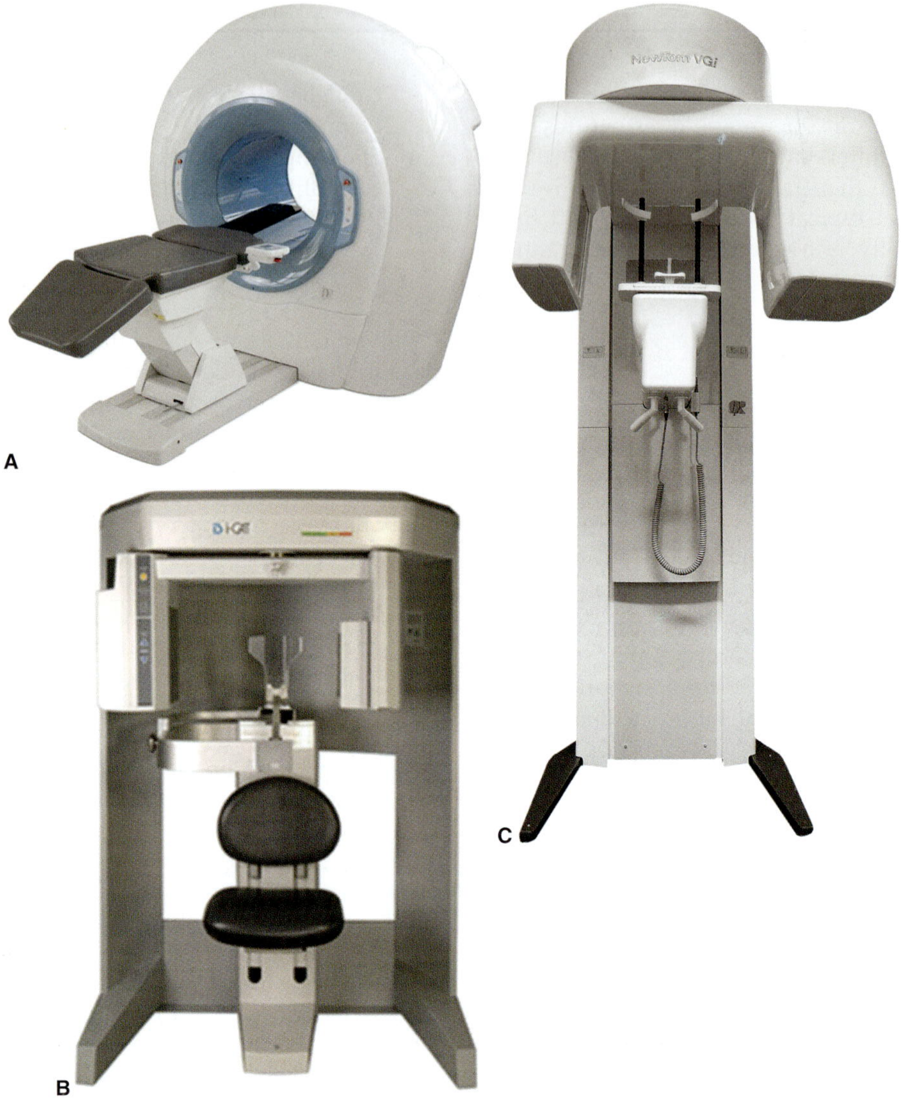

Figure 2.3 Examples of CBCT units with different patient positioning. *A:* Supine patient position, CBCT (NewTom 5G). *B:* Sitting patient position, CBCT (iCat NG). *C:* Both sitting and standing patient position, CBCT (NewTom VGi). (Images courtesy of the manufacturers.)

Table 2.2 Small to medium FOV CBCT units.

Manufacturer	Jmorita			Carestream Dental	PreXion Inc.	PreXion Inc.
Scanner	Veraviewepocs 3D	Veraviewepocs 3De	3D Accuitomo 80	Kodak 9000 3D and 9000c 3D	PreXion 3D	PreXion 3D Elite with CLEARimage scanning
Voxel size	0.125 mm	0.125 mm	0.080 mm, 0.125 mm, 0.16 mm	0.076 mm	0.2 mm	0.147, 0.101 mm
Reconstruction time	30–60 seconds	30–60 seconds	NA	Kodak 9000 3D = less than 2 minutes Kodak 9000c 3D = depends on the PC	N/A	30 seconds
Grayscale	13 bit	13 bit	13 bit	14 bit	16 bit	13 bits
Image detector	CMOS flat panel detector (FPD)	FPD	FPD with CsI[a] scintillator	CMOS sensor with optical fiber	CsI[a] FPD	FPD
Patient positioning	Standing	Standing	Seated	Seated/standing/ wheelchair	Seated	Seated
Scan time	Approximately 9.4 seconds (3D image)	Approximately 9.4 seconds (3D image)	18 seconds or less	13.2 to 13.9 seconds	19 seconds standard, 37 seconds HD (fixed X-ray source)	RAPID = 8.6 seconds (217° rotation) HD = 16.8 seconds (360° rotation) ULTRA HD = 33.5 seconds (360° rotation)
Field of view (FOV)	4 × 4 cm (D × H) 4 × 8 cm (D × H) 8 × 8 cm (D × H)	4 × 4 cm (D × H) 4 × 8 cm (D × H)	4 × 4 cm (D × H) 6 × 6 cm (D × H) 8 × 8 cm (D × H)	5 × 3.8 cm single 9 × 7 × 3.75 cm stitched	8.1 × 7.5 cm	8.1 × 7.5 cm 5.6 × 5.2 cm
Bundled software	i-Dixel One Data Viewer	i-Dixel One Data Viewer	i-Dixel viewer software	Kodak imaging software	PreXion 3D viewer software	PreXion3D viewer software

[a]Cesium iodide.

Source: Compiled and adapted from http://www.conebeam.com/cbctchart and manufacturer advertised specifications on the Web.

Table 2.3 Medium to large FOV CBCT units.

Manufacturer	Imaging Sciences International	QR S.r.l.	QR S.r.l.	Sirona Dental Systems	Gendex	Sirona Dental Systems	Myray	Vatech America	Vatech America	Soredex
Scanner	i-CAT Precise	NewTom Vgi	NewTom Vgi Flex[a]	GALILEOS Comfort	Gendex CB-500 & CB-500 HD	GALILEOS Compact	SkyView	PaX – Reve 3D	PaX-Duo 3D PLUS	Scanora 3D
Voxel size	0.4, 0.3, 0.25, 0.2, 0.125 mm	Standard scan: 0.075, 0.10, 0.125, 0.15 mm Boosted scan: 0.15, 0.20, 0.25, 0.30 mm HiRes scan: 0.15, 0.20, 0.25, 0.30 mm	Standard scan: 0.075, 0.10, 0.125, 0.15 mm Boosted scan: 0.15, 0.20, 0.25, 0.30 mm HiRes scan: 0.15, 0.20, 0.25, 0.30 mm	0.3/0.15 mm	0.4,0.3, 0.25, 0.2, 0.125 mm	0.3 mm	0.33 mm (FOV 15 cm) 0.23 mm (FOV 11 cm) 0.17 mm (FOV 7 cm)	0.08–0.25 mm	0.12–0.4 mm changes by field of view size	0.13, 0.20, 0.25, 0.30, 0.35 mm
Reconstruction time	Less than 20 seconds (standard mode) Less than 95 seconds (extended diameter scan[EDS] mode)	Approximately 1 minute	Approximately 1 minute	2.5–4.5 minutes	Less than 20 seconds (standard mode) Less than 95 seconds (EDS mode)	4.5 minutes	30–70 seconds	Less than 1 minute	18–59 seconds	1–2 minutes
Grayscale	14 bit	14-bit scanning, 16-bit reconstruction	14-bit scanning, 16-bit reconstruction	12 bit	14 bit	NA	12 bit	14 bit	14 bit	12 bit
Image detector	Amorphous silicon flat panel with CsI scintillator	Amorphous silicon flat panel 20×25 cm field of view	Amorphous silicon flat panel 20×25 cm field of view	Image intensifier CCD	Amorphous silicon flat panel	Image intensifier CCD	High resolution image intensifier digital CCD sensor	Amorphous flat panel detector	Amorphous flat panel sensor	CMOS flat panel 12.4× 12.4 cm
Patient positioning	Seated	Standing or seated and wheelchair accessible	Seated/ standing	Standing/seated	Seated	Standing/ seated, chin rest/bite block head fixing system	Supine	Seated/ wheelchair accessible	Standing/ wheelchair accessible	Seated

Scan time	4.8 seconds (0.3 and 0.4 voxel, standard mode) 8.9 seconds (0.3 and 0.4 voxel, standard/EDS mode) 12.6 seconds (0.125, 0.2 and 0.25 voxel, standard mode) 23 seconds (0.125, 0.2 and 0.25 voxel, standard/EDS mode)	18 to 26 seconds(X-ray emission time 3.6–5.6 seconds) pulsed X-ray	18–26 seconds (X-ray emission time 3.6–6.7 seconds) pulsed X-ray	14 seconds/ (exposure 2–6 seconds)	8.9 sec (0.3 and 0.4 voxel, standard/EDS mode) 23 sec (0.125, 0.2, and 0.25 voxel, high resolution scans) (pulsed X-ray)	14 seconds/ (exposure 2–6 seconds)	10,15, 20,30 seconds	15–24 seconds	15–24 seconds	10–26 seconds (exposure time 2.5–6 seconds)
Field of view	8 cm (D) and 14 cm (D) Fully adjustable height between 2 and 8 cm	Standard scan: 15×15, 15×12, 12×8 cm (D×H) Boosted scan: 8×8 cm (D×H) HiRes scan: 12×8, 8×8, 6×6 cm (D×H)	Standard scan: 15×15, 15×12, 12×8 cm (D×H) Boosted scan: 8×8 cm (D×H) HiRes scan: 12×8, 8×8, 6×6 cm (D×H)	15×15×15 cm	**CB-500** 8×8 cm (DxH), standard mode 14×8 cm (DxH), EDS mode **CB-500 HD** 8 cm diameter and 14 cm diameter Fully adjustable height between 2 and 8 cm	12×15× 15 cm	15 cm (9″ detector) 11 cm (6″ detector) 7 cm (H.R. zoom 4″)	5×5 to 15×15 cm (15×19 cm optional)	5×5, 8×5, 8.5×8.5, 12×8.5 cm	6×6 cm (H×D) 3D Small 7.5×10 cm (H×D) 3D Medium 7.5×14.5 cm (H×D) 3D Large 13×14.5 cm (H×D) 3D XL
Bundled software	Tx Studio™ treatment software Free i-CATVision™ viewing and sharing	NNT™ with free viewer and sharing application	NNT™ with free viewer and sharing application	GALAXIS/ SIDEXIS/ GALELIOS Implant	Free i-CAT Vision™ viewing and sharing software included	GALAXIS/ SIDEXIS/ GALELIOS Implant	SkyView software	EasyDent/ Ez3D2009	EasyDent/ Ez3D2009	3D visualization software

Source: Modified from http://www.conebeam.com/cbctchart and compiled from manufacturer advertised specifications.
[a]The NewTom VGi Flex only portable CBCT scanner available.

Table 2.4 Extended FOV CBCT units suitable for craniofacial imaging.

Manufacturer	Imaging Sciences International	QR S.r.l.	KaVo	IMTEC	Carestream Dental	Vatech America	Hitachi Medical Systems
Scanner	Classic i-Cat	NewTom 3G	3D eXam	ILUMA® CBCT Scanner ILUMA LFOV	Kodak 9500 3D	Picasso Master 3D	CB MercuRay
Voxel size	0.125, 0.2, 0.25, 0.3, 0.4 mm	0.2–0.4 mm	0.125–0.4 mm	Standard = 0.4 mm Normal = 0.3 mm High = 0.2 mm Ultra high = 0.09 mm	Up to 0.20 mm	0.164, 0.2, 0.3, 0.4 mm	0.2 to 0.376 mm
Reconstruction time	1.5 minutes	2 minutes	<1 minute	Two minutes or greater	2 minutes 20 seconds (depends on computer configuration)	Less than 2 minutes (option 29 seconds)	6 minutes
Grayscale	14 bit	12 bit	14 bit grayscale	16 bit (16,384 grayscales)	16 bit	14 bit	12 bit
Image detector	Amorphous silicon flat panel FPD	Image intensifier CCD	Amorphous silicon flat panel 20 × 25 cm	Amorphous silicon flat panel	Amorphous silicon flat panel	FPD	CCD camera
Patient positioning	Seated	Reclining	Seated	Seated with rear head stabilization and chin support	Seated/ standing/ wheelchair	Seated/ standing/ wheelchair	Seated
Scan time	10, 20, 40 seconds pulsed X-ray	36 seconds pulsed X-ray	8.5 and 26 seconds pulsed X-ray	Variable scan times Between 20 to 40 seconds per single 360° rotation and 7.8 seconds per single 190° rotation	NA	15 seconds/24 seconds	10 seconds
Field of view (FOV)	16 × 13 to 22 cm (D × H)	20 × 20 cm (D × H) 15 × 20 cm (D × H) 10 × 20 cm (D × H)	Standard and high resolution: 16 × 13 cm (D × H) Ultra high resolution: 8 × 8 cm (D × H) Cephalometric mode: 23 × 17 cm (D × H)	(Cylindrical) up to 21.1 × 14.2 cm	Medium 15 × 9 cm Large 20 × 18 cm	20 × 15 cm 20 × 19 cm	25 × 15 cm 25 × 30 cm
Bundled software	i-CatVision	NNT™ with free viewer and sharing application	NA	DigiGuide™ MDI	Kodak imaging software	Picasso CT and 3D software	CB Works

Source: Modified from http://www.conebeam.com/cbctchart using current manufacturers advertised specifications.

Table 2.5 CBCT units with wide range of FOV.

Manufacturer	QR S.r.l.	Imaging Sciences International	Planmeca USA	Planmeca USA	Planmeca USA	Jmorita	Vatech America
Scanner	Newtom 5G	i-CAT Next Generation	Promax 3D	Promax 3D mid	Promax 3D Max	3D Accuitomo 170	PaX – Zenith 3D
Voxel size	0.3, 0.25, 0.2, 0.15 mm Standard and boosted scan 0.15, 0.125, 0.1, 0.075 HiRes scan	0.4, 0.3, 0.25, 0.2, 0.125 mm	0.1, 0.2, 0.4 mm	0.1×0.1×0.1 mm, isotropic 0.15×0.15×0.15 mm, isotropic 0.2×0.2×0.2 mm, isotropic 0.4×0.4×0.4 mm, isotropic 0.6×0.6×0.6 mm, isotropic	0.10, 0.15, 0.2, 0.4, 0.6 mm	0.08, 0.125, 0.16, 0.2, 0.25 mm	Selectable/ 0.08–0.3 mm
Reconstruction time	Less than 1 minute	Less than 30 seconds	15–60 seconds	15 seconds at minimum	15 seconds at minimum	65 seconds (4×4 cm, 360° scan at highest resolution of 0.08 mm)	10–221 seconds
Grayscale	14-bit scanning, 16-bit reconstruction	14 bit	15 bit	15 bit	15 bit	14 bit	14 bit
Image detector	Amorphous silicon flat panel	Amorphous silicon flat panel with CsI scintillator	Flat panel	Flat panel	Flat panel	Flat panel detector	Amorphous flat panel sensor
Patient positioning	Supine, motorized patient table + laser	Seated	Seated/standing/ wheelchair	Seated/standing/ wheelchair	Seated/standing/ wheelchair	Seated	Seated/ wheelchair

(Continued)

Table 2.5 (*Continued*)

Manufacturer	QR S.r.l.	Imaging Sciences International	Planmeca USA	Planmeca USA	Planmeca USA	Jmorita	Vatech America
Scanner	Newtom 5G	i-CAT Next Generation	Promax 3D	Promax 3D mid	Promax 3D Max	3D Accuitomo 170	PaX – Zenith 3D
Scan time	18 to 36 seconds/ (X-ray emission time 3.6 to 6.7 seconds) pulsed X-ray	5, 8.9, or 26.9 seconds pulsed X-ray	18 seconds pulsed X-ray	18–26 seconds pulsed X-ray	18–26 seconds pulsed X-ray	**Mode: (360°/180°)** Standard mode: 17.5/9.0 sec. Hi-Fi mode: 30.8/15.8 sec. Hi-Res mode: 30.8/15.8 sec. Hi-Speed mode: 10.5/5.4 sec	15–24 seconds
Field of view	Standard scan: 18×16 cm (D×H) Boosted scan: 15×12, 12×8, 8×8 (cm) (D×H) HiRes scan: 15×5, 12×8, 8×8, 6×6 (cm) (D×H)	Standard scan: 4, 6, 8, 10, 13 cm (H) ×16 cm (D), 8×8 cm (H×D) Custom mode: any height from 2 to 13 cm(H) ×16 cm (D) Extended field of view (cephalometric): 17×23 cm (H×D)	Volume (child mode) Single:8×8 cm (6.8×6.8 cm) (D×H) 8×5 cm (6.8×4.2 cm) (D×H) 4×8 cm (3.4×6.8 cm) (D×H) 4×5 cm (3.4×4.2 cm) (DxH) Stitched: 14.4×10.5×8 cm	Volume (child mode) 4×5 cm (3.4×4.2 cm) (D×H) 4×7 cm (3.4×6 cm) (D×H) 7×5 cm (6×4.2 cm) (D×H) 7×7 cm (6×6 cm) (D×H) 9×5 cm (7.5×4.2 cm) (D×xH) 9×9 cm (7.5×7.5 m) (D×H) 16×5 cm (16×5 cm) (D×H) 16×9 cm (16×9 cm) (D×H) 16×16 cm (16×16 cm) (D×H)	Volume size (child mode) 5×5.5 cm (4.2×5.0 cm) (D×H) 10×5.5 cm (8.5×5.0 cm) (D×H) 10×9.0 cm (8.5×7.5 cm) (D×H) 13×5.5 cm (11×5 cm) (D×H) 13×9.0 cm (11×7.5 cm) (D×H) 10×13 cm (8.5×11 cm) (D×H) 13×13 cm (11×11 cm) (D×H) 13×16 cm (11×13.6 cm) (D×H) 23×16 cm (D×H) 23×26 cm (D×H)	17×12 cm (DxH) 17×5 cm (DxH) 14×10 cm (DxH) 14×5 cm (DxH) 10×10 cm (DxH) 10×5 cm (DxH) 8×8 cm (DxH) 6×6 cm (DxH) 4×4 cm (DxH)	Free FOV 5 × 5 to 21 × 19 cm
Bundled software	NNT™ with free viewer and sharing application	Included	Romexis	Romexis	Romexis	i-Dixel 2.0 One Data Viewer	EasyDent/ Ez3D2009

Source: Modified from http://www.conebeam.com/cbctchart and compiled from manufacturer advertised specifications.

It should be noted that there is no standardized terminology for using the size of FOV for classification of the CBCT units. Extended, large, medium, and small FOV are the terms often used; however, their exact range of FOV is manufacturer defined. For example, a large FOV for one manufacturer may be of similar size to an extended FOV for another manufacturer (Table 2.2, Table 2.3, Table 2.4, and Table 2.5). FOV is usually mentioned in a range of dimensions and the volume scanned by the unit may vary from 4 × 4 cm to 25 × 30 cm depending on the FOV settings and the machine chosen. In general, a unit with large or extended FOV that also has capabilities of using smaller FOVs when desired would be preferable for orthodontic applications.

Earlier generation CBCT scanners either had fixed FOV or limited capabilities for adjusting the FOV. Currently, several manufacturers provide multiple FOV settings to incorporate flexibility in use (Table 2.2, Table 2.3, Table 2.4, and Table 2.5). Some newer units such as i-CAT Next Generation (NG), i-CAT Precise, and PaX-Reve 3D have fully adjustable FOV heights, contributing to an increase in flexibility of the units. Also, as discussed below and elsewhere (Chapter 3), FOV settings affect image quality and radiation exposure.

OTHER KEY ATTRIBUTES OF CBCT SCANNERS

Imaging protocols

Manufacturers currently are expanding protocols to enhance the utility and flexibility of CBCT units; however, all imaging protocols do not yield the same result in terms of radiation exposure and image quality. A clinician may choose to use specific protocols for different applications such as maxillofacial imaging, orthodontics, implant, periapical diagnosis, or endodontics.

FOV selection is one of the key elements of the clinical protocol and, in turn, is an important parameter that determines the volume of tissue scanned, radiation exposure, and image quality. In general, a small FOV increases the image resolution and reduces the overall radiation dose (Loubele *et al.*, 2008). Since the edge of FOV is prone to increased scatter radiation and artifacts, however, images of structures close to edges may have limited diagnostic utility. Also, choosing a smaller FOV may cause a failure to capture the ROI, which may result in the need for re-exposure (Suomalainen *et al.*, 2009). On the other hand, use of large FOV increases the radiation exposure and reduces the image quality while reducing the likelihood of missing the ROI. Also since a broad area is covered, the edge-related artifacts have less chance of interfering with the diagnostic accuracy of the scan. Thus, appropriate trade-offs have to be considered while planning the scan protocol for obtaining the desired image quality.

Image quality

High image quality results from the composite effect of high resolution, low noise, and fewer artifacts and is measured in both subjective and objective ways. Subjective methods include visual examination, while objective methods include measurement of accuracy, contrast resolution, spatial resolution, and absence of artifacts. CBCT images have high resolution due to smaller voxel size, but greater noise and lower LCD than MSCT images. A few studies report that CBCT images may be better than MSCT images (Liang *et al.*, 2010), but this may not always be true. For soft tissues, MSCT images are more accurate, diagnostically superior, and have higher contrast resolution compared with CBCT images (Miracle & Mukherji, 2009a, 2009b). Imaging of hard tissues is comparable in both systems (Liang *et al.*, 2010).

Image quality may vary significantly between various CBCT systems, especially with regard to quality and visualization of anatomic structures (Loubele *et al.*, 2007; Kwong *et al.*, 2008; Alqerban *et al.*, 2011). However, due to wide variation in the imaging protocols used and the difference in hardware and software functions (e.g., use of filters, reconstruction kernels), it is difficult to compare the image quality of any two units directly. A radiologist or technician should strive to attain the best image quality by adjusting the unit's parameters for the best outcome.

Subjective image quality

Limited data currently are available on image quality comparison between various CBCT units.

However, among the available studies, Liang and colleagues (2010) concluded that 3D Accuitomo was superior to MSCT and all other CBCT systems in depicting anatomical structures, while MSCT was superior to all other CBCT systems in terms of reduced image noise (Accuitomo 3D, i-CAT, NewTom 3G, Galileos, Scanora 3D).

Kamburoğlu and Kursun (2010) compared Iluma (ultra-resolution, high-resolution, low-resolution) with 3D Accuitomo (6 × 6 cm, 8 × 8 cm FOV) for the detection of simulated root resorption defects in extracted teeth. They concluded that ultra- and high-resolution Iluma and Accuitomo CBCT images were superior to low-resolution Iluma images in the detection of simulated internal resorption. Kamburoğlu *et al.* (2011) compared Veraviewepocs 3D model X550, Iluma Ultra, Kodak 9000, and Vatech PanX-Duo3D Pano/CBCT. They concluded that Veraviewepocs 3D had the highest quality images for most of the assessed features (Table 2.6).

Alqerban and associates (2011) compared the subjective image quality of 3D Accuitomo-XYZ Slice View Tomograph, Scanora 3D, Galileos® 3D Comfort, Picasso Trio, ProMax 3D, and Kodak 9000 3D for evaluation of root resorption craters. When assessing contrast and image quality, ProMax images were rated the best, followed by Galileos®. ProMax also had the highest imaging area and radiation dose, which approximates that of a four-slice CT scan. It should be noted that when using such CBCT scanners, the operator can adjust the settings to reduce the exposure, yet maintain the image quality. For example, reducing the tube current-time product (mAs) by half also reduces the radiation dose by half, while contrast-to-noise ratio (CNR) is reduced only by the square root of two (Suomalainen *et al.*, 2009). Finally, it has been demonstrated that familiarity and experience with the software increases the comfort level of the operator and may increase the operator's diagnostic ability (Alqerban *et al.*, 2011).

Objective image quality

CBCT systems are known to have high accuracy, sensitivity, and specificity. When compared with actual measurements of skulls or measurements on MSCT, it has been demonstrated that CBCT tends to slightly underestimate both linear distances and volume (Loubele *et al.*, 2006). However, there may be differences in the accuracy of the measurements when comparing various CBCT units among themselves. Loubele and colleagues (2006) demonstrated that Accuitomo 3D, NewTom 9000 DVT, and i-CAT all were able to segment the bone phantom with submillimeter accuracy, but were less accurate compared with MSCT for evaluation of bone thickness. CBCT images underestimated bone thickness with the exception of the NewTom

Table 2.6 Efficacy of CBCT units in identifying anatomic landmarks (Kamburoğlu *et al.*, 2011).

Parameter	Rating
Caries assessment	Veraviewepocs 3D > Kodak 9000 > Vatech > Iluma
Amalgam assessment	Vatech > Veraviewepocs 3D > Kodak 9000 > Iluma
Final implant drill	Veraviewepocs 3D > Vatech > Iluma > Kodak 9000
Root canal filling	Veraviewepocs 3D > Vatech > Kodak 9000 > Iluma
Metal crown	Vatech > Veraviewepocs 3D > Iluma > Kodak 9000
Mandibular canal	Veraviewepocs 3D > Vatech > Kodak 9000 > Iluma
Mental foramen	Veraviewepocs 3D > Vatech > Kodak 9000 > Iluma
Tooth	Veraviewepocs 3D > Vatech > Kodak 9000 > Iluma
Trabecular pattern	Veraviewepocs 3D > Kodak 9000 > Vatech > Iluma
Soft tissue	Veraviewepocs 3D > Vatech > Iluma > Kodak 9000

9000 DVT, which overestimated the thickness. However, the difference was less than a millimeter for most areas, making the difference clinically acceptable. In addition, a Gaussian smoothing kernel could be used to reduce the difference in the measurements between the units, except in NewTom 9000 DVT (Loubele *et al.*, 2006). In another in vitro study, Loubele *et al.* (2008) concluded that among NewTom 3G, i-CAT, and MercuRay CB, i-CAT had the highest accuracy for segmentation of mandible (protocols I2 and I3) combined with a low radiation dose.

When comparing the resolution of various CBCT units, Suomalainen and colleagues (2009) found that 3D CCD Accuitomo provided the highest resolution (0.8 lp/mm at 0.1 MTF) under simulated clinical conditions. However, 3D Accuitomo CCD/3D Accuitomo FB also had the lowest CNR, thus limiting the image quality; ProMax 3D had the highest CNR (Suomalainen *et al.*, 2009). Despite the low CNR, 3D Accuitomo CCD/3D Accuitomo FB provided diagnostically adequate images of the craniofacial region. Other studies have shown different resolving power under actual clinical conditions; 1 lp/mm at 0.5 MTF for Ortho CT unit (Arai *et al.*, 1999) and 2.3 lp/mm at 0.1 MTF in the dental mode for CB MercuRay (Araki *et al.*, 2004).

Radiation dose

Radiation dose depends on many factors, including kVp, mAs, FOV, voxel size, tissue volume to be scanned, and scanner-related parameters. The latter include scanning time, receptor sensitivity, number and degree of rotations, collimators, and filters used. Different CBCT units also have different geometries and protocols for scanning the patient and deliver different amounts of radiation dose per scan accordingly. Despite the low dose of many new CBCT units, strict adherence to "as low as reasonably achievable" (ALARA) guidelines is recommended strongly when imaging patients. Hence, as stated elsewhere (Chapters 1 and 6), CBCT use should be limited for cases in which specific clinical and/or imaging findings indicate that it could be beneficial to the patient's treatment. Its use as a screening diagnostic tool in dentistry is fundamentally incorrect (Angelopoulos *et al.*, 2012).

Degrees of rotation

The geometry of the scanner, including rotation arc, affects the radiation dose. While many scanners irradiate through a full 360° rotation, some, such as the ProMax 3D or Galileos®, expose for only part of a rotation (191° and 210°, respectively; Ludlow & Ivanovic, 2008). This potentially reduces the scan time and, thereby, radiation dose. However, images produced by this method may have greater noise and suffer from reconstruction interpolation artifacts (Scarfe & Farman, 2008). CBCT scanners such as PreXion 3D high resolution use two 360° rotations to increase basic images and, thereby, resolution (Ludlow & Ivanovic, 2008). Other units, for example, NewTom Vgi, Gendex CB-500, i-CAT Next Generation, and Promax 3D Max, use pulsed X-ray output to reduce the exposure time, which leads to a reduction in radiation dose (Ludlow *et al.*, 2006). Alternatively, altering the exposure settings to reduce the scan to 180° instead of the usual 360° turns can be used to reduce the radiation exposure without compromising the image quality (Durack & Patel, 2011).

Field of view (FOV)

FOV has a strong correlation with radiation dose and exposure. In general, increasing the FOV increases the exposure because a larger area is scanned. As the FOV is increased from the smallest (40 mm × 40 mm) to a large FOV (170 mm × 120 mm), scatter increases by a factor of 4.5 (SEDENTEXCT, 2012; Figure 2.4). Alternatively, decreasing the FOV from 12 inches (300 mm) to 9 inches (230 mm) lowers the effective dose by 17% to 49% (Suomalainen *et al.*, 2009); reducing the FOV from 9 to 6 inches (150 mm) may reduce the exposure by up to 42%. The relationship between FOV and effective radiation exposure is complicated further by the fact that effective doses for the same or similar FOVs can vary substantially between units from different manufacturers (Table 2.7; Ludlow & Ivanovic, 2008; see also Chapter 3). The use of different protocols in the same scanner also can change the exposure drastically. For example, a 500% increase in dose occurs when "ultra" setting is used in Iluma instead of "standard" exposure. This change usually is related to increase in mAs and/or reduction in voxel size (Ludlow & Ivanovic, 2008).

Loubele and associates (2008) compared i-CAT, NewTom 3G, Accuitomo 3D, and MercuRay CB units and found that NewTom 3G delivered the highest dose of radiation while Accuitomo 3D delivered the lowest. However, when the radiation was standardized by the volume of the region scanned, the radiation dose of Accuitomo 3D was highest while i-CAT and NewTom 3G provided equal doses. Suomalainen and coworkers (2009) concluded that among ProMax 3D, 3D Accuitomo CCD, 3D Accuitomo FP, and Scanora 3D CBCT units, the ProMax 3D scanner not only imaged the largest height, but also delivered the highest radiation dose; Accuitomo provided the lowest dose due to small FOV. Even after standardization of the imaging area, the dose of the ProMax was two to four times higher than other CBCT units compared in the study. Pauwels and colleagues (2012) performed a comprehensive review of the radiation dosage of various machines at different protocols. They found that at large FOV, the dose varied from 83 μSv (i-CAT NG and NewTom VG) to 368 μSv (Iluma Elite; Table 2.8). In medium FOV, the radiation dose varied from a low of 45 μSv (i-CAT NG and Scanora 3D) to a high of 265 μSv (NewTom VGi; Table 2.9); in small FOV, the dose ranged from 19 μSv (Kodak 9000 3D) to 44 μSv (Pax-Uni 3D; Table 2.10).

Theodorakou and coworkers (2012) compared i-CAT NG, NewTom VG, Kodak 9000C 3D, ProMax 3D, and 3D Accuitomo 170 and found the pediatric organ effective doses in the following order:

- *Small FOV*: Kodak 9000C 3D < ProMax 3D < Accuitomo 170 < i-CAT NG < NewTom VG
- *Medium to large FOV*: NewTom VG < i-CAT NG < 3D Accuitomo 170

Since CBCT is a high-scatter environment, measurement of scatter and environmental radiation also are important considerations. The review by

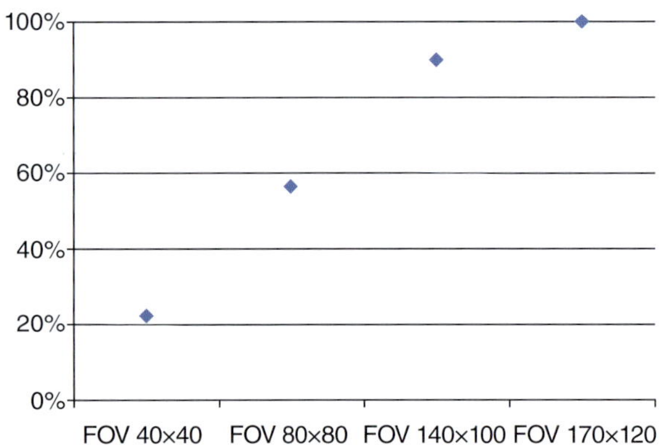

Figure 2.4 Effect of FOV on scatter dose for 3D Accuitomo 170 depicted relative to the maximum of 100% (*y*-axis) for the largest FOV. (Reprinted with permission from SEDENTEXCT, 2012.)

Table 2.7 Maximum and minimum FOV-dependent effective radiation dose variations between units from different manufacturers using ICRP 2007 (Ludlow & Ivanovic, 2008).

FOV	Maximum effective radiation (μSv)	Minimum effective radiation (μSv)
Large	CB MercuRay maximum quality 1073 μSv	Newtom 3G 68 μSv
Medium	CB MercuRay 560 μSv	Classic i-Cat 69 μSv
Small	Promax 3D large adult dose 652 μSv	PreXion 3D standard exposure 189 μSv

Table 2.8 Effective radiation exposure with large FOV (maxillofacial) protocols for different CBCT scanners (Pauwels *et al.*, 2012).

	Galileos® Comfort	i-Cat NG	Iluma Elite	Kodak 9500	NewTom VG	NewTom VGi	Scanora 3D	SkyView
Effective dose (μSv)	84	83	368	136	83	194	68	87

Table 2.9 Effective radiation exposure with medium FOV (dentoalveolar or single jaw) protocols for different CBCT scanners (Pauwels *et al.*, 2012).

	3D Accuitomo 170	i-Cat NG	Kodak 9500	New Tom VGi	Picasso Trio		ProMax 3D		Scanora 3D			Vera-viewepocs 3D
Protocol/ site	Upper jaw	Dentoalveolar (both jaws)			High dose	Low dose	High dose	Low dose	Upper jaw	Lower jaw	Both jaws	Dentoalveolar (both jaws)
Effective dose (μSv)	54	45	92	265	123	81	122	28	46	47	45	73

Table 2.10 Effective radiation exposure with small FOV (localized) protocols for different CBCT scanners (Pauwels *et al.*, 2012).

	3D Accuitomo 170	Kodak 9000 3D	Kodak 9000 3D	Pax-Uni 3D
Site	Lower jaw, molar region	Upper jaw, front region	Lower jaw, molar region	Upper jaw, front region
Effective dose (μSv)	43	19	40	44

SEDENTEXCT (2012) concluded that radiation dose per scan at 1 m from the isocenter of the CBCT was lowest for Kodak 9000 3D (4.1 μSv) and maximum for the ProMax 3D (12.2 μSv; Figure 2.5).

ROLE OF SOFTWARE FUNCTIONS IN IMAGE INTERPRETATION

Advanced software functions are capable of handling large amounts of data with great ease and allow visualization of volumetric data acquired from CBCT scanners in different display modes. Enhanced presentation and life-like volume-rendered images are of particular interest to nonradiologists mainly because of the ease of interpretation. Because of the advances in computer software technology and computing power, image reconstruction now is faster, more intuitive, user-friendly, and, in some cases, almost instant compared with what it was just a few years ago (see Chapter 5). The important reconstruction types include multi-planar reconstruction (MPR; Figure 2.6), maximum intensity projection (MIP; Figure 2.7), curved planar reconstruction (CPR; Figure 2.8), and volume rendering technique (VRT; Figure 2.9).

A common problem with image rendering techniques is that they are prone to artifacts and loss of data. Thus, undisplaced fractures or those lesions that do not involve the cortex can be overlooked easily when using rendering techniques such as VRT and surface rendering (SR). Such findings, however, may be observed in the source images or in MPR where there is no loss of information. Therefore, it should be emphasized that a clinician should review all images, not just VRT images, when making a diagnosis.

Although 3D image reconstruction techniques are improving rapidly, one must realize their advantages and limitations. Currently, 3D reconstruction is mostly carried out using a volume rendering technique because of its inherent advantages over the surface rendering techniques. Surface rendering has its own advantages, such as rapid data processing. However, its drawbacks include the inability to highlight subsurface details accurately and lack of image fidelity due to loss of significant amount of data during rendering. Volume rendering, on the other hand, has two distinct advantages over surface rendering. First, it uses percentage classification, which provides a physically realistic depiction of volume-averaged CT data. Also, volume rendering uses the complete dataset contained in the volume, which makes the reconstruction more accurate. Volume-rendered images better

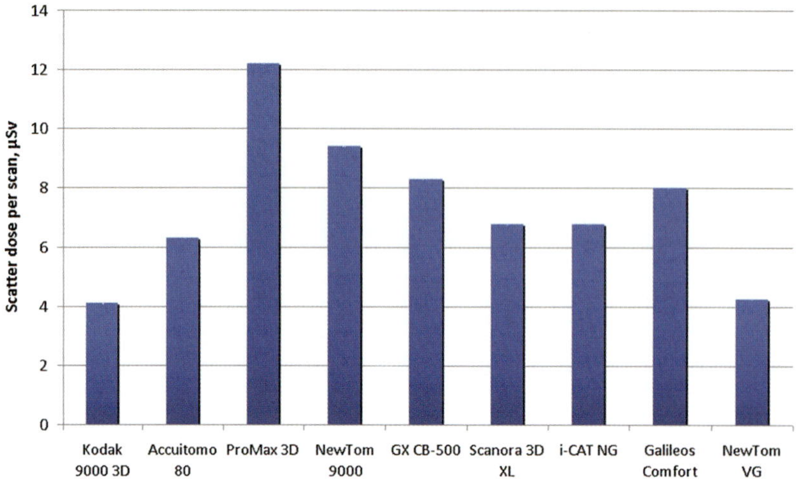

Figure 2.5 Comparison of maximum scatter per scan at 1 m for several CBCT models. (Reprinted with permission from SEDENTEXCT, 2012.)

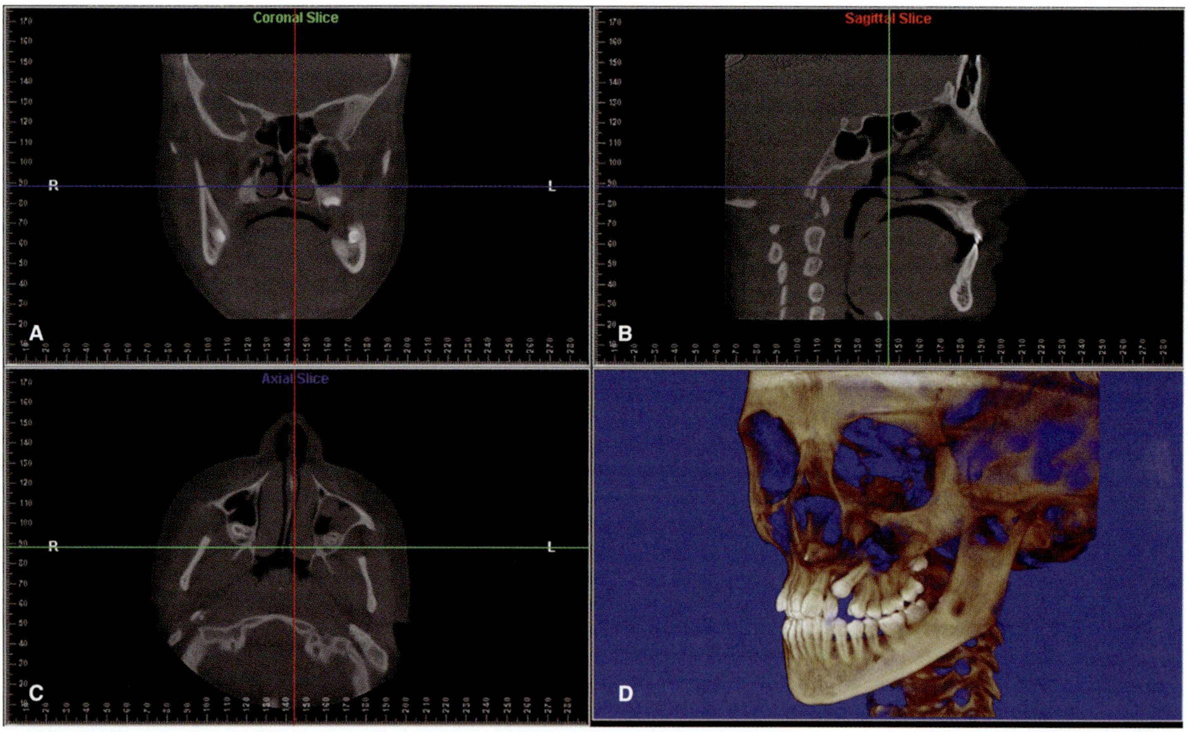

Figure 2.6 Orthogonal MPR and 3D reconstruction using CBCT data. *A*: Coronal slice. *B*: Sagittal slice. *C*: Axial slice. *D*: Volumetric reconstruction. Data processing and reconstruction done with Dolphin 3D imaging software 11.5 (Dolphin Imaging, Chatsworth, California).

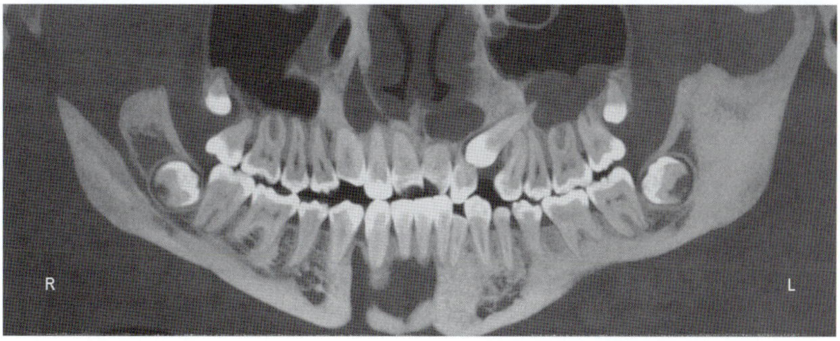

Figure 2.7 Maximum intensity projection (MIP) of curved planar reconstruction (CPR) image. In the MIP, the highest attenuation voxels are selected along lines projected through the volume dataset. Data processing and reconstruction done with Dolphin 3D imaging software 11.5.

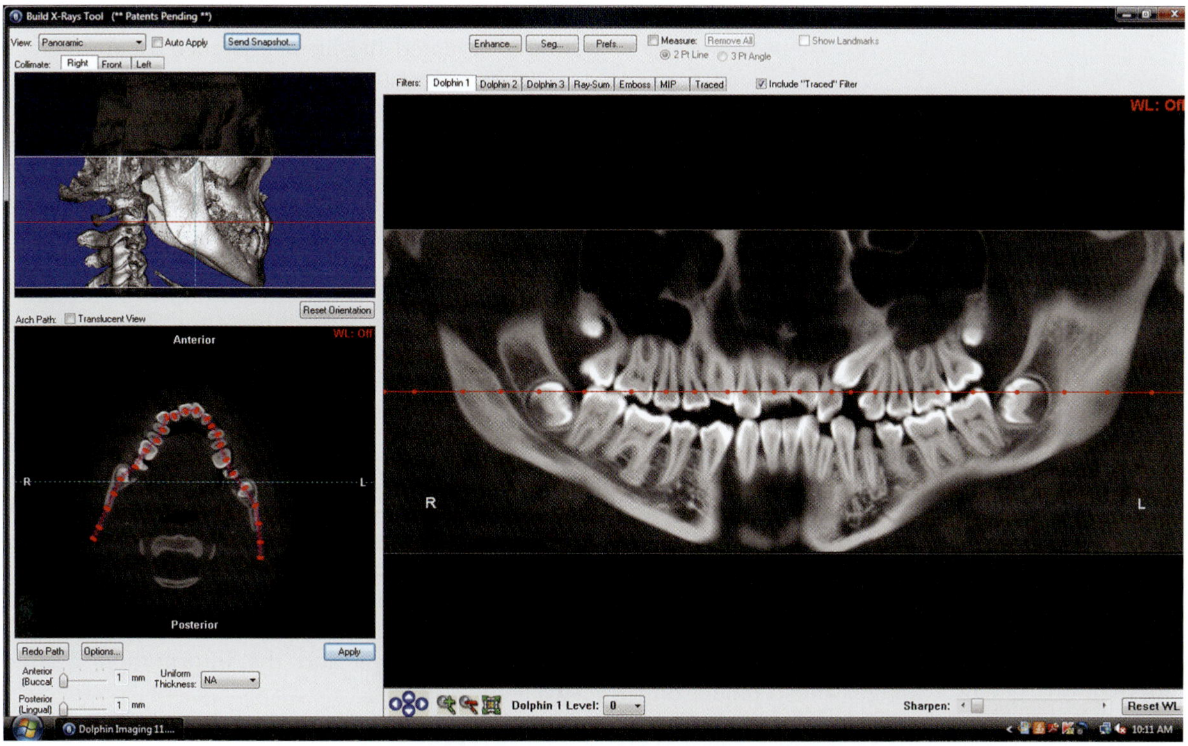

Figure 2.8 Curved planar reconstruction (CPR) from a CBCT dataset at the field of interest (FOI). *A*: 3D-rendered image craniofacial region with the FOI shown by the central horizontal line. *B*: Axial slice of FOI with desired focal trough. *C*: Curved planar tomograph (CPT) showing panoramic view of the focal trough. Data processing and reconstruction done with Dolphin 3D imaging software 11.5.

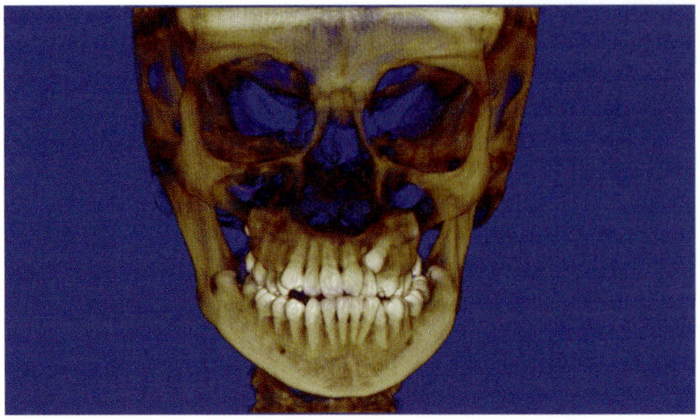

Figure 2.9 Volume rendering reconstruction of the craniofacial region using CBCT data set. Data processing and reconstruction done with Dolphin 3D imaging software 11.5.

highlight subsurface structures, and the displayed intensity is related to the amount of bone encountered along a line extending through the volume (Etlik *et al.*, 2004). This is especially significant when one needs to evaluate subcortical bony pathologies such as cysts or tumors. Finally, in a few instances, the 3D-rendered images may not provide the exact nature of details sought by the clinician. Therefore, it should be emphasized that a clinician should review all images, not just VRT images, when making a diagnosis.

Accuracy of measurements

Landmark identification and accuracy of 3D software reconstruction has been documented in many studies. In general, linear measurements on 3D reconstruction have been found to be more accurate than on 2D CBCT images and cephalograms. CBCT measurements, however, tend to underestimate the actual distance, which, although statistically significant, may not be relevant clinically. Lagravère and associates (2008) found that measurements on 3D images obtained with the NewTom 3G and reconstructed using AMIRA software (MercuRay Computer Systems, Berlin, Germany) were accurate within clinically tolerable limits. They noted variations of up to 0.6 mm in linear measurements in FOVs of 9 and 12 inches. The angular measurements also showed differences of not more than 1° from the gold standard. Berco and coworkers (2009) used i-CAT unit with Dolphin 3D™ imaging software (Dolphin Imaging, Chatsworth, CA) and demonstrated a linear accuracy within 0.3 mm on reconstructed 3D images, which was lower than the resolution of the scan. They also showed that alterations in skull position prior to image acquisition did not influence the accuracy of virtual linear measurements. Thus, CBCT imaging has a significant advantage over traditional 2D skull films in which changes in patient position affect linear and angular measurements. Periago and colleagues (2008) using CBCT images obtained from i-CAT system with XoranCat acquisition software and imported into Dolphin 3D software found that the 3D CBCT images underestimated the linear distance by an average of 1.13%. Most of the deviations occurred within 2 mm of the actual measurement. This was similar to the accuracy obtained with MSCT units, which showed the mean differences between measured and actual dimensions as 0.38 mm ± SD 1.14 (Williams & Richtsmeier, 2003).

Selection of voxel size is important for planning a scan as it affects the amount of radiation, image quality, and scanning time. Damstra and associates (2010) concluded that a voxel size of 0.4 mm is adequate for measurement of craniofacial structures (measurement error = 0.05 mm). An increased voxel resolution (0.25 mm) did not increase the accuracy of the surface models (measurement error = 0.07 mm). However, the risk of misdiagnosis must be weighed, suggesting that a scanning protocol with a 0.4 mm voxel size might not be suitable for every patient. Thus, selection of the voxel size should be based on the patient's problems and the information desired from the scan.

Effect of patient positioning on craniometric measurements

Hassan and coworkers (2009) compared the effect of patient positioning on the accuracy of CBCT image using linear and angular variables. They found that in the ideal position, the largest deviation of CBCT measurement from actual measurement was less than 0.5 mm for 3D reconstruction, less than 1 mm for 2D tomographic slices, and less than 5 mm for 2D cephalometric (lateral and postero-anterior [PA]) projection images. When the measurements were performed in rotated skull position, the 3D and 2D tomographic scans were accurate in measurement, while the lateral and PA cephalometric projections showed significant differences of up to 10 mm. It was concluded that analysis performed with 3D reconstructions was more accurate than that with 2D cephalometric projections.

Maret and colleagues (2010) compared CBCT 3D reconstruction images (9000 3D Kodak, AMIRA software) with those from a high-resolution peripheral micro-CT scanner (XtremeCT, Scanco Medical, Bassersdorf, Switzerland). They found a strong correlation coefficient between the micro-CT and CBCT volumes. For posterior teeth, micro-CT and CBCT volume measurements were not different significantly from one another, while the anterior teeth showed a small but statistically significant difference. They noted that CBCT images did show a slight underestimation of the volume of interest compared with micro-CT. Liu and coworkers (2010) concluded that volume measurements of teeth derived from CBCT deviated slightly from their physical volumes by 4–7%. Moreover, smoothing reduced volume measurements on CBCT reconstructions by 3–12%.

OTHER CONSIDERATIONS

Flexibility and multimodality

Manufacturers currently offer scanners with enhanced capability and flexibility in clinical applications. For example, the same unit may be used for both panoramic imaging and small to medium FOV CBCT imaging, thus reducing the need for two separate scanners.

ProMax 3D was the first scanner to incorporate a small FOV 3D sensor to their ProMax digital panoramic machine (Scarfe *et al.*, 2009). Interestingly, ProMax 3D offers the ability to be upgraded from an existing panoramic platform to a CBCT scanner. Examples of other hybrid units are Veraviewepocs 3D, Kodak Dental Imaging 9000 DS, and Picasso Trio.

Calibration

Calibration is performed to align the sensors of the scanner for efficient use of incident radiation and to reduce the generation of image artifacts. For example, scanners such as i-CAT require daily or twice daily calibration, while Accuitomo and ProMax do not require calibration. This may become an important consideration for busy practices because a frequent need for calibration may lead to reduced productivity (Miles & Danforth, 2007).

Flexibility of imaging protocol

Currently, most units offer only fixed protocols that are preset by the manufacturer. Accuitomo and MercuRay, however, allow the operator to alter mA and kVp settings to customize a protocol (Lofthag-Hansen *et al.*, 2011). For example, the exposure can be increased where requirements dictate, such as for periapical imaging for endodontic purposes, or reduced for planning implant placement. Similarly, increased exposure for the lower jaw compared with the upper can be planned even while limiting the arc of rotation to 180° instead of 360°. While these features can be useful for optimization of radiation exposure, they also can be counterproductive in the hands of an inexperienced operator.

CT scanners also use a variety of reconstruction filters that can alter post-exposure image processing according to the needs of the operator (see Chapter 5) and that allow the same image to be optimized for visualizing different tissues, such as soft tissues or bone (Loubele *et al.*, 2008).

CONCLUSIONS

The emergence of the cone beam concept from multiscan technology is a big leap forward in medical and dental imaging. Technological advances in imaging sensors from CCD to flat panel, their quality control, introduction of pulsed radiation, limited scan arc, overall reduction in the bulk of the machine, and portability has enhanced the comfort and uses of CBCT for patient care and research. The image processing and manipulation are software functions that have been enhanced greatly, enabling rapid processing and the ability to view images in multiple modes ranging from a 2D to a volume-rendered image.

When selecting a unit for orthodontic imaging, several factors need to be considered, including FOV and its customizability, radiation exposure, positioning of patient, ease of use, image quality, footprint, scan time, reconstruction time, and grayscale. Although different manufacturers offer scanners and software functions with a range of capabilities, it truly is the end user's decision regarding what equipment meets the specific needs of his or her practice and patient care.

References

Akpek, S., Brunner, T., Benndorf, G., *et al.* (2005) Three-dimensional imaging and cone beam volume CT in C-arm angiography with flat panel detector. *Diagnostic and Interventional Radiology (Ankara, Turkey)*, 11 (1), 10–13.

Alqerban, A., Jacobs, R., Fieuws, S., *et al.* (2011) Comparison of 6 cone beam computed tomography systems for image quality and detection of simulated canine impaction-induced external root resorption in maxillary lateral incisors. *American Journal of Orthodontics and Dentofacial Orthopedics*, 140 (3), e129–e139.

Angelopoulos, C., Scarfe, W.C., & Farman, A.G. (2012) A comparison of maxillofacial CBCT and medical CT. *Atlas of the Oral and Maxillofacial Surgery Clinics of North America*, 20 (1), 1–17.

Arai, Y., Tammisalo, E., Iwai, K., *et al.* (1999) Development of a compact computed tomographic apparatus for dental use. *Dentomaxillofacial Radiology*, 28 (4), 245–248.

Araki, K., Maki, K., Seki, K., *et al.* (2004) Characteristics of a newly developed dentomaxillofacial X-ray cone beam CT scanner (CB MercuRay): system configuration and physical properties. *Dentomaxillofacial Radiology*, 33 (1), 51–59.

Barrett, J.F. & Keat, N. (2004) Artifacts in CT: recognition and avoidance. *Radiographics*, 24 (6), 1679–1691.

Berco, M., Rigali, P.H., Jr, Miner, R.M., *et al.* (2009) Accuracy and reliability of linear cephalometric measurements from cone beam computed tomography scans of a dry human skull. *American Journal of Orthodontics and Dentofacial Orthopedics*, 136 (1), 17. e1–e9.

Broderick, M., Menezes, G., Leech, M., *et al.* (2007) A comparison of kilovoltage and megavoltage cone beam CT in radiotherapy. *Journal of Radiotherapy in Practice*, 6 (3), 173–178.

Damstra, J., Fourie, Z., Huddleston Slater, J.J.R., *et al.* (2010) Accuracy of linear measurements from cone beam computed tomography-derived surface models of different voxel sizes. *American Journal of Orthodontics and Dentofacial Orthopedics*, 137 (1), 16. e1–e6.

Dörfler, A., Struffert, T., Engelhorn, T., *et al.* (2008) Rotational flat-panel computed tomography in diagnostic and interventional neuroradiology. *RoFo*, 180 (10), 891–898.

Durack, C. & Patel, S. (2011) The use of cone beam computed tomography in the management of dens invaginatus affecting a strategic tooth in a patient affected by hypodontia: a case report. *International Endodontic Journal*, 44 (5), 474–483.

Etlik, O., Temizöz, O., Doğan, A., *et al.* (2004) Three-dimensional volume rendering imaging in detection of bone fractures. *European Journal of General Medicine*, 1 (4), 48–52.

Ghosh, S., Kharbanda, O.P., Kapila, S.D., *et al.* (2013) Three-dimensional imaging in orthodonics. In Kharbanda, O.P. (ed.), *Orthodontics: Diagnosis and Management of Malocclusion and Dentofacial Deformities*. 2nd ed. New Delhi: Elsevier India.

Goldman, L.W. (2007) Principles of CT: radiation dose and image quality. *Journal of Nuclear Medicine Technology*, 35 (4), 213–225.

Goldman, L.W. & Fowlkes, J.B. (eds.) (2000) *2000 Syllabus: Categorical Course in Diagnostic Radiology Physics: CT and US Cross-Sectional Imaging*. Radiological Society of North America, Oak Brook, IL.

Hassan, B., van der Stelt, P., & Sanderink, G. (2009) Accuracy of three-dimensional measurements obtained from cone beam computed tomography surface-rendered images for cephalometric analysis: influence of patient scanning position. *European Journal of Orthodontics*, 31 (2), 129–134.

Hounsfield, G.N. (1976) Picture quality of computed tomography. *American Journal of Roentgenology*, 127 (1), 3–9.

Kamburoğlu, K. & Kursun, S. (2010) A comparison of the diagnostic accuracy of CBCT images of different voxel resolutions used to detect simulated small internal resorption cavities. *International Endodontic Journal*, 43 (9), 798–807.

Kamburoğlu, K., Murat, S., Kolsuz, E., *et al.* (2011) Comparative assessment of subjective image quality of cross-sectional cone beam computed tomography scans. *Journal of Oral Science*, 53 (4), 501–508.

Kau, C.H., Božič, M., English, J., *et al.* (2009) Cone beam computed tomography of the maxillofacial region: an update. *International Journal of Medical Robotics and Computer Assisted Surgery*, 5 (4), 366–380.

Kwong, J.C., Palomo, J.M., Landers, M.A., *et al.* (2008) Image quality produced by different cone beam computed tomography settings. *American Journal of Orthodontics and Dentofacial Orthopedics*, 133 (2), 317–327.

Lagravère, M.O., Carey, J., Toogood, R.W., *et al.* (2008) Three-dimensional accuracy of measurements made with software on cone beam computed tomography images. *American Journal of Orthodontics and Dentofacial Orthopedics*, 134 (1), 112–116.

Liang, X., Jacobs, R., Hassan, B., *et al.* (2010) A comparative evaluation of cone beam computed tomography (CBCT) and multi-slice CT (MSCT). Part I: on subjective image quality. *European Journal of Radiology*, 75 (2), 265–269.

Liu, Y., Olszewski, R., Alexandroni, E.S., *et al.* (2010) The validity of *in vivo* tooth volume determinations from cone beam computed tomography. *Angle Orthodontist*, 80 (1), 160–166.

Lofthag-Hansen, S., Thilander-Klang, A., & Gröndahl, K. (2011) Evaluation of subjective image quality in relation to diagnostic task for cone beam computed tomography with different fields of view. *European Journal of Radiology*, 80 (2), 483–488.

Loubele, M., Maes, F., Schutyser, F., *et al.* (2006) Assessment of bone segmentation quality of cone beam CT *versus* multislice spiral CT: a pilot study. *Oral Surgery, Oral Medicine, Oral Pathology, Oral Radiology, and Endodontics*, 102 (2), 225–234.

Loubele, M., Guerrero, M.E., Jacobs, R., *et al.* (2007) A comparison of jaw dimensional and quality assessments of bone characteristics with cone beam CT, spiral tomography, and multi-slice spiral CT. *International Journal of Oral & Maxillofacial Implants*, 22 (3), 446–454.

Loubele, M., Jacobs, R., Maes, F., *et al.* (2008) Image quality *vs* radiation dose of four cone beam computed tomography scanners. *Dentomaxillofacial Radiology*, 37 (6), 309–318.

Ludlow, J.B. & Ivanovic, M. (2008) Comparative dosimetry of dental CBCT devices and 64-slice CT for oral and maxillofacial radiology. *Oral Surgery, Oral Medicine, Oral Pathology, Oral Radiology, and Endodontics*, 106 (1), 106–114.

Ludlow, J.B., Davies-Ludlow, L.E., Brooks, S.L., *et al.* (2006) Dosimetry of 3 CBCT devices for oral and maxillofacial radiology: CB MercuRay, NewTom 3G and i-CAT. *Dentomaxillofacial Radiology*, 35 (4), 219–226.

Mahesh, M. (2009) *MDCT Physics. The Basics: Technology, Image Quality and Radiation Dose*. Lippincott Williams & Wilkins, Philadelphia.

Maret, D., Molinier, F., Braga, J., *et al.* (2010) Accuracy of 3D reconstructions based on cone beam computed tomography. *Journal of Dental Research*, 89 (12), 1465–1469.

Miles, D.A. & Danforth, R.A. (2007) A Clinician's Guide to Understanding Cone Beam Volumetric Imaging (CBVI). Available at http://www.ineedce.com/courses/1413/PDF/A_Clin_Gde_ConeBeam.pdf, accessed October 7, 2012.

Miracle, A.C. & Mukherji, S.K. (2009a) Conebeam CT of the head and neck. Part 1: physical principles. *American Journal of Neuroradiology*, 30 (6), 1088–1095.

Miracle, A.C. & Mukherji, S.K. (2009b) Conebeam CT of the head and neck. Part 2: clinical applications. *American Journal of Neuroradiology*, 30 (7), 1285–1292.

Molen, A.D. (2011) Comparing cone beam computed tomography systems from an orthodontic perspective. *Seminars in Orthodontics*, 17 (1), 34–38.

Mozzo, P., Procacci, C., Tacconi, A., *et al.* (1998) A new volumetric CT machine for dental imaging based on the cone beam technique: preliminary results. *European Radiology*, 8 (9), 1558–1564.

Orth, R.C., Wallace, M.J., & Kuo, M.D. (2008) C-arm cone beam CT: general principles and technical considerations for use in interventional radiology. *Journal of Vascular and Interventional Radiology*, 19 (6), 814–820.

Pauwels, R., Beinsberger, J., Collaert, B., *et al.* (2012) Effective dose range for dental cone beam computed tomography scanners. *European Journal of Radiology*, 81 (2), 267–271.

Periago, D.R., Scarfe, W.C., Moshiri, M., *et al.* (2008) Linear accuracy and reliability of cone beam CT derived 3-dimensional images constructed using an orthodontic volumetric rendering program. *Angle Orthodontist*, 78 (3), 387–395.

Scarfe, W.C. & Farman, A.G. (2008) What is cone beam CT and how does it work? *Dental Clinics of North America*, 52 (4), 707–730.

Scarfe, W.C., Levin, M.D., Gane, D., *et al.* (2009) Use of cone beam computed tomography in endodontics. *International Journal of Dentistry*, article ID 634567.

SEDENTEXCT (2012) Safety and Efficacy of a New and Emerging Dental X-Ray Technology. Available at http://www.sedentexct.eu/system/files/SEDENTEXCT%20D2.2%20v1%20FINAL_0.pdf, accessed July 8, 2012.

Suomalainen, A., Kiljunen, T., Käser, Y., *et al.* (2009) Dosimetry and image quality of four dental cone beam computed tomography scanners compared with multislice computed tomography scanners. *Dentomaxillofacial Radiology*, 38 (6), 367–378.

Theodorakou, C., Walker, A., Horner, K., *et al.* (2012) Estimation of paediatric organ and effective doses from dental cone beam CT using anthropomorphic phantoms. *British Journal of Radiology*, 85 (1010), 153–160.

Williams, F.L. & Richtsmeier, J.T. (2003) Comparison of mandibular landmarks from computed tomography and 3D digitizer data. *Clinical Anatomy (New York, N.Y.)*, 16 (6), 494–500.

Yu, L., Vrieze, T.J., Bruesewitz, M.R., *et al.* (2010) Dose and image quality evaluation of a dedicated cone beam CT system for high-contrast neurologic applications. *American Journal of Roentgenology*, 194 (2), W193–W201.

3 Cone Beam Computed Tomography in Orthodontics: Perspectives on Radiation Risk

Sharon L. Brooks, DDS, MS, and John B. Ludlow, DDS, MS

As orthodontists and other dental specialists learn to take advantage of the benefits that three-dimensional (3D) imaging through cone beam computed tomography (CBCT) can bring for their patients, questions arise regarding the radiation risks associated with using this technology. Opinions within the profession and the public range from belief that the risk from CBCT is insignificant to great concerns about all types of radiological examinations, but particularly those used in dentistry. Claus and colleagues (2012) reported a relationship between the history of dental bitewing radiographs and brain tumors. More specifically, they noted that individuals who recalled having multiple sets of bitewings had two times greater risk of developing this type of tumor than those who had no or less frequent bitewings. This article was distributed widely via the Internet, newspapers, and magazines, resulting in many patients expressing great anxiety about the use of X-rays on themselves or their children. Although this study has been criticized due to its methodology of asking subjects about their history of dental radiographic examinations and the inherent problem of recall bias, the issues it raised ought to be of concern to every clinician who uses ionizing radiation, particularly on children.

In response to earlier criticisms in the press regarding the possible overuse of diagnostic imaging, particularly computed tomography (CT) and specifically in children, the medical profession has made a concerted effort to evaluate its approach to the utilization of imaging and put forth recommendations to guide clinicians regarding the most appropriate use of radiographic imaging. As such, the American College of Radiology has adopted the Image Wisely and Image Gently campaigns in order to obtain all the benefits of diagnostic imaging while minimizing risks. The Image Wisely program (http://www.imagewisely.org) provides guidance on selecting the most appropriate imaging examinations for specific clinical problems, while the Image Gently program (http://www.imagegently.org), developed by the Alliance for Radiation

Cone Beam Computed Tomography in Orthodontics: Indications, Insights, and Innovations, First Edition. Sunil D. Kapila.

Safety in Pediatric Imaging (Goske *et al.*, 2008) specifically focuses on imaging in children. Many professional organizations, including the American Academy of Oral and Maxillofacial Radiology, have endorsed the Image Gently campaign. Because a large proportion of an orthodontic practice involves children and adolescents, the issues of radiation dose and risk to this vulnerable population should be of great interest to orthodontists.

The purpose of this chapter is to provide the orthodontist with the necessary information to: (1) be able to select the appropriate imaging parameters to meet the goals of the diagnostic imaging examination, (2) understand the risks associated with these choices, and (3) be comfortable explaining the risks and benefits to patients and their parents. The chapter begins with a review of the basics of radiation biology and dose measurement in order to provide the necessary foundation for the discussion of these issues with regard to the use of CBCT and other imaging examinations in orthodontics. Information on doses from a variety of CBCT machines then is presented, along with a discussion of the factors that affect these doses, particularly those that the user can change. Since dose alone is not sufficient for the selection of an imaging technique, this section is followed by a short discussion on the relationship between image quality and radiation dose, and image quality and imaging goals. Finally, the chapter highlights the general radiation risk assessment for orthodontic imaging.

RADIATION EFFECTS

It did not take long after the discovery of X-rays for the first incidents of radiation injury to be reported. In those days, little information was available about how this new technology worked, either physically or biologically; early users exposed themselves, colleagues, and patients to large doses of radiation. Because X-rays are invisible, it was easy to think that nothing was happening—until tissue burns and other evidence of necrosis occurred. Early exposures were large, requiring 30 minutes or more to obtain a suitable image, and injury, at least in the form of skin reddening, was not uncommon.

As knowledge grew and the technology of image capture (film systems) and radiation shielding improved, the incidence of obvious radiation injury declined. Years after radiation was used commonly for conditions as diverse as ankylosing spondylitis, mastitis after childbirth, ringworm, tonsillitis, and acne, however, an increase in cancer incidence in tissues irradiated during these procedures was observed (National Research Council, 2006). Subsequently, research on the effects of ionizing radiation and attempts to try to minimize these effects by controlling radiation dose for diagnostic imaging increased dramatically following the aftermath of the atomic bombs dropped on Hiroshima and Nagasaki in World War II.

All forms of ionizing radiation, including X-rays, have the potential to cause cellular and tissue damage. The type and extent of damage depend on many factors, including:

(1) The type of radiation
(2) The amount or dose of radiation
(3) The size of the beam
(4) The radio-sensitivity of the tissues irradiated
(5) How the radiation is delivered (dose rate, fractionation)
(6) Sex and age of the patient
(7) The adequacy of the repair mechanisms of the organism.

Some consequences of radiation, such as carcinogenesis, are thought to require the interaction of radiation with other initiators and/or promoters for cancer to occur. There may be a long latent period between the time the radiation injury occurs and the time the signs or symptoms are observable. For many cancers, the latent period may be 20–30 years, making it difficult to determine the cause for any specific case of cancer. This latency also may make it easier to dismiss the idea that radiation exposure to the head during a childhood orthodontic examination might be the cause of the cancer.

Much of the basic radiation biology information currently available has been obtained through animal and tissue culture studies, while much of the information on human effects of radiation comes from case reports and epidemiologic studies of subjects who have been exposed to large doses of radiation. More recently, there have been studies looking at subjects exposed to much lower doses of radiation, such as those used in diagnostic imaging (Preston-Martin & White, 1990; Claus *et al.*, 2012).

Much of the radiation damage to cells and tissues is a direct effect of X-ray energy on the cells, leading to ionization of molecules, along with the disruption of molecular bonds and the reformation of those bonds that often does not occur correctly. Radiation also may cause effects indirectly by ionizing other molecules in the tissue (e.g., water), leading to the production of free radicals, which then can interact with adjacent molecules to produce damage. Most of the radiation effects occur as a result of damage to the DNA that, depending on the specific injury, may lead to cell death, heritable mutations, or carcinogenesis. The body has a number of mechanisms to repair damage to DNA, but the repair is not always successful, particularly when a break in the double strand of the DNA occurs.

Radiation damage frequently is described in terms of two major types of effects: deterministic and stochastic. Deterministic effects are a result of killing of a large number of cells and typically have a threshold below which no damage is seen. Once the threshold is reached, the *severity* of effect is proportional to the dose. However, the *probability* of an effect occurring is independent of dose: once the threshold is reached, which may differ between individuals, damage will occur. Common types of deterministic effects include skin reddening, mucosal ulceration, salivary dysfunction, and cataract formation, but these typically have large thresholds and likely are seen only in large doses of radiation, such as might occur in radiation therapy or nuclear accident. It is unlikely that the doses used in diagnostic imaging, including CBCT, will cause deterministic effects.

The other major category of radiation effects, stochastic, is of concern with the use of diagnostic imaging because in this case, the *probability* of the effect is proportional to the dose. Stochastic effects occur as a result of sublethal damage to DNA. The cells are not killed outright, but the DNA is damaged and may not be repaired correctly. The more radiation the cells receive, the more likely nonreparable or improperly repaired damage will persist. There is no guarantee that the radiation will cause an observable effect (e.g., cancer or a heritable mutation), but the probability for these effects increases with the amount of radiation received. The *severity* of the effect is independent of the dose, but the probability is not. Once cancer occurs as a result of radiation, for example, the severity of the cancer is related to which cells are affected, not to the total amount of radiation. There is no threshold for stochastic effects: theoretically, a tiny amount of radiation is enough to lead to cancer, given the presence of other initiator and/or promoter factors and the lack of repair of the DNA damage.

Most biologic effects of radiation, whether deterministic or stochastic, are due to damage to the DNA, whereas a much larger dose is required to damage the non-nuclear cell cytoplasmic contents, which are more resistant to radiation. Sublethal damage to DNA can lead to mutations that vary in significance, depending on the cell type exposed. The term "genetic mutation" is used to describe alterations in the DNA occurring in reproductive cells. These mutations can be passed on to future offspring of the irradiated person, hence causing heritable mutations. Genetic mutations are not considered to be a significant risk in dental imaging because the gonads are not in the primary beam and the gonadal dose is extremely low, on the order of background radiation.

The term "somatic mutation" is used to describe DNA damage occurring in any other cells of the body (somatic cells). This damage is passed on to other cells in the same cell line, but not to offspring of the irradiated person. For example, exposure of the bone marrow can lead to the development of leukemia in the affected person, but it will not affect that person's future children. Because leukemia is a stochastic effect, however, the exposure may not cause any problems at all; rather, it may only increase the risk of complications occurring.

Because stochastic effects involve a chance of damage occurring after irradiation, the only way to determine whether these effects occur in humans is by looking at large numbers of exposed persons, since it is unethical to expose humans deliberately or experimentally. Over the years, a large number of epidemiologic studies have been performed to evaluate the effects of radiation dose. Much of our current knowledge has been derived from the study of the people in Hiroshima and Nagasaki, Japan, who were present when the atomic bombs were dropped at the end of World War II (National Research Council, 2006). Information from radiation doses, known or calculated, and incidence of cancer in a population typically are evaluated statistically to develop a model that can then be used to predict cancer incidence from other doses, extrapolating from high doses to low doses. The choice of a statistical model then will affect the prediction of risk from radiation. It should be emphasized that this statistically derived *population* risk cannot be (or should not be) used to specify the risk for an individual person exposed to a certain dose. The most commonly used model is that of the linear, no threshold model, which states that the radiation risk is proportional directly to the radiation dose without a threshold. Theoretically, any dose above zero carries some risk, although the risk is small at low doses. Typically, the risk is expressed as "x" number of additional cancers beyond the normal cancer rate per million individuals per specific radiation dose, usually 1 Sievert (Sv). Some scientists feel that there are so many uncertainties in the models that the risk of cancer from low doses can be considered negligible with no cause for concern at these dose levels (Preece, 1997).

In addition to the total amount of radiation received, the way the radiation is received also may influence the amount of damage that occurs. Radiation can be delivered acutely, that is, in a relatively short period of time, such as during a dental radiographic examination, which typically requires less than 1 second for an intraoral radiograph. There can also be chronic radiation, where the dose is delivered over long periods of time; background radiation is the best example of this type of chronic radiation exposure. Humans are exposed on a continual basis to background radiation, including cosmic radiation from outer space and a variety of naturally occurring radioactive materials in the soil, building materials, food, and air. The average background radiation dose in the United States is ~3.1 mSv/year or ~0.008 mSv/day (8 μSv/day; National Council on Radiation Protection and Measurements [NCRP], 2009). Radiation risks from diagnostic imaging sometimes have been compared to equivalent days of background radiation, but this can be problematic due to the acute nature of diagnostic radiation exposure versus the chronic nature of background exposure. Acute exposure can overwhelm the DNA repair mechanism, leading to a higher risk of unrepaired damage than may arise from the same amount of radiation given in a low dose rate manner, as in background radiation.

The type of tissue exposed also contributes to the amount of damage occurring from a specific radiation dose. With respect to deterministic effects, the most sensitive cells are those that divide rapidly, have the longest dividing future, and are the most undifferentiated (least specialized) due to the primary effect of the radiation being on the DNA. Because of their rapidly dividing cells and long life expectancy, children are considered to have a three to five times higher risk than adults for the same radiation dose (International Commission on Radiological Protection, 1991).

With respect to radiation carcinogenesis, various tissues are more susceptible than others: colon, stomach, lung, bone marrow, and the female breast are considered highly susceptible to radiation-induced cancer; bone surface, brain, salivary glands, and skin are considered to be of low susceptibility. Other tissues are of intermediate susceptibility (White & Pharoah, 2009).

RADIATION DOSE MEASUREMENT

To determine radiation risks, information on radiation doses is needed. At first, that would seem to be a relatively simple task: place some type of a meter in the X-ray beam during exposure. This is a straightforward procedure for standard dental imaging, such as intraoral bitewing or lateral cephalometric radiographs. In both of these situations, there is a single exposure of the film or image receptor. However, the amount of radiation recorded on the meter does not account for the size of the X-ray beam or the type of tissue exposed, just the amount hitting the surface of the tissue. In addition, there is a slight difference between the amount of exposure and the amount actually absorbed by the tissues, although this frequently is ignored and the total amount of exposure is assumed to be absorbed.

Measuring the radiation exposure is more problematic when the X-ray beam is moving around the patient's head over a period of several seconds, as occurs in standard dental panoramic radiography or CBCT. This is because the tissues receive variable amounts of radiation depending on their location, with no tissue receiving the entire exposure.

For these complex types of imaging examinations, radiation doses for various tissues typically are measured with a special phantom equipped with thermoluminescent dosimeters (TLDs). These devices, which are made of radiation-sensitive chemicals in the form of small chips or strips of material, absorb radiation energy and undergo a change in electron structure in the process. Later they are heated and give up the stored energy in the form of light, which can be measured and used to calculate the dose. Thus, the *absorbed dose* to various tissues and organs can be measured, even with a moving X-ray beam. The *equivalent dose* is obtained by weighting the absorbed dose by a factor related to the type of radiation used, thus allowing for mixed radiation exposure. The weighting factor for X-rays is 1. The unit for equivalent dose is Sievert (Sv), with smaller doses being designated in milliSievert (mSv, 10^{-3}Sv) or microSievert (μSv, 10^{-6}Sv).

While the equivalent dose is useful if someone wants to know the dose to a specific tissue (e.g., the brain), it can be confusing to have a long list of individual tissue/organ doses to deal with. The *effective dose* combines all the equivalent doses into one single term, by weighting the equivalent dose to specific tissues with a factor accounting for the radiosensitivity of the tissue and then summing the weighted doses. In a simplistic way, the effective dose can be considered almost a weighted average of the radiation dose over the entire body.

The International Commission on Radiological Protection (ICRP) has determined the weightings of the various tissues and decided which tissues should be included in the calculation of the effective dose. While the ICRP is an advisory body whose opinions do not have force of law, the scientific community nevertheless has accepted their recommendations; the effective doses for CBCT reported later in this chapter are based on the 2007 ICRP report (International Commission on Radiological Protection, 2008). Their earlier report (International Commission on Radiological Protection, 1991) was used for many years and many dose studies were published using their weighting factors. In their 2007 recommendations, which are in current use, some of the tissue weights were changed, but the biggest change affecting effective dose calculations for dental imaging arose from the reconfiguration of what is called "the remainder." This is a collection of all tissues that do not have individual weights assigned. Also significant in the 2007 changes was the addition of the salivary glands as a weighted tissue. Since the salivary glands are in the direct X-ray beam during dental radiography, including CBCT, the effect of this change was to increase the effective dose for all dental radiographic examinations (Ludlow & Ivanovic, 2008). Thus, in comparing radiation doses from a variety of imaging techniques, such as bitewings and CBCT, it is important to know which ICRP weighting scheme was used in the calculations, 1990 or 2007, and to make sure that the data being compared use the same approaches.

DOSES FOR VARIOUS CBCT MACHINES

CBCT units produce a range of sizes of field of view (FOV) from volumes as small as 4 cm × 4 cm to ones that provide complete visualization of the head and neck area (see also Chapters 1 and 2). Although there is no standard classification scheme for FOV size, it is useful to categorize fields into four ranges: large (>15 cm), medium (10–15 cm), small (8–10 cm), and dentoalveolar (4–6 cm). While some CBCT units provide a single-size FOV, others permit a variety of fields and some allow adjustable vertical collimation of the field (see Chapter 2). When other acquisition variables are held constant, reduction of the FOV results in a reduction of dose. However, there are a number of acquisition variables that, when adjusted in different combinations, can contribute to a large range in resulting dose. Table 3.1 illustrates reported ranges of effective dose from CBCT scans grouped according to FOV. Table 3.2 provides effective doses measured on a sample of CBCT units with medium and large FOVs, which most commonly are used in orthodontic diagnosis.

Table 3.1 Range of doses by field of view size for selected CBCT units.

Field of view	Effective dose 2007 ICRP calculation
Large (>15 cm)	68–1073 μSv
Medium (10 to 15 cm)	69–560 μSv
Small (8 to 10 cm)	189–652 μSv

Factors affecting dose: technical factors

mAs, pulsed and continuous exposure, number of basis images

X-ray dose is of interest in the context of how much exposure is required to provide needed image quality for the diagnostic task and to what potential risk the patient may be subjected from the dose associated with that exposure. Examining the effect

Table 3.2 Examination doses for a sample of large and medium CBCT units.

Technique	Effective dose in μSv—ICRP 2007 Calculation	Reference
Large FOV		
NewTom3G, large FOV	68	Davies-Ludlow & Ludlow, 2009
CB Mercuray, "facial" FOV (maximum quality)	1073	Ludlow *et al.*, 2008
CB Mercuray, "facial" FOV (standard quality)	569	Ludlow *et al.*, 2008
i-CAT classic extended field	70	Ludlow *et al.*, 2008
Next Generation i-CAT portrait mode	74	Ludlow *et al.*, 2008
Iluma (standard)	98	Ludlow *et al.*, 2008
Iluma (ultra)	498	Ludlow *et al.*, 2008
Kodak 9500, large field, medium adult	163	Ludlow, 2011a
SCANORA 3D dual scan	125	Ludlow, 2009b
Promax Mid, stiched scan, medium adult	345	J.B. Ludlow, unpublished data
Medium FOV		
CB Mercuray, "panoramic" FOV	560	Ludlow *et al.*, 2008
Classic i-CAT, standard scan	69	Ludlow *et al.*, 2008
Next Generation i-CAT landscape mode	87	Ludlow *et al.*, 2008
Galileos (default exposure)	70	Ludlow, 2011b
Galileos (maximum exposure)	128	Ludlow, 2011b
SCANORA 3D, large FOV	76	Ludlow, 2009b
Newtom VG	109	Davies-Ludlow & Ludlow, 2009
CS 9500, medium field, medium adult	98	Ludlow, 2011a
CS 9300, 17 × 13.5 cm medium adult, standard quality	198	J.B. Ludlow, unpublished data
NewTom VGi, 15 cm, standard resolution	99	Ludlow, 2012b

of radiographic parameters on dose, a number of relationships stand out. The most important of these are the traditional measures of radiographic exposure: time (s) and tube current (mA). The product of these factors (mAs) is a good starting point for estimating dose differences between otherwise comparable examinations. mAs is not always self-evident when looking at a list of operating specifications for a CBCT unit. Scanning time, for example, is the time from first to last exposure, but is not necessarily the exposure time. Flat panels and the complementary metal oxide semiconductor (CMOS) and charge-coupled devices (CCDs) used in image intensifier receptors do not acquire information during short phases of the imaging cycle when the charge in the receptor is integrated and sent to the frame grabber for storage. Because of this, some manufacturers pulse X-ray output, turning the beam off during the integration/data transmission phase of image acquisition. If the X-ray source is left on during this period when no new data can be acquired, the exposure is wasted and contributes unnecessarily to patient dose. The difference between pulsed exposure and scanning times can be large. For instance, the NewTom 3G (QR srl, Verona, Italy) has a 36-second scan time, but a typical large FOV (20 cm) adult exposure is only 5.4 seconds (Ludlow & Ivanovic, 2008). The almost sevenfold difference between scan and exposure times also represents a sevenfold difference in dose. Even with short scan times, pulsing is an effective method of reducing dose. The CS 9300 (Carestream Dental, Rochester, NY) fast scan mode has a 12-second scan time, but produces only 6.4 seconds of exposure. When pulsing of the X-ray source is utilized, the time of exposure of a single projection typically is constant. In this case, tube current is modulated to adjust for differences in patient size.

CBCT image volumes are produced from computer reconstruction of data from a series of two-dimensional (2D) images, called basis images, acquired as the X-ray beam revolves around the patient's head. The number of basis images acquired for an image volume are established by the manufacturer. In some units, standard quality and "high quality" image options are available. Typically, high quality is reflected as a 60–100% increase in the number of basis images rather than a change in pixel size, mA, or exposure time for an individual projection. In this situation, there is a direct correspondence in the percentage change in number of basis images, mAs, and patient dose. Figure 3.1 illustrates this linear relationship of mAs and dose.

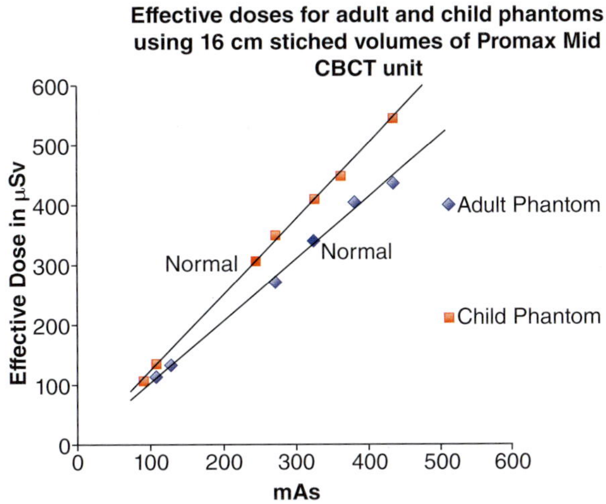

Figure 3.1 Relationship of mAs to patient dose over range of available settings for 16 cm stitched FOV of Promax Mid CBCT unit.

Volume size

The second most important determinant of patient dose is volume of the tissue that is irradiated directly. Size of FOV is proportional to dose when other factors are held constant. However, it should be noted that other factors, such as pixel size or number of basis images, may be altered automatically when FOV is reduced. Reduction in pixel size for many small FOV scanners is the principal reason for the higher range of doses for devices providing these fields (Table 3.1).

Pixel size

Pixel size of the detector has a direct influence on dose when manufacturers increase exposure to achieve an equivalent signal-to-noise ratio as pixel size is decreased. Because pixels in CBCT images are square, pixel dimensions commonly are reported with a single measurement value. The

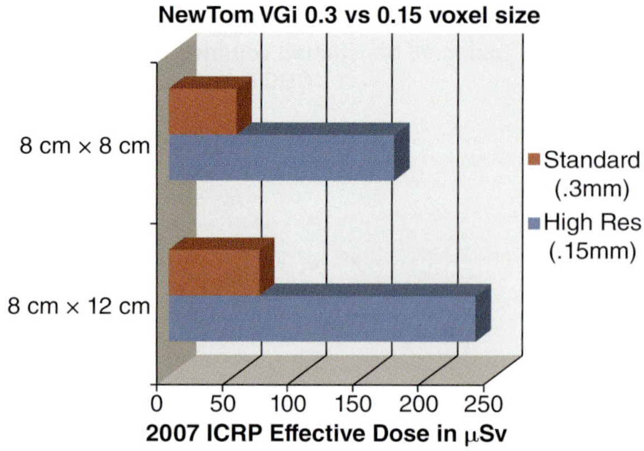

Figure 3.2 Relationship of pixel size and dose for a constant volume size.

Table 3.3 Example of dose reduction using vertical collimation of beam for a unilateral TMJ examination using the Orthophos XG 3D.

Region	Setting	Small adult effective dose	Change from standard centered view (%)
Central	Full 8 cm × 8 cm	64 μSv	0
TMJ	Full 8 cm × 8 cm	56 μSv	13
	Collimated 8 cm × 6 cm	20 μSv	69

third dimension of a pixel (voxel) also has the same measure as the other dimensions and is termed *isotropic*. Figure 3.2 provides an example of the relationship of pixel size to dose. The NewTom VGi (QR srl) demonstrates a 70% reduction in dose when using standard resolution (0.3 mm voxel) rather than high resolution (0.15 mm voxel).

Reduction in pixel size in image acquisition may occur in conjunction with reduction in the size of FOV. For some units, this is automatic or reflected in the default settings for the scanner. Coupling of pixel size to field size is universal for scanners using image-intensifier technology. Image intensifiers take a desired field size and focus this on a CCD or CMOS detector of fixed dimensions. The effective image pixel size is a function of the ratio of X-ray field and the detector area; larger fields result in larger pixels and reduced resolution for the same receptor matrix. For instance, a 20 cm FOV with a 0.4 mm voxel size acquired with the NewTom 3G using an adult ATOM phantom resulted in a 36 μSv effective dose. Effective dose for the same phantom scanned with a 15 cm FOV and 0.3 mm voxels was 70 μSv (J.B. Ludlow, unpublished data). A caveat to the general rule of resolution increasing with field reduction is the use of field collimation in some CBCT units. In this case, both the X-ray field and the image matrix are reduced while maintaining resolution. The potential effect of collimation is illustrated by its use for a unilateral temporomandibular joint (TMJ) examination with the Orthophos XG 3D where a 25% reduction in the vertical dimension of the scan results in a 64% reduction in effective dose (Table 3.3).

CBCT scanners using flat panel detectors are unable to increase or reduce the size of the FOV optically in the way that image intensifier systems can. In some units, field size is increased by acquiring scan projections that use an eccentric center of rotation. With this approach, the first half of the scan covers the anterior aspect of the patient and the second half of the scan covers the posterior aspect. This technique works because only 180° of data are required for computer algorithms to reconstruct a volume completely. No change in pixel size occurs when the FOV is increased in this way. FOV also can be reduced using beam collimation. When a reduced area of the flat panel is used, resolution does not change unless the detector is capable of unbinning pixels. Flat panel matrices often are operated by combining (binning) adjacent groups of pixels. For instance, an image matrix of 512 × 512 0.4 mm pixels might be reconstructed from a physical panel matrix of 1024 × 1024 0.2 mm pixels. The technical advantages of binning include a higher signal-to-noise ratio from averaging over four pixels and less computational time due to dealing with a dataset that is one quarter of the alternate size. Of course, an added benefit is that less exposure is required for acceptable image quality. If higher resolution is desired, pixels can be unbinned prior to image reconstruction. This must be planned prior to imaging of the patient because greater exposure will be needed to achieve an adequate signal-to-noise ratio in the individual pixels.

Sometimes manufacturers will couple pixel size changes with smaller FOV automatically. A clinical rationale for this approach is that practitioners using smaller fields typically look for diagnostic signs that benefit from increased resolution. Endodontic detection of narrow canals and nondisplaced root fracture are examples of tasks that may benefit from greater resolution and require relatively small FOV. On the other hand, tasks such as planning for single implant placement or assessment of the position of an impacted tooth may not require the increase in resolution or elevated dose that accompanies this increase.

Mean kV, beam filtration

Increases in peak tube voltage (kVp) and beam filtration have the potential to reduce dose by reducing the number of low energy photons in the X-ray beam. Low energy photons that have high probability of being absorbed in the patient contribute little diagnostic information while adding to patient dose, regardless of the absorption characteristics of the tissue. As an example, adjustments made by increasing beam filtration with 0.4 mm of copper and increasing kVp by 10–16 kV were shown to reduce dose by an average of 44% for both large and medium FOV and all adult default settings for the CS 9500 (Ludlow, 2011a). Similar reductions in dose have been demonstrated when filtration has been added to other CBCT units (Qu *et al.*, 2010). Because it also requires change in the reconstruction algorithm, the manufacturer rather than the end user must make a change in the amount of filtration offered with the unit (Ludlow, 2011a).

Receptor technology

The shape of the FOV related to detector technology influences dose to peripheral tissues. Image intensifiers utilize a vacuum tube with a circular face. Circular images acquired with this device are reconstructed into a sphere (Figure 3.3). Flat panels acquire rectangular images, which are reconstructed into a cylinder. A sphere tends to increase brain and thyroid exposures in large FOVs, while

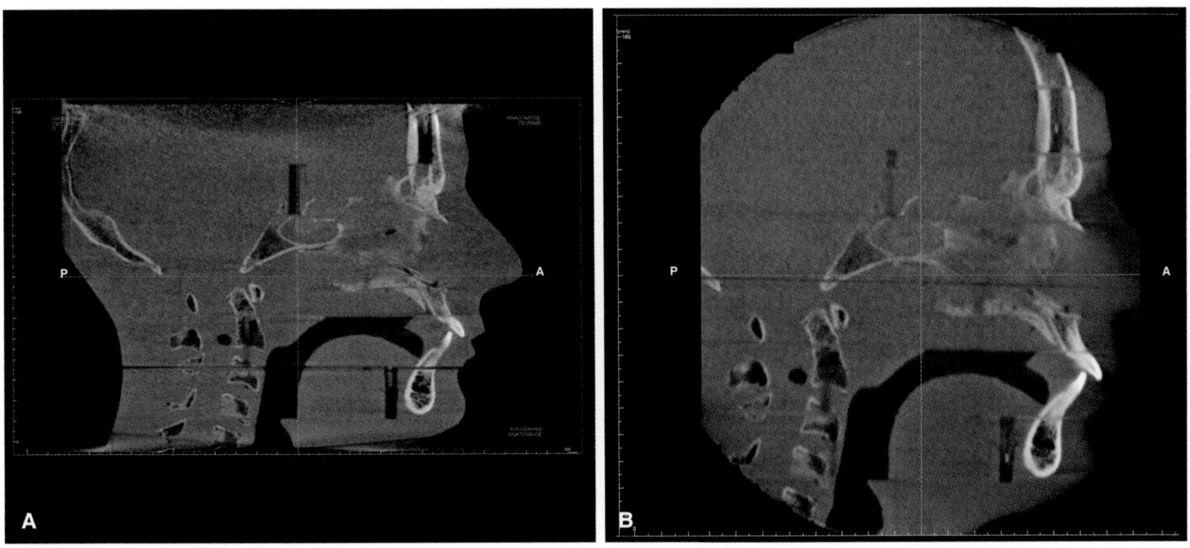

Figure 3.3 Comparison of differences in FOV shape. *A*: Flat panels acquire rectangular fields, which are assembled into cylindrical volumes. *B*: Image intensifiers acquire round fields, which are assembled into spherical volumes. Images of midsagittal sections of comparable fields from a cylinder (*A*; iCAT portrait view) and a sphere (*B*; NewTom 3G large field). Note the additional areas of brain and thyroid that are exposed in the spherical acquisition.

a carefully collimated cylinder can image the anatomy between the condyles and chin with a reduced vertical beam height.

Phosphor coating

Sodium iodide is the most commonly used phosphor coating for both image intensifier and flat-panel technologies. Some manufacturers have used alternate coatings, such as gadolinium oxybromide. Selection of the type and thickness of a phosphor coating is important for both detector efficiency and image quality. Thicker coatings of material are more efficient absorbers of X-rays; however, greater diffusion of photons with increasing coating thickness results in loss of spatial resolution. Research into more efficient phosphor materials is ongoing; this is a potential area for increased image quality and reduced dose in the future (see Chapter 5).

Patient-related factors

Volume location

The location of the FOV also has a significant impact on dose. Although the location effect is most apparent with smaller FOVs, even large FOVs may produce differing patient risks depending on how peripheral tissues and organs (e.g., the thyroid and pituitary glands) are positioned with respect to direct exposure from the X-ray beam. Lower positioning of the FOV may result in direct exposure of the thyroid gland. Because the thyroid gland has a weighting factor of 0.04 (International Commission on Radiological Protection, 2008), it makes a significant contribution to the total effective dose calculation, and even a small amount of direct exposure can cause a significant increase in effective dose. Susceptibility of measurement of thyroid dose to even subtle differences in patient positioning has been shown, where a rotation of even 10° in a RANDO (radiation analog dosimetry system; Nuclear Associates, Hicksville, NY) phantom position can result in a 92% difference in thyroid dose for a large FOV scan (Ludlow, 2009a). Differences of 29% in total effective dose from the same CBCT protocol have been attributed to small changes in phantom positioning (Ludlow, 2012a). For most diagnostic tasks, the thyroid gland is below the anatomical region of interest and can be placed beyond the field of direct exposure with careful patient positioning. This is more challenging for pediatric patients, in whom the thyroid anatomy is closer to the lower border of the mandible, than for adult patients. Thyroid shields and careful positioning strategies may reduce patient dose, but must be applied in such a way as to not reduce image quality of regions of diagnostic importance.

Given a choice, dentists prefer images with technical factors that provide high signal-to-noise ratios and high resolution. Dentists requesting images from an imaging center or providing examinations in their own offices may not understand the risk implications of using higher doses to obtain image volumes. While it is clear that quantitative and qualitative differences in image quality can be related to dose, little data exist documenting the diagnostic importance of these differences. Image quality thresholds in terms of resolution and signal-to-noise ratios need to be established for many diagnostic tasks. Until that research is available, the clinician must be guided by clinical judgment. The principle of "as low as reasonably achievable" (ALARA) always should be part of that judgment.

If "pretty pictures" are being obtained when what really is needed is an image of diagnostic quality, we are doing the patient a disservice. Further complicating this picture, general dentists referring patients to imaging centers may not communicate clearly the diagnostic reason for the scan, or the radiographic technician lacking the training of a registered radiologic technologist may not be aware of the differences in image quality/resolution that are required for such varied tasks as investigating possible vertical root fracture versus orthodontic diagnosis.

RISK ESTIMATES FOR CBCT

Given the radiation dose for diagnostic imaging expressed in terms of effective dose, it should be a straightforward process to develop risk estimates that can be shared with patients. However, there is no uniform agreement on the best way to do this. Methods that commonly have been used include:

(1) Expressing the risks in terms of predicted number of cancers that could occur as a result of the exposure
(2) Comparing the risk of the X-ray exposure to that from a certain number of days of background radiation with the same overall risk
(3) Comparing risks from radiation exposure to other risks with which the patient may be familiar
(4) Categorizing risks into levels of zero, minimal, low, medium, and high risk, based on radiation dose, as recommended by the American College of Radiology (ACR; http://www.acr.org/~/media/ACR/Documents/AppCriteria/RRLInformation.pdf).

Each of these methods has advantages and disadvantages; the selection of one over another may be a personal choice. However, in all except the last method listed above, the issue of acute exposure present during diagnostic imaging versus chronic exposure, such as in background radiation, is not resolved—and frequently is ignored in the calculations.

Another problem with risk estimation from radiation exposure is that most of the methods are suited only for population risks, not individual risks, and most of the scientific bodies recommend against using some of the methods to predict a risk for an individual patient from a specific exposure. However, they do not offer useful alternatives, other than the categorization model from the ACR.

Even though the excess cancer risk estimation is not considered by many to be an appropriate way of estimating risks for individuals, it still is used frequently and will be presented here.

It has been estimated (International Commission on Radiological Protection, 2008) that the overall detriment-adjusted risk factor for the population as a whole is $5.7 \times 10^{-2} Sv^{-1}$, with $5.5 \times 10^{-2} Sv^{-1}$ of that from cancer and $0.2 \times 10^{-2} Sv^{-1}$ from heritable effects. This implies that for every Sievert of radiation exposure, 0.055 cancers would be expected. Obviously, since fractional cancers cannot occur, this way of risk estimation is not suitable for use with individuals. This risk estimate should be multiplied by a factor of three for children under age 10 and by two for children ages 10 to 20 (International Commission on Radiological Protection, 1991). When these figures are coupled with doses for varying imaging techniques, it should be simple to calculate a cancer risk for any dental imaging examination. The probability of fatal cancers per million examinations ranges from 0.1 (single periapical or bitewing radiograph with digital imaging and rectangular collimation) to 21 (full-mouth intraoral survey [FMX] with D-speed film and round collimation, a common but not recommended technique). Cancer risks for CBCT are in the range of 1 to 59×10^{-6}, depending on technique, with most at the lower end. For example, a machine with an effective dose of 70 μSv has a cancer risk of approximately 4×10^{-6} (four per million examinations).

While these calculations can be performed, are they helpful in explaining risks to patients? Do clinicians and patients have an intuitive feel for what a risk of 4×10^{-6} really means? For most people, the answer probably is no.

Another common way of expressing radiation risk is in terms of days of background radiation. Using the calculated effective dose and the average annual background exposure of 3.1 mSv (3100 μSv), the number of background days with the equivalent risk of the radiation exposure can be computed. With the doses provided in Table 3.2, the number of background days' equivalence ranges from 8 to 126 days for large FOV machines, with most being at the lower end of this range. This can be compared to the background equivalent of 1 day for a single digital bitewing radiograph, 2 days for a digital panoramic, and 14 hours for a digital cephalometric radiograph.

This may be the easiest way for patients to understand radiation risks, but there still is the unresolved issue of acute versus chronic exposure. It also can be observed that a full FOV CBCT generally produces a higher risk than a conventional panoramic and cephalometric radiograph for orthodontic diagnosis.

What about comparing radiation risks to other common risks, such as smoking, driving, and flying across the country? One-in-a-million risks of dying have been calculated as smoking 1.4 cigarettes (cardiovascular disease, cancer), driving 300

Table 3.4 Relative radiation level for diagnostic imaging.

	Effective dose estimated range (mSv)	
	Adult	Child
None	0	0
Minimal	<0.1	<0.03
Low	0.1–1.0	0.03–0.3
Medium	1.0–10.0	0.3–3.0

Source: American College of Radiology (ACR). Appropriateness Criteria, 2011 (http://www.acr.org/~/media/ACR/Documents/AppCriteria/RRLInformation.pdf).

miles (fatal accident), or flying 6000 miles (cosmic radiation; Cohen, 1991). Thus, a typical CBCT could have the equivalent risk of dying as a few cross-country airplane trips. This approach has been criticized in that it is easier for people to appreciate the benefits of these activities and to diminish the perceived risks (e.g., "I am a good driver and have never had an accident") than for radiation, which frequently is misunderstood and feared.

Another way to describe risks from radiation exposure is to divide them into several basic categories, each with a corresponding dose range for adults and children. This approach has been used by the ACR to derive relative radiation levels (Table 3.4).

Imaging techniques with no risk are those that do not use ionizing radiation, namely, magnetic resonance imaging (MRI) and ultrasonography. Imaging examinations classified with minimal risk have effective doses of <0.1 mSv (100 μSv) for adults and 0.03 mSv (30 μSv) for children. The low-risk category includes a dose range of 0.1–1.0 mSv (100–1000 μSv) for adults and 0.03–0.3 (30–300 μSv) for children. Using the data on CBCT doses in Table 3.2, most of the large FOV scans fall into the minimal-to-low-risk category for adults, but in the low-to-medium-risk category for children. The combined use of panoramic and cephalometric radiographs places risk in the minimal category.

Although a problem with using this system is that each person must decide what a minimal, low, or medium risk is and how it compares with other risks of everyday life that he or she is willing to accept, it does provide a framework that may be helpful to clinicians in discussing radiation issues with their patients.

REDUCING RADIATION RISK WITH CBCT

The most important dose-limiting factor for radiographic examinations is appropriate selection of patients for CBCT imaging (see also Chapters 1 and 6). If the examination is not beneficial (i.e., it does not affect the diagnosis, treatment, and/or management of the patient), the radiation risk can be considered too high. As CBCT is a relatively new and rapidly evolving technology, there is little evidence-based information on the appropriate or best use of CBCT imaging for many, if not most, diagnostic tasks. Selection criteria have been developed by a panel of experts for endodontic imaging (American Association of Endodontics & American Academy of Oral and Maxillofacial Radiology, 2011) and implant imaging (Tyndall *et al.*, 2012)). The American Dental Association (2012a, 2012b) also has updated its imaging recommendations and developed guidelines on CBCT uses in general. These guides will be helpful in directing use of CBCT technology while emphasizing the ALARA principle, which applies to all radiographic imaging.

Once a decision is made that a CBCT scan will be beneficial for a specific patient, the clinician then should select the imaging parameters that will provide the needed diagnostic information for the lowest possible dose compatible with the imaging task (see also Chapters 1, 6, and 8). One important aspect of this selection process is choosing the right imaging volume, something that is easy to ignore with the idea that more information is better. For example, if the diagnostic task is determining the exact position of an impacted canine so that the best outcome of treatment can occur, is it necessary to expose the entire head? If a full FOV is deemed necessary for orthodontic treatment planning, can the image height be limited, particularly in small children, to avoid exposing the entire skull and brain?

The principles espoused by the Alliance for Radiation Safety in Pediatric Imaging in their Image Gently campaign noted below have particular relevance for orthodontics and should be integrated into CBCT imaging of orthodontic patients:

CT helps us save kids' lives! This may be more applicable to medical CT used to explore serious conditions, but it also could be relevant to orthodontics.

(1) But, when you image, radiation matters!
(2) Children are more sensitive to radiation.
 (a) What *we* do now lasts for *their* lifetime.
 (b) So, when you image, image gently.
(3) More usually is *not* better. When CT is the right thing to do:
 (a) Child-size the kV and mA.
 (b) One scan is usually enough.
 (c) Scan only the indicated area.

CONCLUSIONS

CBCT technology provides significant advantages in orthodontics and its appropriate use should be welcomed. However, it also entails risks, particularly for children, that must be considered and minimized whenever possible. Careful selection of cases for imaging and careful selection of imaging parameters will allow both clinicians and patients to benefit from the technology.

References

American Association of Endodontics & American Academy of Oral and Maxillofacial Radiology (2011) Use of cone-beam computed tomography in endodontics: joint position statement of the American Association of Endodontics and the American Academy of Oral and Maxillofacial Radiology. *Oral Surgery, Oral Medicine, Oral Pathology, Oral Radiology, and Endodontics*, 111 (2), 234–237.

American Dental Association, Council on Scientific Affairs (2012a) The use of cone-beam computed tomography in dentistry: an advisory statement from the American Dental Association Council on Scientific Affairs. *Journal of the American Dental Association*, 143 (8), 899–902.

American Dental Association, Council on Scientific Affairs (2012b) Dental Radiographic Examinations: Recommendations for Patient Selection and Limiting Radiation Exposures. Available at http://www.ada.org/sections/professionalResources/pdfs/Dental_Radographic_Examiations_2012.pdf.

Claus, E.B., Calvocoressi, L., Bondy, M.L., *et al.* (2012) Dental X-rays and risk of meningioma. *Cancer*, 118 (18), 4530–4537.

Cohen, B.L. (1991) Catalogue of risks extended and updated. *Health Physics*, 61 (3), 317–335.

Davies-Ludlow, L. & Ludlow, J. (2009) Dosimetry comparison of the NewTom 3G and the NewTom VG. *Journal of Dental Research*, 88 (Spec Iss A). Abstract #1955. Available at http://iadr.confex.com/iadr/2009miami/webprogram/Paper116961.html.

Goske, M.J., Applegate, K.E., Boylan, J., *et al.* (2008) The "Image Gently" Campaign: increasing CT radiation dose awareness through a national education and awareness program. *Pediatric Radiology*, 38 (3), 265–269.

International Commission on Radiological Protection (1991) 1990 recommendations. ICRP publication 60. *Annals of ICRP*, 21, 1–201.

International Commission on Radiological Protection (2008) 2007 recommendations. ICRP publication 103. *Annals of ICRP*, 37, 1–332.

Ludlow, J.B. (2009a) Dose and risk in dental diagnostic imaging with emphasis on dosimetry of CBCT. *Korean Journal of Oral and Maxillofacial Radiology*, 39 (4), 175–184.

Ludlow, J.B. (2009b) Dosimetry of small FOV tomography using OP 200 VT & Scanora 3D. 60th annual session of the American Academy of Oral and Maxillofacial Radiology (AAOMR), Louisville, KY, October 22.

Ludlow, J.B. (2011a) A manufacturer's role in reducing the dose of CBCT examinations: effect of beam filtration. *Dentomaxillofacial Radiology*, 40, 115–122.

Ludlow, J.B. (2011b) Dose reduction from maxillary/mandibular collimation using Galileo's comfort and compact CBCT. 61st annual session of the American Academy of Oral and Maxillofacial Radiology (AAOMR), Chicago, IL.

Ludlow, J.B. (2012a) Comment on "Effective dose range for dental cone beam computed tomography scanners." *European Journal of Radiology*. 81 (12), 4219–4220.

Ludlow, J.B. (2012b) Effective doses of NewTom VGi variable volume dental CBCT unit. Annual meeting of the American Association of Dental Research (AADR), Tampa, FL, March 21–24.

Ludlow, J.B. & Ivanovic, M. (2008) Comparative dosimetry of dental CBCT devices and 64 row CT for oral and maxillofacial radiology. *Oral Surgery, Oral Medicine, Oral Pathology, Oral Radiology, and Endodontics*, 106 (1), 930–938.

Ludlow, J.B., Davies-Ludlow, L.E., & White, S.C. (2008) Patient risk to common dental radiographic examinations: the impact of 2007 ICRP recommendations regarding dose calculation. *Journal of the American Dental Association*, 139 (9), 1237–1243.

National Council on Radiation Protection and Measurements (NCRP) (2009) Ionizing Radiation Exposure of the Population of the United States. Report No. 160. Bethesda, MD.

National Research Council (2006) *Health Risks from Exposure to Low Levels of Ionizing Radiation. BEIR VII Phase 2*. National Academies Press, Washington, DC.

Preece, J.W. (1997) Isn't it about time we changed our perception of diagnostic risks? *Oral Surgery, Oral Medicine, Oral Pathology, Oral Radiology, and Endodontics*, 84 (4), 329.

Preston-Martin, S. & White, S.C. (1990) Brain and salivary gland tumors related to prior dental radiography: implications for current practice. *Journal of the American Dental Association*, 120 (2), 151–158.

Qu, X.M., Li, G., Ludlow, J.B., *et al.* (2010) Effective radiation dose of ProMax 3D CBCT scanner with different dental protocols. *Oral Surgery, Oral Medicine, Oral Pathology, Oral Radiology, and Endodontics*, 110 (6), 770–776.

Tyndall, D.A., Price, J.B., Tetradis, S., *et al.* (2012) Position statement of the American Academy of Oral and Maxillofacial Radiology on selection criteria for the use of radiology in dental implantology with emphasis on cone beam computed tomography. *Oral Surgery, Oral Medicine, Oral Pathology, Oral Radiology*, 113, 817–826.

White, S.C. & Pharoah, M.J. (2009) *Oral Radiology Principles and Interpretation*. 6th ed. Mosby-Elsevier, St. Louis, MO.

4 Rational Basis for Transitioning from 2D to 3D Radiographic Imaging in Orthodontic Practice and Research

Birte Melsen, DDS, Certified Specialist in Orthodontics, Dr. Ordont., and Michel Dalstra, MSc, PhD

INTRODUCTION

The orthodontic profession has been successful in merging the dental, technical, and medical worlds. Publications in dental journals initially transferred one clinician's experiences about treatment technologies to his or her colleagues. The "fathers of orthodontics" further developed the profession by sharing their experiences and descriptions of techniques without applying any basic rules of research.

Although clinicians initially attempted to raise the level of treatment through clinical trials, a research- or evidence-based approach to clinical practice did not exist yet. Indeed, of the approximately 50,000 papers with the keywords *orthodontic* or *orthodontics* published between 1912 and 2012, fewer than 6,000 were retrieved when the search was limited to clinical trials, randomized clinical trials, or animal experiments. The majority of the remaining manuscripts were written by orthodontists who were reporting their experiences or describing new clinical methods.

Following the introduction of the cephalostat in the United States by Broadbent (1931) and in Europe by Hofrath (1931), cephalometric studies dominated the literature. Almost 6,000 studies reported results from clinical trials, prospective or retrospective, and rarely randomized controlled studies, all based on cephalometric analyses. However, the two-dimensional (2D) measurements on which this research was based had inherent errors related to the 2D imaging of three-dimensional (3D) structures, as well as the projection of bilateral structures with different magnification onto one image. Thus the larger the distance from the anode to the film compared with that of the object to the film, the smaller the error. Due to the need to minimize irradiation and the footprint of the unit, however, the anode to film distances have been reduced from 240 cm to 190 cm to as low as 150 cm for most of the cephalostats used in the orthodontist's offices today, while maintaining the object-to-film constant at 10 cm with each of these configurations. Thereby

Cone Beam Computed Tomography in Orthodontics: Indications, Insights, and Innovations, First Edition. Sunil D. Kapila.

both types of flaws related to the images were increased.

The panoramic radiograph was the second contributor as a source of information on which the orthodontic problem list was developed and soon became a standard component of the diagnostic material. However, panoramic images also have caveats such as distortions and differences in magnification of the two sides resulting from the dissimilarities in object-film distance caused by asymmetry or asymmetrical positioning of the patient (Schulze *et al.*, 2000).

After cephalograms were introduced into practice, a variety of analyses were developed in which measurements typically were performed on midsagittal structures and generally were limited to angles or proportions in order to minimize the influence of the inherent bias (Athanasiou, 1995). Norms for different populations made it possible to classify patients with malocclusions into different categories according to their skeletal and dentoalveolar presentation or future development. A number of databases were generated and consisted of cephalograms taken of untreated individuals annually or biannually; these recently were made available for public use by the American Association of Orthodontists Foundation (AAOF) Craniofacial Growth Legacy Collection (http://www.cril.org/aaof/aaof_home.asp).

By superimposing on the stable structures, it was possible to perform longitudinal studies illustrating normal and atypical growth patterns. It was, however, not until stable indicators were inserted into the maxilla and the mandible that it was possible to differentiate between displacements of the jaw due to sutural and condylar growth, and modeling of the individual bones and intramaxillary tooth movements. The detailed description of a series of radiographs of untreated individuals with the Bjork indicators deepened the understanding of the factors contributing to the post-natal development of the craniofacial skeleton, specifically in the sagittal plane of space (Bjork & Skieller, 1972). The transverse development was studied on postero-anterior (PA) headfilms (Athanasiou *et al.*, 1992; Kapila *et al.*, 2011), but few standard analyses have been developed specially for these projections. An attempt to obtain 3D information was proposed by combining the occlusal image of the study casts or virtual models with the profile image, but it still was far from the true 3D situation (Bjork & Skieller, 1974, 1977). Frontal and axial exposures were recommended when specific information in these planes of space was required and a reduction of the distortion of the lateral structures could be obtained by a 45° image in which the body of the mandible was positioned parallel to the film (Sakima *et al.*, 2004).

In spite of the questionable validity and the low reproducibility of many of the applied variables, treatment plans traditionally have been developed based on a cephalometric analysis and study casts.

Although there are limitations related to the 2D imaging of 3D structures, several attempts to obtain 3D information by stereometry were made, although the approach never became part of a clinical routine (Baumrind *et al.*, 1983a, 1983b). The need for real 3D images remained an important objective, however, and the use of fan-beam computed tomography (CT) was reported for specific problems such as treatment planning of patients suffering from craniofacial anomalies or particular types of ectopic teeth (Ericson & Kurol, 1987). Both the high doses of radiation and high costs limited the use of this method, but these concerns have been mitigated substantially when cone beam computed tomography (CBCT) was introduced to the dental community (Mozzo *et al.*, 1998). As a result, CBCT is becoming an important component of the orthodontic armamentarium. Its role still is not well defined and there is little consensus regarding the indications for CBCT imaging within the field of orthodontics (Kapila *et al.*, 2011; Halazonetis, 2012; Larson, 2012).

The purpose of this chapter is to present an objective assessment on the utility of CBCT imaging for clinical and research applications in orthodontics. More specifically, we discuss whether (1) CBCT can replace the conventional set of radiographs, (2) CBCT will lead to improvements in treatment relative to that performed with conventional radiography, (3) research based on CBCT will change the treatment approach, and (4) the fusion of CBCT with other 3D visualization modalities can enhance treatment and research.

CAN CBCT REPLACE THE CONVENTIONAL SET OF RADIOGRAPHS?

The dynamic character of the CBCT image allows for the generation of distortion-free images in user-defined planes of space. Additionally, the parameters defined in the midsagittal plane of space from a lateral cephalometric radiograph obviously can be replicated by the CBCT images (Adams *et al.*, 2004). The question then arises whether all parameters derived from 2D cephalometric images can be measured on reconstructions made from CBCT scans (Farman & Scarfe, 2006; Cattaneo *et al.*, 2008). As the CBCT images allow for measurements of true distances and undistorted angles, the answer to the above question definitely is "yes," but the question could be rephrased by replacing the word "can" with "should." In that case, should a new set of cephalometric analyses be developed? Our answer here is "no." To replace all headfilms indiscriminately with CBCT scans would be not only costly but also unethical. It also should be mentioned that anatomy is taught based on the observation of 3D structures and the education in cephalometrics is focused on describing 3D structures in 2D. Keeping the original anatomy intact rather than reducing it to a 2D derivation contributes to a better understanding of the CBCT image as well as that of the true anatomy and relationships of the craniofacial structures.

Although it has been almost universally accepted that orthodontic treatment is based on a plan that is generated following a clinical, a model, and a cephalometric analysis, the value of the latter has been questioned from time to time. Nijkamp and coworkers, (2008) demonstrated that important decisions regarding treatment rarely were influenced by cephalometric parameters. The ability to acquire valid 3D information, therefore, should not lead to the routine use of CBCT, which, as with cephalometric analyses of 2D headfilms, may be superfluous in making treatment decisions. The availability of undistorted 3D measurements should not necessarily call for a repetition of the multiplicity of analyses that describe morphological characteristics of various populations and/or determine the effects of different appliances with similar but true absolute values obtained from the 3D images.

Radiographs should be taken only when the findings are likely to have a decisive impact on the patient's treatment plan (see Chapter 6). In other cases, the clinician should refrain from taking both conventional headfilm and CBCT. In this context, Kapila and colleagues (2011) listed the types of cases that could benefit from CBCT imaging, which include those requiring (1) precise assessment of root morphology and length, (2) detailed information regarding morphology of alveolar bone and interdental relationship, (3) morphometric analysis of craniofacial anomalies, (4) specific analysis of TMJ in health and disease, and (5) assessment of the airways. These recommendations, however, do not justify a routine replacement of headfilms with CBCT in clinical orthodontics today. As Kapila and associates (2011) suggested in concordance with several others (Kau *et al.*, 2006, 2009; Hussain *et al.*, 2008; DeVos *et al.*, 2009), the possibility of obtaining 3D information should lead the orthodontist to define a new set of rules identifying where this type of imaging can benefit the individual patient. These sets of rules are discussed in depth elsewhere in this textbook (Chapters 1 and 6).

WILL CBCT LEAD TO IMPROVEMENT OF TREATMENT?

In relation to an orthodontic treatment, information derived from CBCT could influence the problem list, the treatment plan, and the evaluation of the treatment result. Specifically, CBCT can be valuable in refining or optimizing a problem list in several types of cases, including those requiring (1) information on the alveolar bone and risks of fenestrations that might result from eventual expansion (Figure 4.1; see also Chapter 14), (2) localization of ectopic teeth (Figure 4.2; see also Chapters 8 and 16), (3) determination of the cause of unexplainable symptoms (Figure 4.3), (4) assessment of morphology and position of the condyles in patients with temporomandibular joint disorders (TMJDs) and in the localization of asymmetries (Figure 4.4; see also Chapters 12 and 21),

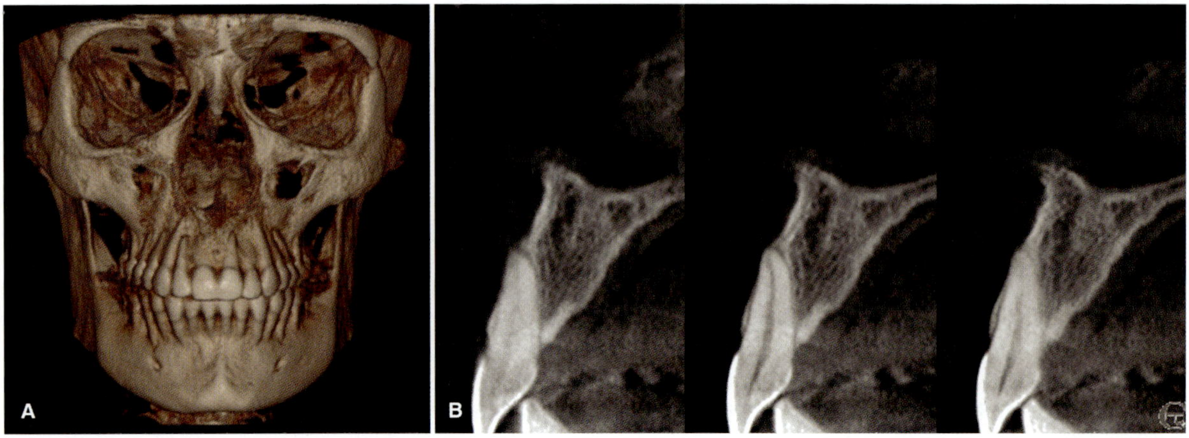

Figure 4.1 *A*: CBCT image illustrating an example of how indiscriminant leveling and expansion has led to tipping of teeth through the buccal bone. *B*: Three sagittal sections of alveolar bone and central incisor before treatment. Note that fenestrations and dehiscences already are present, indicating that further expansion would not be advisable.

(5) description and quantification of anomalies in the craniofacial skeleton in all three planes of space using appropriate 3D coordinates (Figure 4.5; see also Chapter 23), and (6) the assessment of whether a skeletal problem can be camouflaged or needs surgery (Figure 4.6).

With regard to its applications to treatment planning, CBCT will be useful when defining the changes planned in 3D, whether dental, dentoalveolar, or skeletal. For dental movements, once these are defined in 3D, the force system needed can be determined and the biomechanically correct appliance designed as demonstrated for impacted teeth elsewhere in this book (Chapter 16). In cases of surgical interventions, a definition of the displacement of the bony units in 3D likewise can be of considerable help in the treatment planning process (see below and also Chapters 20 and 22).

In relation to quality control or assessing to what degree the chosen treatment approach has achieved the treatment goal, this is possible only if the treatment goal has been proactively defined, which frequently is not the case. CBCT or other 3D imaging technologies are likely to be the method of choice in future clinical studies in which 3D rather than 2D images will provide the required information on whether a pre-specified treatment goal has been achieved.

WILL CBCT-BASED RESEARCH CHANGE THE TREATMENT APPROACH?

Many prospective and numerous retrospective studies using cephalometrics have focused on comparing treatment results obtained from different treatment approaches. Due to ethical reasons including radiation exposure, many of these studies probably are not repeatable with CBCT imaging. However, the magnification and other adjustments necessary for performing valid comparisons between conventional and CBCT-constructed cephalometric images are possible. As the longitudinal radiographic records of the AAOF Legacy Project never will be repeated, the information held in this database regarding normal growth and development will serve as a valuable basis with which the results of CBCT-based trials can be compared.

Although cephalometric studies that assess the effect of various interventions can be repeated with a smaller error of the method, these studies should be performed only where it is expected that the data derived will be substantially more precise than what currently are available and would have a significant impact on clinical practice. On the other hand, it should not be considered *lege artis* to perform new clinical studies based on

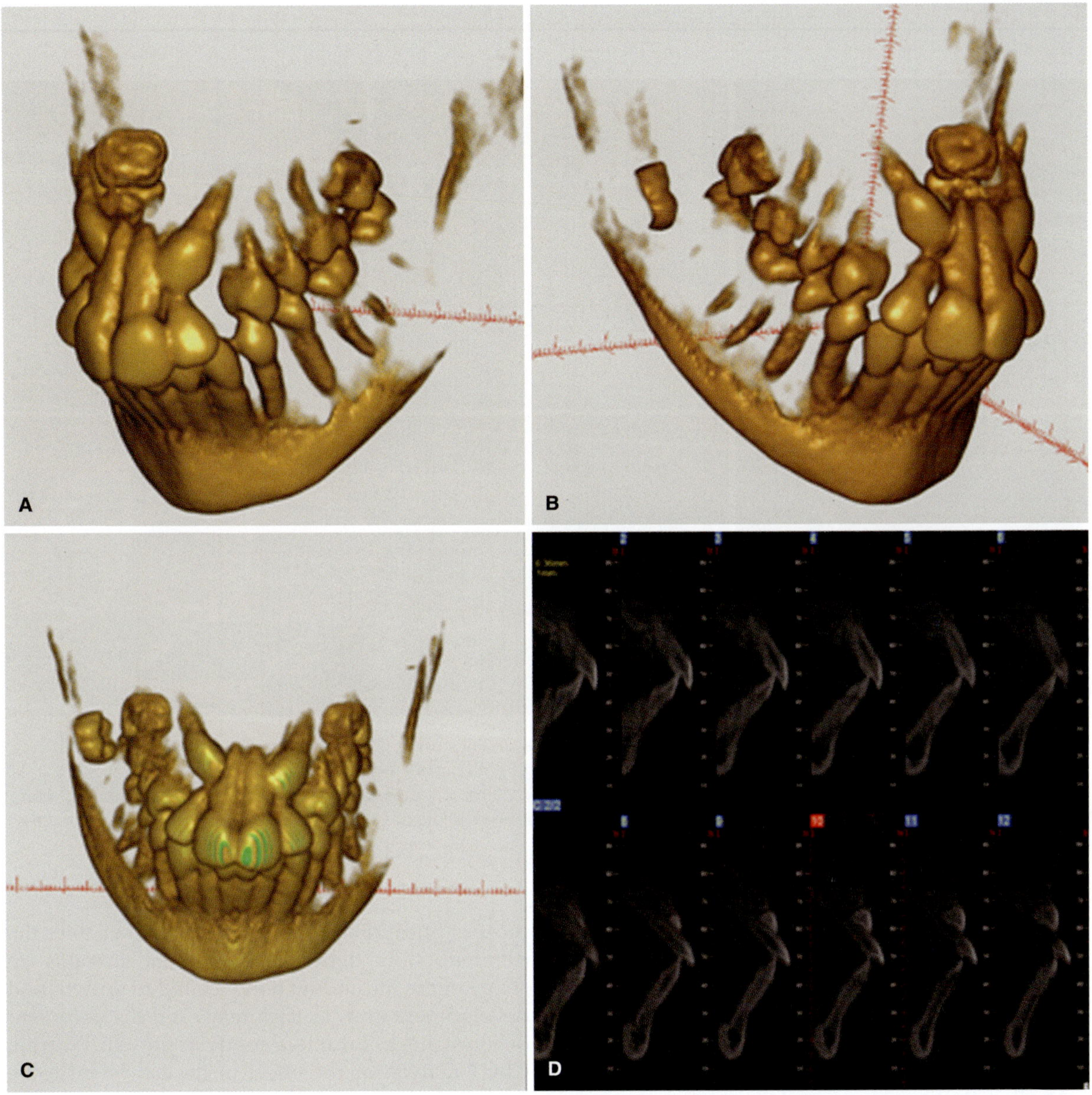

Figure 4.2 Volumetrically rendered image (*A–C*) and sagittal sections (*D*) of ectopic canines, demonstrating the precise localization of these teeth in 3D, making it easier to design the optimal biomechanical system for treatment.

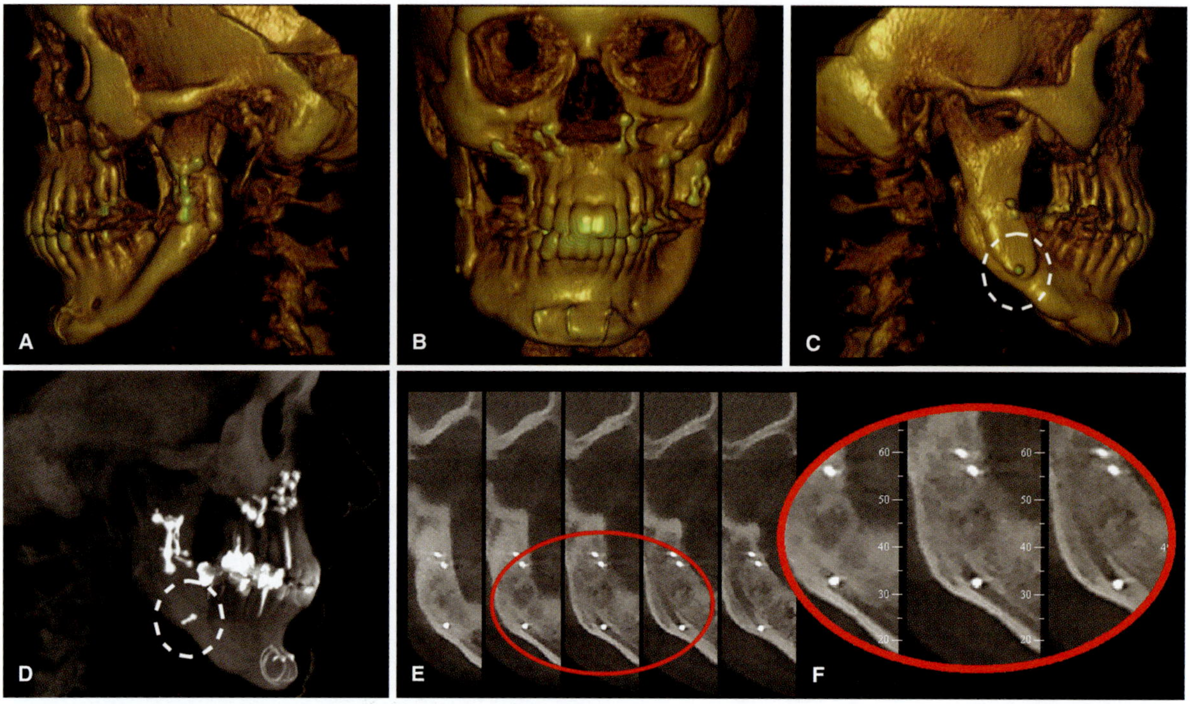

Figure 4.3 Example demonstrating the diagnosis of unexplainable findings using CBCT imaging. The patient had severe symptoms in the right side of the face. Volumetric images (*A–C*) and a reconstructed cephalometric image (*D*) localized a surgical screw in the lower boundary of the right mandibular body. *E* and *F*: Further analysis using tomograms generated from the CBCT image revealed that the surgical screw used for stabilization of bilateral sagittal split osteotomy was placed directly in the mandibular canal.

conventional 2D headfilms. Whereas an indiscriminate use of CBCT for routine clinical use can be questioned seriously, there is no doubt that clinical research that evaluates the results of different approaches to treatment will benefit from a well-planned prospective and, if possible, randomized controlled studies using CBCT images.

Until this point, CBCT imaging has had only limited impact on research. Most studies have been focused on the technology and its possible clinical uses; only a few randomized clinical trials have been published. Tai and colleagues (2010, 2011) analyzed the 3D changes generated with Schwartz appliances; Botticelli and coworkers (2011) assessed the influence of the 3D image on the treatment plan in a clinical trial on unerupted canines; and Cattaneo and associates (2011) performed a randomized clinical trial comparing the results of two different bracket systems on the expansion of the upper arch. Because CBCT imaging also allows for the identification of stable structures, it enables the differentiation between modeling, changes in shape of the individual bone related to growth and development and/or treatment, and displacement of bones due to sutural or condylar growth. Overall, CBCT allows for the effect of the treatment to be analyzed in great detail since orthopedic and orthodontic effects can be differentiated by superimposing on both internal and external stable structures (Cevidanes *et al.*, 2005, 2009).

CAN THE FUSION OF CBCT WITH OTHER 3D VISUALIZATION MODALITIES ENHANCE TREATMENT AND RESEARCH?

Despite the advantages and new possibilities of CBCT imaging as a diagnostic, treatment planning, and evaluation tool, there are some inherent

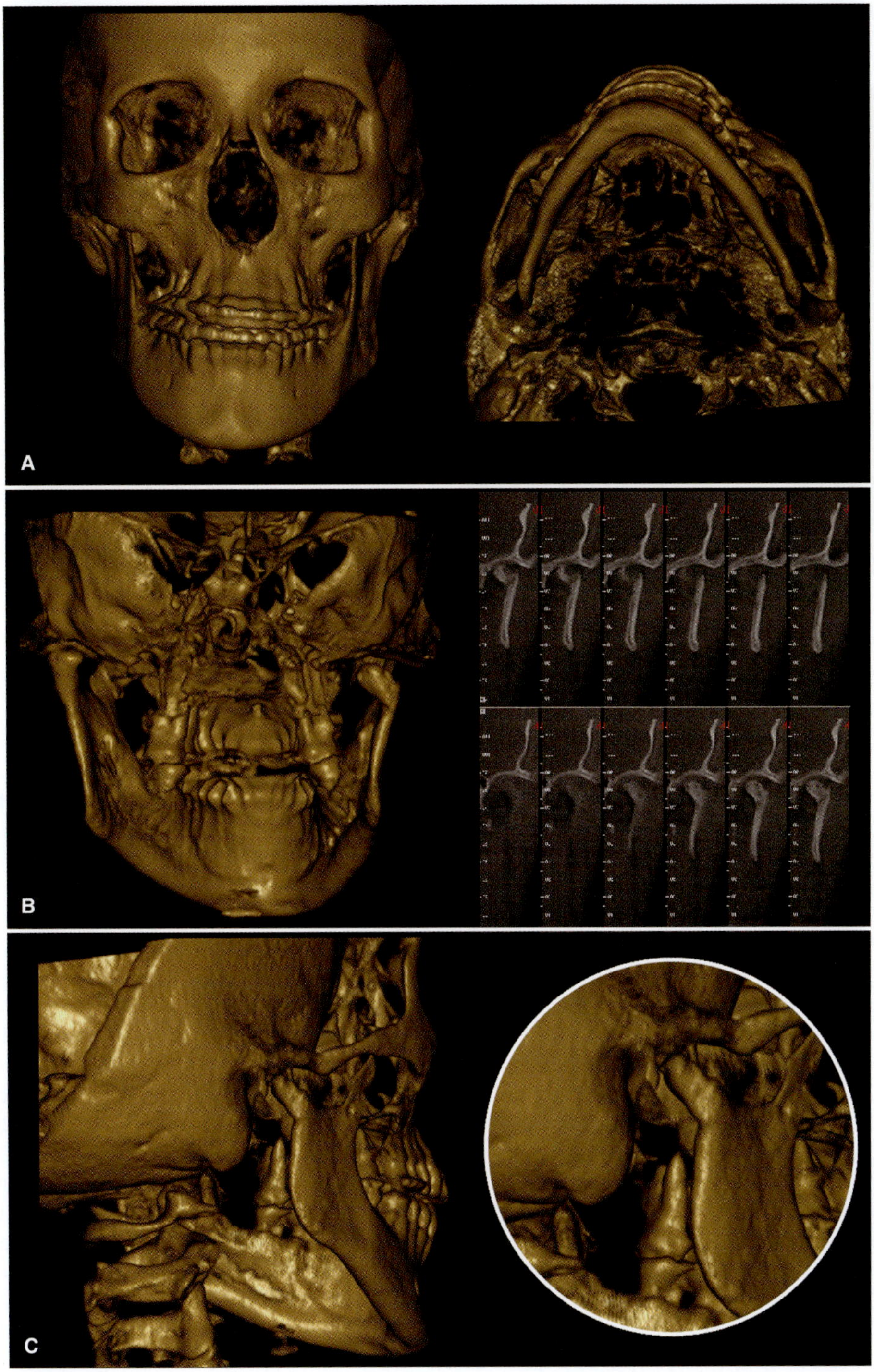

Figure 4.4 Following a trauma to the mandible, the patient complained of pain in the right condylar area and difficulties in lateral movement of the mandible to the right side with pain in the left side. The extraoral examination revealed a facial asymmetry with the menton displaced toward the left side. *A*: On the frontal and submental volumetric images, a shortening of the right side could be verified. *B*: This shortening of the right side of the mandible is more obvious when evaluating volumetric reconstruction from the posterior, which together with planar views demonstrates that the right condyle is displaced medially. *C*: A postero-lateral view of the volumetric reconstruction confirmed that the condyle was displaced medially following a fracture, thereby preventing translation in the left joint.

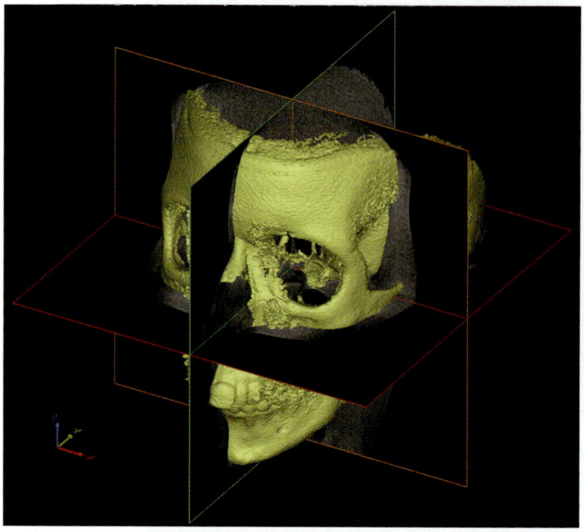

Figure 4.5 A 3D coordinate system that can be used as a reference to assess select parameters for craniofacial anomalies and developmental defects.

problems with CBCT scans. The most important is the inability to create smooth surfaces of anatomical structures in 3D reconstructions. The lower depth and contrast in gray values, as compared with conventional CT, makes it harder to distinguish between the different tissues. As a consequence, isolation of a particular tissue by segmentation of the gray values can result in surfaces that do not correspond to the true anatomy. This could be due to the presence of noise when the threshold value is set too low or holes when the threshold is too high. When making a 3D reconstruction of a skull from a CBCT dataset, a typical problem is that when a threshold value that gives a fair representation of the dental surfaces is chosen, it leads to underestimation of the trabecular volume in the condyles. On the other hand, a threshold value that optimizes the representation of the condyles results in overestimated and bloated surfaces of the crowns. Additionally, the presence of artifacts due to amalgam fillings and/or metal orthodontic brackets hampers the presentation of the crown surfaces in an anatomically correct manner. As opposed to the caveats of global thresholding, local thresholding might provide an optimal solution (Burghardt *et al.*, 2007; Plooij *et al.*, 2011), but this requires more user interaction and consequently longer reconstruction times. Another solution is to fuse CBCT datasets with other 3D visualization modalities, which can better represent the structures for which CBCT is not optimal or requires substantial manipulation. These techniques for fusing different images for orthodontics and orthognathic surgery are presented in a systematic review by Plooij and colleagues (2011). Fusion with digital models thus can be used to obtain smooth and correct dental surfaces anatomically, while fusion with 3D photography would provide an accurate description of the surface of the face. Theoretically, magnetic resonance imaging (MRI) also could qualify as a fusion modality in the case of patients for whom a detailed 3D representation of the musculature of the skull is required.

CBCT AND DIGITAL MODELS

Maxillofacial and orthognathic surgery planning is a prime candidate for the application of fusing CBCT and digital models for virtual treatment planning and splint fabrication. In order to be successful in these endeavors, it is important to simulate the occlusion and have a good representation of the crown surfaces (Figure 4.7), which, as discussed above, cannot be achieved with CBCT alone. An additional advantage of virtual surgery planning is the ability to bypass the indirect procedure of facebow transfer, which is employed in conventional pre-operative planning when mounting plaster models in an articulator. This facebow transfer serves for the positioning of the maxillary dentition in a correct relationship to a defined horizontal reference plane (Walker *et al.*, 2008).

Facebow transfers are prone to several errors that contribute to complications during surgery and may compromise treatment results. Facebows are designed with the assumption that the Frankfort Horizontal Plane (FHP) will be identical to the upper cross member of the articulator. Several studies have shown, however, that the plane defined on the articulator does not correspond accurately to the anatomical planes (Ellis *et al.*, 1992; Sharifi *et al.*, 2008; Barbenel *et al.*, 2010; Zizelmann *et al.*, 2012). Consequently, the position of the maxilla as defined by the articulator and facebow registration will vary considerably in relation to

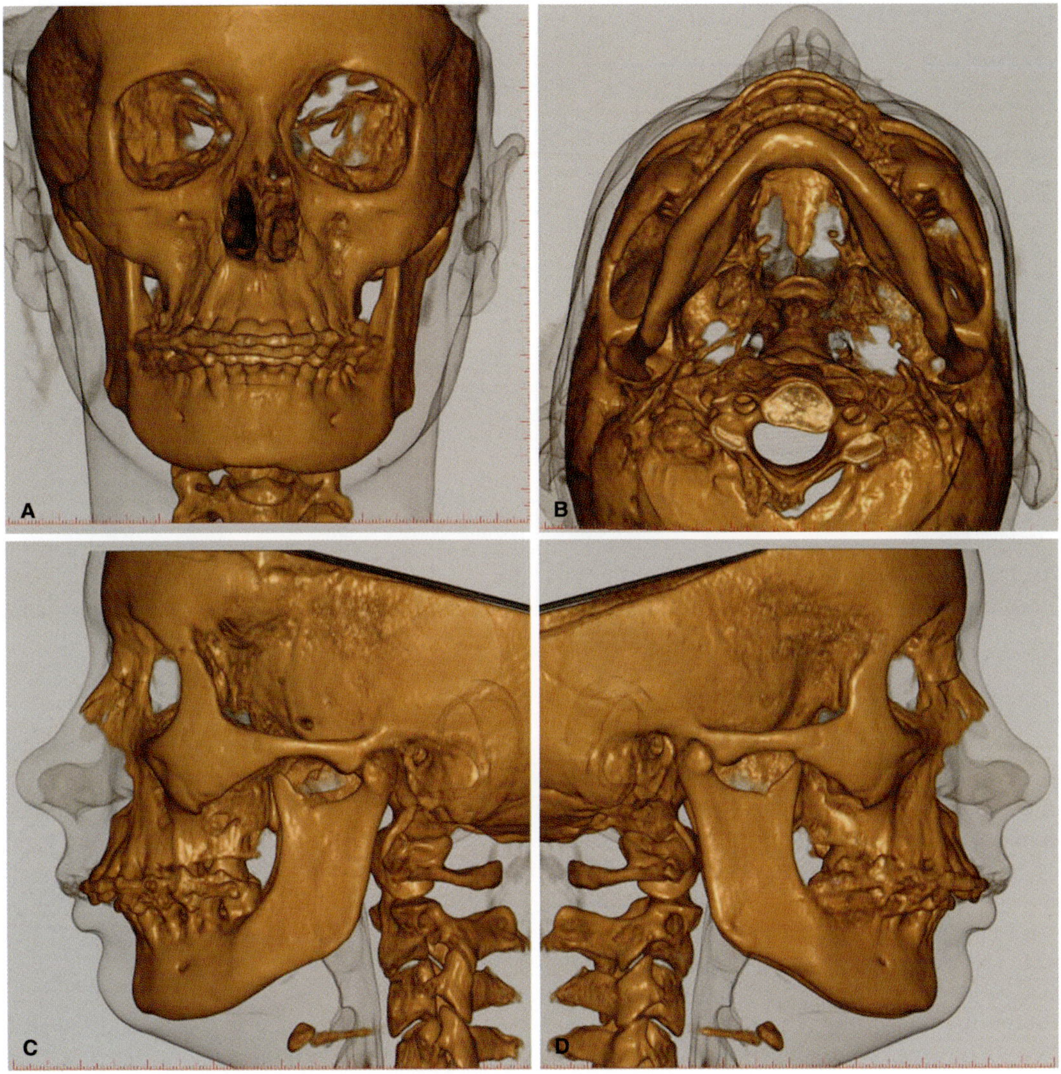

Figure 4.6 *A–D*: CBCT images to help determine the choice between camouflage or surgical treatment options. Determination of both the skeletal relationship and the structure and quality of the alveolar bone will help to clarify how the problem can be handled, whether by camouflage treatment or a surgical intervention.

the true anatomical position of the maxilla, leading to errors in the model surgery and the resulting surgical wafers that, in turn, will influence the final surgical outcome. Ellis and coworkers (1992) assessed the reproducibility of placement of the maxilla in an articulator and found a difference of up to 25° in the cant of the occlusal plane when measured on the lateral headfilm and on the articulator. The selection of the type of facebow also may influence the result (Freeland, 2012). When studying the envelopes of movement resulting from two different facebow systems, Bamber and associates (1996) found significant differences in the distances between the articulator mounting ring and reference points in the horizontal and vertical planes. The coefficients of variation in their study ranged

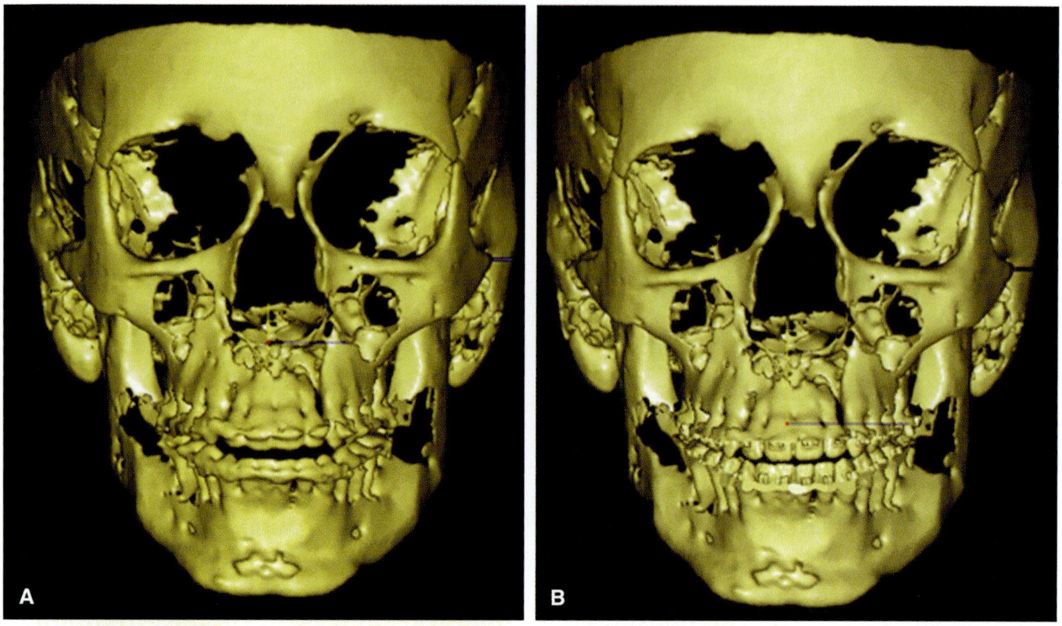

Figure 4.7 Comparison of a 3D reconstruction of a skull without (*A*) and with (*B*) fused digital models.

from 9 to 82%, which was well above the 5–8% normally considered acceptable for biometrics.

In addition to the errors related to model surgery itself, Barbenel and colleagues (2010) demonstrated that the result of orthognathic surgery may differ significantly from the planned outcome based on articulator mounted study casts. They also showed that both forward and upward maxillary movement was more pronounced than planned and that the planned maxillary impaction was achieved in only half of the cases. On the other hand, when planning for forward and downward maxillary movement, a smaller advancement resulted than originally planned, indicating the need for development of more accurate procedures for translating the planned surgical procedure to the one that actually is performed.

Virtual treatment planning of maxillofacial surgery involving the integration of 3D CT/CBCT datasets with digital study models has been proposed as a solution to this problem (Gateno *et al.*, 2003; Swennen *et al.*, 2007a). Digital 3D models are accurate (Dalstra & Melsen, 2009) but do not have the same coordinate system as the CBCT dataset. The 3D models, therefore, need to be integrated into the coordinate system of the CBCT dataset. Different mathematical routines and algorithms can be used to register 3D datasets, based on a point-to-point algorithm, the correspondence of anatomical features, or a combination thereof (Cevidanes *et al.*, 2005, 2009; Swennen *et al.*, 2007a, 2007b, 2009a, 2009b). The so-called triple-scan procedure presented by Swennen and associates (2009a) presently is the most accurate with a maximum variability of less than 0.10 mm. However, this method requires the patients to be exposed to extra radiation as they are scanned twice during the procedure, albeit the second time with a lower dosage. A different methodology that can help facilitate virtual orthognatic surgery on the composite 3D image of CBCT and the digital models is to combine the two images using common reference points. This approach has been adopted for the virtual surgery procedure (O3DM Surgery), which has been developed as a collaborative effort of the Section of Orthodontics, Department of Dentistry, Aarhus University (Aarhus, Denmark), OrtoLab Sp. z o.o. (Czestochova, Poland), and QR Verona (Verona, Italy). The consecutive steps of this procedure are described below in detail.

Step I: Import and segmentation of CBCT/CT data

The main 3D model of the skull is based either on CBCT or conventional CT scanning. The latter modality has a better depth of gray values, but as it exposes the patient to a much higher radiation dose (Roberts *et al.*, 2009), CBCT scanning usually is preferred. Both modalities have the capability of exporting the scanned data into a DICOM format, which can be interpreted by virtual surgery simulation software.

The imported DICOM data represent the voxel data in gray values. In order to make virtual cuts, these data first need to be segmented (i.e., divided into voxels), which, according to their density, represent *bone* and *nonbone*. The threshold for the gray values that determine this differentiation is set by the operator. The selection of this threshold value is subjective and interactive in principle; by sliding the mouse over the histogram of the gray values, the operator can see the resulting surface representation for a given threshold value immediately. The higher this value, the fewer voxels are set to *bone* (Figure 4.8). From the voxels, which are set to *bone*, a surface representation is made consisting of thousands of triangles.

The registration procedure (Step III) is based on the identification of corresponding points on the crowns of the teeth of the CBCT image. These points are presented in the DICOM format and on the crowns in the digital models. A threshold value is chosen for this procedure, allowing for a good representation of the enamel of the crowns, even if this means that the bone appears to have disappeared in the surface reconstruction of regions with low-density bone (e.g., the condyles).

After setting the threshold, many separate 3D objects will be created because many bony parts are not connected (e.g., the hyoid bone and the vertebrae); there also are many isolated noise particles. The software features a split function that will remove all the isolated objects that are not connected to the main 3D object (i.e., the skull). Due to the low density of the condylar bone, the condyles also are not visualized, resulting in a lack of contact between the mandible and the skull in the TMJ regions after segmentation. However, due to the occlusal contacts, the mandible will remain connected to the rest of the main 3D object despite the split function.

The final phase of this step is to define the anatomical coordinate system. The operator is asked to identify the left orbitale, the left and right porions, and the nasion. The first three points define the FHP. The frontal plane is defined by the left and right porions and is perpendicular to the FHP. The midsagittal plane is defined by the nasion and is perpendicular to both the FHP and the frontal plane.

Step II: Import of the digital model

Digital models are generated from 3D intraoral laser scanning of the surfaces of the teeth, from impressions or plaster models, or from detailed industrial CT scannings of the impression or plaster models. A 3D model typically is built up as a cloud of thousands of points located on the surface of the crowns and gingiva. Each of these points then is connected to neighboring points in a triangulated format. Although the various manufacturers of digital models produce their own 3D models in a format specific to their own visualization and analysis software, the company-specific format usually can be exported in a generally accessible STL format, originating from CAD/CAM. Because the coordinate system of the STL models does not correspond to that of the CBCT dataset, a registration procedure is necessary to transfer the models to their anatomical correct position (Figure 4.9).

Step III: Registration of CBCT and digital models

Several algorithms can be used for 3D registration of the CBCT scan and 3D models. The most straightforward is a point-to-point procedure, which is based on the fact that at least three corresponding points are required to superimpose two common objects in a 3D space. Theoretically, the distances between these three points on both objects should be exactly the same; however, due to inaccuracies in selecting the points (error of the method) and the surface description of the skull, which is dependent on the threshold setting (see

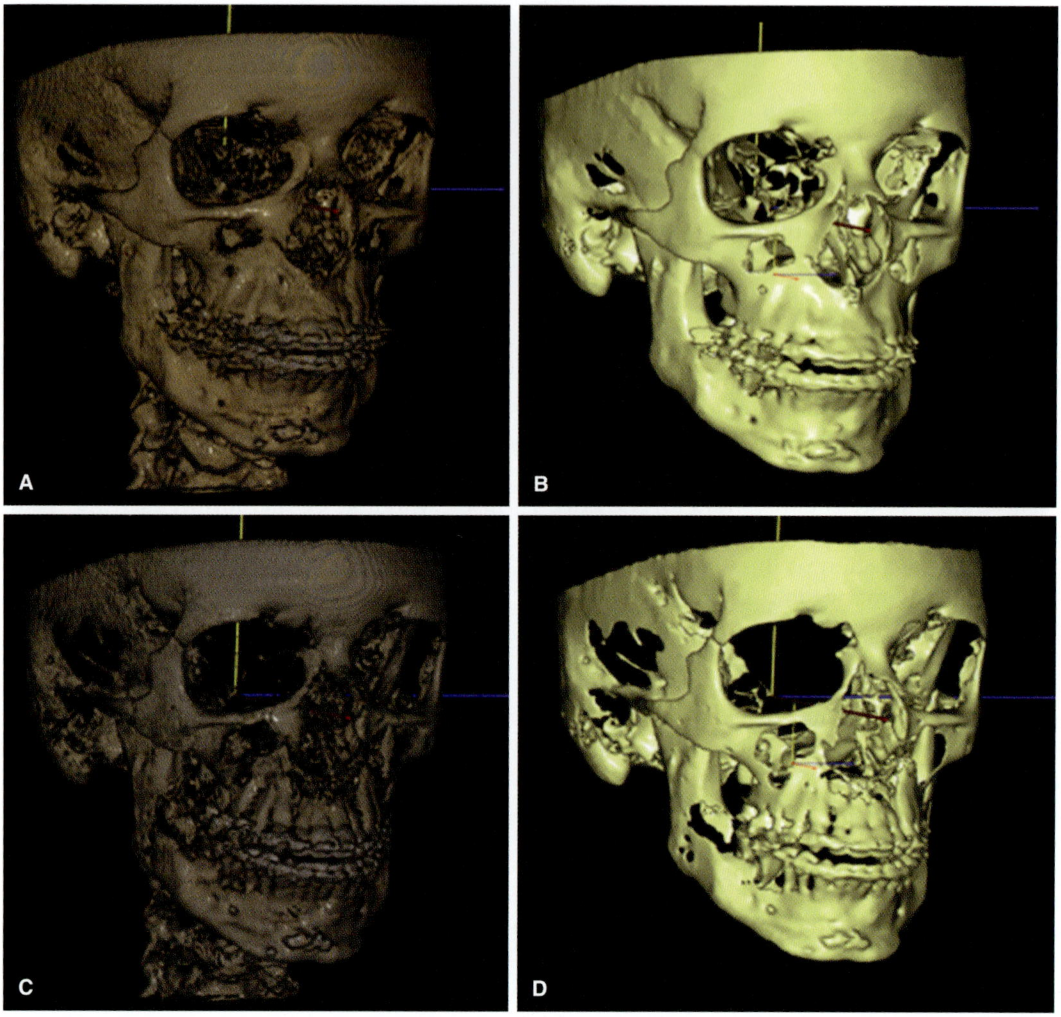

Figure 4.8 Voxel-based (*A* and *C*) and surface-based (*B* and *D*) 3D reconstructions of a skull, segmented at a low (*A* and *B*) and a high (*C* and *D*) threshold value.

Step I), errors will occur. A least-squares algorithm is applied to minimize these errors when determining the final positioning of the registered object (in this case the digital models) by the point-to-point procedure. The selection of points that are identifiable on both the digital models and on the 3D objects is critical to the accuracy of this procedure. Theoretically, one could select more than three points in order to minimize the overall error by averaging out the error described above over a larger number of points. However, the more pairs of corresponding points selected, the more difficult it is to find new and easily identifiable points; thereby, new errors could be introduced. A study of double measurements of various numbers of pairs of corresponding points for the registration on six patients revealed a minimal overall translational error of 0.2 mm and rotational error of 1.0° (Figure 4.10) for five pairs of corresponding points. In the software, the number of pairs of matching points is not fixed and the operator decides how many points should be selected. Visual feedback of

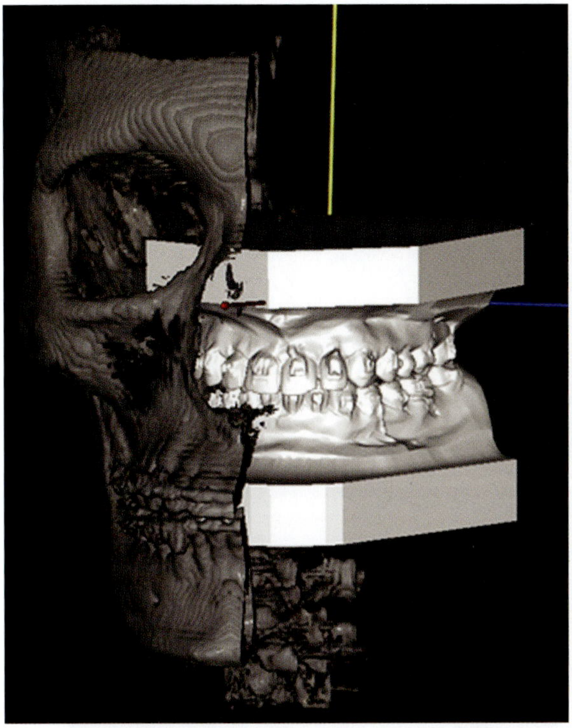

Figure 4.9 Import of a digital model into a CBCT dataset. The initial misalignment of the digital model has to be corrected by performing a registration. For visualization purposes, only half of the skull is shown.

the location to which the digital models will move after each set of matching points has been indicated will help guide the operator, who then can decide whether or not an extra set of points will be required to improve the accuracy of the registration.

Whether both upper and lower teeth from the models are registered together or separately should be determined on a case-by-case basis. Registering them together is quicker, but requires that the patient presents with the exact same occlusion in the CBCT scan as when the impression for the digital models was taken. Therefore, impression and CBCT ideally should be performed on the same day and a wax-bite should be used to maintain the identical bite during the scan and transfer of the models to the CBCT image.

Step IV: Removal of CBCT teeth and model bases

Once the digital models are placed into the CBCT reconstruction, both the DICOM teeth of the CBCT dataset and the model bases can be removed. Using the cutting tools of the software, a "cutting box" following the gingival margin of the digital models can be drawn and everything inside this box will

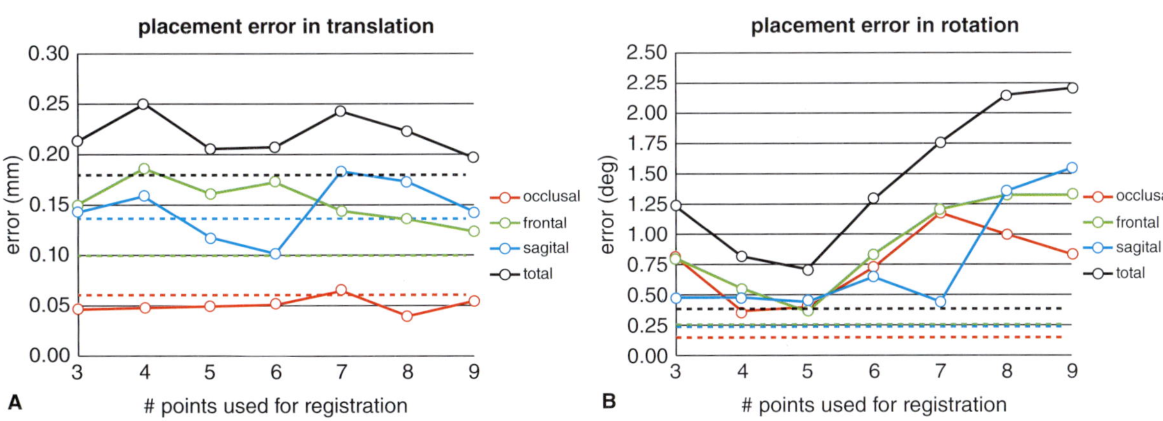

Figure 4.10 Translational (*A*) and rotational errors (*B*) depending on the number of pairs of corresponding points used for the point-to-point registration process.

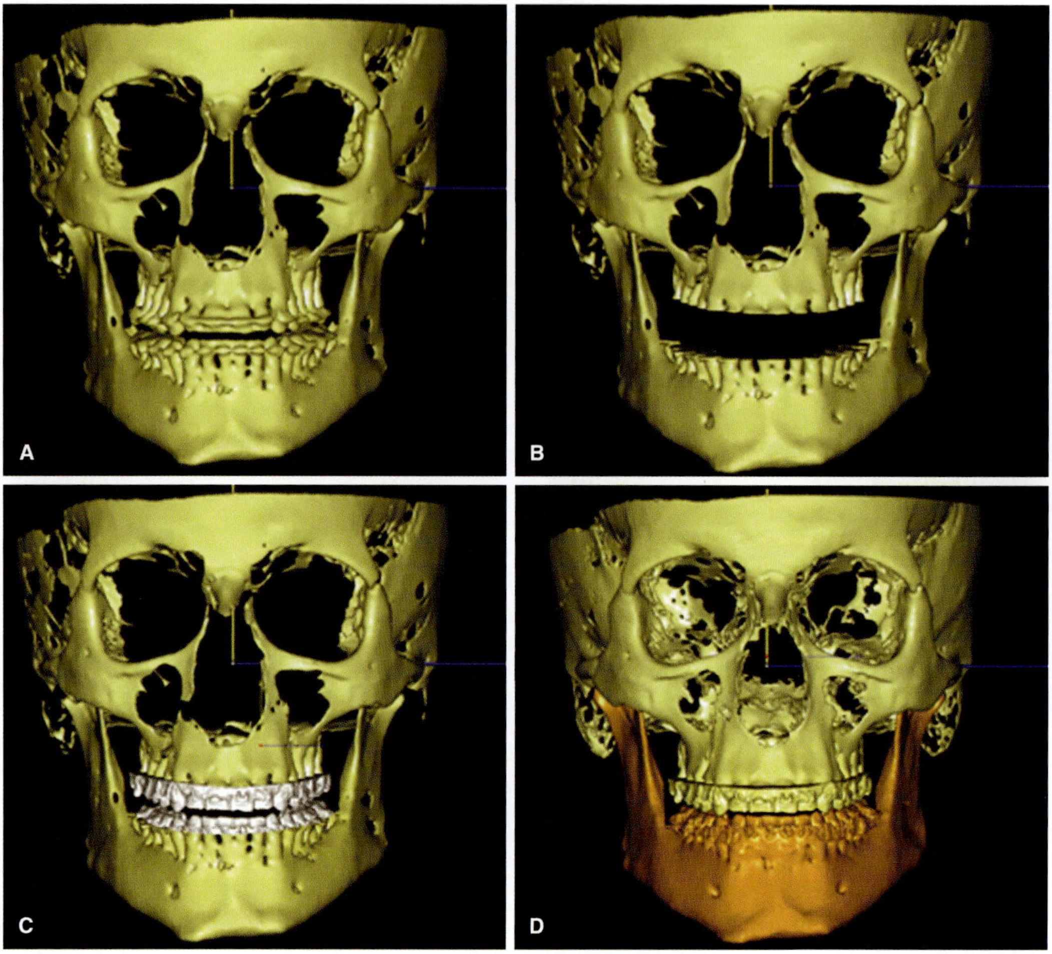

Figure 4.11 The steps for replacing the CBCT crowns with those of the digital models. *A*: Intact CBCT of the craniofacial skeleton with DICOM crowns. *B*: Removal of the DICOM crowns. *C*: Crowns from the digital models in position. *D*: Merging of the maxillary crowns to the skull and the mandibular crowns to the mandible.

be removed from the dataset. The same cut will be used to separate the bases from the digital dental surfaces, thus ensuring a continuous transition from the skull to the model dental surfaces (Figure 4.11). The removal of the DICOM teeth from the CBCT image will leave the skull and the mandible as two separate 3D objects, as the only contact between the skull and mandible has been the teeth in occlusion (see Step II). Consequently, the maxillary and mandibular teeth from the 3D models are merged with the 3D skull object and mandible object, respectively.

Step V: Set-up of the virtual articulator

With the mandible virtually separated from the skull, the physiological movements of the mandible relative to the skull can be prescribed using a virtual articulator, which is incorporated in the simulation software. Activation of the virtual articulator will display two ellipsoids, representing the left and right TMJ, which can be dragged to their corresponding anatomical positions (Figure 4.12). Once the anatomical position is established, any physiological movement of the lower jaw can be

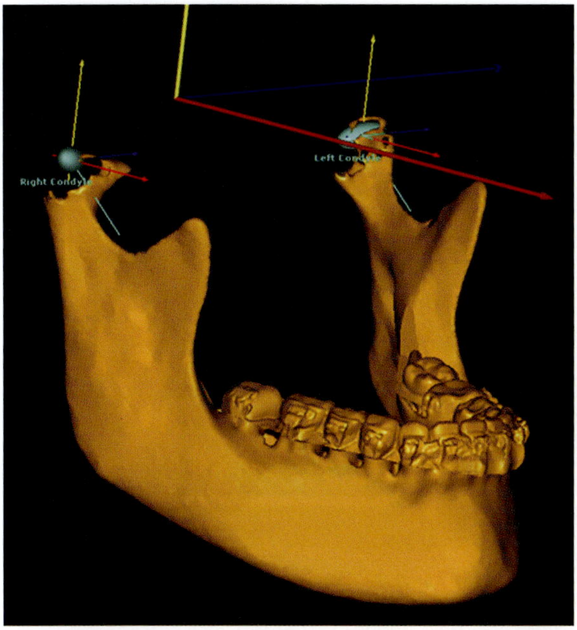

Figure 4.12 Mandible with the ellipsoids representing the location of the TMJs for use in simulating mandibular movements on a virtual articulators.

simulated, including autorotation and translation of the mandible.

Step VI: Virtual surgery

After the model is prepared, simulation of the surgery can begin. The surgical cuts are simulated using the cutting tool of the software in the form of a "cutting box." When the "cutting box" has been defined, the object(s) inside the box is/are separated from the object(s) outside the box. For identification purposes, the cut objects are assigned a different color. All standard surgical procedures can be performed virtually. Once an object has been cut loose from the main 3D object, it can be repositioned with all six degrees of freedom according to the operator's wishes. When the displaced object is selected from the object list, the amount of rotation and translation for that object will be displayed relative to the three anatomical planes. Another way to keep track of the amount of displacements of the individual bony elements is to make a copy of the displaced objects and leave this copy at its original position. Distances between user-defined common points on both the original object and its copy (e.g., a cusp of a crown) can be measured and are updated each time the object is repositioned. Several examples of virtual surgical procedures are shown in Figure 4.13. In the final phase of repositioning the loose segment(s), the operator performs a visual check of the new relationship between the maxillary and mandibular teeth and their occlusion. If the operator is satisfied with the result, a detailed quantitative analysis of the occlusion is performed next.

Step VII: Occlusion check

Once the object's parts are transferred to their desired position during virtual surgery, the software features an occlusal viewing mode. In this mode, distances between the upper and lower crowns with a distance of less than 0 mm are shown in bright blue, indicating that this occlusion is not possible in reality and requires further adjustment. Alternatively, these "hard contacts" also can be accepted for the moment and subsequently can be corrected by grinding down the tooth structure during the actual surgery. Fine-tuning adjustments can be performed manually, but the software also offers the option of calculating an optimal occlusion. By specifying which components of translation and rotation the software is allowed to vary and the step-size of these variations, the software then will calculate all possible solutions and finally present one in which the overall distance distribution of occlusal contacts is minimal, yet excludes "penetrations" between occlusal contacts (Figure 4.14).

Step VIII: Generating the surgical splint

In the case of a single-jaw surgery, the new occlusion is checked and approved by the operator and a surgical wafer or splint has to be produced. The first step is to open the bite by simulating a slight posterior rotation of the mandible around the condyles (0.5 or 1.0°), thus leaving just enough space between the teeth in the upper and lower arches

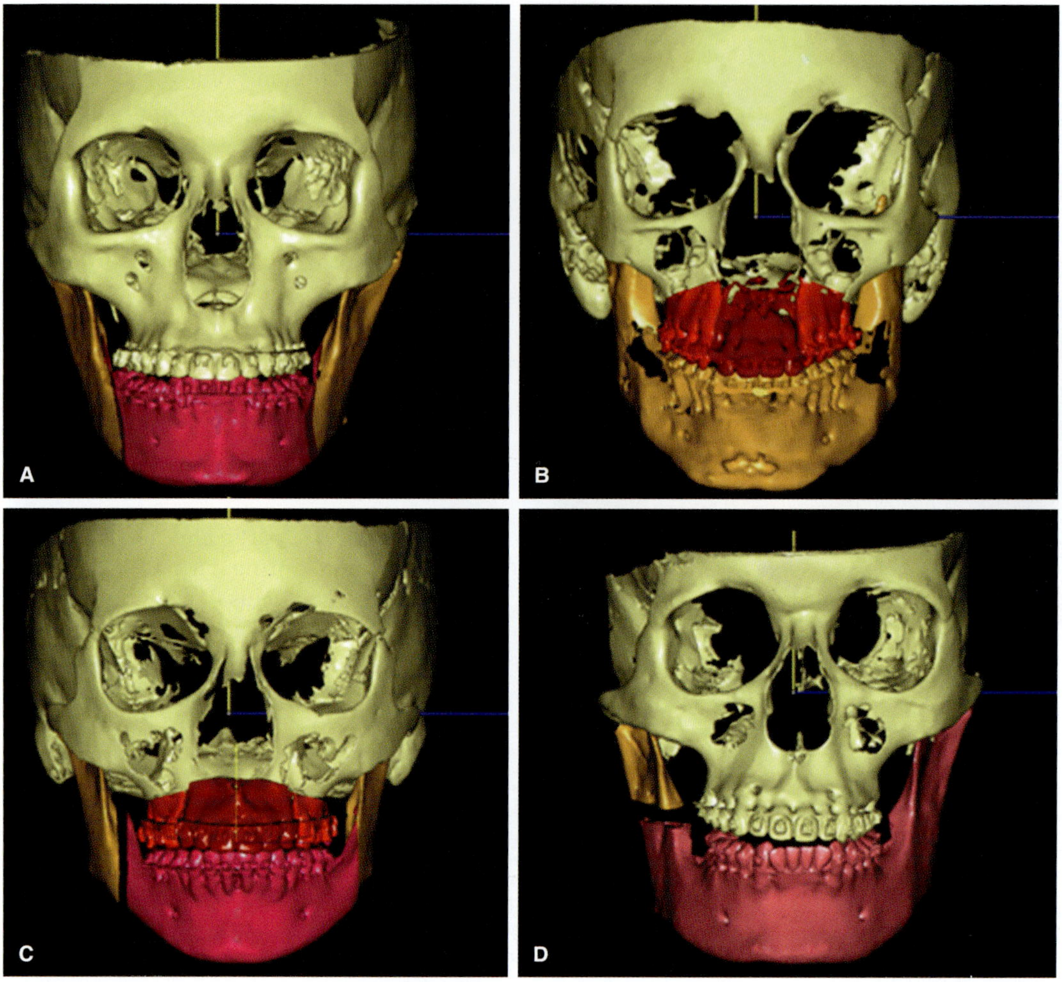

Figure 4.13 Examples of different surgical procedures performed virtually. *A*: Mandibular advancement. *B*: LeFort I osteotomy. *C*: Double jaw procedure. *D*: Unilateral right mandibular distraction osteotomy in which the gap between the right ramus and the rest of the mandible will be filled up by osteogenesis.

for the wafer. By activating the wafer function, a default box automatically will be placed around the upper and lower dentitions. The height of this box can be adjusted separately for the maxillary and mandibular arches. The operator also can adjust the box manually to the inclination of the occlusal plane or the curve of Spee. Once satisfied with the position of this box, the final wafer, following the contours of the crowns, will be created as a separated 3D object, which then can be exported into an STL format (Figure 4.15). The STL file of the wafer then can be printed in acrylic on a 3D printer or milled on a milling machine. In the case of a double procedure, two splints are produced: one as a temporary wafer between the new position of the mandibular teeth and the pre-op position of the maxillary teeth (provided the mandible is operated on first), and the final wafer between the new positions of both mandibular and maxillary teeth.

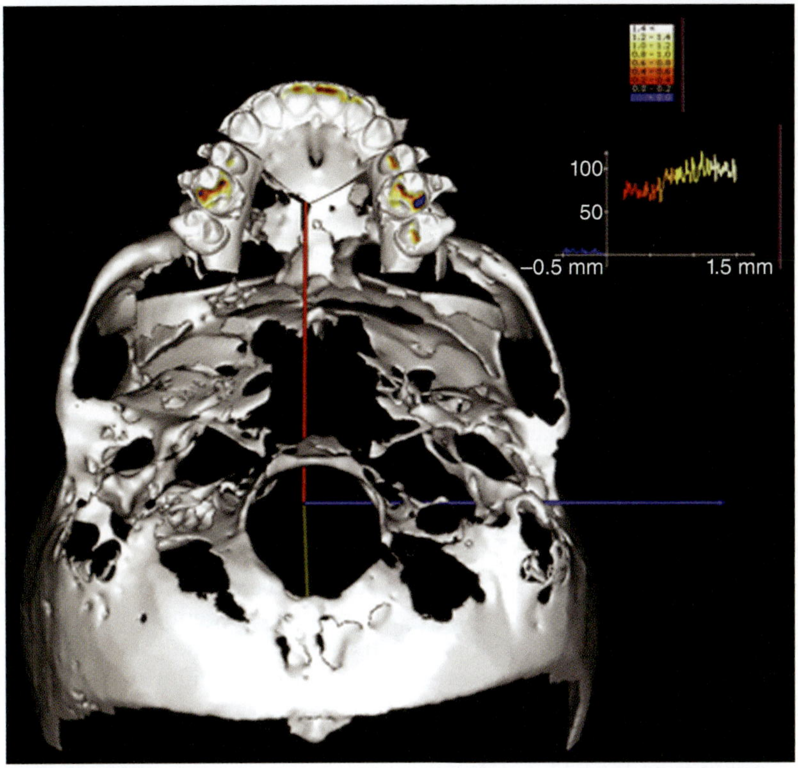

Figure 4.14 Occlusal view showing color distribution of occlusal contacts on the occlusal surfaces.

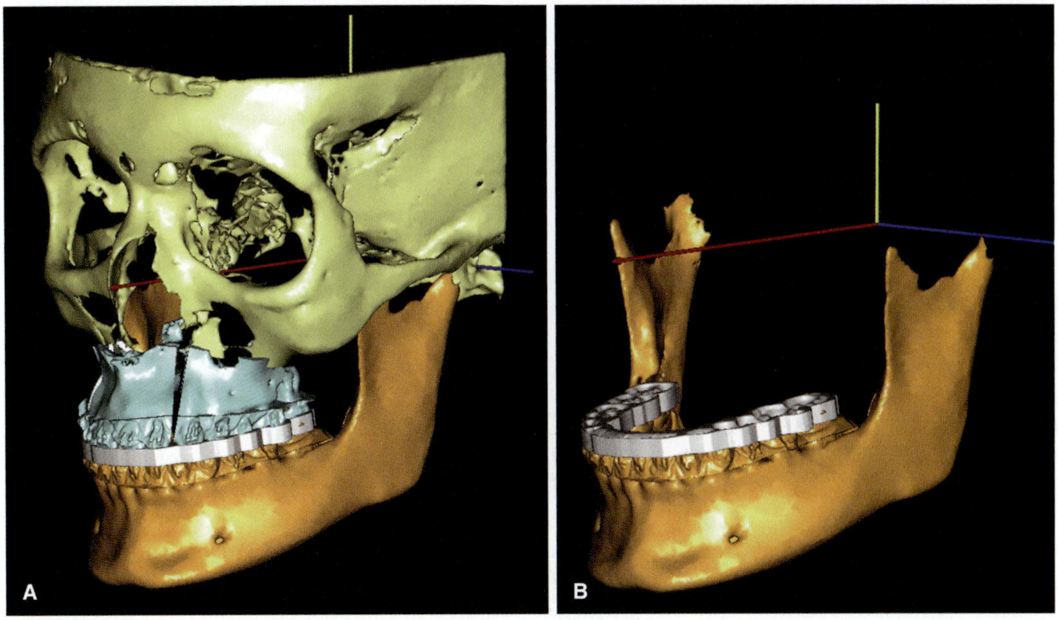

Figure 4.15 A model with a virtual surgical wafer (*A*) and with the skull removed (*B*).

CBCT AND 3D PHOTOGRAPHY

Following surgery, the treatment result can be assessed on a post-surgery CBCT scan, where the treatment objective and actual results can be superimposed on the cranial base, thus making it possible to quantify changes (Cevidanes *et al.*, 2005). However, this approach enables evaluation of surgical changes only in hard tissues and their relationship to the desired goals of the virtual surgery. Generally, however, the main concern of the patients is the expected soft tissue changes that would result from the surgery.

One method to evaluate the outcome of orthodontic or surgery treatment on the soft tissue changes is to analyze the changes of the face over the course of treatment. This could be taken a step further by proactively predicting the changes to the shape of the face in the treatment planning phase, thus virtually trying out different treatment options and comparing the various predicted outcomes. Such a prediction would require a segmentation of the skin from the CBCT dataset, but as with the dental surfaces mentioned previously, a smooth surface can be difficult to achieve. In recent years, 3D facial photography has progressed from a somewhat cumbersome laboratory technique to an easily applicable clinical tool. The combination of synchronous laser scanning and dual angle photography produces triangulated data, representing the surface of the face, which can be mapped with photorealistic skin (Figure 4.16). Similar to digital models, data can be exported in STL format and thus fused with the CBCT's DICOM data.

The steps for importing and registration of both DICOM and 3D photography datasets are comparable to the fusing of DICOM and digital models. The area between the eyebrows and bridge of the nose usually is utilized for superimposition. When importing both pre- and post-treatment 3D photography datasets into the same CBCT dataset, Boolean tools, which normally come with the software, can be used to visualize and quantify the facial changes that have occurred during treatment. In order to predict soft tissue changes, the software requires an algorithm, which can compute these changes given the prescribed displacements of the bones of the skull and mandible; a mass-spring model typically forms the basis of this algorithm. Here the triangles, making up the surface of the face, are given a spring constant, representing the tangential (in-plane) elasticity of the skin. Furthermore, another spring constant is given to the nodes on the skin surface; its nearest neighbors on the underlying bony surfaces represent the perpendicular (in-depth) elasticity of the soft tissue (Schendel & Lane, 2009). In the pre-operative model, no residual forces are assumed to be present in the spring elements. When surgery is simulated and a section of the bony surface of the skull or mandible has been moved, the distance of its surface points to their neighboring points on the skin will be altered; therefore, forces are being developed locally in the spring elements. Given the tangential and perpendicular elasticity, the points on the free skin surface will move to their new equilibrium positions (the situation where the sum of all residual forces is minimal) and the shape of the new skin surface can be calculated. However, changes in function that may lead to enhancement or weakening of certain muscle groups (e.g., a change from a lip catch to a normal swallowing pattern) are not taken into consideration. For this reason, care must be taken when interpreting the results of these predictions, particularly when sharing this information with the patients, as it might lead them to have unrealistically high expectations that cannot be fulfilled. Nevertheless, the approach has its merits as a tool for expeditiously modeling and visualizing different treatment alternatives and will form the basis for further research on soft tissue adaptation following surgery.

CONCLUSIONS

When a new product is marketed, it generates a reaction that can vary from refusal to a wait-and-see attitude to total adoption, depending on the individual user's traits and comfort. This attitude most likely will depend on an understanding of the new device's advantages and disadvantages. Any change in established patterns of practice or where additional skillsets are required will be met with initial obstruction and hesitation that slowly will

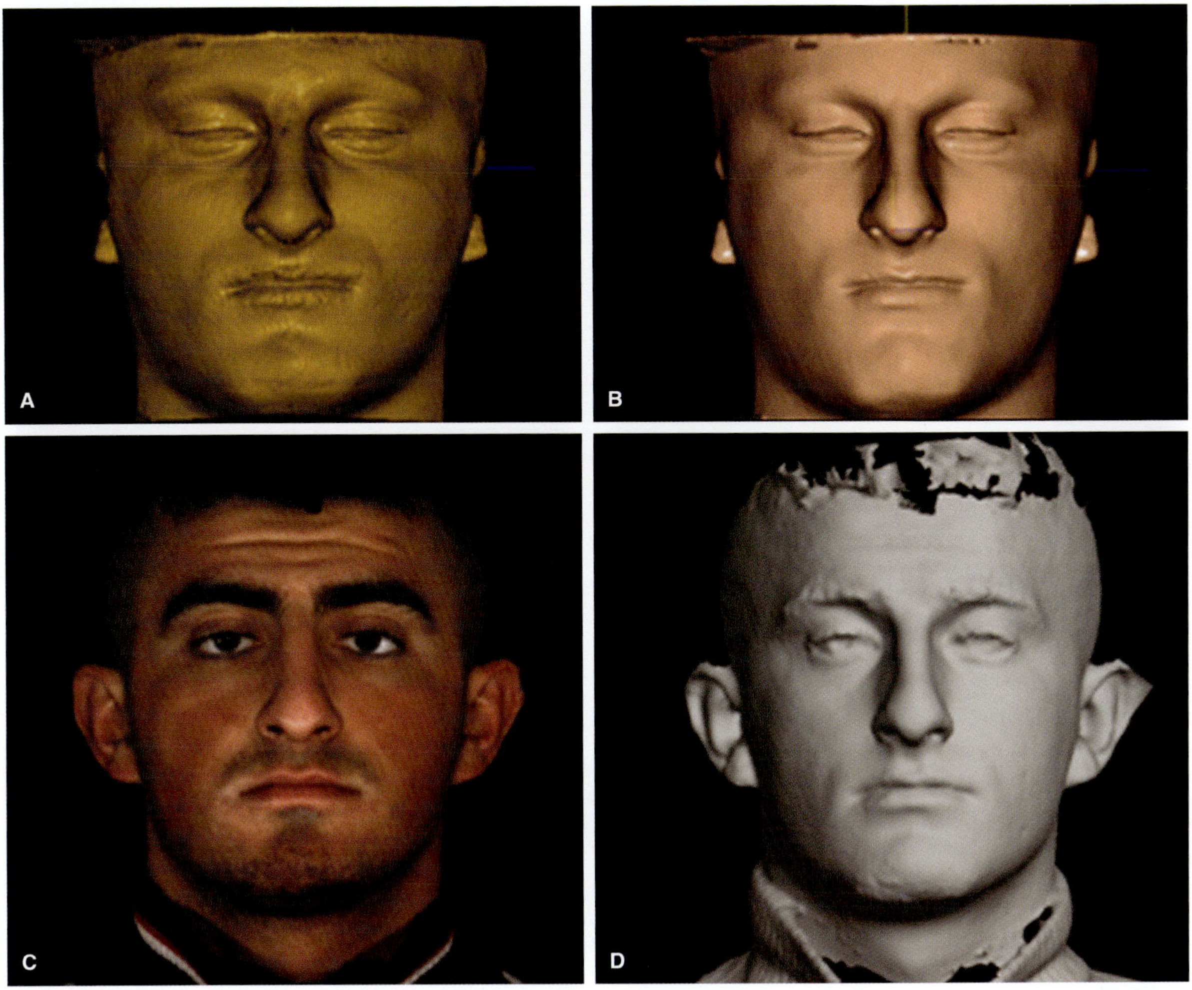

Figure 4.16 Soft tissue representation. *A*: Voxel-based CBCT. *B*: Surface-based CBCT. *C*: 3D photography with photorealistic representation. *D*: 3D photography with surface representation.

change into acceptance if the device indeed proves to enhance patient care.

The goal of this chapter has been to show how access to CBCT images has had an impact on the process of diagnosis and treatment planning. The decision to utilize this new technology most likely originates from the feeling of inadequacy in decision making for specific patients for whom the additional CBCT-derived information could be of clinical benefit. This is true particularly when planning surgical treatments, for which the initial results suggest that CBCT and 3D imaging can contribute to more efficient planning by facilitating the transfer of virtually planned displacements and interventions to the patient in the operating theater.

References

Adams, G.L., Gansky, S.A., Miller, A.J., *et al.* (2004) Comparison between traditional 2-dimensional cephalometry and a 3-dimensional approach on human dry skulls. *American Journal of Orthodontics and Dentofacial Orthopedics*, 126 (4), 397–409.

Athanasiou, A.E. (1995) *Orthodontic Cephalometry*. 1st ed. Mosby-Wolfe, London.

Athanasiou, A.E., Droschl, H., & Bosch, C. (1992) Data and patterns of transverse dentofacial structure of 6- to 15-year-old children: a posteroanterior cephalometric study. *American Journal of Orthodontics and Dentofacial Orthopedics*, 101 (5), 465–471.

Bamber, M.A., Firouzai, R., Harris, M., *et al.* (1996) A comparative study of two arbitrary face-bow transfer systems for orthognathic surgery planning. *International Journal of Oral and Maxillofacial Surgery*, 25 (5), 339–343.

Barbenel, J.C., Paul, P.E., Khambay, B.S., *et al.* (2010) Errors in orthognathic surgery planning: the effect of inaccurate study model orientation. *International Journal of Oral and Maxillofacial Surgery*, 39 (11), 1103–1108.

Baumrind, S., Moffitt, F.H., & Curry, S. (1983a) The geometry of three-dimensional measurement from paired coplanar X-ray images. *American Journal of Orthodontics*, 84 (4), 313–322.

Baumrind, S., Moffitt, F.H., & Curry, S. (1983b) Three-dimensional X-ray stereometry from paired coplanar images: a progress report. *American Journal of Orthodontics*, 84 (4), 292–312.

Bjork, A. & Skieller, V. (1972) Facial development and tooth eruption: an implant study at the age of puberty. *American Journal of Orthodontics*, 62 (4), 339–383.

Bjork, A. & Skieller, V. (1974) Growth in width of the maxilla studied by the implant method. *Scandinavian Journal of Plastic and Reconstructive Surgery*, 8 (1–2), 26–33.

Bjork, A. & Skieller, V. (1977) Growth of the maxilla in three dimensions as revealed radiographically by the implant method. *British Journal of Orthodontics*, 4 (2), 53–64.

Botticelli, S., Verna, C., Cattaneo, P.M., *et al.* (2011) Two- versus three-dimensional imaging in subjects with unerupted maxillary canines. *European Journal of Orthodontics*, 33 (4), 344–349.

Broadbent, H.B. (1931) A new X-ray technique and its application to orthodontia. *Angle Orthodontist*, 1 (2), 45–66.

Burghardt, A.J., Kazakia, G.J., & Majumdar, S. (2007) A local adaptive threshold strategy for high resolution peripheral quantitative computed tomography of trabecular bone. *Annals of Biomedical Engineering*, 35 (10), 1678–1686.

Cattaneo, P.M., Bloch, C.B., Calmar, D., *et al.* (2008) Comparison between conventional and cone-beam computed tomography-generated cephalograms. *American Journal of Orthodontics and Dentofacial Orthopedics*, 134 (6), 798–802.

Cattaneo, P.M., Treccani, M., Carlsson, K., *et al.* (2011) Transversal maxillary dento-alveolar changes in patients treated with active and passive self-ligating brackets: a randomized clinical trial using CBCT-scans and digital models. *Orthodontics & Craniofacial Research*, 14 (4), 222–233.

Cevidanes, L.H., Bailey, L.J., Tucker, G.R., Jr., *et al.* (2005) Superimposition of 3D cone-beam CT models of orthognathic surgery patients. *Dentomaxillofacial Radiology*, 34 (6), 369–375.

Cevidanes, L.H., Heymann, G., Cornelis, M.A., *et al.* (2009) Superimposition of 3-dimensional cone-beam computed tomography models of growing patients. *American Journal of Orthodontics and Dentofacial Orthopedics*, 136 (1), 94–99.

Dalstra, M. & Melsen, B. (2009) From alginate impressions to digital virtual models: accuracy and reproducibility. *Journal of Orthodontics*, 36 (1), 36–41.

DeVos, W., Casselman, J., & Swennen, G.R. (2009) Cone-beam computerized tomography (CBCT) imaging of the oral and maxillofacial region: a systematic review of the literature. *International Journal of Oral and Maxillofacial Surgery*, 38 (6), 609–625.

Ellis, E., III, Tharanon, W., & Gambrell, K. (1992) Accuracy of face-bow transfer: effect on surgical prediction and postsurgical result. *Journal of Oral and Maxillofacial Surgery*, 50 (6), 562–567.

Ericson, S. & Kurol, J. (1987) Incisor resorption caused by maxillary cuspids: a radiographic study. *Angle Orthodontist*, 57 (4), 332–346.

Farman, A.G. & Scarfe, W.C. (2006) Development of imaging selection criteria and procedures should precede cephalometric assessment with cone-beam computed tomography. *American Journal of Orthodontics and Dentofacial Orthopedics*, 130 (2), 257–265.

Freeland, T.D. (2012) Articulators in orthodontics. *Seminars in Orthodontics*, 18, 51–62.

Gateno, J., Xia, J., Teichgraeber, J.F., *et al.* (2003) A new technique for the creation of a computerized composite skull model. *Journal of Oral and Maxillofacial Surgery*, 61 (2), 222–227.

Halazonetis, D.J. (2012) Cone-beam computed tomography is not the imaging technique of choice for comprehensive orthodontic assessment. *American Journal of Orthodontics and Dentofacial Orthopedics*, 141 (4), 403, 405, 407.

Hofrath, H. (1931) Die Bedeutung der Röntgenfern- und Abstandsaufnahme fur die Diagnostik der Kieferanomalien. *Fortschitte der Orthodontik*, 1, 232–258 (in German).

Hussain, A.M., Packota, G., Major, P.W., *et al.* (2008) Role of different imaging modalities in assessment of temporomandibular joint erosions and osteophytes: a systematic review. *Dentomaxillofacial Radiology*, 37 (2), 63–71.

Kapila, S., Conley, R.S., & Harrell, W.E., III (2011) The current status of cone-beam computed tomography imaging in orthodontics. *Dentomaxillofacial Radiology*, 40 (1), 24–34.

Kau, C.H., Zhurov, A., Richmond, S., *et al.* (2006) Facial templates: a new perspective in three dimensions. *Orthodontics & Craniofacial Research*, 9 (1), 10–17.

Kau, C.H., Bozic, M., English, J., *et al.* (2009) Cone-beam computed tomography of the maxillofacial region: an update. *International Journal of Medical Robotics + Computer Assisted Surgery*, 5 (4), 366–380.

Larson, B.E. (2012) Cone-beam computed tomography is the imaging technique of choice for comprehensive orthodontic assessment. *American Journal of Orthodontics and Dentofacial Orthopedics*, 141 (4), 402, 404, 406.

Mozzo, P., Procacci, C., Tacconi, A., *et al.* (1998) A new volumetric CT machine for dental imaging based on the cone-beam technique: preliminary results. *European Radiology*, 8 (9), 1558–1564.

Nijkamp, P.G., Habets, L.L., Aartman, I.H., *et al.* (2008) The influence of cephalometrics on orthodontic treatment planning. *European Journal of Orthodontics*, 30 (6), 630–635.

Plooij, J.M., Maal, T.J., Haers, P., *et al.* (2011) Digital three-dimensional image fusion processes for planning and evaluating orthodontics and orthognathic surgery: a systematic review. *International Journal of Oral Maxillofacial Surgery*, 40 (4), 341–352.

Roberts, J.A., Drage, N.A., Davies, J., *et al.* (2009) Effective dose from cone beam CT examinations in dentistry. *British Journal of Radiology*, 82 (973), 35–40.

Sakima, M.T., Sakima, C.G., & Melsen, B. (2004) The validity of superimposing oblique cephalometric radiographs to assess tooth movement: an implant study. *American Journal of Orthodontics and Dentofacial Orthopedics*, 126 (3), 344–353.

Schendel, S.A. & Lane, C. (2009) Orthognathic surgery simulation using image fusion. *Seminars in Orthodontics*, 15, 48–56.

Schulze, R., Schalldach, F., & Hoedt, B. (2000) Effect of positioning errors on magnification factors in the mandible in digital panorama imaging. *Mund Kiefer Gesichtschirurgie*, 4 (3), 164–170 (in German).

Sharifi, A., Jones, R., Ayoub, A., *et al.* (2008) How accurate is model planning for orthognathic surgery? *International Journal of Oral and Maxillofacial Surgery*, 37 (12), 1089–1093.

Swennen, G.R., Barth, E.L., Eulzer, C., *et al.* (2007a) The use of a new 3D splint and double CT scan procedure to obtain an accurate anatomic virtual augmented model of the skull. *International Journal of Oral and Maxillofacial Surgery*, 36 (2), 146–152.

Swennen, G.R., Mommaerts, M.Y., Abeloos, J., *et al.* (2007b) The use of a wax-bite wafer and a double computed tomography scan procedure to obtain a three-dimensional augmented virtual skull model. *Journal of Craniofacial Surgery*, 18 (3), 533–539.

Swennen, G.R., Mollemans, W., De Clercq, C.C., *et al.* (2009a) A cone-beam computed tomography triple scan procedure to obtain a three-dimensional augmented virtual skull model appropriate for orthognathic surgery planning. *Journal of Craniofacial Surgery*, 20 (2), 297–307.

Swennen, G.R., Mommaerts, M.Y., Abeloos, J., *et al.* (2009b) A cone-beam CT based technique to augment the 3D virtual skull model with a detailed dental surface. *International Journal of Oral and Maxillofacial Surgery*, 38 (1), 48–57.

Tai, K., Hotokezaka, H., Park, J.H., *et al.* (2010) Preliminary cone-beam computed tomography study evaluating dental and skeletal changes after treatment with a mandibular Schwarz appliance. *American Journal of Orthodontics and Dentofacial Orthopedics*, 138 (3), 262–263.

Tai, K., Park, J.H., Mishima, K., *et al.* (2011) 3-dimensional cone-beam computed tomography analysis of transverse changes with Schwarz appliances on both jaws. *Angle Orthodontist*, 81 (4), 670–677.

Walker, F., Ayoub, A.F., Moos, K.F., *et al.* (2008) Face bow and articulator for planning orthognathic surgery: 1 face bow. *British Journal of Oral and Maxillofacial Surgery*, 46 (7), 567–572.

Zizelmann, C., Hammer, B., Gellrich, N.C., *et al.* (2012) An evaluation of face-bow transfer for the planning of orthognathic surgery. *Journal of Oral and Maxillofacial Surgery*, 70 (8), 1944–1950.

5 The Future of Cone Beam Computed Tomography and 3D Imaging in Orthodontics

Michael W. Vannier, MD, and Bin Jiang, MD

Computed tomography (CT) is the cornerstone of the modern radiology department, often the first and only examination required for diagnosis, treatment planning, or follow-up for medical and surgical diseases. The scans depict bone and soft tissue structures, often after administration of oral enteric and intravenous iodinated contrast agents. CT was adopted and has become available widely for many biomedical disciplines, especially for oromaxillofacial imaging and otolaryngology, neuroimaging, orthopedic, cardiovascular, thoracic, abdominopelvic, radiotherapy, and whole body applications. CT scanning technology has evolved with many generations of advances from the slow mechanical systems of the mid-1970s to the current state-of-the-art scanners that can freeze cardiac motion with subsection 3D acquisitions (Kalender, 2011).

For orthodontics, CT imaging more recently has been adopted based on the development of compact inexpensive specialized systems that employ cone beam geometry for examinations limited to the oromaxillofacial structures (Merrett *et al.*, 2009; Kapila *et al.*, 2011; Van Vlijmen *et al.*, 2012). Similar scanners are used for otolaryngology (Hodez *et al.*, 2011), dental implant, oral surgery, prosthetics, and general dentistry applications (Scarfe & Farman, 2008). Chapter 2 provides a historical perspective on the evolution and current status of this technology for applications in dentistry and specifically in orthodontics.

This chapter evaluates the technologies that will influence the future of CT in the next several years. There are several limitations of current scanners that can be overcome using new technology that already is available in the laboratory or for some specialized applications. To a large degree, the market for CT scanners will determine how quickly the translation of new technology into clinical practice will take place.

In a typical hospital radiology setting, 16- and 64-slice scanners are the norm. These multirow detector spiral CT scanners can acquire and reconstruct several thousand slices from a whole body

Cone Beam Computed Tomography in Orthodontics: Indications, Insights, and Innovations, First Edition. Sunil D. Kapila.

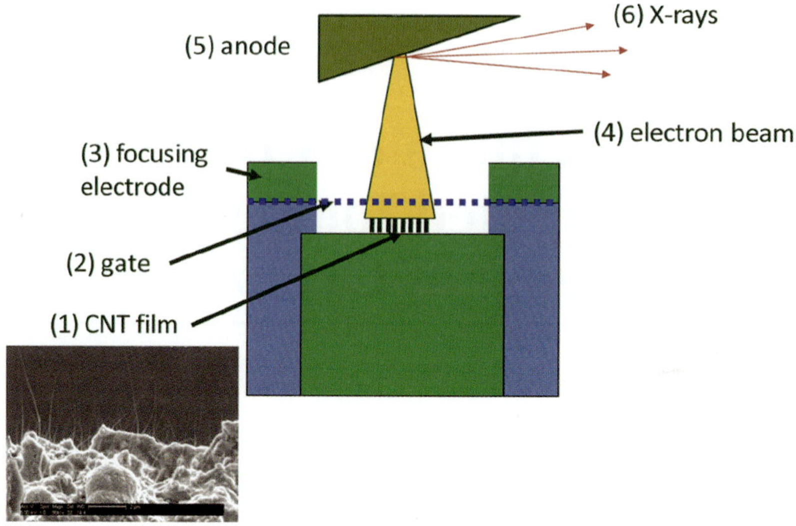

Figure 5.1 Carbon nanotube X-ray source. This cold cathode tube emits electrons from the carbon nanotubes shown in the lower left panel, which strike a tungsten target that emits X-rays. Multiple sources can be constructed in a linear array, for example, so there is no filament and no moving parts. (Reproduced with permission from Sprenger *et al.*, 2011.)

acquisition in less than 2 minutes. A single CT scanner can be used to examine dozens of patients in a single day with a variety of protocols that solve complex diagnostic problems of cancer, cardiopulmonary disease, infection, trauma, and others. Most large hospitals in the United States have several CT scanners in the radiology department, with another (e.g., virtual simulator) in the radiotherapy department.

The technology improvements that motivated the expanded use of CT for whole body applications have not ceased. Future improvements in CT scanning will include new X-ray source, detector, and computational enhancements.

Fundamentally, CT scanning is used to delineate bone and soft tissue. The X-ray attenuation differences at the interface between air and soft tissue as well as between soft tissue structures and bone are high, facilitating post-processing extraction of soft tissue surfaces and bony surfaces for 3D visualization. The soft tissue discrimination of CT is orders of magnitude greater than that found with ordinary radiographs, largely as a result of X-ray collimation, high dynamic range detectors, and reconstruction methods (Hsieh, 2009; Buzug, 2010).

X-RAY SOURCES

Virtually all CT scanners used for biomedical applications employ thermionic emission tungsten target X-ray tubes. These have many similar characteristics to the Crookes tube technology used by Röntgen in 1896 when X-rays were discovered. Despite numerous improvements in X-ray source technology, the fundamental physics of the source remains the same.

In the future, new X-ray source technologies may be adopted. Among the most promising are carbon nanotube (CNT) sources that employ field emission (Xu *et al.*, 2011; Figure 5.1). As cold cathode devices, there is no filament (Lee *et al.*, 2011). They have no moving components and CNT sources can be constructed with a variety of geometries, are significantly less restrictive than the conventional X-ray tube (Wang *et al.*, 2011), and already are in use for animal micoCT (Figure 5.2).

The principal reasons for the continued use of tungsten target tubes today are source brightness, cost, and reliability. Even large patients with transverse body diameters of up to 70 cm and body weight of more than 250 kg can be penetrated

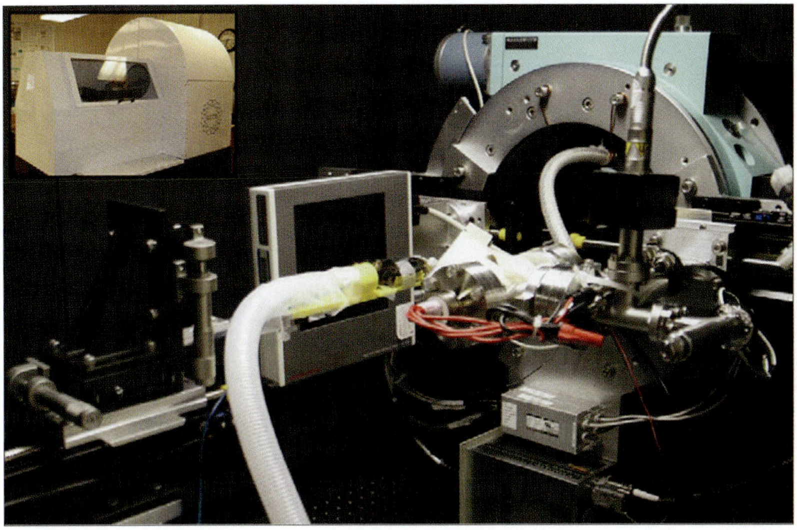

Figure 5.2 Experimental microCT scanner used for animal imaging. This unique device employs a carbon nanotube X-ray source and is housed in an enclosure shown in the upper left panel. (Reproduced with permission from Lee *et al.*, 2011.)

readily to produce high signal-to-noise ratio images with conventional X-ray tubes. This is difficult to achieve with any alternative source. The cost of the tungsten target tube, shielding, and power supply is modest in comparison to any alternative technology.

Modern CT scanners with rotating gantries have a medium frequency power supply and liquid or gas cooled X-ray tube mounted on a frame that rotates around the patient. The mechanical characteristics and weight of this system can tolerate 30 Gs of acceleration when rotated 360° around patients in less than 300 ms. The X-ray source can be operated at 80, 100, 120, or 140 kVp up to 1000 mAs, depending on the patient's body habitus and specific scanning requirements.

DETECTORS

Almost all CT scanners use scintillators linked to photodiodes as detectors. The solid-state systems can be built with sufficient economy and performance to satisfy the demanding requirements of modern scanners. They have significant limitations, however, particularly dose efficiency and electronic noise floor. In the future, direct photon-counting detectors may be perfected and incorporated into CT instruments (Shikhaliev *et al.*, 2009). Photon counting offers significant advantages in low dose performance with reduced electronic noise and the ability to discriminate X-ray energies that carry specific information on the material composition of the imaged objects (Bornefalk, 2011).

Spectral CT

By detecting X-rays with different energies or spectra, it is possible to expand the capabilities of CT, providing better characterization of imaged materials (Figure 5.3 and Figure 5.4). For example, an X-ray beam inspecting a body part may penetrate air, soft tissue, fat, and bone. After administration of intravenous contrast, iodinated agents that enhance blood vessels must be discriminated. Spectral CT can be done at two, three, or more simultaneous energy levels. Using dual energy techniques, it is possible to discriminate structures with calcium, iodinated contrast in vessels, soft tissue, and fat. Beam-hardening artifacts may be suppressed greatly using equivalent monoenergetic CT scan reconstructions reconstructed using dual energy scans (Johnson *et al.*, 2010).

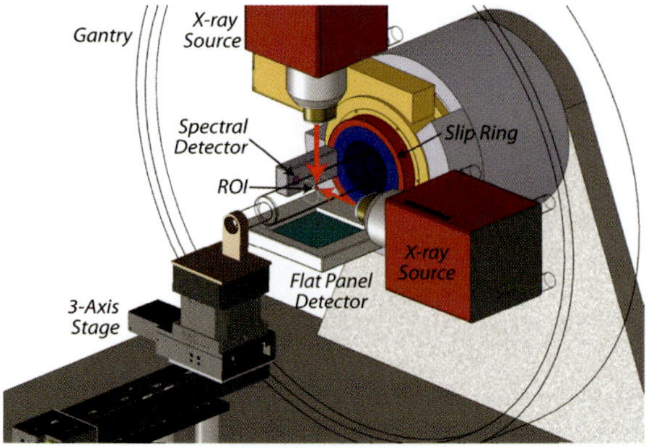

Figure 5.3 Spectral CT scanner with two X-ray sources. One illuminates a flat-panel 2D detector and the other illuminates a spectral detector. The sources and detectors rotate about a three-axis stage. This experimental microCT scanner generates color CT scans that discriminate materials of different composition in addition to attenuation maps that conventional CT scanners produce. (Reproduced with permission from Xu *et al.*, 2012.)

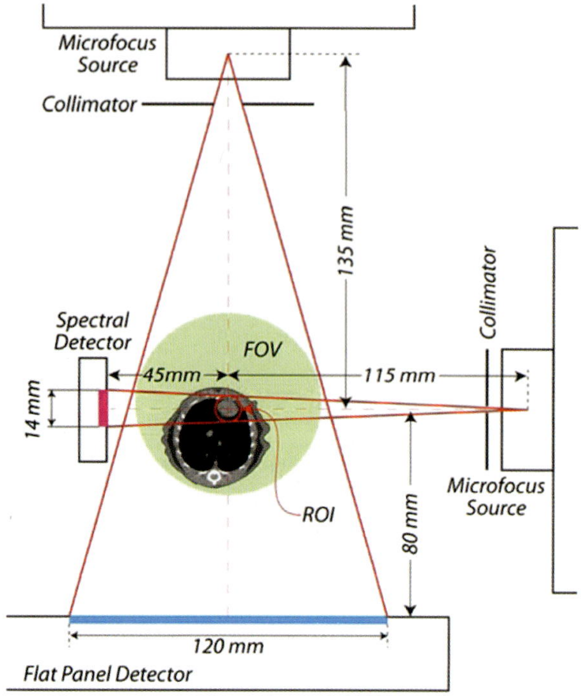

Figure 5.4 Line drawing of the microCT scanner illustrated in Figure 5.3 shows the overall geometry with two X-ray sources and a pair of detectors. The 2D flat-panel detector is similar to conventional CBCT and the spectral detector adds the unique capability to discriminate material composition. (Reproduced with permission from Xu *et al.*, 2012.)

Spectral CT refers to the fact that the X-ray source illuminates body parts with a spectrum of energies that are attenuated differently by structures with varying composition. Spectral CT detectors include the simplest dual energy designs and newer laboratory instruments that can discriminate three, five, or more energy ranges in the detected X-rays. Different materials have variation in X-ray attenuation according to their elemental composition. These can be separated with post-processing image reconstruction to create new CT scan images with a variety of unique and potentially valuable characteristics. For example, the separation of bone and soft tissue can be enhanced. Iodinated contrast within blood vessels can be separated from vascular calcifications due to atherosclerosis in the vessel walls. Artifacts due to metallic appliances can be suppressed. The enhancement of vascular beds by exogenous iodinated contrast can be used to extract CT perfusion parameters such as transit time and blood flow per gram of tissue.

CT image reconstruction

Virtually all biomedical CT scanners have utilized the filtered back-projection method to reconstruct images since the early 1980s when the technique was perfected. Despite years of development, alternative CT reconstruction methods did not become popular until recently (Pan *et al.*, 2009).

Filtered back projection is a technique that modifies the raw projections using a finite impulse response digital filter that can be computed rapidly, followed by a back-projection summation step. This algorithm has been implemented in hardware, and conventional medical scanners that produce a 512 × 512 pixel image matrix can reconstruct up to 40 slices per second on state-of-the-art instruments.

The image quality from filtered back projection has been sufficient to satisfy clinical needs. The computational efficiency of the algorithm and modest implementation cost has resulted in universal adoption of the technique (Hanson, 1980).

The scanner geometry may incorporate a pencil beam, fan beam, or, most recently, cone beam with area detectors, among the most common source-detector geometries that have been implemented. Potentially, all of these can use variations of filtered back projection (Suzuki & Yamaguchi, 1988). For example, the FDK filtered back-projection cone beam reconstruction algorithm (Feldkamp *et al.*, 1984) is used widely because of its computational efficiency and adequate image quality.

Recently, concerns have been expressed regarding the X-ray dose of CT scanning, due to its widespread adoption for medical purposes (Brenner & Hricak, 2010). CT scanning is a high X-ray dose procedure with long continuous exposures at high mAs, delivering much greater radiation dose than static radiography or image-intensified fluoroscopy. Due to the growing popularity of CT, the population dose from this procedure has grown, creating concerns that cancers may result as a consequence of the diagnostic X-ray radiation exposure (Brenner, 2010). These concerns have stimulated the development and incorporation of numerous dose reduction measures into modern CT scanners (Tamm *et al.*, 2011). For example, scanners today have additional shielding, collimation, lower accelerating potentials, and adaptive X-ray dose modulation capability (Halliburton *et al.*, 2011; see also Chapter 3).

There has been major progress in microprocessors used widely in personal computers and workstations. Multicore microprocessors now are commonplace and the computational performance of microprocessors has increased steadily year by year since the initial development of CT. In the early years of CT reconstruction, a minicomputer and later multiple microprocessors were used for image reconstruction, but their performance was insufficient to use algorithms other than filtered back projection. In the past 5 years, the situation has changed and the computational performance of microprocessors now is sufficient to allow much more demanding computational algorithms to be used for practical clinical systems.

So what does this have to do with dose? Using the same set of raw projection data, alternative reconstruction algorithms (e.g., applied to the projection and image spaces) can provide different image quality (Figure 5.5). Thus, substantial image

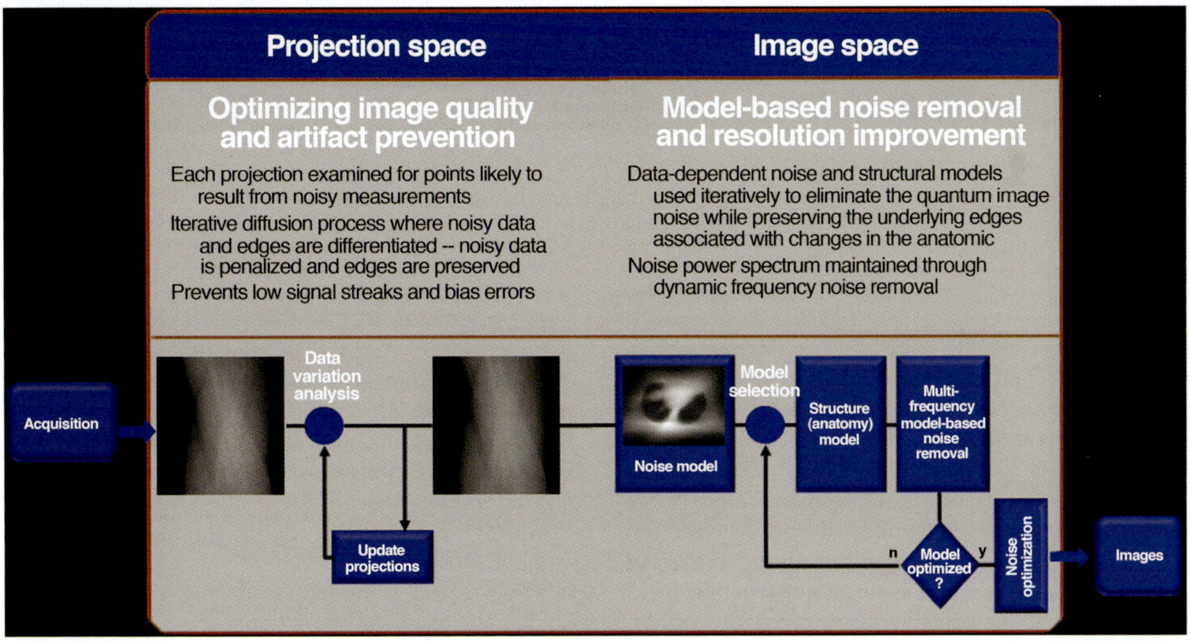

Figure 5.5 Iterative CT reconstruction combines two processes, one performed in projection space and another in image space. Conventional filtered back projection is performed in projection space only. Iterative methods enable greater image quality and artifact suppression, while image space methods suppress noise and can improve resolution. (Reproduced with permission from Philips Healthcare, Inc.)

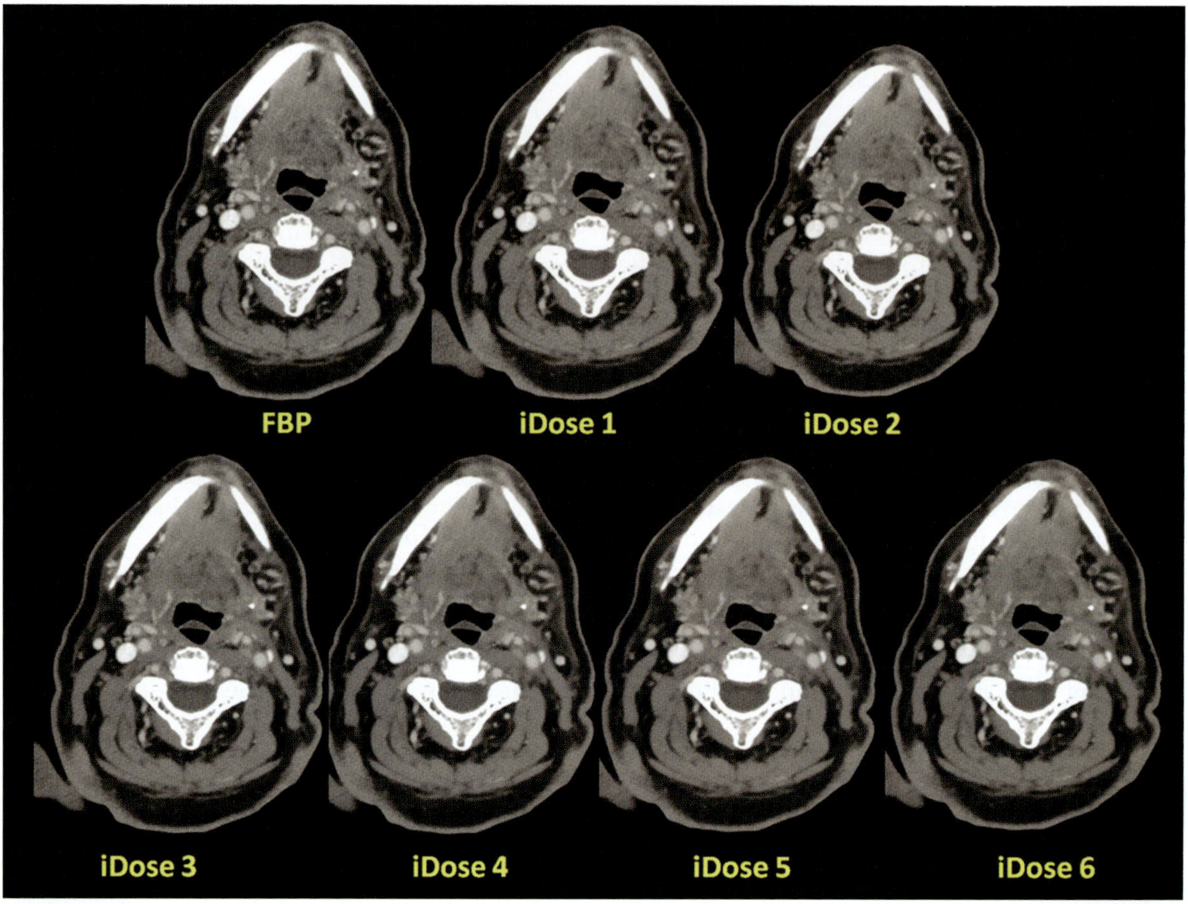

Figure 5.6 Applying an iterative CT reconstruction algorithm to the same CT slice allows noise suppression and resolution enhancement that can be used to reduce X-ray dose requirements substantially, up to 80% without a significant reduction in image quality. Axial CT scan slice through the mandible processed with conventional filtered back projection (FBP) and six levels of iterative construction (iDose levels 1–6). The noise is reduced and apparent detail in images increases proportionately step-by-step with iterative reconstruction.

quality improvements can be made relative to filtered back projection allowing use of lower radiation dose for data acquisition without sacrificing image quality when alternative iterative algorithms are employed. The iterative algorithms make multiple passes through the raw projection data. This increases the computational cost and complexity substantially. New reconstruction techniques, especially based on compressed sensing, promise to reduce computational requirements and to improve image quality in the future (Choi *et al.*, 2009).

A state-of-the-art medical CT scanner in 2014 would include filtered back projection and iterative reconstruction methods as shown in Figure 5.6 and Figure 5.7 with numerous other dose-saving technologies. The dose reduction is difficult to state generally since it depends on the specific patient and CT protocol, but reductions of 80% or more relative to the standard dose only 2 years previously are reported widely (ImPACT, 2011). The improvements in CT technology, which resulted in further dose savings, will continue with the goal of making most CT examinations available in the <1

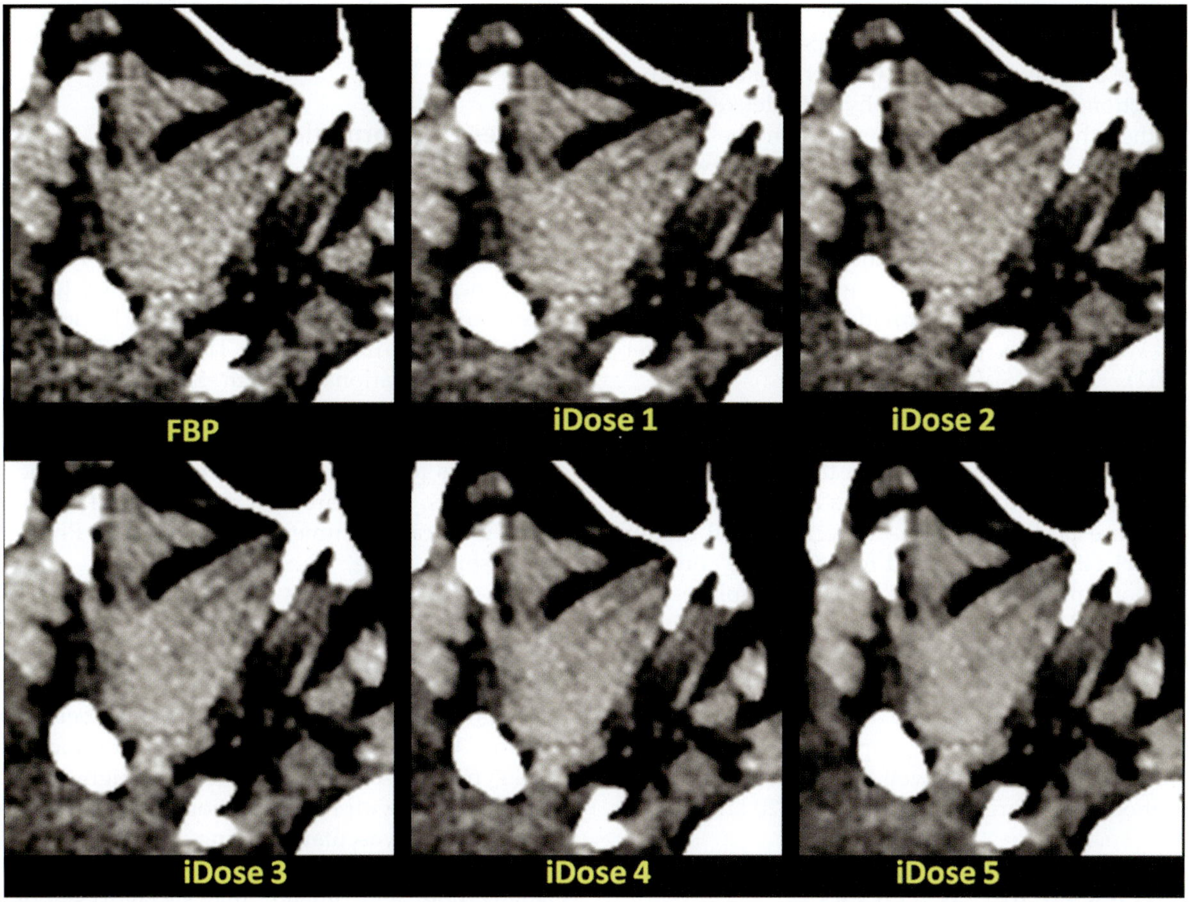

Figure 5.7 By magnifying axial CT images centered on the temporalis fossa, the effect of increasing iterative reconstruction levels can be appreciated. Noise and artifacts are suppressed and soft tissue features appear more homogeneous. Axial CT scans of the left temporalis fossa using a smaller FOV than in Figure 5.6. These images allow detailed comparison of conventional FBP with increasing levels of iterative reconstruction (iDose levels 1–5) and demonstrate step-by-step reduction in noise and artifact suppression.

milli-Sievert (mSv) range. The standard radiation dose from natural sources and cosmic radiation at the Earth's surface is approximately 2–3 mSv per year (World Nuclear Association, 2011), so a sub-mSv CT scan examination of a body part is a major achievement with acceptable safety for many applications.

Post-processing

Medical CT scans rarely are printed on film or other media. Today, most scans are viewed on soft-copy screens throughout the clinical enterprise (Bui & Taira, 2010). Clinicians view CT scans at their office or clinic on ordinary networked PCs. Diagnostic interpretations are rendered with high-resolution monitors at workstations in the radiology department. The images are archived on picture archiving and communication systems (PACS; Huang, 2010), which are ubiquitous in hospitals today. The costs associated with generating, developing, storing, and viewing films have been eliminated (Huang, 2011; Inamura & Kim, 2011; Lemke, 2011).

Visualization and advanced image analysis workstations complement medical CT scanners.

Many procedures have separate reimbursement for post-processing on an independent workstation, especially CT angiography, craniofacial reconstruction, and CT urography (Haidekker, 2010). Rather than process these scans on the scanner itself, an essential resource for collecting new scans, the post-processing is done on a networked workstation (Vannier, 2009) consisting of a PC workstation with high performance display and appropriate software. Enterprise access to visualization and analysis tools now are provided with client/server or Web services technology (Kagadis & Langer, 2011).

Among the most demanding applications for medical CT is cardiopulmonary imaging. Functions to extract the heart from the chest, delineate and label the cardiac chambers and great vessels, measure cardiac function—especially wall motion and ejection fraction—and to extract the coronary tree and measure stenoses are commonplace.

Surgical planning software tools are incorporated in the workstation, for example, to plan radio frequency (RF) ablation of solid tumors or liver metastases, to determine organ volume (sometimes needed in liver transplantation and stereotactic localization), as well as for craniofacial and orthognathic surgery (see Chapters 20 and 23).

OTHER CT APPLICATIONS

In radiotherapy treatment planning, a virtual simulator almost always is employed for dose administration planning. The virtual simulator consists of a specialized CT scanner with treatment planning software on the workstation. The simulator can emulate the setup of the external beam radiotherapy or brachytherapy applicators (Garcia-Ramirez *et al.*, 2002).

Virtually all medical PET scanners sold today include a CT scanner as an integral part of the apparatus. The PET scanners utilize noncontrast CT for attenuation correction and for image overlay correlation with more detailed anatomy.

Portable CT scanners are available widely in tertiary medical centers for use with the ICU patients and in the clinic for orthopedic surgery or otolaryngology (ear, nose, and throat [ENT]). There is a specialized market for compact and inexpensive CT scanners and for oraomaxillofacial imaging with numerous stand-alone instruments.

Sources of information

Simulation frequently is used in the development of new CT reconstruction methods, and several simulators are available on the Internet (Farrell, 2008), including one specifically designed to test cone beam computed tomography (CBCT) methods (Rezvani, 2010; Abbasi, 2011). The ImpaCT^2 project for the UK National Health Service (ImPACT, www.impactscan.org; July 2012) is an important national resource for technology assessments and guidebooks for the worldwide market of medical CT scanners. There are four major manufacturers of the medical instruments: Siemens, GE, Philips, and Toshiba.

High-end CT scanners serve the most demanding applications, principally cardiovascular imaging. These high-end scanners have multirow detectors with relatively wide area coverage. Scanners with between 64 and 320 rows and between 128 and 320 channels are available. They include EKG synchronization accessories and high output X-ray sources, with rapid rotation of the gantry to support cardiovascular imaging. These high-end systems invariably are tied to high-performance visualization and image analysis workstations used to extract the morphologic and functional cardiac information from 4D scanner data sets.

Consumer information regarding the usability and reliability of scanners is provided by organizations such as the ECRI Institute (ECRI Institute, 2012, www.ecri.org; July 2012) and KLAS (Klas, 2012, www.klasresearch.com; July 2012), independent resources that survey and compile the results of experience from the scanner users community.

FUTURE PERSPECTIVES

The growth of CT scanning in the U.S. market has reversed since 2007, as a result of the Deficit Reduction Act (DRA) and healthcare reform measures intended to contain the cost of medical imaging. Many entrepreneurial outpatient facilities with CT scanning have ceased operation as a consequence.

The popularity of CT screening without a specific clinical indication has been slowed—a scenario that probably is applicable to the routine use of CBCT imaging in orthodontics. Despite considerable evidence of potential benefit, CT screening for colon cancer and lung cancer is not reimbursed widely or available. Although these screening techniques potentially may be useful, it is difficult to predict when they will become reimbursable and widely adopted.

The growth of CT scanning in Asia, especially China, has been significant, and numerous designs including specialized instruments built locally have emerged. In the future, CT scanning markets will be based on the reimbursement decisions in each nation's healthcare system as well as potential new markets created by further advances in CT technology and the need to replace older systems to reduce maintenance costs, reduce population dose, or add specialized capabilities such as high-end cardiovascular imaging.

References

Abbasi, N.M. (2011) Computed Tomography Simulation Using the Radon Transform Wolfram Demonstration Project. Available at http://demonstrations.wolfram.com/ComputedTomographySimulationUsingTheRadonTransform/, accessed July 8, 2012.

Bornefalk, H. (2011) Task-based weights for photon counting spectral X-ray imaging. *Medical Physics*, 38 (11), 6065–6073.

Brenner, D.J. (2010) Slowing the increase in the population dose resulting from CT scans. *Radiation Research*, 174 (6), 809–815.

Brenner, D.J. & Hricak, H. (2010) Radiation exposure from medical imaging: time to regulate? *Journal of the American Medical Association*, 304 (2), 208–209.

Bui, A.A.T. & Taira, R. (2010) *Medical Imaging Informatics*. Springer-Verlag, Germany.

Buzug, T.M. (2010) *Computed Tomography: From Photon Statistics to Modern Cone-Beam CT*. Springer-Verlag, Germany.

Choi, J.Y., Kim, M.W., Seong, W., *et al*. (2009) Compressed sensing metal artifact removal in dental CT. In *Proceedings of the IEEE International Symposium on Biomedical Imaging (ISBI), Institute of Electrical and Electronics Engineers (IEE)*, Boston, June 28–July 1, 2009, pp. 334–337.

ECRI Institute (2012) The ECRI Institute. Available at http://www.ecri.org, accessed July 8, 2012.

Farrell, D. (2008) LearnCT: computed tomography image reconstruction interactive simulation. Available at http://homepage.ntlworld.com/jfarrell/javactapp/index.html, accessed May 6.

Feldkamp, L.A., Davis, L.C., Kress, J.W. (1984) Practical cone-beam algorithm. *Journal of the Optical Society of America*, A1, 612–619.

Garcia-Ramirez, J.L., Mutic, S., Dempsey, J.F., *et al*. (2002) Performance evaluation of an 85-cm-bore X-ray computed tomography scanner designed for radiation oncology and comparison with current diagnostic CT scanners. *International Journal of Radiation Oncology, Biology, Physics*, 52 (4), 1123–1131.

Haidekker, M. (2010) *Advanced Biomedical Image Analysis*. Wiley, USA.

Halliburton, S.S., Abbara, S., Chen, M.Y., *et al*. (2011) Society of Cardiovascular Computed Tomography: SCCT guidelines on radiation dose and dose-optimization strategies in cardiovascular CT. *Journal of Cardiovascular Computed Tomography*, 5 (4), 198–224.

Hanson, K.M. (1980) On the optimality of the filtered back projection algorithm. *Journal of Computer Assisted Tomography*, 4 (3), 361–363.

Hodez, C., Griffaton-Taillandier, C., & Bensimon, I. (2011) Cone-beam imaging: applications in ENT. *European Annals of Otorhinolaryngology, Head and Neck Diseases*, 128 (2), 65–78.

Hsieh, J. (2009) *Computed Tomography: Principles, Design, Artifacts, and Recent Advances*, 2nd ed, vol. PM188. SPIE Press, Washington.

Huang, H.K. (2010) *PACS and Imaging Informatics: Basic Principles and Applications*, 2nd ed. Wiley-Blackwell, USA.

Huang, H.K. (2011) Short history of PACS. Part I: USA. *European Journal of Radiology*, 78 (2), 163–176.

ImPACT (2011) ImPACT: imaging performance assessment of CT scanners evaluation center. Available at http://www.impactscan.org/, accessed July 8, 2012.

Inamura, K. & Kim, J.H. (2011) History of PACS in Asia. *European Journal of Radiology*, 78 (2), 184–189.

Johnson, T., Fink, C., Schönberg, S.O., *et al*. (2010) *Dual Energy CT in Clinical Practice*. Springer-Verlag, Germany.

Kagadis, G.C. & Langer, S.G. (2011) *Informatics in Medical Imaging (Imaging in Medical Diagnosis and Therapy)*. CRC Press, USA.

Kalender, W.A. (2011) *Computed Tomography: Fundamentals, System Technology, Image Quality, Application*. 3rd ed. Wiley-VCH, Germany.

Kapila, S., Conley, R.S., & Harrell Jr, W.E. (2011) The current status of cone beam computed tomography imaging in orthodontics. *Dentomaxillofacial Radiology*, 40 (1), 24–34.

KLAS (2012) Klas Enterprises. Available at http://www.klasresearch.com/, Orem, UT, accessed July 10, 2012.

Lee, Y.Z., Burk, L., Wang, K.H., *et al.* (2011) Carbon nanotube based X-ray sources: applications in pre-clinical and medical imaging. *Nuclear Instruments and Methods Physics Research. Section A*, 648 (Suppl. 1), S281–S283.

Lemke, H.U. (2011) Short history of PACS. Part II: Europe. *European Journal of Radiology*, 78 (2), 177–183.

Merrett, S.J., Drage, N.A., & Durning, P. (2009) Cone beam computed tomography: a useful tool in orthodontic diagnosis and treatment planning. *Journal of Orthodontics*, 36 (3), 202–210.

Pan, X., Sidky, E.Y., & Vannier, M. (2009) Why do commercial CT scanners still employ traditional, filtered back-projection for image reconstruction? *Inverse Problems*, 25 (12), 1230009.

Rezvani, N. (2010) OSCaR: An Open-Source Cone-Beam CT Reconstruction Tool for Imaging Research. Available at http://www.cs.toronto.edu/~nrezvani/OSCaR.html, accessed July 8, 2012.

Scarfe, W.C. & Farman, A.G. (2008) What is cone-beam CT and how does it work? *Dental Clinics of North America*, 52 (4), 707–730.

Shikhaliev, P.M., Fritz, S.G., & Chapman, J.W. (2009) Photon counting multienergy X-ray imaging: effect of the characteristic x rays on detector performance. *Medical Physics*, 36 (11), 5107–5119.

Sprenger, F., Calderon, X., Gidcumb, E., *et al.* (2011) Stationary digital breast tomosynthesis with distributed field emission X-ray tube. *Proceedings of SPIE*, 7961, 878280.

Suzuki, S. & Yamaguchi, S. (1988) Comparison between an image reconstruction method of filtering backprojection and the filtered back projection method. *Applied Optics*, 27 (14), 2867–2870.

Tamm, E.P., Rong, X.J., Cody, D.D., *et al.* (2011) Quality initiatives: CT radiation dose reduction: how to implement change without sacrificing diagnostic quality. *Radiographics*, 31 (7), 1823–1832.

Van Vlijmen, O.J., Kuijpers, M.A., Bergé, S.J., *et al.* (2012) Evidence supporting the use of cone-beam computed tomography in orthodontics. *Journal of the American Dental Association*, 143 (3), 241–252.

Vannier, M.W. (2009) Medical imaging workstations: what is missing and what is coming? *Archives of Pathology & Laboratory Medicine*, 133 (4), 542–546.

Wang, S., Calderon, X., Peng, R., *et al.* (2011) A carbon nanotube field emission multipixel X-ray array source for microradiotherapy application. *Applied Physics Letters*, 98 (21), 213701.

World Nuclear Association (2011) Nuclear Radiation and Health Effects. Available at http://www.world-nuclear.org/info/inf05.html, accessed November 11, 2012.

Xu, Q., Yu, H., Bennett, J., *et al.* (2012) Image reconstruction for hybrid true-color micro-CT. *IEEE Transactions on Bio-medical Engineering*, 59 (6), 1711–1719.

Xu, X., Kim, J., Laganis, P., *et al.* (2011) A tetrahedron beam computed tomography benchtop system with a multiple pixel field emission X-ray tube. *Medical Physics*, 38 (10), 5500–5508.

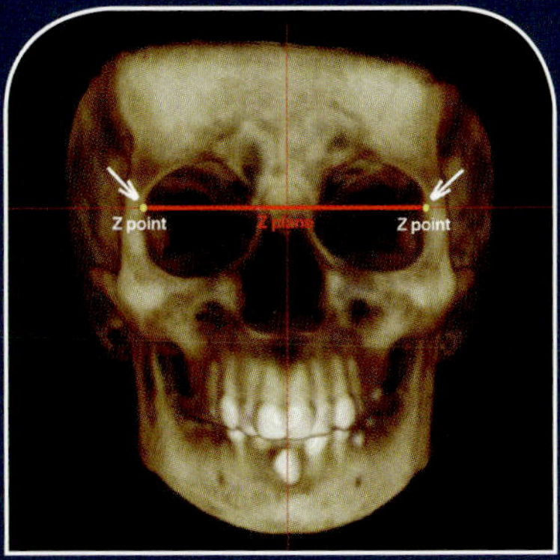

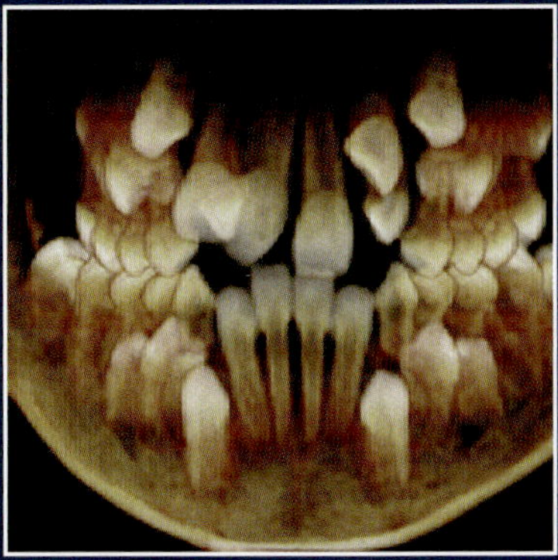

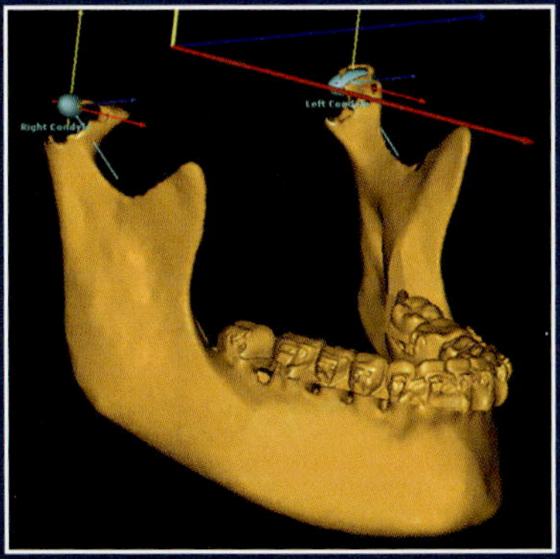

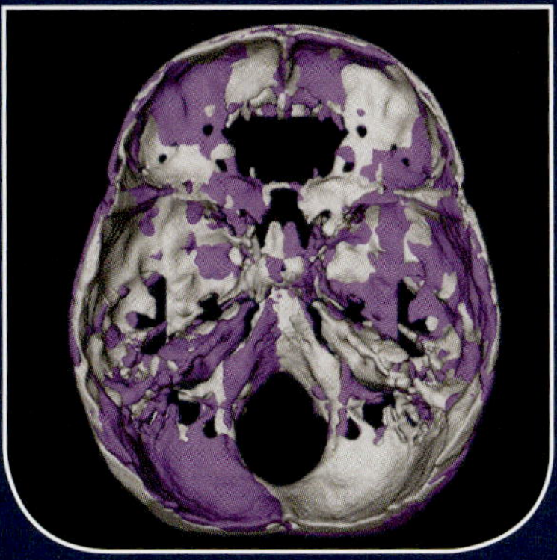

PART 2

Protocols and Principles for Cone Beam Computed Tomography Imaging in Orthodontics

6

Development of Evidence-Based Selection Criteria for Cone Beam Computed Tomography in Orthodontics

William C. Scarfe, BDS, FRACDS, MS, Kirt E. Simmons, DDS, PhD, and Carla A. Evans, DDS, DMSc

INTRODUCTION

The deficiencies of two-dimensional (2D) extraoral radiography for maxillofacial assessment in orthodontics have been recognized for decades (Baumrind *et al.*, 1976; Moyers & Bookstein, 1979; Johnston, 2011; see also Chapters 1 and 4). Thus, while demonstrating a composite of anterior-posterior and vertical relations, 2D extraoral radiography, in particular lateral cephalometric imaging, provides limited information on unilateral or transverse aspects of malocclusions or craniofacial anomalies. To choose the most appropriate therapy from the increasing number of treatment options available, orthodontic planning and management will require an appreciation of the complex anatomic relationships and surrounding structures of the maxillofacial skeleton in specific cases. The introduction of cone beam computed tomography (CBCT) to dentistry at the start of the 21st century has provided orthodontists with a relatively low-cost, in-office, diagnostic imaging technology capable of demonstrating these relationships in the third dimension.

A dramatic increase in the use of CBCT imaging has occurred in the field of dentistry over the last decade. This technology has found particular application in the assessment of orthodontic conditions in both adult and pediatric patients (Hechler, 2008; Kapila *et al.*, 2011). There now are more than 30 different units approved by the U.S. Food and Drug Administration (FDA) for maxillofacial use (Figure 6.1; see also Chapter 2).

This technology has been embraced in orthodontics to the extent that some professionals advocate replacement of traditional cephalometry with CBCT imaging. This often is proposed based on illustrative, but anecdotal, case reports without consideration of the appropriate evidence base in support of such practice or addressing the possible risks involved (Hechler, 2008; Silva *et al.*, 2008; Mah *et al.*, 2010).

Dental practitioners have a professional obligation not only to become familiar with the technical

Cone Beam Computed Tomography in Orthodontics: Indications, Insights, and Innovations, First Edition. Sunil D. Kapila.

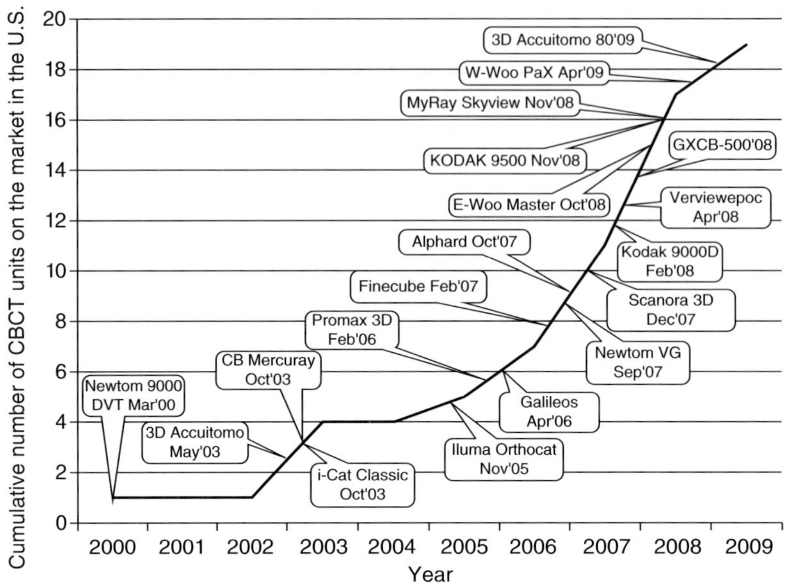

Figure 6.1 Trend for the number of 510(K) FDA approvals for CBCT units in the United States from 2000 to 2010.

and operational aspects of CBCT, but also to understand the scientific validity and health risks of its use in specific applications. As an individual practitioner, this can be a daunting task at a time when information and evidence-based consensus may be conflicting and still evolving. Therefore, the development of clinical use guidelines based on current evidence and best practices can serve an important role in selecting appropriate situations for the use of CBCT. This chapter reviews the development of such clinical use guidelines for the field of orthodontics.

ADVANTAGES AND RISKS OF CBCT IMAGING IN ORTHODONTICS

Advantages of CBCT in orthodontics

There is no doubt that CBCT offers advantages over conventional extraoral imaging, including panoramic and lateral cephalometric radiography, for the visualization of specific clinical conditions, especially when surgical options are considered. These situations, detailed in several other chapters (Chapters 12 and 14–23), include:

(1) Maxillofacial dysmorphology associated with either craniofacial conditions or severe facial asymmetry where orthognathic surgery or distraction osteogenesis is anticipated
(2) Temporomandibular joint (TMJ) articulation issues in patients with diminishing quality of life issues, such as persistent pain or limited opening, or with severe TMJ dysmorphology
(3) Anomalies of the dentition such as impacted teeth and supernumerary teeth and third molars
(4) Maxillary transverse discrepancies if rapid maxillary expansion (RME) is considered
(5) Establishment of dentoalveolar boundaries for orthodontic tooth movement in certain patients such as those with bimaxillary protrusion
(6) Dental alveolar morphology for patients who are potential candidates for dental implants, bone grafts, or temporary anchorage devices (TADs; White & Pae, 2009; Mah *et al.*, 2010; Kapila *et al.*, 2011).

In addition, CBCT may be useful in assessing the treatment outcomes of orthognathic surgery, grafting procedures, and use of nonsurgical devices to affect significant sagittal, vertical or transverse discrepancies (Merrett *et al.*, 2009; Mah *et al.*, 2010; Kapila *et al.*, 2011; see also Chapters 17, 19, 22, and 23).

Many technical and practical issues regarding CBCT operation in orthodontics still remain, however, as applications are evolving and technology is maturing. These include the most appropriate choice of field of view (FOV) and the optimal radiological exposure settings of different scanners to provide diagnostic images for similar tasks (Kwong *et al.*, 2008). Additional controversies related to CBCT use include technical difficulties associated with the fusion of CBCT and surface scan data, the necessity for use of multiple CBCT scans, lack of and utility of three-dimensional (3D) norms, the lack of evidence qualifying the impact of CBCT imaging on treatment outcome, clarification of the responsibility for the diagnosis of incidental findings and pathology, and calibration and maintenance of the equipment (Palomo *et al.*, 2008). Several of these controversies are discussed in further detail in other chapters (Chapters 1, 4, 7, and 10).

Risks involved with CBCT imaging for orthodontics

CBCT imaging uses ionizing radiation; therefore, clinical benefits should be balanced against the potential radiation risks, incorporating an understanding of the relative sensitivity of those who are imaged.

The long-term risks associated with diagnostic radiographic imaging are related to radiation-induced carcinogenesis among patients (see also Chapter 3). Any radiation exposure must be justified clinically and principles and procedures must be applied that minimize patient radiation exposure while optimizing maximal diagnostic benefit. This concept is known as "as low as reasonably achievable" (ALARA; Gelskey & Baker, 1984). The risk of cancer development over a lifetime is determined from absorbed radiation dose in combination with other factors that account for variations in specific tissue radiosensitivity and general patient susceptibility factors (e.g., sex and age).

Effective dose (E) is the currently accepted index used to calculate whole-body dose and measure relative risk from exposure to ionizing radiation. E is calculated by multiplying actual organ doses in specific susceptible tissues by "risk-weighting factors"—which give each organ's relative radiosensitivity to developing cancer—and adding up the total of all the numbers; the sum of the products is the "effective whole-body dose," or simply "effective dose" (International Commission on Radiological Protection, 1991). The estimated risk-weighting factors for specific tissues have been revised recently, and a number of additional tissues found in the head and neck region have been included, most importantly the salivary glands, lymphatic nodes, muscle, and oral mucosa (ICRP, 2007). These modifications have resulted in substantial increases in radiation effective doses for specific maxillofacial radiographic procedures, ranging from 32 to 422% (Ludlow *et al.*, 2008).

The actual risk for maxillofacial radiographic procedures, including CBCT, is difficult to assess, and estimates are based on conservative assumptions. Although radiation may cause cancers at high doses and high-dose rates, no data exist currently to establish unequivocally the occurrence of cancer following exposure to low doses and low-dose rates (below about 100 milliSievert [mSv]). Below this level, in the realm of dental diagnostic radiology, a linear, nonthreshold (LNT) dose-response relationship describing the relation of radiation dose with cancer occurrence currently is the model adopted by regulatory agencies for human radiation exposure in the United States (Preston *et al.*, 2003; National Research Council of the National Academies, Committee to Assess Health Risks from Exposure to Low Levels of Ionizing Radiation, 2006; ICRP, 2007; United Nations Scientific Committee on the Effects of Atomic Radiation, 2008). Acceptance of this dose-response hypothesis implies that any increase in dose, no matter how small, results in an incremental increase in risk (ICRP, 2007); therefore, there is no safe limit or "safety zone" for radiation exposure in orthodontic diagnostic imaging. Every exposure cumulatively increases the risk of cancer induction.

Since the adoption of the new tissue-weighting factors for the calculation of effective dose (ICRP, 2007), numerous authors have reported on the dose

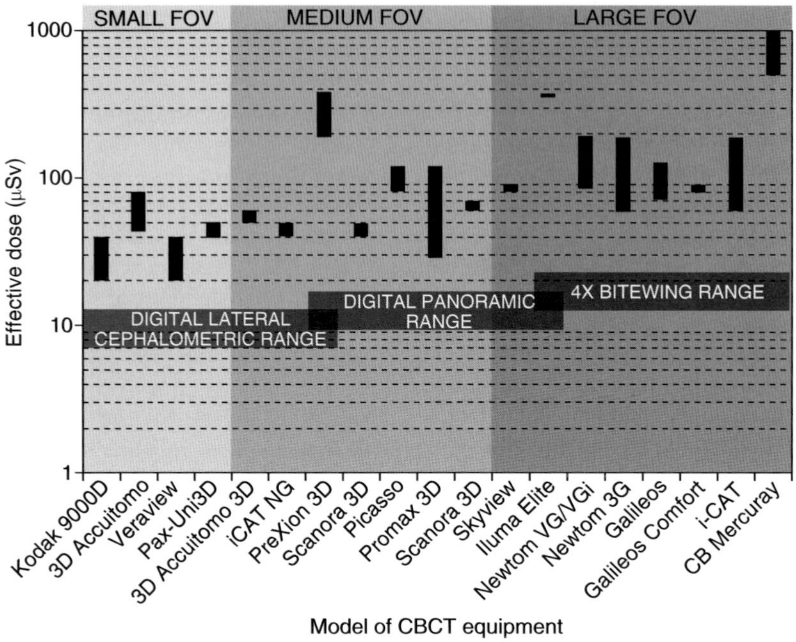

Figure 6.2 Comparison of the range of published effective dose (E_{2007}) for various CBCT units available in the United States according to field of view (FOV; μSv, microSievert). Vertical bar, plotted in a log scale, indicates range of reported values from different studies or different scan parameters for the same unit. Published dose range for extraoral (digital lateral cephalometric and panoramic radiography) and four-image bitewing series are superimposed as horizontal bars for comparison.

of various CBCT systems (Figure 6.2; Coppenrath *et al.*, 2008; Hirsch *et al.*, 2008; Lofthag-Hansen *et al.*, 2008; Loubele *et al.*, 2008; Ludlow & Ivanovic, 2008; Palomo *et al.*, 2008; Silva *et al.*, 2008; Okano *et al.*, 2009; Roberts *et al.*, 2009; Carrafiello *et al.*, 2010; Pauwels *et al.*, 2010; Davies *et al.*, 2012); these are described further in Chapters 2 and 3.

As a trend, the larger the FOV of the CBCT unit, the greater the effective dose to the patient. However, comparable FOV units produce a range of effective doses. Almost all CBCT units impart higher doses than the range reported from digital panoramic, lateral cephalometric, or four-image, bitewing, intraoral radiography (Ludlow *et al.*, 2008; Gavala *et al.*, 2009).

The effective dose for CBCT is an especially important consideration in orthodontics because the modal age for initiating orthodontic treatment occurs in the pediatric age group. For pediatric patients, exposure to ionizing radiation is of particular concern for four reasons:

(1) Younger patients are more radiosensitive than adults. This implies the cancer risk per unit dose of ionizing radiation is higher for younger patients (National Research Council of the National Academies, Committee to Assess Health Risks from Exposure to Low Levels of Ionizing Radiation, 2006).
(2) Younger patients have a longer expected lifetime for the effects of radiation exposure to manifest as cancer.
(3) Organ doses, particularly the salivary glands, and effective doses for children are on average 30% higher than for adolescents with the same exposure (Theodorakou *et al.*, 2012).
(4) Use of equipment and exposure settings designed for adult use can result in excessive radiation exposure for a smaller patient.

Children may be two to ten or more times sensitive to radiation carcinogenesis than mature adults (Brenner *et al.*, 2001; Smith-Bindman *et al.*,

2009). This translates to a mortality risk to children of three to five times that of adults for the same exposure (International Commission on Radiological Protection, 1991; National Research Council of the National Academies, Committee to Assess Health Risks from Exposure to Low Levels of Ionizing Radiation, 2006). As a result of these considerations, the American College of Radiology (2011, 2012) has incorporated considerations of the pediatric effective dose estimate range for specific medical imaging procedures. In addition, there are at least two national radiation safety initiatives to raise awareness of using lower radiation doses to image children: Image Gently™ (The Alliance for Radiation Safety in Pediatric Imaging, 2011) and the National Children's Dose Registry (American College of Radiology, 2012).

SELECTION CRITERIA FOR CBCT IMAGING IN ORTHODONTICS

Fundamentals of criteria development

Clinical practice guidelines are "systematically developed statements to assist practitioner and patient decisions about appropriate health care for specific clinical circumstances" (Field & Lohr, 1990). The statements are intended to be "a distillation of current evidence and opinion on best practice" (Grimshaw & Russell, 1994). In the United States, the term "selection criteria" has been adopted for use in oral and maxillofacial radiology to identify the concept of appropriate diagnostic imaging selection based on patient presentation with specific clinical conditions. This concept promulgates one of the guiding ALARA principles in that there should be a clinically derived rationale for all exposures to ionizing radiation; this concept is referred to as justification. The medical radiography profession, specifically the American College of Radiography (ACR), has applied this concept in their Appropriateness Criteria (Cascade, 1994, 2000). It is important to highlight that selection criteria are but one component of good healthcare decision making, which also should take into account patients' preferences and values, clinicians' values and experience, and the available resources.

The initial recommendations for appropriate radiographic examinations in dentistry in the United States resulted from a panel convened by the FDA in 1983. These initially were published by Matteson and coworkers (1987), and the latest version was published by the U.S. Department of Health and Human Services (Council of Scientific Affairs, 2012). However, these documents provide no clinical protocols for radiography in patients with growth or dental anomalies presenting for orthodontic treatment. Both the European Union (European Commission, 2004, 2012) and the United Kingdom (Isaacson *et al.*, 2008) have dental imaging guidelines stating there are *no* indications for routine radiographs for all orthodontic patients. In the United Kingdom, clinical decision algorithms are used for orthodontic radiography based on the age of the patient and clinical presentation.

Optimal patient care is predicated on applying research-based evidence to clinical practice. The development and adoption of evidence-based practice guidelines often are viewed with skepticism by practicing clinicians. Many perceive that reimbursement decisions by government and/or third-party payers often are based on a prescriptive formula. However, integral to evidence-based practice is the concept that while a particular diagnostic modality may be indicated based on application of a specific clinical algorithm, choice of imaging strategy, treatments, or management plans must be personalized to reflect the specific characteristics of individual clinical circumstances and must be based on professional judgment.

The evidence base for CBCT imaging in orthodontics

Fundamental to evidence-based guidelines development are systematic reviews of the published literature. Systematic reviews use well-defined and reproducible literature search strategies to identify evidence that is directed toward the use of a modality for a specific clinical problem. Evidence then can be graded according to its level, methodological rigor (or quality), relevance, and strength (National Health and Medical Research Council of Australia, 1999).

Van Vlijmen and colleagues (2012) used a search strategy for identifying all CBCT-related articles in orthodontics for six literature databases for the period up to and including March 10, 2010, and found 550 articles. After applying inclusion (human participants only, case series with a sample size of five or more) and exclusion criteria (reviews, letters, and case reports), they found only 50 articles that satisfied adequate scientific rigor. Using a scale of methodological soundness, they reported that quality averaged 53% (range = 15–77%) of the maximum score (100%) and concluded there was limited evidence that CBCT confers an advantage in diagnostic potential, treatment planning, or treatment outcomes. They categorized and reported the frequency of publication of previous research under seven categories:

(1) Assessment of interradicular space, cortical bone thickness, and palatal bone thickness in regard to TAD placement (26%)
(2) Comparison of CBCT-derived and conventional cephalometry in regard to head orientation, orientation of 3D images, and anthropometric analyses (20%)
(3) Orthodontic surgical treatments, specifically with respect to 3D CBCT evaluations of surgically assisted RME, voxel-based superimposition of pre- and post-treatment 3D models, and condylar position after orthodontic surgical treatment (12%)
(4) Airway measurements focusing on airway volume in 3D and comparisons between the airway area in 2D and 3D (10%)
(5) Tooth position, impaction and root resorption before and during orthodontic treatment (12%)
(6) Cleft lip and palate (6%)
(7) Other topics including incidental findings with CBCT, the quality of CBCT images, and the justification and indication for CBCT (14%).

Considering the additional radiation exposure and risks with CBCT, they concluded that the use of CBCT should be justified by further rigorous research to quantify the effects of CBCT on procedures, outcome monitoring, and treatment results.

The need for guidelines

Best practice in orthodontics requires a judicious and, in the void of evidence, conservative approach to imaging based on the use of imaging selection criteria. The choice of modality used for imaging an orthodontic patient should be based on research-supported clinical judgment as to whether the examination is likely to provide a clinical benefit for the patient, in addition to an assessment of the risk. Guidelines for the use of CBCT in orthodontics may be developed with particular consideration to the three-fold increased risk associated with radiation exposure to the largely pediatric patient population. Factors that may be considered in developing guidelines include:

(1) Basing the decision to order a CBCT scan on the patient's history, clinical examination, and the presence of a clinical condition, assuring that the benefits to the patient outweigh the potential risks of exposure to radiation, especially in the case of a child or young adult
(2) Using CBCT only when the clinical question for which imaging is required cannot be answered adequately by lower-dose conventional dental radiography or alternate nonionizing imaging modalities
(3) Avoiding the use of CBCT solely to facilitate the placement of orthodontic appliances such as aligners and computer-bent wires
(4) Creating CBCT protocols that are task-specific and incorporating the imaging goal for the patient's specific presenting circumstances. Such protocols may include considerations of exposure (mA and kVp), minimum image-quality parameters (e.g., number of basis images, resolution), and restriction of the FOV to visualize adequately the region of interest as discussed elsewhere in this book (Chapters 1–3)
(5) Using CBCT solely to generate 2D projected images (e.g., lateral cephalometric, panoramic images) when not otherwise indicated
(6) Refraining from re-exposure of the patient solely to provide 2D images when a previous CBCT scan is available from which these images can be produced.

DETERMINING PATIENT RADIATION DOSE RISK

Orthodontists should be knowledgeable of the radiation risk when performing CBCT imaging and be able to communicate this risk clearly to their patients before imaging. The specific radiation risk of CBCT units in dentistry has been determined most often by comparing CBCT effective-dose estimation to other imaging modalities (e.g., multiples of typical panoramic images or a multislice CT), background equivalent radiation time (e.g., days of background), or radiation detriment (e.g., probability of x per million of stochastic/cancer effect). The failing of this approach is that the base unit for these comparisons (typical panoramic dose, per capita background radiation, weighted probabilities of fatal and nonfatal cancer) often is not absolute and is variable. This means that depending on what panoramic image dose is used for the comparison (e.g., equipment manufacturer and model, film vs. digital acquisition), for example, the risk for CBCT can be over- or underestimated as compared with panoramic radiography.

Because there is a wide range of radiation exposures associated with different diagnostic procedures, the ACR has proposed the use of a Relative Radiation Level (RRL) when considering radiation risk for imaging examinations (Table 6.1; American College of Radiology, 2011, 2012). The RRL levels are based on data from the BEIR VII report (National Research Council of the National Academies, Committee to Assess Health Risks from Exposure to Low Levels of Ionizing Radiation, 2006), wherein it is estimated that approximately one in 1,000 individuals will develop cancer from an exposure of 10 mSv (ICRP, 2007).

Most important for orthodontics, the RRL also includes considerations for pediatric patients. The RRL provides a meaningful method of reporting radiation dose risk, independent of relative benchmark, and is useful for determination of orthodontic radiation dose risk. Therefore, the RRL for various imaging protocols incorporating CBCT at various treatment phases for either a single examination or multiple exposures over a course of orthodontic treatment can be assessed for adults and children using published effective dose calculations (Coppenrath *et al.*, 2008; Hirsch *et al.*, 2008;

Table 6.1 Estimations of relative radiation level designations for children and adults for orthodontics.

Relative Radiation Level	Effective Dose Estimate Range (μSv)	
	Adult	Child
0	0	0
☢	<100	<30
☢☢	100 to 1,000	30 to 300
☢☢☢	1,000 to 10,000	300 to 3,000
☢☢☢☢	10,000 to 30,000	3,000 to 10,000

Source: Reprinted with permission from the American College of Radiology (ACR), 2012. Some of the information in this document was provided with permission from ACR and taken from the ACR Appropriateness Criteria. The ACR is not responsible for any deviations from original ACR Appropriateness Criteria content.

Lofthag-Hansen *et al.*, 2008; Loubele *et al.*, 2008; Ludlow & Ivanovic, 2008; Ludlow *et al.*, 2008; Palomo *et al.*, 2008; Silva *et al.*, 2008; Gavala *et al.*, 2009; Okano *et al.*, 2009; Roberts *et al.*, 2009; Carrafiello *et al.*, 2010; Pauwels *et al.*, 2010; Davies *et al.*, 2012). For example, if a typical imaging protocol for an episode of orthodontic treatment for a child (<18 years) incorporates three digital (Orthophos XG) panoramic images (initial diagnostic and mid- and post-treatment) with 14.2 μSv of effective dose for each exposure (totaling 42.6 μSv; Ludlow *et al.*, 2008) and two digital (photo-stimulable storage phosphor) lateral cephalometric images (initial and post-treatment) with 5.6 μSv for each exposure (totaling 11.2 μSv; Ludlow *et al.*, 2008), then the total equivalent dose over the entire course of treatment can be calculated to be 53.8 μSv. This represents an RRL of ☢☢. This dose can be compared with that from an imaging protocol for an imaging series for a child (<18 years) incorporating a large-FOV CBCT (NewTom VGi) pre-treatment image (194 μSv; Pauwels *et al.*, 2010), two comparable digital (Orthophos XG) panoramic images at mid- and post-treatment at 14.2 μSv for each exposure (totaling 28.4 μSv; Ludlow *et al.*, 2008), and one post-treatment digital (photo-stimulable storage phosphor) lateral cephalometric image at 5.6 μSv (Ludlow *et al.*, 2008), for a cumulative equivalent dose over the entire course of treatment of 228 μSv.

While this is almost four times the absolute dose, radiation risk for a child as estimated by RRL level remains the same (☢☢). This approach underlines the principle that every effort should be made to reduce the effective radiation dose to the patient not only for a single exposure, but more so for the cumulative dose over a course of orthodontic treatment.

MINIMIZING PATIENT RADIATION EXPOSURE

The basic tenet in using ionizing radiation is to minimize patient risks associated with radiation exposure. This can be accomplished through the development of selection criteria. Images of varying dimensions also can be produced by CBCT to cover specific regions of interest by collimating the X-ray beam to expose various FOV volumes. In addition, the operator can adjust exposure settings and resolution, depending on the equipment type and operator preferences. Different CBCT units vary dose by as much as ten-fold for an equivalent FOV examination (Ludlow & Ivanovic, 2008). Additionally, adjustments of exposure factors to improve image quality are available in many CBCT units and can cause as much as seven-fold differences in dose (Ludlow & Ivanovic, 2008). All of these parameters affect the resultant total radiation dose to the patient. Avoiding regions of high relative radiation risk (eyes, thyroid glands) also can reduce the risk to patients. Approaches for minimizing patient radiation exposure are discussed in greater detail in Chapter 3.

Not all available CBCT units currently are capable of implementing exposure reduction techniques to accommodate the difference in exposure risk between children and adults. Recently the U.S. FDA announced that it is seeking public comment on a proposal recommending that manufacturers design new X-ray imaging devices with protocols and instructions that address use on pediatric patients (U.S. Department of Health and Human Services, Food and Drug Administration, Center for Devices and Radiological Health, 2012); this proposal specifically covers dental CBCT devices. Furthermore, it proposes that manufacturers who do not demonstrate adequately that their new X-ray imaging devices are safe and effective in pediatric patients should include a label on their device that cautions against use in children.

CONCLUSIONS

Clinical guidelines to assist dental practitioners on the appropriate use of CBCT in orthodontics must address considerations of clinical presentation, justification, optimization to minimize radiation risk, and practitioner competence. As of 2012, the scientific evidence base is deficient to establish CBCT imaging as a replacement for extraoral (lateral cephalometric and panoramic) radiography in orthodontics. Therefore, as recently stated by the American Dental Association, "CBCT should be considered as an adjunct to standard oral imaging modalities." Furthermore, the ADA states that "CBCT may supplement or replace conventional (two dimensional or panoramic) dental radiography for the diagnosis, monitoring and treatment of oral disease or the management of oral conditions when, in the clinician's decision-making process, he or she determines that oral anatomical structures of interest may not be captured adequately by means of conventional radiography" (American Dental Association Council on Scientific Affairs, 2012). As evidence evolves, a number of general recommendations for prudent use of CBCT in orthodontics should be made, as children have a three to five times greater radiation risk than adults for the same exposure. Specific recommendations should be based on such variables as phase of treatment, clinically assessed treatment difficulty, presence of dental and/or skeletal modifying conditions, and pathology. Guidance should be directed toward the overall appropriateness of CBCT based on current evidence and include suggested appropriate imaging parameters. Practitioners have an obligation to be mindful of the radiation risk of individual imaging exposures, as well as cumulative effective doses related to an episode of orthodontic care, and to relate these to the evidence-supported benefits of imaging on an individual basis, with full patient participation in the decision process.

ACKNOWLEDGMENTS

We are indebted to our colleagues Drs. Lucia Cevidanes, Martin Palomo, Stu White, John Ludlow, and Mansur Ahmad for the opportunity to discuss and develop many of the concepts related to CBCT selection criteria in orthodontics presented in this chapter. Some of the information in this document was provided with permission from the ACR and taken from the ACR Appropriateness Criteria. The ACR is not responsible for any deviations from original ACR Appropriateness Criteria content.

References

American Academy of Oral and Maxillofacial Radiology (2013) Clinical recommendations regarding use of cone beam computed tomography in orthodontics [corrected]. Position statement by the American Academy of Oral and Maxillofacial Radiology. *Oral Surgery, Oral Medicine, Oral Pathology, Oral Radiology*, 116 (2), 238–257. Erratum in *Oral Surgery, Oral Medicine, Oral Pathology, Oral Radiology*, 116 (5), 661.

American College of Radiology (2011) ACR Appropriateness Criteria®: Rating Round Information. Available at http://www.acr.org/~/media/ACR/Documents/AppCriteria/RatingRoundInfo.pdf, accessed September 23, 2011.

American College of Radiology (2012) ACR Appropriateness Criteria®: Radiation Dose Assessment Introduction. Available at https://nrdr.acr.org/Portal/QuIRCC/Main/page.aspx, accessed January 7, 2013.

American Dental Association Council on Scientific Affairs (2012) The use of cone-beam computed tomography in dentistry: an advisory statement from the American Dental Association Council on Scientific Affairs. *Journal of the American Dental Association* 143 (8), 899–902.

Baumrind, S., Miller, D., & Molthen, R. (1976) The reliability of head film measurements. 3: tracing superimposition. *American Journal of Orthodontics and Dentofacial Orthopedics*, 70 (6), 617–644.

Brenner, D.J., Elliston, C.D., Hall, E.J., *et al.* (2001) Estimated risks of radiation-induced fatal cancer from pediatric CT. *American Journal of Roentgenology*, 176 (2), 289–296.

Carrafiello, G., Dizonno, M., Colli, V., *et al.* (2010) Comparative study of jaws with multislice computed tomography and cone-beam computed tomography. *La Radiologia Medica*, 115 (4), 600–611.

Cascade, P.N. (1994) Setting appropriateness guidelines for radiology. *Radiology*, 192 (1), 50A–54A.

Cascade, P.N. (2000) The American College of Radiology: ACR appropriateness criteria project. *Radiology*, 214 (Suppl), 3–46.

Coppenrath, E., Draenert, F., Lechel, U., *et al.* (2008) Cross-sectional imaging in dentomaxillofacial diagnostics: dose comparison of dental MSCT and NewTom 9000 DVT. *RoFo*, 180 (5), 396–401 (in German).

Council of Scientific Affairs, American Dental Association, Food and Drug Administration, U.S. Department of Health and Human Services (2012) Dental Radiographic Examinations: Recommendations for Patient Selection and Limiting Radiation Exposure: Revised 2012. Available at http://www.fda.gov/downloads/Radiation-EmittingProducts/RadiationEmittingProductsandProcedures/MedicalImaging/MedicalX-Rays/UCM329746.pdf accessed January 6, 2013.

Davies, J., Johnson, B., & Drage, N.A. (2012) Effective doses from cone beam CT investigation of the jaws. *Dentomaxillofacial Radiology*, 41 (1), 30–36.

European Commission (2004) Radiation Protection 136 European Guidelines on Radiation Protection in Dental Radiology: The Safe Use of Radiographs in Dental Practice. Available at http://ec.europa.eu/energy/nuclear/radioprotection/publication/doc/136_en.pdf, accessed January 6, 2012.

European Commission (2012). Radiation Protection No 172. Cone Beam CT for Dental and Maxillofacial Radiology: Evidence Based Guidelines. Available at http://ec.europa.eu/energy/nuclear/radiation_protection/doc/publication/172.pdf, accessed January 6, 2013.

Field, M.J. & Lohr, K.N. (1990) *Clinical Practice Guidelines: Directions for a New Program*. Institute of Medicine, National Academy Press, Washington, DC.

Gavala, S., Donta, C., Tsiklakis, K., *et al.* (2009) Radiation dose reduction in direct digital panoramic radiography. *European Journal of Radiology*, 71 (1), 42–48.

Gelskey, D.E. & Baker, C.G. (1984) The ALARA concept: population exposures from x rays in dentistry: as low as reasonably achievable? *Journal of the Canadian Dental Association*, 50 (5), 402–403.

Grimshaw, J.M. & Russell, I.T. (1994) Achieving health gain through clinical guidelines. II: ensuring guidelines change medical practice. *Quality in Health Care*, 3 (1), 45–52.

Hechler, S.L. (2008) Cone-beam CT: applications in orthodontics. *Dental Clinics of North America*, 52 (4), 753–759.

Hirsch, E., Wolf, U., Heinicke, F., *et al.* (2008) Dosimetry of the cone-beam computed tomography

Veraviewepocs 3D compared with the 3D Accuitomo in different fields of view. *Dentomaxillofacial Radiology*, 37 (5), 268–273.

International Commission on Radiological Protection (1991) The 1990 Recommendations of the International Commission on Radiological Protection, ICRP Publication 60. *Annals of the International Commission on Radiological Protection*, 21, 1–3.

International Commission on Radiological Protection (2007) The 2007 Recommendations of the International Commission on Radiological Protection. ICRP Publication 103. Valentin, J. ed. *Annals of the International Commission on Radiological Protection* 37 (2–4).

Isaacson, K.G., Thom, A.R., Horner, K., *et al.* (2008) *Orthodontic Radiographs: Guidelines for the Use of Radiographs in Clinical Orthodontics*. 3rd ed. British Orthodontic Society, London.

Johnston, L.E. Jr. (2011) A few comments on an elegant answer in search of useful questions. *Seminars in Orthodontics*, 17, 13–14.

Kapila, S., Conley, R.S., & Harrell, W.E. Jr. (2011) The current status of cone beam computed tomography imaging in orthodontics. *Dentomaxillofacial Radiology*, 40 (1), 24–34.

Kwong, J.C., Palomo, J.M., Landers, M.A., *et al.* (2008) Image quality produced by different CBCT settings. *American Journal of Orthodontics and Dentofacial Orthopedics*, 133 (2), 317–327.

Lofthag-Hansen, S., Thilander-Klang, A., Ekestubbe, A., *et al.* (2008) Calculating effective dose on a cone-beam computed tomography device: 3D Accuitomo and 3D Accuitomo FPD. *Dentomaxillofacial Radiology*, 37 (2), 72–79.

Loubele, M., Van Assche, N., Carpentier, K., *et al.* (2008) Comparative localized linear accuracy of small-field cone-beam CT and multislice CT for alveolar bone measurements. *Oral Surgery, Oral Medicine, Oral Pathology, Oral Radiology, and Endodontics*, 105 (4), 512–518.

Ludlow, J.B. & Ivanovic, M. (2008) Comparative dosimetry of dental CBCT devices and 64-slice CT for oral and maxillofacial radiology. *Oral Surgery, Oral Medicine, Oral Pathology, Oral Radiology, and Endodontics*, 106 (1), 930–938.

Ludlow, J.B., Davies-Ludlow, L.E., & White, S.C. (2008) Patient risk related to common dental radiographic examinations: the impact of 2007 International Commission on Radiological Protection recommendations regarding dose calculation. *Journal of the American Dental Association*, 139 (9), 1237–1243.

Mah, J.K., Huang, J.C., & Choo, H. (2010) Practical applications of cone-beam computed tomography in orthodontics. *Journal of the American Dental Association*, 141 (Suppl 3), 7S–13S.

Matteson, S.R., Joseph, L.P., Bottomley, W., *et al.* (1987) *The Selection of Patients for X-Ray Examinations: Dental Radiographic Examinations*. Center for Devices and Radiological Health, U.S. Department of Health and Human Services, Public Health Service, Food and Drug Administration, Washington, DC.

Merrett, S.J., Drage, N.A., & Durning, P. (2009) Cone beam computed tomography: a useful tool in orthodontic diagnosis and treatment planning. *Journal of Orthodontics*, 36 (3), 202–210.

Moyers, R.E. & Bookstein, F.L. (1979) The inappropriateness of conventional cephalometrics. *American Journal of Orthodontics and Dentofacial Orthopedics*, 75 (6), 599–617.

National Health and Medical Research Council of Australia (1999) A Guide to the Development, Implementation and Evaluation of Clinical Practice Guidelines. Available at http://www.nhmrc.gov.au/_files_nhmrc/publications/attachments/cp30.pdf, accessed September 23, 2011.

National Research Council of the National Academies, Committee to Assess Health Risks from Exposure to Low Levels of Ionizing Radiation (2006) *Health Risks from Exposure to Low Levels of Ionizing Radiation: BEIR VII—Phase 2*. The National Academies Press, Washington, DC.

Okano, T., Harata, Y., Sugihara, Y., *et al.* (2009) Absorbed and effective doses from cone beam volumetric imaging for implant planning. *Dento Maxillo Facial Radiology*, 38 (2), 79–85.

Palomo, J.M., Rao, P.S., & Hans, M.G. (2008) Influence of CBCT exposure conditions on radiation dose. *Oral Surgery, Oral Medicine, Oral Pathology, Oral Radiology, and Endodontics*, 105 (6), 773–782.

Pauwels, R., Beinsberger, J., Collaert, B., *et al.* (2010) Effective dose range for dental cone-beam computed tomography scanners. *European Journal of Radiology*, 81 (2), 267–271.

Preston, D.L., Shimizu, Y., Pierce, D.A., *et al.* (2003) Studies of mortality of atomic bomb survivors. Report 13: solid cancer and non-cancer disease mortality: 1950–1997. *Radiation Research*, 160 (4), 381–407.

Roberts, J.A., Drage, N.A., Davies, J., *et al.* (2009) Effective dose from cone-beam CT examinations in dentistry. *British Journal of Radiology*, 82 (973), 35–40.

Silva, M.A., Wolf, U., Heinicke, F., *et al.* (2008) Cone-beam computed tomography for routine orthodontic treatment planning: a radiation dose evaluation. *American Journal of Orthodontics and Dentofacial Orthopedics*, 133 (5), 640.

Smith-Bindman, R., Lipson, J., Marcus, R., *et al.* (2009) Radiation dose associated with common computed tomography examinations and the associated lifetime attributable risk of cancer. *Archives of Internal Medicine*, 169 (22), 2078–2086.

The Alliance for Radiation Safety in Pediatric Imaging (2011) Image Gently™. Available at http://www.imagegently.org, accessed December 21, 2011.

Theodorakou, C., Walker, A., Horner, K., *et al.* (2012) Estimation of paediatric organ and effective doses from dental cone-beam CT using anthropomorphic phantoms. *British Journal of Radiology*, 85 (1010), 153–160.

United Nations Scientific Committee on the Effects of Atomic Radiation (2008) *Effects of Ionizing Radiation: United Nations Scientific Committee on the Effects of Atomic Radiation: UNSCEAR 2006 Report, Volume 1: Report to the General Assembly, with Scientific Annexes A and B*. United Nations, New York.

U.S. Department of Health and Human Services, Food and Drug Administration, Center for Devices and Radiological Health (2012) Draft Guidance for Industry and Food and Drug Administration Staff: Pediatric Information for X-Ray Imaging Device Premarket Notifications. Available at http://www.fda.gov/MedicalDevices/DeviceRegulationandGuidance/GuidanceDocuments/ucm300850.htm, accessed May 12, 2012.

van Vlijmen, O.J.C., Kuijpers, M.A.R., Berge, S.J., *et al.* (2012) Evidence supporting the use of cone-beam computed tomography in orthodontics. *Journal of the American Dental Association*, 143 (3), 241–252.

White, S.C. & Pae, E.-K. (2009) Patient image selection criteria for cone-beam computed tomography imaging. *Seminars in Orthodontics*, 15, 19–28.

7 To Scan or Not to Scan: Medico-Legal Implications

Bernard Friedland, BChD, MSc, JD

INTRODUCTION

The question of whether or not to perform a particular diagnostic or treatment procedure on a specific patient is a complex one involving clinical findings, patient preferences—which may include family, social, and cultural considerations, religious beliefs, and ability to pay, among others—and the standard of care. While cone beam computed tomography (CBCT) has been in clinical use since the early 2000s (Sukovic, 2003), for most practitioners it is still in a relatively nascent stage with respect to its use in orthodontics and cannot be said to constitute the standard of care at the present time. Opinions run the gamut from advocating the use of CBCT on every patient to the view that it has a limited role to play in the average orthodontic patient. "To scan or not to scan" thus is a question currently facing all orthodontists. Although evidence-based selection criteria are being developed (see Chapters 1 and 6) and will continue to evolve, the answer to this question is much in flux and is in large part unanswerable currently. However, two points can be made with near certainty. First, it is not appropriate to scan every orthodontic patient; to argue otherwise is to demonstrate a fundamental misunderstanding of the difference between a diagnostic test and a screening procedure (Grimes & Schulz, 2002). Second, it is equally wrong to assert that no patient should be scanned, for some surely will benefit from the information provided. The challenge for the orthodontic profession is to establish selection criteria between these two extremes in such a manner that it is useful clinically.

For the individual orthodontist, when deciding whether or not to take a CBCT scan on a patient, the issue comes down to the standard of care. This chapter is not a discussion of any individual's opinion of whether and when a CBCT scan

Cone Beam Computed Tomography in Orthodontics: Indications, Insights, and Innovations, First Edition. Sunil D. Kapila.

is indicated for the orthodontic patient. Neither is it an in-depth discussion on how the specialty of orthodontics should decide that question, although that will be mentioned briefly. Rather this chapter explores: (1) how the standard of care is determined and to which sources practitioners may turn for guidance during the nascent stage of a new technology, and (2) what the "average qualified" or "reasonably prudent" practitioner should do when there is no clearly defined standard based on common usage or as defined by the courts. The chapter concludes by examining some associated ethical and regulatory issues regarding the clinical use of CBCT, thus providing insights on how an individual orthodontist might determine whether a CBCT scan is or has become the standard of care and, if so, when he or she ought to order a scan for a particular patient. The information provided in this chapter is supplemented elsewhere in this book (Chapters 1 and 6) by the emerging evidence-based and case-based selection criteria that emphasize the need to determine the benefit-to-risk ratio prior to CBCT scanning of any given patient.

This chapter addresses only one of the medico-legal aspects related to clinical uses of CBCT, namely, whether or not to scan a patient. There is a multitude of other medico-legal and legal issues related to the CBCT. These include matters related to the purchasing and ownership of a CBCT machine (e.g., what are the legal issues if you choose to buy one in conjunction with a physician?) and the responsibility for interpreting the images. The latter itself raises a plethora of issues, among them being where the radiologist who is interpreting the images needs to licensed if a clinician opts to send a CBCT scan to be read by an out-of-state radiologist. An additional legal issue arises when dentists including orthodontists seek to limit their liability for reading CBCT scans, especially when they read the images themselves, by asking patients to sign a waiver of liability. Of practical importance too is whether a dentist's malpractice insurance carrier will cover a dentist who owns a machine and takes CBCT scans and interprets them for other dentists. For these and other medico-legal issues, the reader is referred to an article in which these issues are discussed in depth (Friedland, 2009).

STANDARD OF CARE

Why is the standard of care relevant or important?

Clinicians typically think most explicitly and consciously about the standard of care when they find themselves at the receiving end of a malpractice suit. Subconsciously, however, they apply the standard of care every time they contemplate whether or not to render treatment or perform a diagnostic test (henceforth referred to collectively as procedure[s]) and, if so, how to undertake it appropriately. Thus, the standard of care's primary purpose is not medico-legal in nature; rather, it is indispensable to the everyday practice of the profession. It is used on a daily basis in deciding what the appropriate course of action is for a particular patient and what to include in the informed consent discussion. Without a standard of care, it would be difficult at best for an individual clinician to know what the appropriate diagnostic and treatment choices are. At a minimum, it serves as a starting point for considering which procedures are appropriate in a given situation. The standard of care has implications beyond the primary aforementioned medical purpose. For example, it may determine whether insurers will cover the cost of care, something that obviously is of concern to both the patient and the clinician.

How does a procedure become the standard of care?

Practitioners often perceive incorrectly that the standard of care is a legally mandated standard set by the court or somehow mandated by their medical malpractice carrier. With this mind, we shall examine some issues related to the standard of care. Who and what determine the standard of care? How would an orthodontist know if and when a procedure, in this case CBCT, is the standard of care?

Unlike drugs, which are introduced into the market upon acceptance by the Food and Drug Administration (FDA), there is no overarching governmental organization that approves or provides for an orderly process for the introduction of new procedures. There also is no private group or organization, no matter how well respected in the profession, that is recognized as having the *legal* authority to establish the standard of care or to mandate a formal mechanism by which a new procedure becomes the standard of care. At one time, it had been suggested that a government agency, the National Center for Health Care Technology (NCHCT), could assume the role of the FDA vis-à-vis medical procedures. Whether this would have proved practical or had any effect is a moot point as the NCHCT was relatively short-lived, having been in existence from only 1979 to 1982 (http://healthaffairs.org/blog/2009/01/22/the-national-center-for-health-care-technology-lessons-learned/, accessed January 5, 2013).

Only rarely is the standard of care established in an instant. In the overwhelming majority of cases it is a slow, imperceptible process, and the time at which a procedure or test became the standard of care often may be recognized only in hindsight. There are a number of ways in which something may become or get recognized as the standard of care. Necheles (1982) explored a few different procedures and how each one came to be accepted as the standard of care. He described how renal transplantation came to be accepted as the standard of care in an unusual manner, namely, through the political process, before it became accepted as such by the medical profession. This resulted from a decision by Congress to enact 42 U.S.C. §426-1, the end-stage renal disease program, an act that still remains in effect (Eggers, 2000). As explained by Necheles (1982), although the decision by Congress was supportable on scientific grounds, it was *Congress's* decision that led to the acceptance of kidney transplants as a routine medical procedure.

During and after an investigational phase, a procedure may hover at the margin of clinical acceptance before becoming the standard of care or falling into abeyance. It may make the jump to clinical practice based on one or more respected institution's decisions to offer the procedure as routine medical care or as a result of the procedure's endorsement by practitioners who are regarded highly by their peers. Alternatively, a procedure may evolve from an experimental stage to a clinically accepted standard of care when third-party payers decide to cover the cost of such care. This is especially true of Medicare and Medicaid's decisions to cover the cost of procedures. Private payer's decisions as to whether to cover a procedure often follow a decision by Medicare and Medicaid to cover that procedure (http://www.prgweb.com/resources/key_elements_of_reimbursement.php, accessed January 5, 2013; http://www.emersonconsultants.com/_assets/document/Fundamentals_of_Reimbursement_Chapter.pdf, accessed January 5, 2013). In its early days, Medicare and Medicaid's decisions often were based on flimsy evidence. Fink (1981) describes how, as a just graduated second-year medical student in the early days of Medicare, he made coverage decisions for Medicare based on talking to physicians who had done the new procedure, as well as to experts in the field. In those days, that was the sum total of the evidence used to make a decision, at least by Medicare and Medicaid.

Decisions by payers, whether governmental or private, are not dispositive of whether a procedure constitutes the standard of care. However, a decision to pay would be some indication of a procedure's acceptance by the insurance community and, thus, more meaningful than a decision not to cover a procedure, since the latter may be motivated primarily as a cost-containment measure. In dentistry, in particular, where the use of the word "insurance" really is a misnomer (Weiss *et al.*, 2003), a decision not to cover a procedure frequently involves primarily or exclusively financial considerations for insurers. Thus, the decision to cover a procedure in dentistry is far more meaningful than a decision not to cover it.

In one of the rare instances in which a test or procedure became the standard of care overnight, the Washington state supreme court held that an ophthalmologist was liable for a patient who developed glaucoma at a much younger age than what is typical. The patient had seen the ophthalmologist for several years, beginning in her thirties. The experts for both the plaintiff and defendant testified that the standard of ophthalmologic care did not require routine pressure tests for glaucoma on patients younger than 40 years of age, since the condition is so rare prior to that age. Despite this expert testimony, the court held the ophthalmologist liable, thereby making testing for glaucoma in even young patients the standard of care overnight. The court based its finding on the fact that the test is simple, relatively inexpensive, objective, and definitive in diagnosing the condition and that development of the condition is devastating (*Helling v. Carey*, 1974). It is rare indeed for a court to hold that an entire profession was practicing negligently, but the case illustrates one way in which a procedure may become a standard of care. Interestingly, despite the court's decision, ophthalmologists did not begin administering the test to everyone under age 40 automatically. Subsequent to the court's decision, the Washington legislature passed a statute in an attempt to have the standard of care revert to what it had been previously, a standard which will be examined below. Although not relevant to this discussion here, there are interesting subsequent Washington state cases discussing whether the language in the statute accomplished the legislature's intent.

In the overwhelmingly majority of cases—indeed, almost universally so—the standard of care is determined by what clinicians actually do in practice. For example, Massachusetts holds that the standard of care is determined by the degree of care and skill of the average qualified practitioner (*Brune v. Belinkoff*, 1968), while Washington state pronounced that a professional's conduct is to be measured against that of a reasonably prudent practitioner (*Harris v. Groth*, 1983). While the precise wording of courts may differ, the intent and effect is the same, namely, it is the professionals "in the field" who set the standard of care. The *Brune* court refers to the care and skill of the *average* qualified practitioner. Clearly, the court could not have meant this statement literally as, by definition, a good many practitioners fall below the standard of the *average* qualified practitioner. Keeton and associates (1984) explained the court's intent by stating, "It is not the middle but the minimum common skill." The *Brune* court added to its enunciated standard the phrase, "Taking into account the advances in the profession." The latter is an affirmation that one cannot keep doing things only the way one was taught—one must keep up with the times, which is highly relevant to the utilization of CBCT in orthodontics. Continuing education and updating curriculum in teaching programs is, of course, the key to staying current.

In the setting of a trial, a jury typically hears from the plaintiff's and the defendant's experts as to what is the standard of care. These experts may base their opinions on experience, knowledge of clinical practice, and texts, treatises, articles, and professional guidelines that the judge, in his or her discretion, may admit into evidence. All of these may be introduced only through an expert witness who must validate or establish the publication as authoritative before it will be allowed into evidence. It then is up to the jury to decide what and whom to believe. It is critical to understand that an expert witness cannot testify to what he or she thinks the standard of care *should* be, only to what it *is*, or at least what he or she thinks it is. And what it *is* depends on what the average qualified practitioner does. To reiterate, the standard of care is set by the profession itself through its practitioners and not by one or more trial experts or by a judge or jury.

NEW PROCEDURES

A difficult dilemma for the practicing clinician regarding the standard of care

The issue of whether something constitutes the standard of care is vexing particularly with regard to a new procedure. Clearly, the majority of "average qualified practitioners" do not adopt a new procedure at the same time. Some will be early adopters; the majority will follow later; a few will follow much later; and some perhaps not at all. In determining the standard of care, courts look to the numbers of practitioners who use the procedure. Thus, practitioners who are or who consider themselves to be at the cutting edge theoretically may place themselves at risk of being accused of substandard care when they are early adopters. However, courts also look to the credentials of those who use a procedure, affording the procedure greater status if the adopters, even though a minority, are respected within the profession. Some jurisdictions explicitly follow the "respectable minority" rule (Cramm *et al.*, 2002), which states, "A physician does not incur liability merely by electing to pursue one of several recognized courses of treatment" (*Downer v. Veilleux*, 1974). Thus, courts accept that there may be a range of acceptable practices. Not all states recognize the rule explicitly, but many, perhaps even a majority, apply it *sub silentio*. The latter means that even though a court or legislature of a state has not mentioned explicitly that it recognizes the respectable minority rule, the rule is implied. This implication usually is evident from the instructions to or decisions of the jury, which appellate courts subsequently have tended to uphold. The rule often is invoked as a defense. To the extent the author is aware, a practitioner has not invoked this rule as a defense with regard to a new, supposedly superior technology or procedure. Most commonly, the rule is invoked when a practitioner uses one of two lesser-used procedures, both of which have been in use for some time. Unfortunately, courts have not defined what they mean by the term "respectable." It could refer to the number of individuals as in "a respectable number of people attended the concert," or it may refer to the esteem in which people are held, as in "they are respectable members of the community." Most commentators assume the standard to incorporate elements of both number and reputation.

The professional guidelines mentioned above are "systematically developed statements to assist practitioners and patient decisions about appropriate health care for specific circumstances" (Field & Lohr, 1990) and are a source to which courts may look in an attempt to define the standard of care. Although still not followed widely by either courts (Hyams *et al.*, 1996) or practitioners (Cabana *et al.*, 1999), these may be helpful especially with the introduction of a new technology, when its use is still in a state of great flux. As such, practice parameters deserve special consideration for our discussion, which involves CBCT, a new technology.

Practice parameters

Professional guidelines are known variously as position statements, practice guidelines, practice parameters, parameters of care, and algorithms, among others (Hastings, 1993). Practice parameters that are promulgated by professional organizations may take on greater significance when a new or emerging test or technology is at issue, since initially there is little evidence of what the "average qualified practitioner" is doing. At the present time, a few orthodontists take CBCT scans on all or just about all patients, while others utilize them rarely. This state of affairs is consistent with findings over decades for even well-established diagnostic and treatment modalities, namely, that there is wide variation in their use, even within the same geographic area (Havighurst, 1991). Since the standard of care is determined by what the average qualified practitioner does, this leaves the orthodontist in a quandary as to just what the standard is. Ironically, this quandary is partly of the profession's own making, since the profession embraces the court's notions that the standard should be determined by what the average qualified practitioner does and not by some other perhaps more objective and definable standard. Apart from this downside to the practitioner, another disadvantage of the standard is that it is "so imprecise and variable as to leave juries wide discretion in imposing liability" (Havighurst, 1991).

Different jurisdictions are inconsistent with respect to whether and to what extent they admit practice parameters into evidence. Some courts have applied them as "two-way streets," by both plaintiffs and defendants, while others are more likely to allow plaintiffs to use the guidelines as swords than to allow defendants to use them as shields (Hyams *et al.*, 1996). In the latter case, if a practitioner does not follow the guidelines, a court will allow the plaintiff to present that to the jury, while it may not allow the practitioner to present his compliance with the guidelines as a defense. Thus, a court may allow a breach of the guidelines to serve as conclusive evidence of negligence or only as some evidence of negligence. If it follows the former rule, then a showing by the plaintiff that the practitioner breached the guidelines would end the inquiry and the practitioner would be liable for negligence. If a court follows the latter rule, then following the plaintiff's showing that the practitioner breached the guidelines, the practitioner would be able to rebut the assumption of negligence. This can be done, for example, by showing that special circumstances dictated a departure from the guidelines. Most people find it fairer if a court follows the rule that breach of the guidelines is some evidence of negligence and not conclusive proof of it.

Generally, compliance by the practitioner with the guidelines does not shield him or her from liability, although a few jurisdictions have adopted this posture, at least on a trial basis (Hyams *et al.*, 1996). A court may allow compliance with guidelines by a practitioner to be used as some evidence of meeting the standard of care, but this is an inference that may be rebutted by the plaintiff.

Practice parameters have been criticized on a number of fronts for their shortcomings. Professional organizations have been accused of using parameters to protect practitioners by setting the lowest level of care. Parameters of care have been criticized for being used to achieve cost control (Grogan *et al.*, 1994) or for being nothing more than the practice of medicine-by-numbers (Genuis, 2005). Perhaps a more valid criticism is that practice parameters are not updated frequently enough. With today's rapid changes in technology, guidelines that are updated only on an occasional basis may not reflect the standard of care at a given time. Also of great importance is the process by which the guidelines are produced. This refers especially to which individuals and organizations are involved in formulating the guidelines, as well as from whom they receive input. That the process is critical in order for the guidelines to be accepted by practitioners is illustrated by two sets of dental guidelines that have been published. A unilateral position paper on the need for pre-operative cone beam scanning prior to implant placement by the American Academy of Oral and Maxillofacial radiology (AAOMR; Tyndall & Brooks, 2000) was criticized roundly by an oral surgeon (Larson, 2001). The criticism was based on a number of grounds, including the fear that "A report such as this will find its way to an elevated status with regard to establishing a standard of care." Rightly or wrongly, the criticism further opined that the AAOMR was arrogating unto oral and maxillofacial radiologists the sole right to perform the majority of diagnostic procedures, pointing out another criticism that may be leveled at an organization that publishes practice parameters, namely, that it is doing so for the self-serving purposes of its members. Contrast the above-referenced AAOMR guidelines with those on the use of CBCT in endodontics, published jointly by the AAOMR and the American Association of Endodontists (Use of Cone-Beam Computed Tomography in Endodontics, 2011). In this situation, the endodontists' own society participated in the decision-making process and endorsed the findings, making any potential criticism of the guidelines by an endodontist more muted and less credible. The AAOMR and the American Association of Orthodontists (AAO) had been working on guidelines on the use of CBCT in orthodontics. Although members of the working group from each organization agreed on a set of guidelines, which was approved by the AAOMR, the AAO did not accept the guidelines, as was reported at the annual meeting of the AAOMR in Savannah, GA, in November 2012. Thus, unfortunately, orthodontists currently do not have a set of guidelines on which they can rely. This setback should spur practicing orthodontists to redouble the effort to come up with practice parameters, something that is done best by a group representing the members whom it proposes to influence, in this case, the AAO.

What to do? Practical considerations

When all is said and done, what is an orthodontist to do? Years from now, once CBCT has been in use for some time, it should be obvious as to what the appropriate indications are for CBCT: practitioners could ask fellow practitioners what they do, attend continuing education courses, listen to experts, and read journals. In the absence of evidence as to what the average qualified practitioner is doing, a situation faced by orthodontists in the immediate to short term, practice parameters, if and when they become available, would be helpful. To what extent courts will pay deference to any guidelines that may be promulgated will have to await a legal decision.

There are other considerations, which are an unfortunate side-effect of private dental practice and of the American malpractice system, that drive the use of technologies and that factor into an orthodontist's consideration of whether to embrace a new technology. While usually of great benefit to society, the commercial aspect of dentistry also serves as a driver for practitioners to adopt new technologies even if they have not been proven to be clinically or cost-effective, simply because other dentists have adopted the technology. If they do not adopt the technology, so the thinking of practitioners goes, patients will think that they are not keeping current; this is a shortcoming of the commercial aspect of dentistry.

As far as the malpractice system is concerned, a practitioner is far less likely to get sued for *using* technology as opposed to being sued for *not* using it. Thus, the tendency to use CBCT, like all technologies, is driven in part by the medico-legal climate. In the context of CBCT, that same medico-legal system, however, also has elements that should give an orthodontist pause before using CBCT routinely. When a CBCT is taken, the practitioner is responsible for reading the entire volume and not just that part of the anatomy related to the reason for the scan or to his or her area of expertise (Friedland, 2009). Thus, he or she will be liable for the consequences of missing or misdiagnosing any pathology that appears on the scan. On the other hand, should pathology that might have been seen in an "orthodontic CBCT," had it been taken, come to light later either clinically or radiographically, the practitioner should not be held liable if the original CBCT had not been indicated for orthodontic reasons. An orthodontist's duty does not extend to a fishing expedition to find pathology unrelated to the reason for treatment; he or she would be ill advised to embark on one. Those practitioners who insist that all orthodontic patients should get a CBCT because it may show undiagnosed pathology, even that unrelated to orthodontic diagnosis and treatment (Baumrind *et al.*, 2003; Kau *et al.*, 2005; Nordstrom, 2009), are conflating a diagnostic test with a screening procedure (Grimes & Schulz, 2002). As defined by Grimes & Schulz (2002), *screening* is the testing of seemingly healthy people to find those at increased risk of having a disease or disorder. A *diagnostic test*, on the other hand, is used to confirm a suspected condition based on a patient's signs or symptoms. An orthodontist who fails to take a CBCT and who faces legal action on that basis may find a safe harbor if he or she follows any established guidelines when they do not call for a CBCT in the particular patient's circumstances. In the future, this may change depending on what the "average qualified orthodontist" does, but for now there is little better advice than to follow the guidelines if and when they are released. Of course, one almost certain way for an orthodontist who takes a scan on every patient to avoid legal liability for the reading of a scan is to engage the services of a medical or an oral and maxillofacial radiologist to report on each scan.

ASSOCIATED ETHICAL, LEGAL, AND REGULATORY ISSUES

Although this chapter addresses medico-legal issues, I would be remiss in not addressing some associated issues, including ethical and regulatory or other legal concerns.

Ethical concerns

One ethical issue is the financial incentive that the acquisition of a CBCT machine creates for a practitioner. The history of CBCT in implant dentistry is instructive in this regard. I speak from firsthand knowledge of this in the region where I practice. There were and are dentists who get a CBCT scan for every implant site on every patient. Some of them refer patients to imaging centers, while some of them have had their own CBCT machine almost from the first implant that they placed. These dentists have been consistent in their practice; namely, for every implant placed, the patient gets a CBCT scan or, prior to the availability of CBCT, a medical CT scan. Other implant dentists have chosen patients selectively, whom they refer to imaging centers for a CBCT or medical scan. In their opinion, in only a small minority of cases is a CBCT indicated for a proposed implant. Some of these dentists later acquired a CBCT scanner. From the day that they installed the machine, they suddenly discovered that every implant patient now needed a CBCT scan. It could be, of course, that these practitioners bought a CBCT machine because they had decided prior to acquiring it that they should change the way they practice and should get a scan on each implant patient. I know with certainty, however, that for at least some of the dentists in this group, the reverse was, in fact, true; it was the purchase of the machine that led to them to take a CBCT scan on every implant patient. You do not have to accept my anecdotal evidence, however.

This observation is in keeping with years of research showing that when nonradiologist physicians own and operate their own X-ray equipment and have the opportunity to self-refer, their utilization is substantially higher than among physicians who refer their patients for radiologic procedures (Hillman *et al.*, 1990; Levin & Rao, 2004). This clearly is what has happened with some dentists when it comes to implant imaging. The orthodontic profession needs to guard against this taking place in its specialty lest it undermine the specialty's and its practitioners' credibility.

An additional concern, both ethical and practical, is whether CBCT improves the outcome of orthodontic treatment and, importantly, who is in the best position to judge that. Although not every treatment modality needs to be evaluated in a randomized control trial (Smith & Pell, 2003)—sometimes observational data more than suffice—such is clearly not the case with CBCT and orthodontics. On closer examination, even seemingly obvious treatments turn out to not bear the fruits that logic almost certainly dictates they would. Consider the recent case of what in the vernacular is called "clogged arteries." Patients who have atherosclerotic plaques and, thus, narrowing of the internal carotid arteries underwent surgery to bypass the narrowing; the hypothesis is that this would reduce ischemic strokes in these patients. A control group did not undergo surgery. Stroke outcome was compared between the groups. Against all expectations and all logic, no significant difference was seen between the two groups, and, in the authors' words, "The trial was terminated early for futility" (Powers *et al.*, 2011). The researchers considered it unethical to continue the study. It certainly is much less obvious that CBCT would improve a patient's outcome than that eliminating a blockage in the internal carotid arteries would reduce strokes. Thus, whether CBCT should become the standard of care, and for which patients, would be determined best through a formal clinical trial. Anything less may prove unacceptable to patients and regulatory authorities.

It should be mentioned that even at this relatively early stage of CBCT use in orthodontics, there are clinical situations where most practitioners would agree that the use of this modality clearly is justifiable; examples include the localization of certain impacted teeth and many surgical cases as detailed further in Chapters 1 and 6. Beyond these and other limited indications, the universal exposure of a CBCT on every patient should await appropriate evidence based on sound research.

Unless CBCT produces a better result and not only a more accurate diagnosis, it is difficult both ethically and practically to justify its routine use in orthodontics. As to who is in the best position to judge the efficacy of CBCT in orthodontics, it is interesting to look at the literature pertaining to surgery in patients with Down Syndrome. Like patients seeking orthodontic treatment, patients with Down Syndrome may have functional problems, but most of the surgery to their faces is done for cosmetic reasons. Similarly, most orthodontic treatment is done for cosmetic reasons. The success of cosmetic treatment is largely a subjective one. An examination of the "success" of plastic surgery on patients with Down Syndrome is instructive in this regard. Studies performed to evaluate the success of surgery to change the appearance of patients with Down Syndrome show, if not a definitive result, at least a strong common trend, the results of which can be summarized broadly as follows: those treating patients, namely surgeons, think that the surgery has greater benefits than do parents. Among those who are unrelated to the child (e.g., teachers and friends), considerably fewer think that the surgery provides significant benefits (Pueschel *et al.* 1986). In another study, "the perceptions of parents of children who had undergone surgery produced little evidence for the positive impact of the surgery on the parents' perceptions of their children's physical, personal and social functioning compared with the parents of children who had not undergone the surgery" (Kravetz *et al.*, 1992).

Thus, I submit that the decision of whether the financial cost and radiation burden of a CBCT scan produces a better result than what currently is used that would favor its routine use is one that is best decided by patients and/or their parents.

Regulatory and legal concerns

While not likely in the United States, a regulatory or legal concern that we should keep in mind if

CBCT scans come to be used on every orthodontic patient is that states or the federal government will step in and impose regulations on the use of CBCT, at least with respect to children, and possibly also on the purchase and ownership of machines. In Ontario, Canada, the Royal College of Dental Surgeons (2011) has instituted stringent guidelines with respect to large field of view (FOV) CBCT scanners, the kind that orthodontists would use (http://rcdso.org/MemberResourceCentre/Dental%20CT%20Scanners, accessed January 5, 2013).

States could base such limitations on the already expressed concerns of the pediatric medical community in which there is great concern over the increased amount of radiation to which especially children—who are more sensitive to radiation than are adults—are being exposed. In fact, the pediatric community has established the Image Gently movement, to which the AAOMR is a signatory, to bring attention to this matter (http://pedrad.org/associations/5364/ig, accessed January 5, 2013; Colletti, 2011). Parenthetically, note the title of Colletti's article, "Image gently: *go with the guidelines*" (my emphasis).

The ensuing example admittedly is not precise, but it does provide a measure of the potential scope of exposure to the childhood population and the reason for the medical community's concern. It has been estimated that in the United Kingdom, approximately 33% of 11- to 12-year-olds are in objective need of orthodontic treatment (Burdenn & Holmes, 1994). One can assume reasonably that in the United States the demand, if not the need, for orthodontic treatment is higher, but we will assume the number to be 33%. In 2010, there were 53,980,105 children of 5 to 17 years old in the United States (http://www.census.gov/prod/cen2010/briefs/c2010br-03.pdf; accessed January 5, 2013). Assuming that the children are spread equally across all age groups, this amounts to 4,152,316 in each age group, or 8,304,632 children of 11 and 12 years old. If we assume that 33% of them require orthodontic treatment, this amounts to 2,768,211 CBCT examinations annually if literally every orthodontic patient undergoes a scan. This does not take into account that some of these patients will receive more than one scan as an in-treatment or post-treatment scan replaces the traditional lateral cephalogram, at least by some orthodontists. This is a number large enough to catch the attention of public health authorities. Thus, the profession can guard its independence best and stay free of governmental interference through the judicious rather than the indiscriminate use of this enormously useful imaging modality.

It also would behoove us to look to what professional organizations in other countries are doing with regard to the use of CBCT in orthodontics. For example, the British Orthodontic Society's latest guidelines on orthodontic radiographs urge practitioners "to use CBCT with caution" (Isaacson *et al.*, 2008). The society points out that the current literature advocating the routine use of CBCT is dominated by anecdotal reports and calls for more research.

CONCLUSIONS

At the present time, the use of CBCT cannot be said to constitute the standard of care in orthodontics. Whether it evolves to become such, only time will tell. In the absence of evidence as to what the average qualified orthodontist is doing, it would be helpful if the AAO would enact practice parameters, either by itself or preferably in conjunction with the AAOMR, to assist orthodontists in their decision making. The profession would be able to support or reject the routine use of CBCT in orthodontics best by conducting clinical trials comparing the results of orthodontic treatment between patients diagnosed with CBCT and those diagnosed with conventional orthodontic radiographs. Since under our system of jurisprudence it is highly unlikely that orthodontists who routinely utilize CBCT will find themselves facing a malpractice suit, at this stage their decision to use it depends on their subjective belief that it is beneficial to patients.

References

Baumrind, S., Carlson, S., Beers, A., *et al.* (2003) Using three-dimensional imaging to assess treatment outcomes in orthodontics: a progress report from the

University of the Pacific. *Orthodontics and Craniofacial Research*, 6 (Suppl 1), 132–142.

Brune v. Belinkoff, 354 Mass. 102, 235 N.E.2d 793, 1968.

Burdenn, D.J. & Holmes, A. (1994) The need for orthodontic treatment in the child population of the United Kingdom. *European Journal of Orthodontics*, 16 (5), 395–399.

Cabana, M.D., Rand, C.S., Powe, N.R., *et al.* (1999) Why don't physicians follow clinical practice guidelines? A framework for improvement. *Journal of the American Medical Association*, 282 (15), 1458–1465.

Colletti, P.M. (2011) Image Gently: go with the guidelines. *Clinical Nuclear Medicine*, 36 (12), e233–e235.

Cramm, T., Hartz, A.J., & Green, M.D. (2002) Ascertaining customary care in malpractice cases: asking those who know. *Wake Forest Law Review*, 37 (3), 699–756.

Downer v. Veilleux, 322 A.2d 82, 87, Me 1974.

Eggers, P.W. (2000) Medicare's end stage renal disease program. *Health Care Financing Review*, 22, 1–10. Available at http://www.cmms.hhs.gov/Research-Statistics-Data-and-Systems/Research/HealthCareFinancingReview/downloads/00fallpg55.pdf, accessed January 5, 2013.

Field, M.J. & Lohr, K.N. (1990) *Clinical Practice Guidelines: Directions for a New Program*. The National Academies Press, Washington DC.

Fink, D.J. (1981) Technology assessment: then and now. Letter to the editor. *New England Journal of Medicine*, 304b, 918.

Friedland, B. (2009) Medico-legal issues related to cone-beam CT. *Seminars in Orthodontics*, 15, 77–84.

Genuis, S.J. (2005) The proliferation of clinical practice guidelines: professional development or medicine-by-numbers? *Journal of the American Board of Family Medicine*, 18 (5), 419–425.

Grimes, D. & Schulz, K.F. (2002) Uses and abuses of screening tests. *Lancet*, 359 (9309), 881–884.

Grogan, C.M., Feldman, R.D., Nyman, J.A., *et al.* (1994) How will we use clinical guidelines? The experience of medicare carriers. *Journal of Health Politics, Policy and Law*, 19 (1), 7–26.

Harris v. Groth, 99 Wash. 2D 438, 663 P.2d 113, 1983.

Hastings, K. (1993) A view from the Agency for Health Care Policy and Research: the use of language in clinical practice guidelines. *Joint Commission Journal on Quality Improvement*, 19, 335–341.

Havighurst, C.C. (1991) Practice guidelines as legal standards governing physician liability. *Law & Contemporary Problems*, 54, 87–117.

Helling v. Carey, 83 Wash. 2D 514, 519 P. 2d 981, 1974.

Hillman, B.J., Joseph, C.A., Mabry, M.R., *et al.* (1990) Frequency and costs of diagnostic imaging in office practice: a comparison of self-referring and radiologist-referring physicians. *New England Journal of Medicine*, 323 (23), 1604–1608.

Hyams, A.L., Shapiro, D.W., & Brennan, T.A. (1996) Medical practice guidelines in malpractice litigation: an early retrospective. *Journal of Health Politics, Policy and Law*, 21, 289–313.

Isaacson, K.G., Thom, A.R., Horner, K., *et al.* (2008) Orthodontic radiographs: guidelines, 3rd ed. *European Journal of Orthodontics*, 30, 669–670.

Kau, C.H., Richmond, S., Palomo, J.M., *et al.* (2005) Three-dimensional cone beam computerized tomography in orthodontics. *Journal of Orthodontics*, 32 (4), 282–293.

Keeton, W.P., Dobbs, D.B., Keeton, R.E., *et al.* (1984) *Prosser and Keeton on the Law of Torts*. 5th ed. West Publishing Company, St. Paul, MN.

Kravetz, S., Weller, A., Tennenbaum, R., *et al.* (1992) Plastic surgery on children with Down syndrome: parents' perceptions of physical, personal, and social functioning. *Research in Developmental Disabilities*, 13 (2), 145–156.

Larson, P.E. (2001) Oral and maxillofacial radiology parameters of care (letter to the editor). *Oral Surgery, Oral Medicine, Oral Pathology, Oral Radiology, and Endodontology*, 92 (5), 480–481.

Levin, D.C. & Rao, V.M. (2004) Turf wars in radiology: the overutilization of imaging resulting from self-referral. *Journal of the American College of Radiology*, 1 (3), 169–172.

Necheles, T. (1982) Standards of medical care: how does an innovative medical procedure become accepted? *Law, Medicine & Health Care*, 10 (1), 15–18.

Nordstrom, D. (2009) Radiographic exposure guidelines. *American Journal of Orthodontics and Dentofacial Orthopedics*, 134 (5), 597–598.

Powers, W.J., Clarke, W.R., Grubb, R.L., Jr., *et al.* (2011) Extracranial-intracranial bypass surgery for stroke prevention in hemodynamic cerebral ischemia: the carotid occlusion surgery study randomized trial. *Journal of the American Medical Association*, 306 (18), 1983–1992.

Pueschel, S.M., Monteiro, L.A., & Erickson, M. (1986) Parents' and physicians' perceptions of facial plastic surgery in children with Down's syndrome. *Journal of Mental Deficiency Research*, 30 (Part 1), 71–79.

Royal College of Dental Surgeons of Ontario (2011) Standard of Practice: dental CT scanners. April 2011.

Smith, G.C. & Pell, J.P. (2003) Parachute use to prevent death and major trauma related to gravitational challenge: systematic review of randomized controlled trials: review. *British Medical Journal*, 327 (7429), 1459–1461.

Sukovic, P. (2003) Cone beam computed tomography in craniofacial imaging. *Orthodontics & Craniofacial Research*, 6 (Suppl 1), 31–36.

Tyndall, D.A. & Brooks, S.L. (2000) Selection criteria for dental implant site imaging: a position paper of the American Academy of Oral and Maxillofacial Radiology. *Oral Surgery, Oral Medicine, Oral Pathology, Oral Radiology, and Endodontology*, 89 (5), 630–637.

Use of cone-beam computed tomography in endodontics: joint position statement of the American Association of Endodontists and the American Academy of Oral and Maxillofacial Radiology. (2011) *Oral Surgery, Oral Medicine, Oral Pathology, Oral Radiology, and Endodontology*, 111 (2), 234–237.

Weiss, H.S., Hecht, L., & Friedland, B. (2003) Health insurance coverage for oral diseases: toward a more sophisticated model. *Journal of Legal Medicine*, 24 (2), 175–198.

8 Protocols for the Use of Cone Beam Computed Tomography in Orthodontic Practice

Aaron D. Molen, DDS, MS

INTRODUCTION

Since its introduction to orthodontics in 2001, cone beam computed tomography (CBCT) has become a popular and useful tool in the diagnosis and treatment planning of orthodontic cases (Hans *et al.*, 2011). Despite its popularity, a consensus regarding proper protocols for its optimal use has yet to be established. The objective of this chapter is to provide the clinician with practical information on how best to utilize CBCT imaging in the diagnosis and treatment of orthodontic patients. The overall goal is to provide the clinician with a greater understanding of the benefits of CBCT in specific clinical situations as well as how to manipulate and interpret the contents of the scan for optimizing orthodontic treatment. This will establish a foundation that the clinician can build upon during the ongoing dynamic phase in which CBCT imaging continues to evolve as a diagnostic tool.

BENEFITS OF CBCT FOR ORTHODONTISTS

There remains some debate on which types of orthodontic cases warrant a CBCT scan versus the use of traditional two-dimensional (2D) projectional (plain film) radiographs (Halazonetis, 2012; Larson, 2012). In general, each case should be evaluated by the orthodontist to determine if the CBCT scan would provide valuable additional diagnostic information that could enhance or alter the treatment plan. The details of specific selection criteria for the use of CBCT in orthodontics are presented in Chapters 1 and 6.

The three-dimensional (3D) data derived from a CBCT scan can, in specific situations, reduce ambiguity in diagnosis, thereby improving the treatment plan and minimizing the risk of negative sequelae or elongated treatment times. Treatment plans based on incomplete or inadequate

Cone Beam Computed Tomography in Orthodontics: Indications, Insights, and Innovations, First Edition. Sunil D. Kapila.

diagnostic data can result in permanent damage to teeth including an increased risk for decalcification, caries, and root resorption (Motokawa *et al.*, 2011). Each case, therefore, should be evaluated to determine if the additional information available in a CBCT scan will decrease the risks inherent in that specific case. It is important to remember that the treatment and outcome of a case ultimately is only as good as its diagnosis.

In general terms, the benefits of acquiring, but not necessarily the rationale for taking CBCT scans are:

(1) Reduced ambiguity in diagnosis
(2) Minimization of unexpected issues and negative sequelae
(3) Acquisition of more diagnostic information, and/or
(4) Increased treatment efficiency.

Reduced ambiguity

Ambiguity is defined as something that can be understood in two or more possible ways. When developing a problem list for an orthodontic case, the ability to interpret an anatomical feature in more than one way may result in several different treatment plans. Since traditional 2D projectional radiographs are prone inherently to issues such as magnification, artifacts, and superimposition of structures, the risk of having multiple possible interpretations of the anatomical structures increases (Botticelli *et al.*, 2011).

The astute clinician will recognize the presence of ambiguity in a diagnostic image and will consider each possible treatment plan and outcome for each possible interpretation of the ambiguous area of the image. After considering how each interpretation might affect the patient's treatment, the clinician may find that the treatment plan and outcome remains the same regardless of the interpretation. In these situations, the previously acquired imaging is adequate despite the ambiguity. If the clinician determines that different interpretations will result in differing treatment approaches and varying outcomes, however, the acquisition of further imaging then is warranted. The danger occurs when the clinician fails to recognize the areas of ambiguity in the diagnostic imaging and fails to assess their potential ramifications adequately.

Figure 8.1A shows a panoramic radiograph of an Angle Class III patient who displays multiple metallic-like opacities and numerous shadowing artifacts contributing to ambiguity in several areas. It was determined that a CBCT scan was necessary to minimize the ambiguity since several of the small opacities appear in close proximity to the apices of the mandibular teeth that would be undergoing orthodontic movement. Furthermore, a definitive diagnosis of the large opacity inferior to the patient's left ramus could help in determining whether or not orthognathic surgery was a viable option to correct the Class III relationship.

After a CBCT scan was taken, a bullet was localized inferior and posterior of the patient's left ramus (Figure 8.1B) that the patient had failed to disclose on his health history. In addition, shrapnel from the bullet was found throughout the anterior mandible, but none was found blocking the likely paths of roots during orthodontic movements. The CBCT scan also clearly showed the entry point inferior to the mandibular right canine (Figure 8.1C). Using the entry point as a reference point, the bullet's path could be extrapolated to its current resting place (Figure 8.1D). In this case, failure to eliminate the initial ambiguity properly could have resulted in damage to the apices of teeth by being moved into shrapnel or prescribing surgery when it was contraindicated.

Several studies have shown that the introduction of a CBCT scan into the diagnostic imagery of a specific case has resulted in a change in that case's treatment plan (Bjerklin & Ericson, 2006; Botticelli *et al.*, 2011). However, the same studies have shown that some treatment plans remain unchanged despite the inclusion of a CBCT scan. Instead of evaluating the value of CBCT scans in such black or white terms, other studies have emphasized the effect CBCT scans have on a clinician's confidence in the treatment plan (Haney *et al.*, 2010). In essence, findings of increased clinician confidence in treatment planning with CBCT imaging imply a decrease in the ambiguity of recognizing important diagnostic features.

Figure 8.2A shows a panoramic radiograph of a 21-year-old female whose maxillary left canine has failed to erupt. It was unclear from 2D imaging

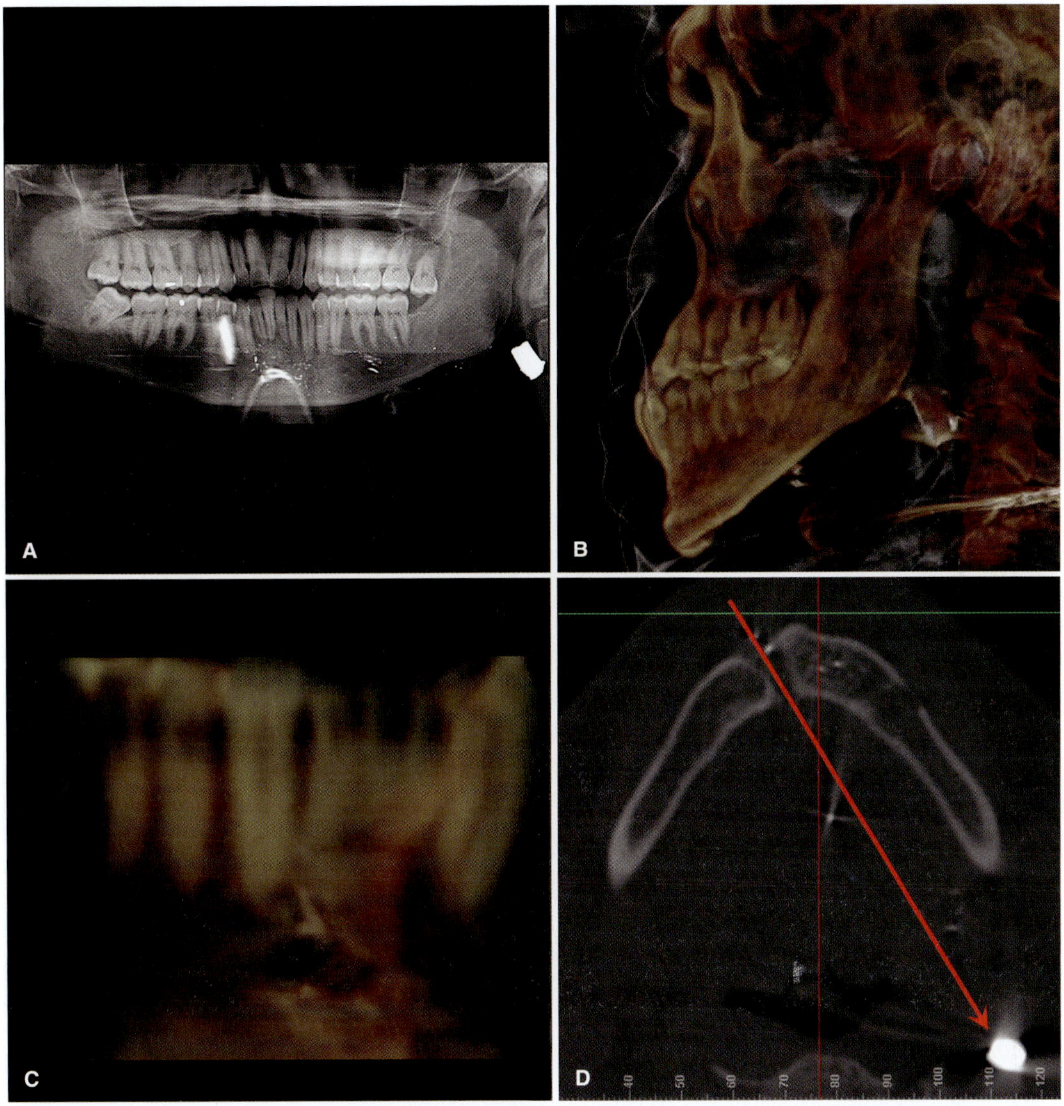

Figure 8.1 *A*: Panoramic radiograph exhibiting several ambiguous opaque artifacts. *B*: Combined surface and volume rendering showing a bullet lodged inferior-posterior to the left ramus. *C*: Volume rendering of the anterior mandible displaying the bullet's entry point inferior to the right canine. *D*: Axial slice through the mandible showing the bullet and its extrapolated path.

why the canine had become ectopic and eventually impacted. However, a CBCT scan revealed that the canine was located in close proximity to a supernumerary tooth that had prevented its eruption (Figure 8.2B,C). The additional information not only answered the question of why the canine had failed to erupt, but also increased the clinician's confidence that once the supernumerary tooth was removed, the canine could be brought into its proper position under orthodontic traction. In this case, the incorporation of CBCT imaging as part of the diagnostic records diminished ambiguity, helped refine the treatment plan, and potentially enhanced treatment outcome.

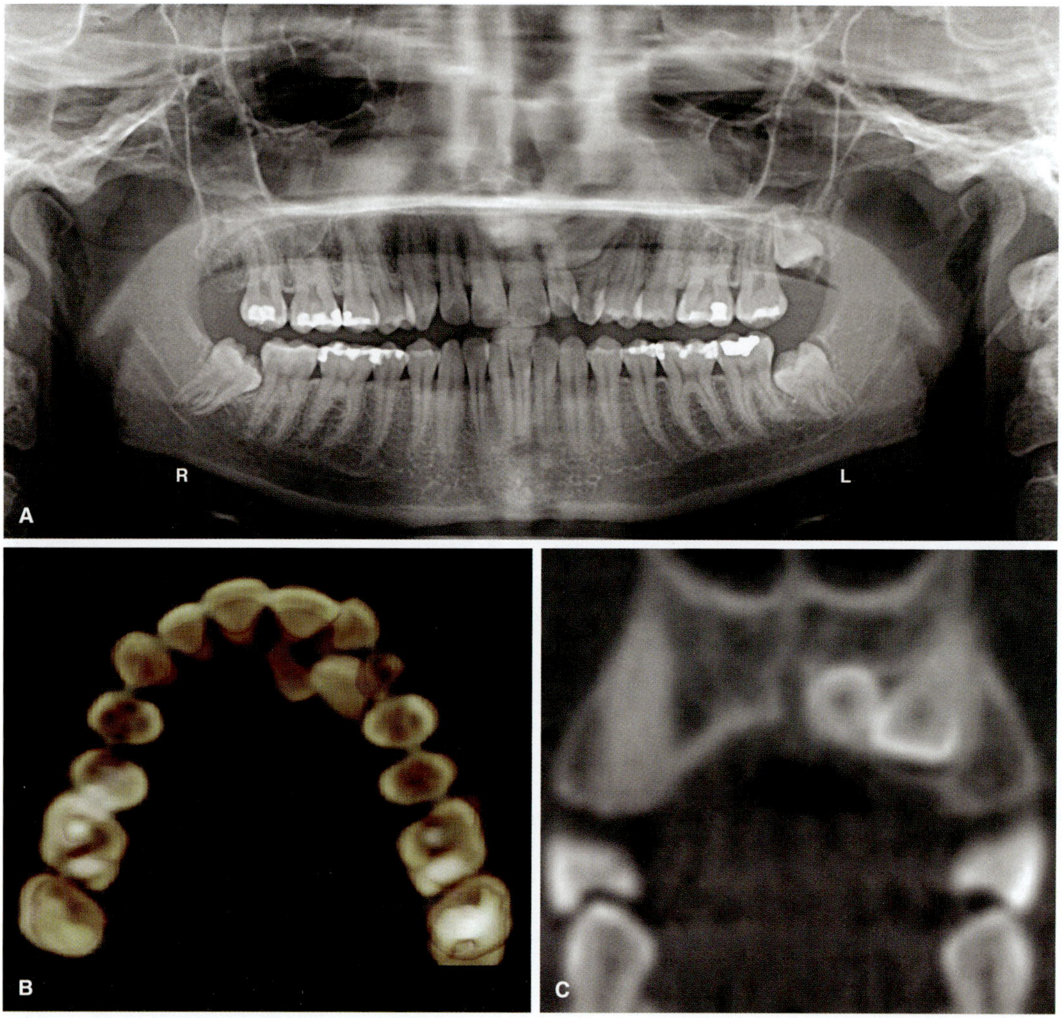

Figure 8.2 *A*: Panoramic radiograph of 21-year-old female showing an unerupted maxillary left canine. *B*: Occlusal view of a volume rendering of the maxillary dentition showing the unerupted left canine lodged against a supernumerary tooth. *C*: Coronal slice showing where the canine and supernumerary tooth contact.

While CBCT imaging is indicated and useful in specific cases such as those described above (see also Chapters 1 and 6), it must be emphasized that if all areas of potential ambiguity can be discerned with a high degree of confidence using 2D projectional radiographs alone, taking a CBCT to reduce ambiguity further would be unjustified. Moreover, the decision to take 2D projectional radiographs as screening tools before determining if a CBCT scan is necessary presently is due to the higher radiation dose associated with CBCT scans versus 2D imaging (see Chapter 3). It is possible that in the future, as the dose associated with CBCT scans decreases to levels equal to or less than 2D imaging, this 3D imaging modality could gain greater acceptance for use as a diagnostic tool during initial orthodontic examination.

Minimization of unexpected issues and negative sequelae

The goal of a problem list is to identify all the current problems of a case. By focusing on the present, however, there may be a tendency to overlook potential future problems or negative sequelae of the treatment plan and its mechanics. One of the most common negative sequelae of orthodontic treatment is root resorption (Motokawa *et al.*, 2011). This is found most commonly on maxillary lateral incisors when a canine has become impacted in close proximity to the incisor root. In addition to resorption on the lateral incisor roots, research conducted using CBCT imaging also has identified resorption on the roots of the central incisors and the first premolars (Walker *et al.*, 2005). This problem can be made worse if care is not taken in determining the proper vector by which to retrieve the impacted canine (Becker *et al.*, 2010a; see also Chapter 16). Thus, if forces are exerted in the wrong direction during canine retrieval, iatrogenic root resorption may result.

An unfortunate example of this point is illustrated in Figure 8.3. It shows an impacted maxillary right canine that has been under orthodontic traction for 19 months. The patient was referred by the orthodontist to an oral surgeon to determine why the tooth had failed to erupt despite being under constant orthodontic traction. The oral surgeon took a CBCT scan to localize the canine and discovered that the canine was not impacted palatally as the orthodontist had assumed, but instead was placed buccally. The utilization of an inappropriate palatal traction vector, possibly due to inadequate diagnostic information, resulted in the proclination of the adjacent lateral incisor, an unnecessary elongation of treatment time and likely iatrogenic root resorption.

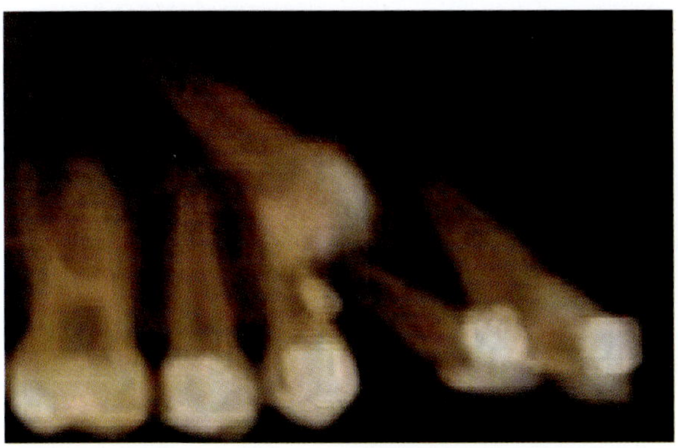

Figure 8.3 Volumetric reconstruction showing a labially displaced maxillary right canine that was placed under orthodontic traction with a palatal vector of pull for 19 months instead of with a more appropriate labial vector of pull.

A close examination of 2D projectional radiographs may reveal a series of recognizable problems. Due to the inherent inadequacies of these radiographs as noted elsewhere (see Chapters 1 and 11), these findings, when identified, may be a reflection of or result from additional significant underlying problems. For example, as with the case described previously where a supernumerary tooth was found contributing to a canine impaction (Figure 8.2), after an ectopic or impacted tooth has been identified, the clinician should focus not solely on determining the solution to the problem, but also on what may have caused the issue to occur in the first place. When the clinician discovers the likely cause of a significant clinical or radiographic finding, the ability to determine the best treatment plan often improves.

The concept described above is demonstrated clearly in the following example of ectopic mandibular left canine (Figure 8.4A). An attempt to determine the reason for the ectopic mandibular left canine from the 2D panoramic radiograph is likely to be nonconclusive. Also note that the mandibular left primary canine exhibits significant root resorption despite the fact that the permanent canine is not in close proximity to its root. To determine the cause of the ectopic canine, a CBCT scan was taken, which revealed a large radiolucent lesion in the left body of the mandible. The lesion had displaced the permanent canine mesially (Figure 8.4B) and labially out from under the primary canine (Figure 8.4C). After the scan was read by an oral radiologist, it was determined that the lesion was fibrous dysplasia, which had contributed to the displacement of the canine. Because orthodontic movement may be compromised in the presence of active fibrous dysplasia, no orthodontic treatment was recommended. In contrast, had the ectopic canine resulted simply due to a

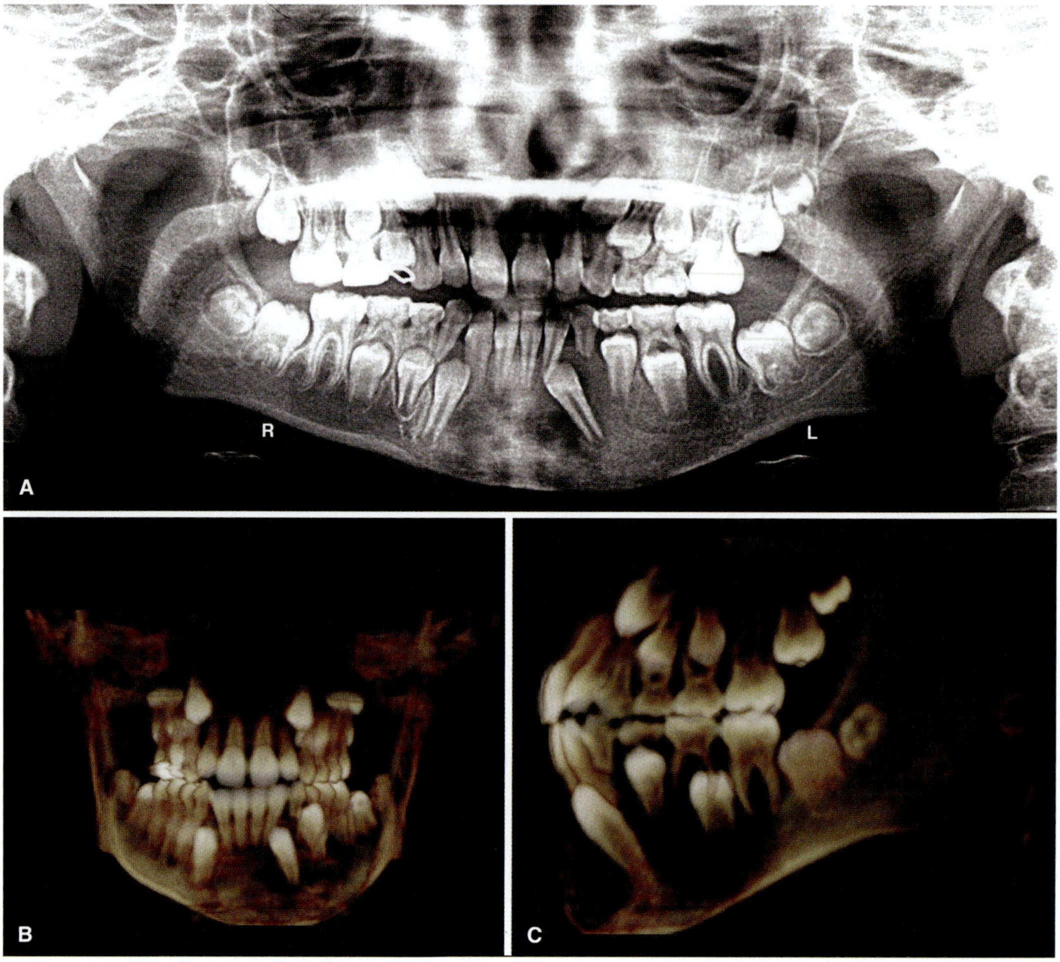

Figure 8.4 *A*: Panoramic radiograph showing an ectopic mandibular left canine. *B*: Frontal view of volume rendering showing a large lucent lesion in the left body of the mandible. *C*: Left lateral view of volume rendering highlighting the size of the lucency and the facial displacement of the mandibular left canine.

deviated eruption path, the treatment would have been different involving orthodontic retrieval of the tooth.

Acquisition of additional diagnostic information

It has been said that a picture is worth a thousand words. In less than a second, a camera can capture more information within a photograph than the human mind can memorize in the same time frame. When compared with conventional 2D projectional radiographs, the same can be said about CBCT. The volume of information contained within all the voxels of a CBCT scan far exceeds that contained within the pixels of a 2D radiograph (Scarfe & Farman, 2008). These additional diagnostic data are helpful, especially in difficult orthodontic cases when determining the best treatment plan.

As 3D beings living in a 3D world, we sometimes have a difficult time interpreting and understanding the context of structures within a 2D image. Cartographers always have understood this

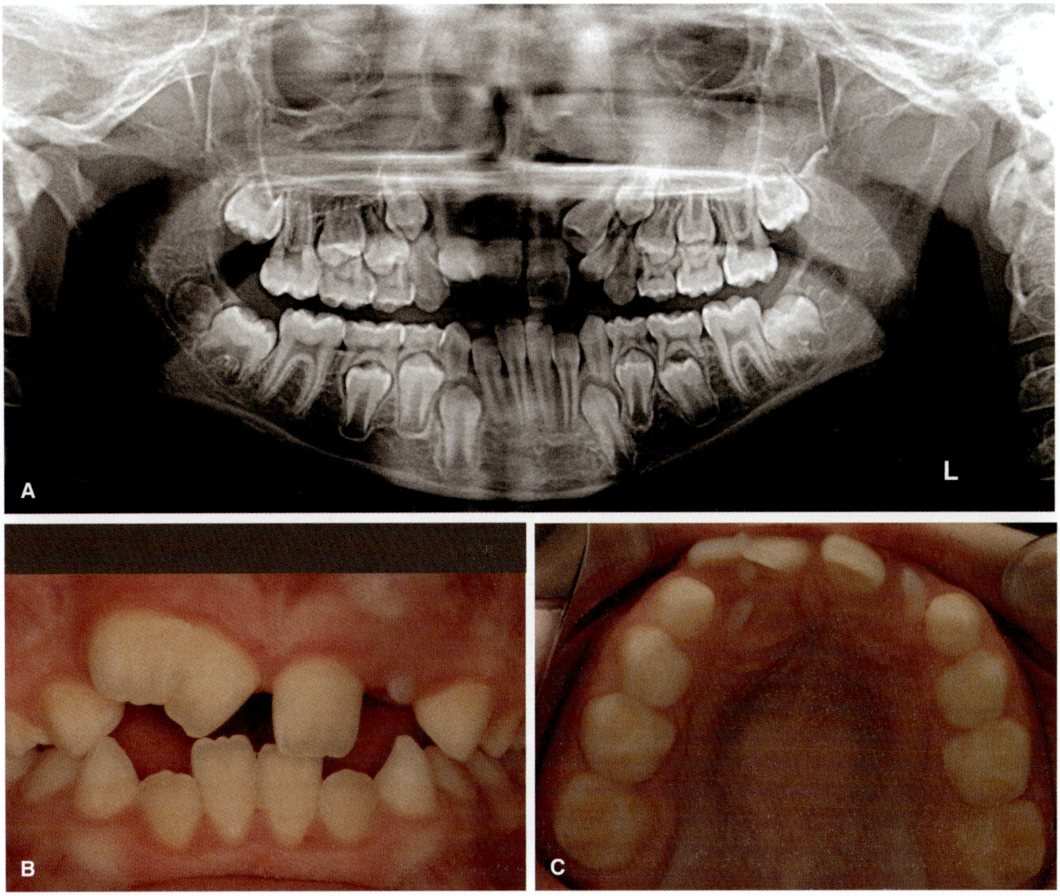

Figure 8.5 *A*: Panoramic radiograph showing two fused maxillary right incisors and several supernumerary teeth. *B*: Frontal intraoral photograph showing fused teeth. *C*: Maxillary occlusal intraoral photo showing fused teeth and erupting supernumerary teeth.

limitation of 2D images. In the book *The Nature of Maps*, the authors state that "The concept of spatial relatedness is a quality without which it is difficult or impossible for the human mind to apprehend anything" (Robinson & Petchenik, 1976). 3D CBCT imaging removes this limitation by giving the clinician the ability to view teeth and their related structures in their natural context while developing an appreciation of how they relate spatially. In difficult orthodontic cases, this additional information and context well may be the difference between an efficient treatment with an ideal outcome and an unnecessarily long treatment with a poor outcome (Becker *et al.*, 2010b).

Complicated orthodontic cases require more information to derive optimal diagnosis than simple cases do (Mah *et al.*, 2010). Figure 8.5 illustrates a complicated orthodontic case consisting of two fused maxillary incisors and some supernumerary teeth. Due to the amount of crowding, it is difficult to ascertain the locations of the supernumerary teeth and the quality of their roots. A CBCT scan taken to determine the best treatment plan for the patient revealed that a supernumerary right maxillary lateral incisor was located palatal to the fused teeth and a supernumerary left maxillary central incisor was located distal and apical to the erupted left maxillary central incisor (Figure

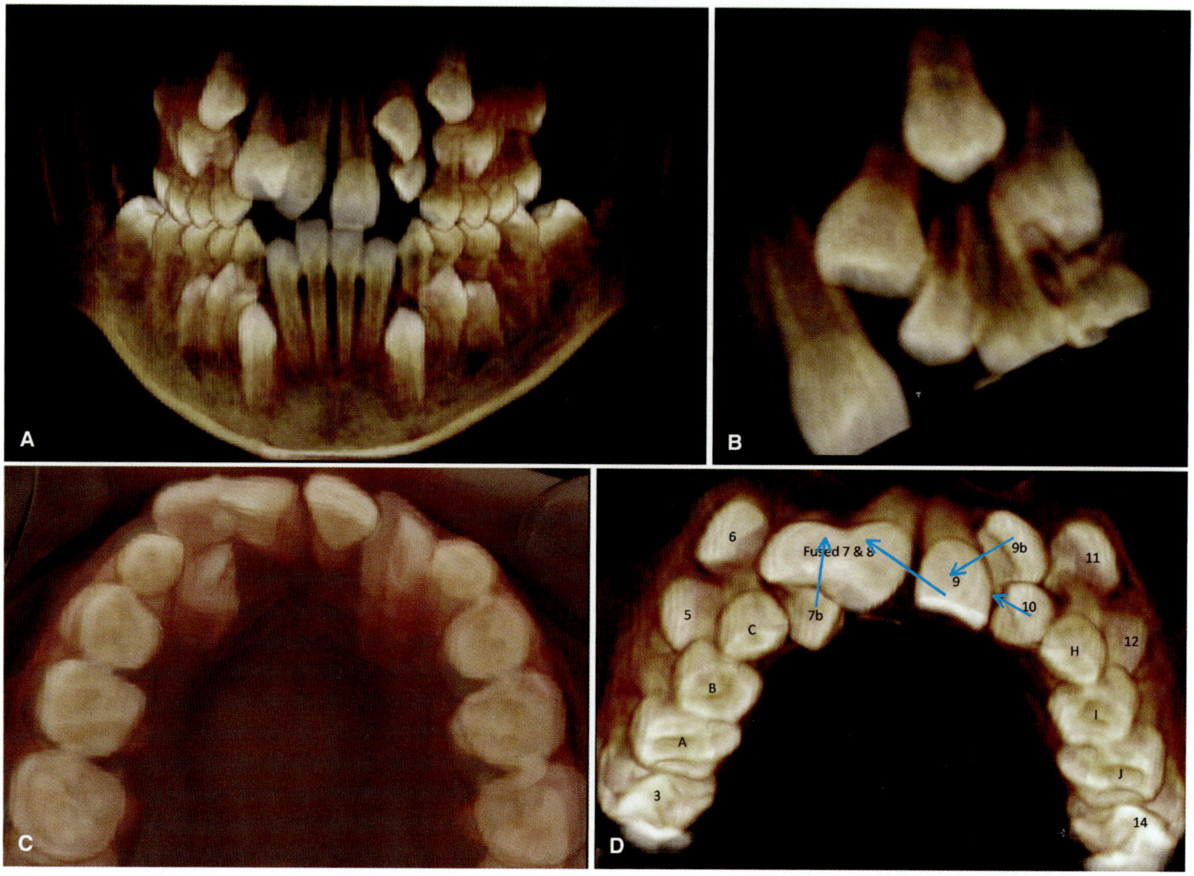

Figure 8.6 *A*: Frontal view of volume rendering showing fused teeth. *B*: Oblique view of volume rendering illustrating the relationship of the supernumerary central incisor to the adjacent teeth. *C*: Superimposition of occlusal intraoral photograph and volume rendering. *D*: Illustration of the proposed treatment plan after the fused teeth are extracted.

8.6A,B). To give further context to the positions of the supernumerary teeth relative to the soft tissue, Adobe Photoshop® was used to superimpose the patient's maxillary occlusal intraoral photograph onto a screenshot of the maxillary dentition rendered from the CBCT scan (Figure 8.6C) and the information used to derive an well-informed treatment plan (Figure 8.6D).

The comprehensive treatment plan depicted in Figure 8.6D involved the extraction of the fused teeth (labeled *Fused 7 & 8*) followed by the bonding of fixed edgewise-orthodontic appliances. The supernumerary right lateral incisor (labeled *7b*) then would be brought labially and the erupted left central incisor (labeled *9*) moved mesially across the midline to replace the extracted fused teeth. The supernumerary left central incisor (labeled *9b*) then would be moved inferiorly and mesially to replace the left central incisor that had been moved across the midline. At a future date, the erupted left central incisor would require an esthetic bonding or veneer to give it the appearance of the missing right central incisor. This treatment plan would allow the patient to keep a full complement of teeth without the need for dental implants or a fixed prosthesis. After 18 months of active orthodontic treatment, the panoramic radiograph shows the improved positions of the teeth (Figure 8.7A); after 22 months of treatment, the dramatic changes could be appreciated clinically (Figure 8.7B,C).

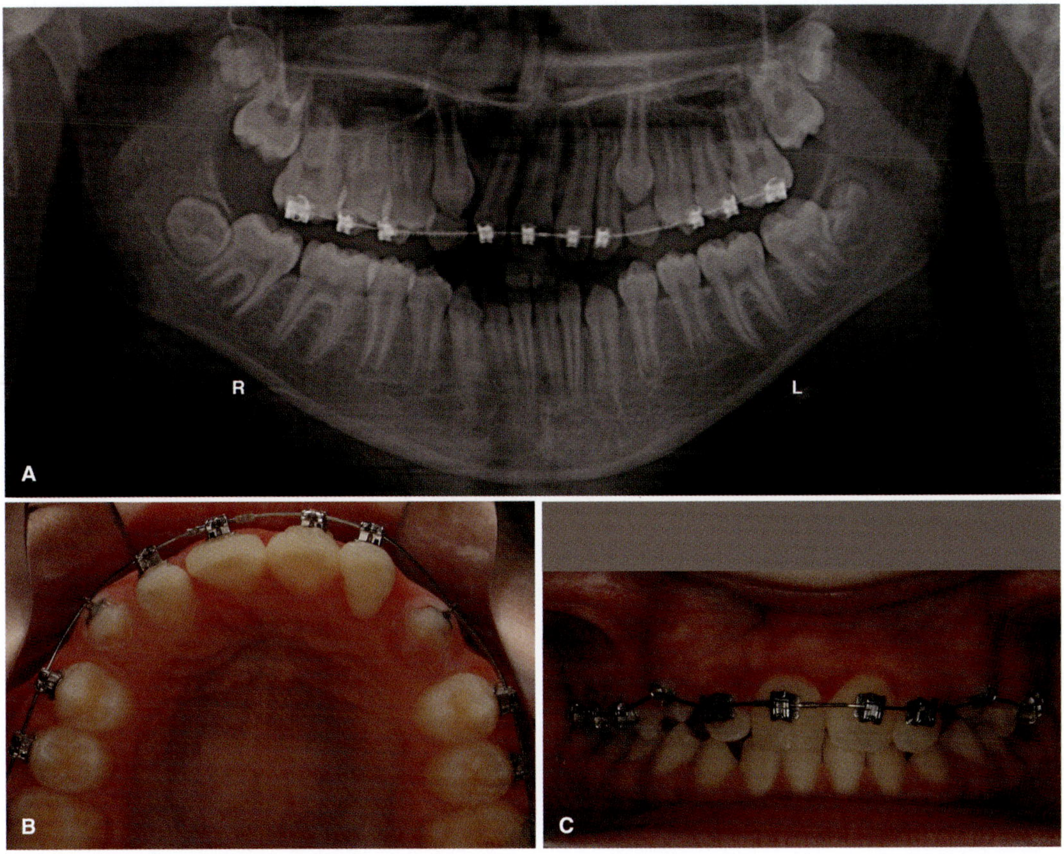

Figure 8.7 *A*: Panoramic radiograph showing treatment progress at 18 months. *B* and *C*: Maxillary occlusal and frontal intraoral intraoral photograph, respectively, showing treatment progress at 22 months.

Increased treatment efficiency

The principle that the shortest distance between two points is a straight line can be applied to orthodontic treatment planning. For a large number of simple cases, an orthodontist's training and experience may suffice to render an efficient treatment plan based on 2D projectional radiographs alone. In cases of facial asymmetries or ectopic, impacted, or supernumerary teeth, however, these traditional projectional radiographs may be insufficient.

The appearance of impacted teeth on panoramic radiographs often can be deceiving (Mah *et al.*, 2003). The goal of taking a CBCT scan in cases of impacted teeth should be to simplify complicated impactions and keep simple impactions from becoming complicated. Often more than one vector of pull is required to bring an impacted tooth in successfully without causing damage to the adjacent teeth (see also Chapter 16). When only one vector of pull is applied, as might happen with inadequate information derived from 2D radiographs, the impacted tooth eventually might be brought into the arch, but may cause iatrogenic root resorption to roots along its path. In some milder cases of impactions, a single vector of pull may be adequate and the CBCT scan simply serves to verify the clinician's treatment plan while increasing his or her confidence in its outcome (Becker *et al.*, 2010a). Ultimately, the treatment plan is only as good as the diagnosis and the diagnosis is only as good as the clinical and radiographic data derived and the tools used to obtain these.

An example of using 3D imaging to create a more efficient treatment plan is demonstrated in the case depicted in Figure 8.8. The panorex (Figure 8.8A) demonstrates an ectopic maxillary right second premolar that is impacted in the mesial furcation of the maxillary right first molar. A CBCT scan was taken to determine the most efficient sequence of vectors by which to deimpact the tooth and bring it into occlusion (Figure 8.8B–D). After only 23 months of active orthodontic treatment, the tooth was brought into functional occlusion without damaging it or the first molar (Figure 8.8E).

Assessing risk

The clinician must evaluate each case to determine if it will benefit from the diagnostic information derived from a CBCT scan. The risks of exposing the patient to additional radiation should be weighed not only against the benefits of acquiring the scan, but also against those of not obtaining additional diagnostic information. It is easy to overlook the increased risk to which the patient may be exposed if we fail to gather adequate diagnostic information and, therefore, fail to diagnose and plan the treatment properly. For example, the patient may be placed at higher risk of developing generalized root resorption due to unnecessarily long treatment times or localized iatrogenic root resorption due to misplaced vectors. In many cases, the ability to reduce ambiguity, minimize negative sequelae, and acquire more diagnostic information will prove invaluable in planning the most efficient treatment with the most ideal outcome for the patient. However, as discussed elsewhere (Chapter 6), CBCT scanning is not recommended for the sole purpose of screening for pathology or when clinical and/or radiographic evaluation do not support its use.

CBCT VOLUME ACQUISITION

Scan settings

Once the clinician has determined that a specific case will benefit from the additional diagnostic information available from a CBCT scan, he or she then must decide which scan settings to prescribe based on the goal of the scan. Most CBCT systems allow the technician to adjust the height and diameter of the scan volume, voxel size, and duration of the scan in seconds, which corresponds to the number of image frames that will be captured (Molen, 2011; see also Chapter 2).

Field of view size

The majority of systems allow the technician to adjust the size of the volume being captured; however, some systems allow only one or two pre-set sizes to be used. The size of the volume is referred to as the field of view (FOV) and should be large enough to capture the clinician's region of interest. For orthodontists, the region of interest can vary from a small region containing an impacted canine to a large region for use in evaluating facial asymmetries (Figure 8.9). Within the dental profession, oral and maxillofacial surgeons and orthodontists are unique in their need to capture the majority of the head occasionally. Even though most orthodontists may not use a large FOV on every patient, it is beneficial to have the capability to take this volume on complicated craniofacial or asymmetry cases.

In general, FOVs can be subdivided into three size categories: large, medium, and small. A large FOV scan will show the roof of the orbits and nasion down to the hyoid bone on a typical adult male. Large FOV scans have a height equal to or greater than 16 cm and are useful for evaluating the entire dentofacial complex for asymmetries.

Medium FOV scans will capture the middle of the orbits down to menton vertically and from condyle to condyle horizontally. Medium FOV scans are useful for reconstructing 2D panoramic radiographs and the localization of multiple impacted, ectopic, or supernumerary teeth. For some adolescents, a medium FOV scan size may be sufficient to capture all of the anatomy usually associated with a large FOV scan. This allows the technician to capture all of the relevant anatomy without having to resort to the greater radiation dose typically associated with large FOV scans.

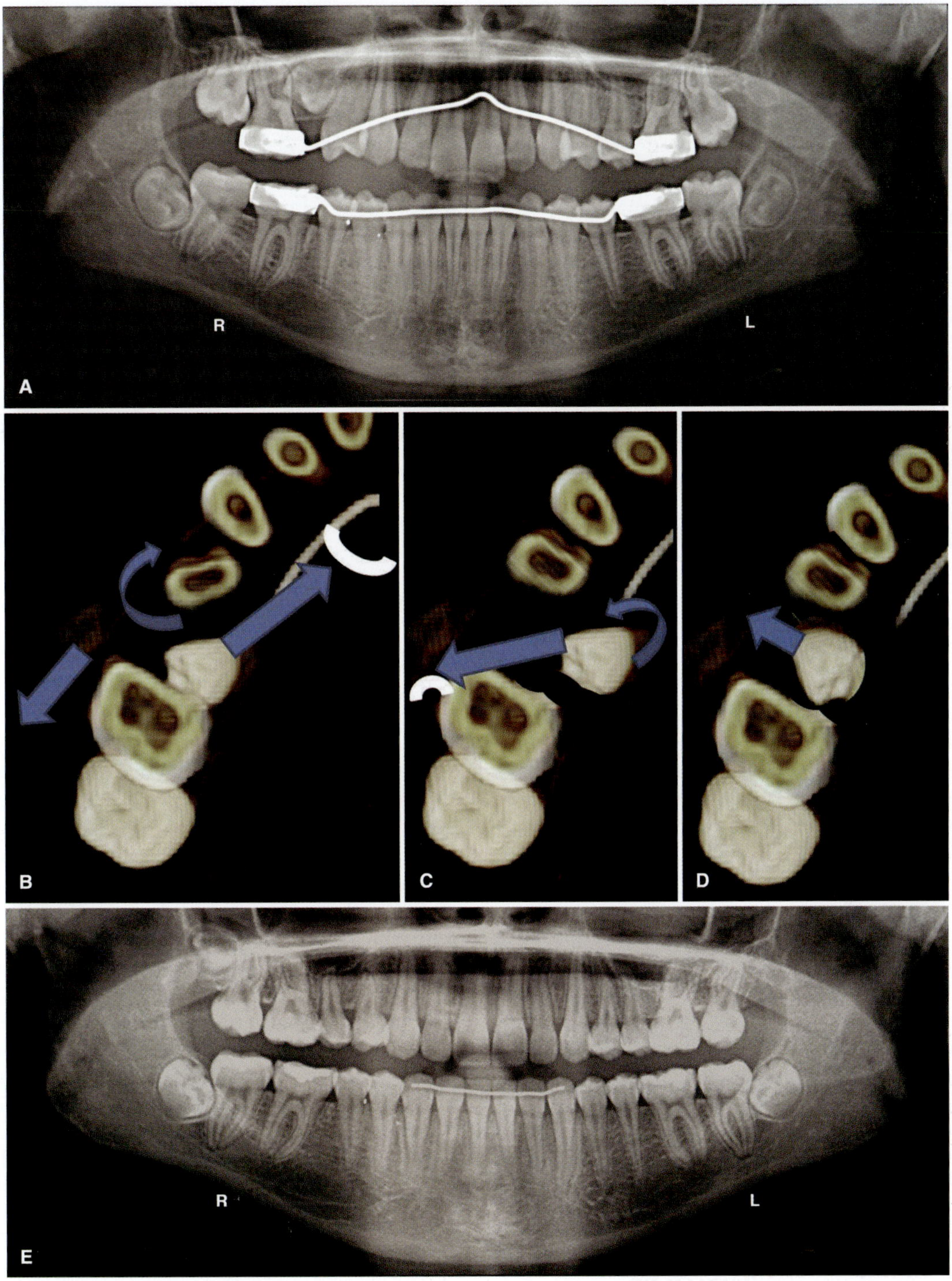

Figure 8.8 *A*: Panoramic radiograph showing the maxillary right second premolar impacted in the furcation of the first molar. *B–D*: Virtual biomechanical planning of the proposed sequence to efficiently de-impact and align the second premolar. This involves (*B*) an initial distal vector of movement for the premolar while developing space by distalizing the molar and derotating the first premolar, followed by (*C*) a disto-buccal movement together with derotation of the impacted second premolar, and finally (*D*) a buccal and extrusive movement to bring the tooth into occlusion. *E*: Panoramic radiograph showing the final position of the second premolar after 23 months of treatment.

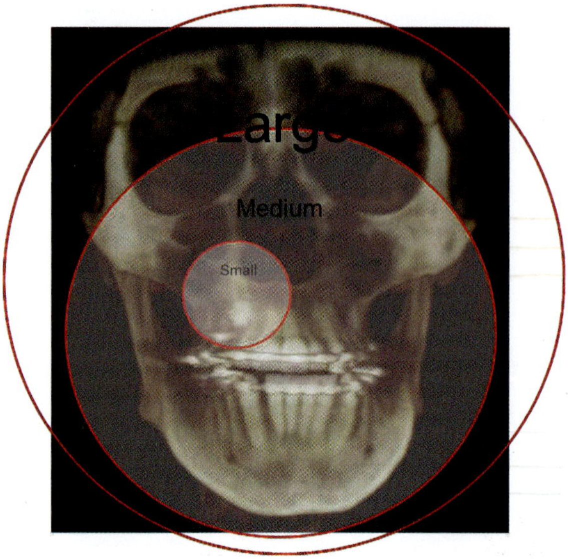

Figure 8.9 Illustration of large, medium, and small FOVs and the anatomy covered.

Small FOV scans capture a user-defined region, usually equal to or less than 10 cm in height. Unlike larger scans, small FOV scans frequently can be collimated horizontally as well as vertically. Small FOV scanners generally are used by orthodontists for the localization of a single impacted, ectopic, or supernumerary tooth.

Voxel size

Another setting that the clinician must prescribe for each scan is the size of the voxel to be used during the scan's acquisition. The characteristic most commonly associated with voxel size is the resolution of the scan. This is a misnomer, however, since the resolution of the reconstructed scan is influenced by several variables. Resolution, more accurately termed angular or spatial resolution, is the minimum distance between distinguishable objects. Though often associated with voxel size, they are not the same. The voxel size represents the dimensions of the volume element into which a volume is being subdivided and usually is measured in millimeters or microns. Each voxel is assigned a value representing the density of the object contained within its boundaries as determined by the attenuation of photons (Molen, 2010; see also Chapter 2).

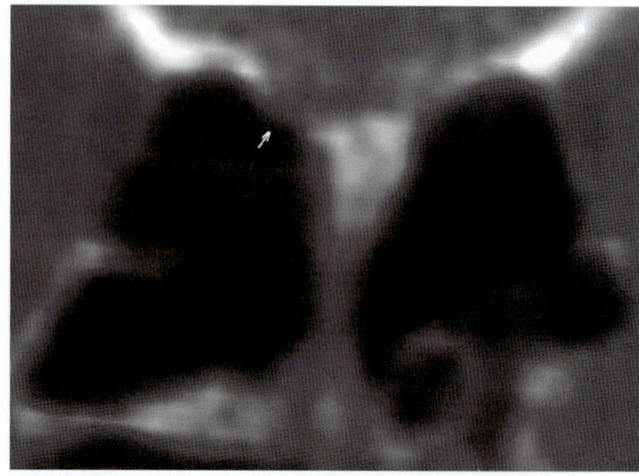

Figure 8.10 Effects of volume averaging in causing the superior wall of the right sphenoid sinus appear to be missing (white arrow).

If the objects contained within a single voxel differ in density, then the average density of the voxel's contents will be used throughout; this process is called volume averaging. The result of volume averaging is that along the periphery of a dense object such as cortical bone, the boundary may be overestimated or appear to be missing depending on the thickness of the bone. Thin bones such as the sphenoid sinus (Figure 8.10), temporal bone, and labial alveolar bone are susceptible especially to volume averaging (Chakeres, 1984).

The use of smaller voxel sizes, therefore, will allow the visualization of smaller variations in density; however, this does not translate directly to spatial resolution. Noise caused by scatter radiation (Endo *et al.*, 2001), volume averaging (Scarfe & Farman, 2008), and artifacts can reduce a scan's spatial resolution. In other words, a scan taken with a 0.3 mm voxel will not result in a spatial resolution of 0.3 mm; rather, it will have a spatial resolution closer to 0.7 mm, depending on the scan settings and CBCT system used (Ballrick *et al.*, 2008).

The ideal way to compare the spatial resolution of CBCT systems is by using a line pair phantom, which are embedded with metallic strips set at

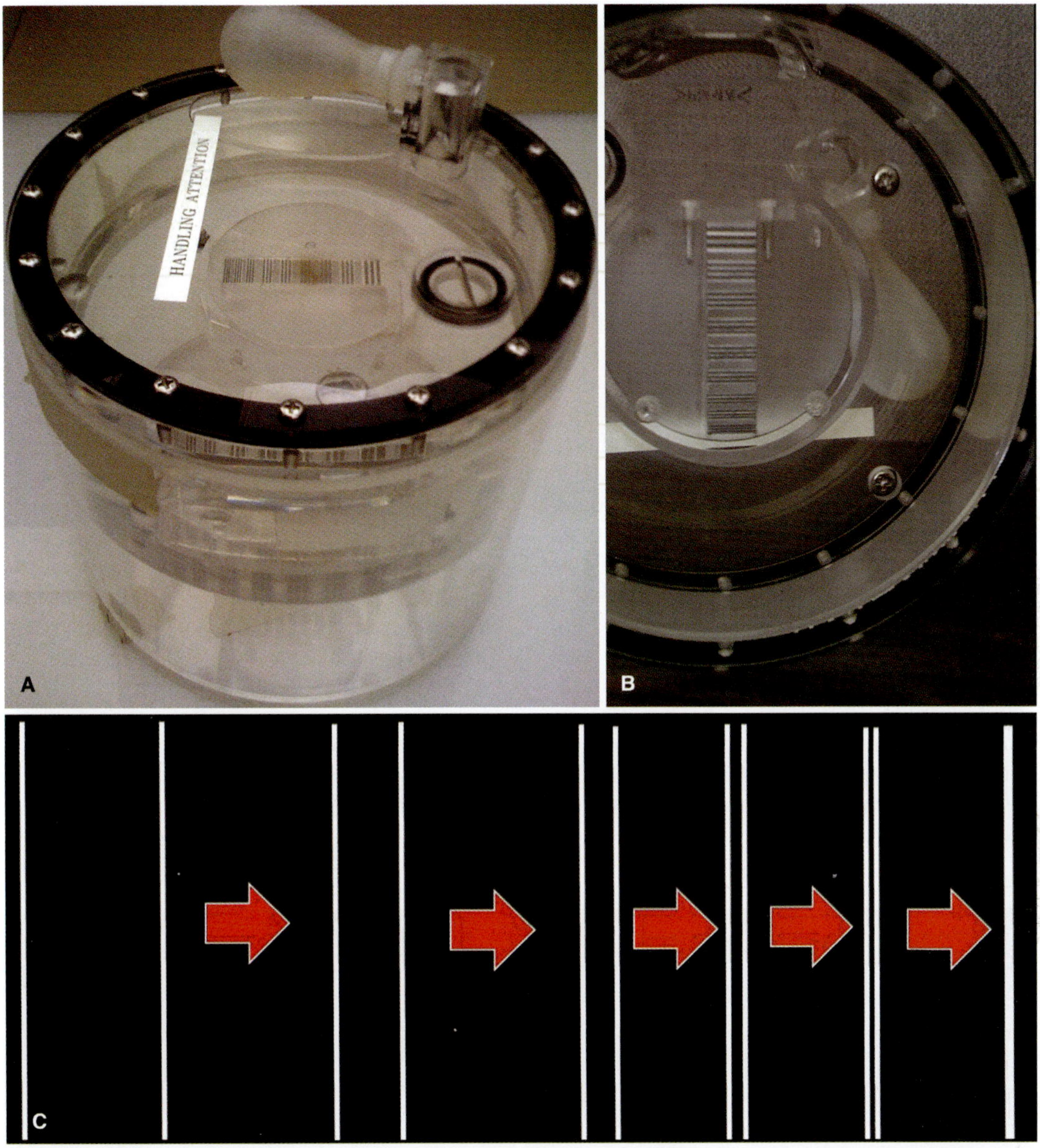

Figure 8.11 *A* and *B*: Example of a line pair phantom. *C*: A demonstration of how line pairs merge into one line, moving from left to right, at the point where their proximity exceeds the viewer's spatial resolution.

ever-decreasing distances from each other (Figure 8.11A,B). The point at which the user no longer can distinguish between two pairs of metallic strips is the point at which the spatial resolution of the scan has been exceeded (Figure 8.11C). The last set of distinguishable metallic strips, therefore, represents the spatial resolution of the scan. When evaluating the results of a line pair test, be aware that since spatial resolution is influenced by voxel size, scan duration (frame acquisition), and FOV, one should compare only the line pair results between scans with similar settings.

Frame acquisition (scan time)

Many systems allow the technician to adjust the number of frames that it will capture during the scan. Since the concept of frame acquisition is somewhat abstract, the setting is referred to more commonly as scan time or scan duration and is measured in seconds. The longer the scan time, the more frames are acquired, the higher the resulting spatial resolution, the better the contrast, but the higher the radiation dose to the patient (Molen, 2010). Inversely, shorter scans acquire fewer frames and expose the patient to less radiation but have less spatial resolution and contrast. For most orthodontic purposes, longer scan times and better spatial resolution do not equate necessarily with greater diagnostic potential. For example, when localizing an impacted tooth, lower scan times with less spatial resolution are adequate to identify the location of the tooth and evaluate its relationship to surrounding structures.

For orthodontic CBCT scans, more spatial resolution is not always better and results in a higher radiation penalty to the patient without a substantial improvement in the scan's diagnostic power. As manufacturers and clinicians alike continue to embrace this concept, we will see an increase in the availability of settings allowing for shorter scan times with less frame acquisition and ultimately a lower radiation dose being delivered to the patient. In the future, this should allow CBCT scans to be performed with radiation doses similar to, or even less than, that of the lateral cephalogram and panoramic projectional radiographs traditionally used for orthodontic screenings.

Patient positioning

Another factor affecting the quality of the resulting scan is how the patient is positioned for the scan. Various systems allow for patients to be seated, standing, or supine. Patient positioning is of paramount importance in CBCT imaging since CBCT scans are sensitive to any patient movement that occurs during the scan (Holberg *et al.*, 2005). Movement artifacts appear as waves within a reconstructed volume (Figure 8.12A) or as the shadowing of structures within the multiplanar reconstructions (Figure 8.12B).

The risk of patient movement artifacts can be decreased by placing the patient in a stable position and by decreasing the duration of the scan. Creating a stable environment for the patient usually requires a seated or supine position, since patients tend to sway or bend their legs when

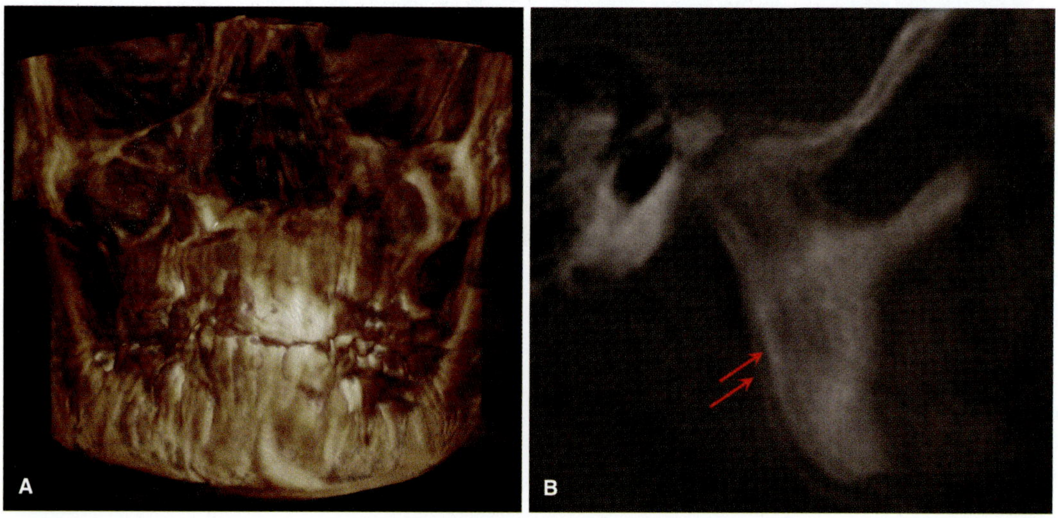

Figure 8.12 *A*: Volume rendering displaying distortion waves due to patient movement during the scan. *B*: Sagittal slice through the ramus exhibiting shadowing along its border (red arrows) due to patient movement during the scan.

standing. Systems that require the patient to be standing can be modified to a seated system simply by having the patient sit on a barstool during the scan. It also is advisable to have the patient close his or her eyes while performing the scan to help him or her resist the urge to follow the rotating arm with eyes and head.

In addition to positioning the patient properly and advising him or her to remain still, the technician should cover the patient with a lead apron. Since a thyroid collar is effective in decreasing the effective dose of CBCT scans (Tsiklakis *et al.*, 2005), it can be used in addition to the lead apron as long as it does not obstruct any anatomy within the region of interest.

ORTHODONTIC EVALUATION OF THE SCAN

The protocols used in several clinical settings and the steps for recognizing normal and abnormal findings in CBCT scans are presented in Chapters 1, 9 and 10. In general, unless the orthodontist is conversant with normal and abnormal anatomy in CBCT images, its assessment for incidental findings, as well as the region of interest, should be performed by an oral maxillofacial or medical radiologist. This assessment should precede any performed by the orthodontist for orthodontic treatment planning. The focus of this section of the chapter is to describe how the orthodontist can utilize CBCT images and the findings to refine diagnosis, treatment plan, and biomechanics.

After the clinician has prescribed the scan settings and the scan has been acquired by the technician, it now must be reconstructed into a 3D volume. CBCT systems themselves perform the primary reconstruction of the volume from all of the captured frames. To truly maximize the diagnostic potential of the scan, however, the clinician or trained technician must perform additional reconstructions and manipulations of the volume using either the proprietary software provided along with the CBCT system or third-party reconstruction software, commonly referred to as either a DICOM reader or a 3D viewer.

It is important for the clinician to have a standardized method by which to evaluate the substantial data contained in a scan. Though the CBCT scan likely was taken to focus on one or two regions of interest, it is important that the clinician who reads the scan avoids getting "tunnel vision." Most important, before any screenshots can be captured, the CBCT volume must be oriented properly in all three planes of space.

Volume orientation

Manual positioning of the head by the technician taking the CBCT scan is not sufficient to ensure that the patient's head has been positioned properly for diagnostic purposes. After the scan has been taken, the volume should be reoriented within the imaging software. To orient the volume, a protocol was developed by this author that involves first viewing the hard tissue volume from the anterior perspective. From the anterior, both zygomatic suture points (Z points), defined by Ricketts and colleagues (1972) as the medial termini of the zygomaticofrontal sutures, are identified. The Z points then are connected together to form the Z plane (Grummons & Kappeyne Van De Coppello, 1987). The Z plane now is used to orient the volume's axial plane and "roll" by aligning it parallel to the floor (Ackerman *et al.*, 2007; Figure 8.13A). The Z plane's location in the superior third of the craniofacial complex distances it sufficiently from the sources of most facial asymmetries and, therefore, presents a stable reference plane (Park *et al.*, 2012).

Next, from the right lateral view, the right side porion and orbitale should be connected together into the Frankfort Horizontal Plane (FHP) and the image adjusted to align this plane parallel to the floor to orient the volume's pitch (Figure 8.13B). Finally, from the inferior view, corresponding points at the medial termini of the zygomaticotemporal sutures, named by this author as the ZT points, should be connected together into the ZT plane and aligned parallel to the base of the computer monitor in order to orient the volume's yaw (Figure 8.13C). After the roll, pitch, and yaw have been oriented, the technician should evaluate the oriented volume for any obvious discrepancies in the orientation (Figure 8.13D). Once the new orientation has been saved, most software will reset the previous Cartesian coordinates to match the new

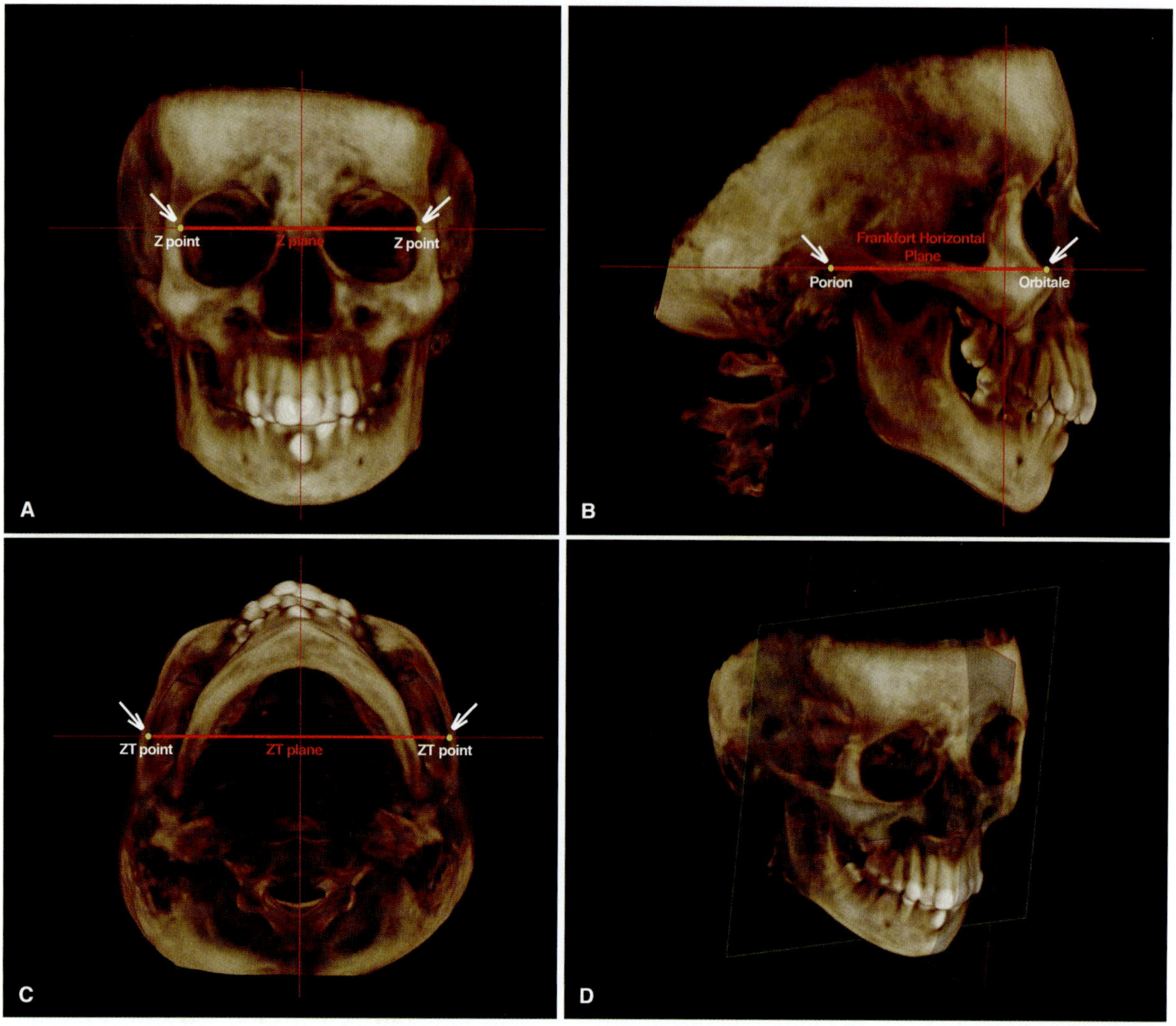

Figure 8.13 Orienting the CBCT volume. *A*: Horizontal alignment of medial termini of the zygomaticofrontal sutures (Z points) to orient the volume's roll. *B*: Horizontal alignment of the right-side porion and orbitale (Frankfort Horizontal Plane) to orient the volume's pitch. *C*: Horizontal alignment of the medial termini of the zygomaticotemporal sutures (ZT points) to orient the volume's yaw. *D*: Volume properly oriented in three planes of space.

orientation while establishing the axial, coronal, and sagittal planes.

Proper set of orientation is important especially if the technician plans on reproducing any traditional 2D views from the 3D volume (Cevidanes *et al.*, 2009). Failure to orient the volume could result in the images displaying erroneous anatomy or becoming distorted similar to their 2D projectional radiograph counterparts.

Standard views

To prevent tunnel vision, it is suggested that a standardized set of images be captured sequentially as screenshots from the oriented volume before focusing on the original region of interest. For example, the protocol used by this author begins by capturing a screenshot of the frontal view of the hard tissue volume (Figure 8.14A). Next, a view of the

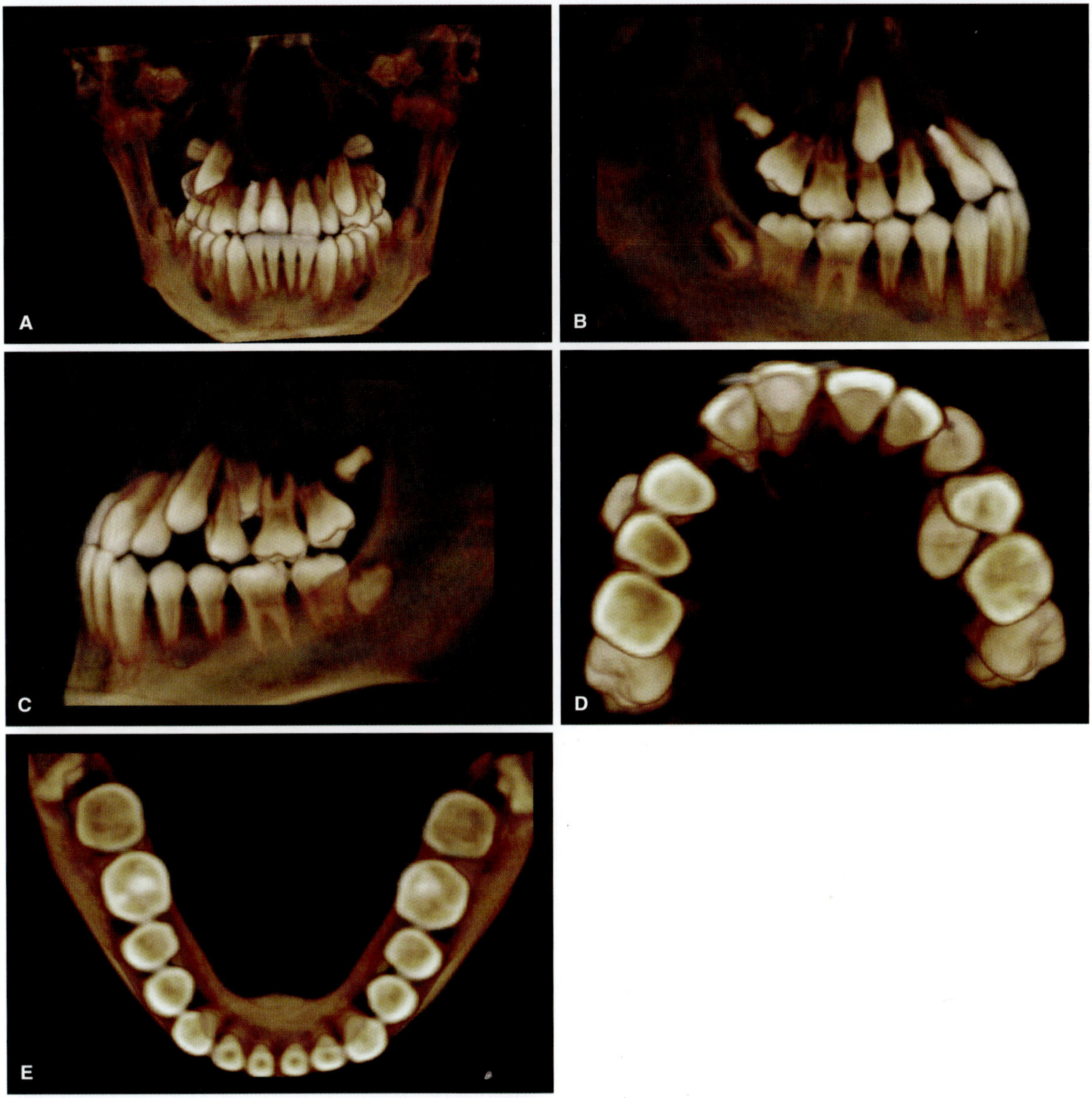

Figure 8.14 *A*: Standard frontal screenshot of the volume rendering. *B*: Standard right lateral screenshot of the volume rendering. Note that the left side of the volume has been removed to prevent the superimposition of structures. *C*: Standard left lateral screenshot of the volume rendering. Note that the right side of the volume has been removed to prevent the superimposition of structures. *D*: Standard maxillary occlusal screenshot of the volume rendering. *E*: Standard mandibular occlusal screenshot of the volume rendering.

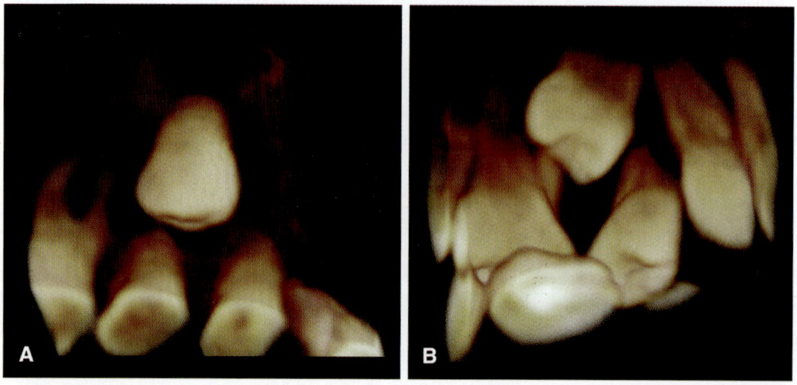

Figure 8.15 *A*: Oblique view of first region of interest of patient shown in Figure 8.14 demonstrating the relationship between the ectopic right canine and the premolars. *B*: Oblique view of second region of interest of the same patient showing the relationship between the impacted second premolar and the surrounding teeth.

right buccal dentition is captured (Figure 8.14B) with the left side clipped from view from the midline over, followed by a view of the left buccal dentition using the same technique (Figure 8.14C). A view of the maxillary dentition is captured by clipping out the anatomy superior to the apices of the roots of the permanent dentition and all of the anatomy inferior to the occlusal surfaces of the maxillary dentition (Figure 8.14D). The same technique is used to acquire an occlusal view of the mandibular dentition (Figure 8.14E). Finally, even if the scan has been read by an oral maxillofacial radiologist, the orthodontist still should scroll through all of the sagittal, coronal, and axial multiplanar slices to get acquainted fully with the scan volume and identify any other potential orthodontic problems.

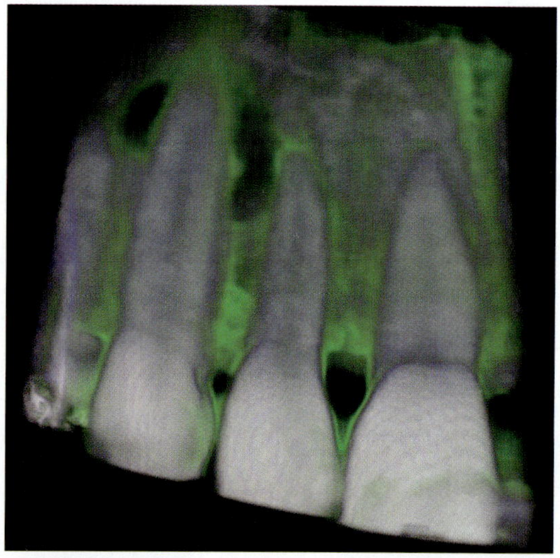

Figure 8.16 Volume rendering with a "moss"-colored filter applied.

Region(s) of interest

Once the standard set of views has been captured, the technician or orthodontist can begin capturing screenshots of the regions of interest. Each region of interest should be viewed from several angles to appreciate the teeth in context fully and localize their relationships with the surrounding structures (Figure 8.15). When the clinician is evaluating the volume, it is advisable to use the static screenshots to obtain an overview of the volume. However, in order to become truly familiar with the contents of the CBCT volume, it should be viewed and manipulated within the 3D volume viewer.

Some reconstruction software also allows the application of various colored filters to be applied to the volume (Figure 8.16). The use of colored filters often can help the human eye better distinguish subtleties within the volume due to the eye's ability to discriminate between millions of colors versus approximately 100 shades of gray.

RECONSTRUCTING 2D RADIOGRAPHS

Since the advent of CBCT, orthodontic practitioners have desired to reconstruct 2D views from the 3D volumes that mimic traditional 2D projectional radiographs in appearance (Moshiri *et al.*, 2007). Before discussing the generation of 2D radiographs, it is important to note that CBCT volumes never should be captured solely for the purpose of generating 2D radiographs. Every CBCT volume should be evaluated in all three planes of space using a volume viewer, multiplanar reconstructions, and 2D reconstructions. Not doing so largely reduces any benefits that could be obtained from 3D dataset to levels similar to information obtained with 2D projectional radiographs while increasing the risk of enhanced radiation.

As discussed previously, when reconstructing conventional 2D radiographs, it is imperative that the 3D volume be oriented in three planes of space first. Failure to orient the volume properly will create the appearance of asymmetries within the radiographs that in reality do not exist. In addition, before reconstructing the radiographs, oversegmenting the hard tissue volume by 10–20% is recommended to ensure that low-density bony structures such as the sella turcica can be visualized adequately post-reconstruction.

Lateral cephalogram reconstruction

The two most commonly reconstructed views are the lateral cephalogram and the panoramic radiograph. When reconstructing a lateral cephalogram from a 3D volume, the left side of the skull can be cropped away to eliminate the superimposition of bilateral structures (Figure 8.17A). This can result in a cleaner looking radiograph (Figure 8.17B) than a standard cephalometric radiograph or one in which the entire volume is used to construct the image. However, this approach has the caveat of eliminating the ability to visualize skeletal asymmetries from a lateral view, which can be compensated for by creating both right and left side lateral cephalograms for comparison.

When using lateral cephalograms generated from CBCT volumes, it is important to remember that the resulting images contain no magnification. This should be kept in mind when interpreting

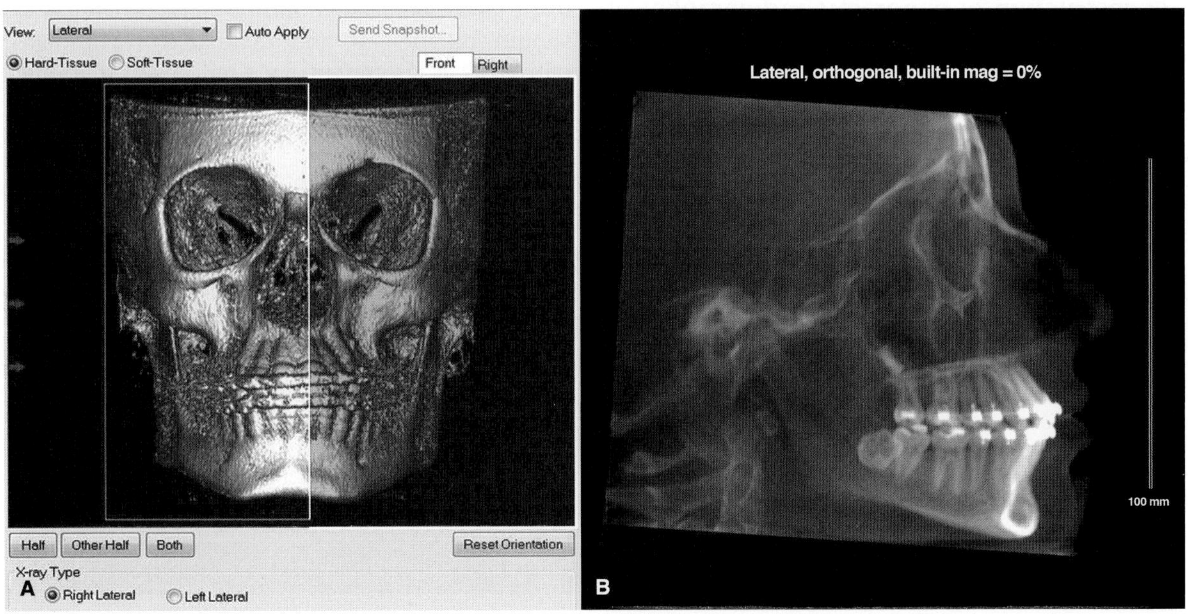

Figure 8.17 *A*: Eliminating the left half of the volume for reconstructing a right side lateral cephalogram, as shown in panel *B*.

cephalometric measurements made on these images since the normal values established using 2D projectional cephalograms are influenced by the presence of magnification (Gribel *et al.*, 2011). Several CBCT software programs allow the user to reintroduce magnification when generating 2D radiographs; however, this author believes that caution should be exercised whenever error is reintroduced intentionally to an image. Ultimately, the clinician should resist the urge to apply orthodontics' previous 2D paradigms to these new 3D volumes.

In response to our ability to visualize the craniofacial complex in 3D, several 3D analyses have been developed and proposed (Swennen, 2005; Faure *et al.*, 2008; Cho, 2009; Farronato *et al.*, 2010). Some of these new analyses reuse landmarks associated with traditional 2D analyses, whereas other analyses propose new landmarks unique to the 3D volume (see Chapter 11). Still other analyses depart completely from the traditional approach of using angles and measurements and instead propose the use of proportions (Jacobson, 2006) or the mirroring of bilateral structures (Cevidanes *et al.*, 2011; Damstra *et al.*, 2011; see also Chapter 21).

Reconstruction of panoramic radiographs

The panoramic radiograph commonly referred to as a Panorex® (or "pano") is a popular screening tool among orthodontists. However, the manner in which it is captured results in several shortcomings. Its primary weakness is the superimposition of structures that makes them appear as if they are overlaying each other when, in reality, they are not. This is simply the result of a 2D radiograph attempting to depict 3D reality. This shortcoming can lead to either the underestimation or overestimation of an orthodontic problem's severity. In addition, due to the curving arc in which the panoramic radiograph is captured, the angulations of the roots often are distorted (Peck *et al.*, 2007; see also Chapter 15). Finally, the need to capture both the maxilla and mandible simultaneously requires that the radiation beam pass through the teeth parallel to the occlusal plane. This beam alignment results in the foreshortening and distortion of any proclined incisors. The need to align the beam parallel to the occlusal plane also requires that the user adjust the volume's pitch from its original orientation (Figure 8.18).

Though substantially more pronounced in plain film panoramic radiographs, the aforementioned 2D shortcomings are also present when generating a panoramic radiograph from a 3D volume. Thus, all of the same cautions should be exercised when evaluating its 3D-generated panoramic radiograph as done when interpreting its traditional projectional counterpart. Also, for this reason, the teeth and their surrounding structures always should be viewed and evaluated within their native 3D environment. This will result in a much greater appreciation of the structures' relationships by the clinician while giving context to their surroundings.

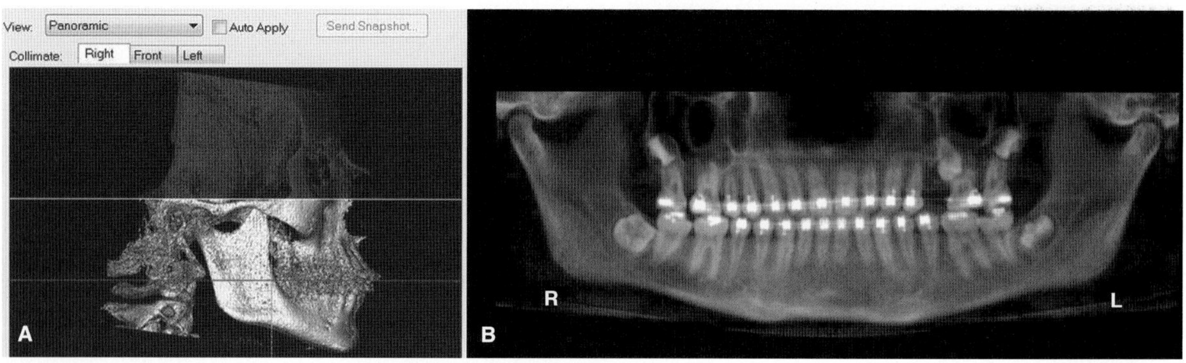

Figure 8.18 *A*: Eliminating the superior and inferior aspects of the volume for reconstructing a panoramic radiograph, as shown in panel *B*. Note that the occlusal plane has been reoriented to be parallel to the ground.

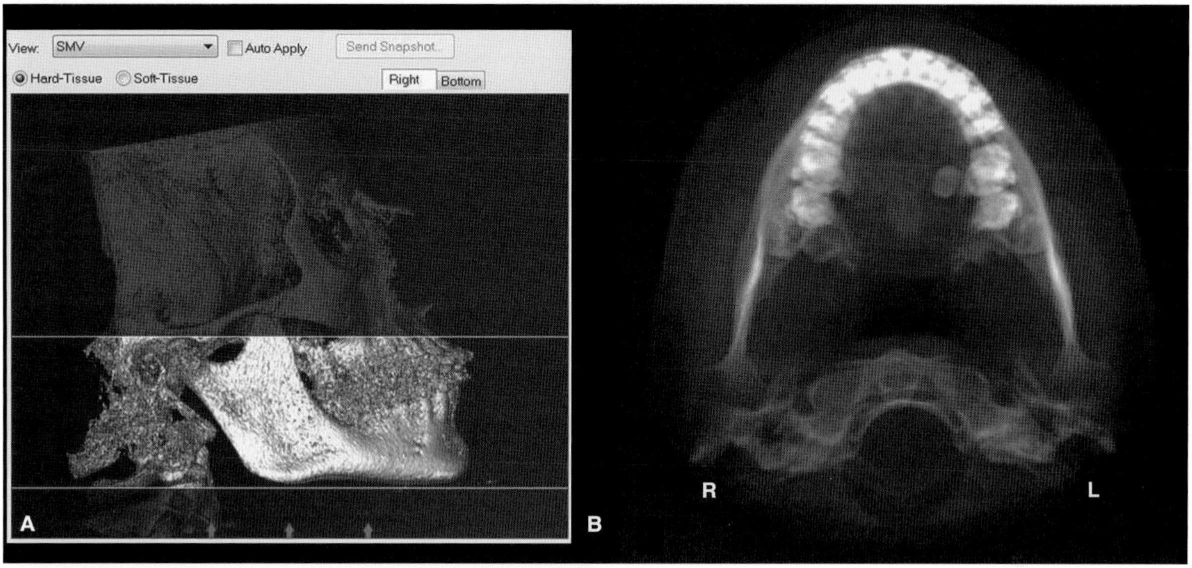

Figure 8.19 *A*: Eliminating the superior and inferior aspects of the volume for reconstructing a submentovertex, as shown in panel *B*.

Reconstruction of submentovertex radiographs

A benefit of CBCT is the ability to reconstruct limitless views of the volume from a variety of angles that often are difficult to capture in real life. For example, the submentovertex view can be helpful particularly in diagnosing asymmetries in the bodies, rami, and condyles of the mandible (Forsberg *et al.*, 1984). However, to maximize its diagnostic potential, the traditional projectional submentovertex should be taken with the radiation beam aligned perpendicular to the angle of the mandible; this is difficult to accomplish in a clinical setting. By comparison, the task of aligning the beam is accomplished indirectly within the CBCT reconstruction software by orienting the volume appropriately prior to reconstructing the projection (Figure 8.19).

Frontal cephalogram reconstruction

Another helpful view in orthodontic diagnosis, but one that is not taken commonly during initial orthodontic screenings, is the frontal cephalogram. Traditionally, this film has been captured with the beam of radiation passing from the posterior to the anterior of the patient and commonly is referred to as a "PA ceph" (Broadbent *et al.*, 1975). However, by using CBCT reconstruction software, this radiograph can be created with ease from either the posterior-anterior or anterior-posterior direction (Kim *et al.*, 2012). In addition, the spine can be cropped out easily to produce a cleaner image (Figure 8.20).

The frontal cephalogram is useful particularly in evaluating patients for the source of facial asymmetries (Athanasiou & Van Der Meij, 1995). Facial asymmetries can be caused by skeletal or dental discrepancies or both; likewise, the origin of the asymmetries can be the maxilla or the mandible or both. Determining whether the asymmetry is skeletal, dental, and maxillary or mandibular in origin is paramount to rendering an accurate diagnosis and, ultimately, an appropriate treatment plan. The prevalence of dentofacial asymmetries in adolescent orthodontic patients has been reported to be as high as 62% (Sheats *et al.*, 1998). Failure to diagnose facial asymmetries properly during the initial

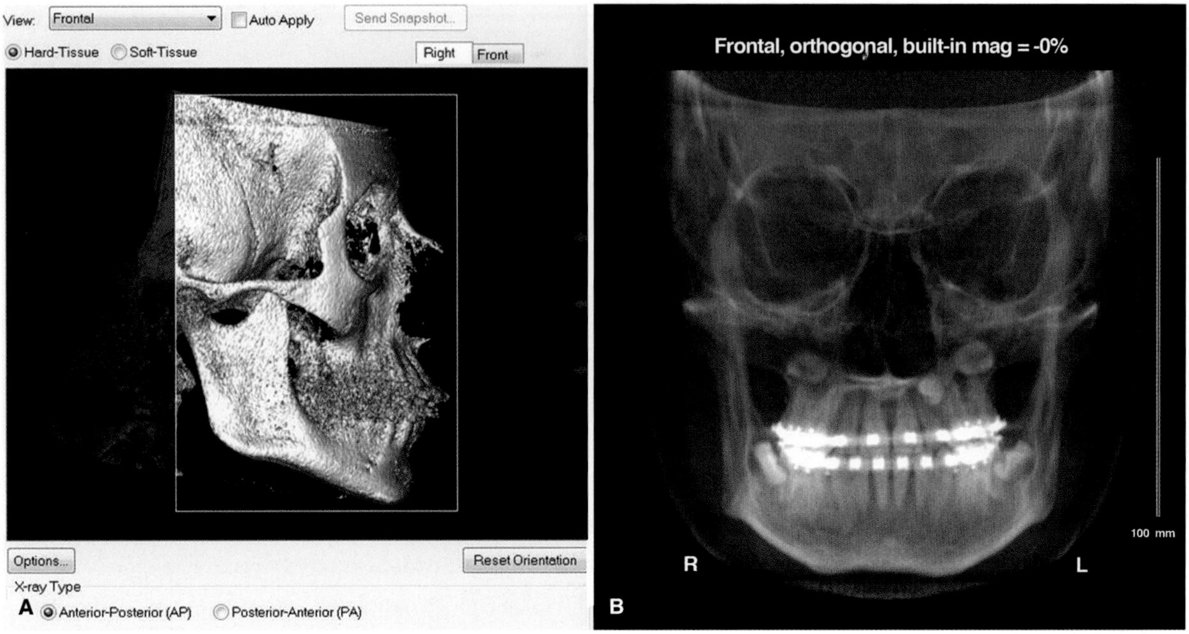

Figure 8.20 *A*: Eliminating the posterior aspects of the volume for reconstructing an anterior-posterior frontal cephalogram, as shown in panel *B*.

treatment plan may result in excessively prolonged orthodontic treatment or compromised final occlusions.

General reconstruction techniques

During the process of reconstructing 2D radiographs from the 3D volume, the technician will be able to apply several algorithm-based filters to create 2D radiographs that emphasize various aspects of the image. Several common rendering filters are ray-sum and maximum intensity projection (MIP). Different filters also allow the viewer to take greater advantage of the CBCT system's grayscale.

CBCT systems currently are available with ranges between 12- and 16-bit grayscale (Hatcher & Aboudara, 2004). Since the human eye cannot distinguish beyond 10-bit grayscale and computer monitors currently are available only in 8- or 10-bit grayscale, it could be assumed that exceeding these thresholds would have little worth (Kimpe & Tuytschaever, 2007). However, that assumption fails to take into account that the reconstruction software uses the increased bit depth to improve its reconstructions, thereby resulting in a cleaner and more defined volume. Most reconstruction software also allows the clinician to change the values of grayscale displayed on the screen using a process referred to as windowing (Buzug, 2008). By scrolling through the various values of gray captured in the scan, the clinician can visualize the volume better, despite the limitations of human eyes and computer monitors. Most reconstruction software allows windowing to be applied to the reconstructed 2D radiographs and also to the multiplanar reconstructions of the volume.

Advanced reconstruction techniques

Beyond simple reconstructions, the various software programs available can perform more advanced manipulations of the volume. For example, algorithms built into the software can identify the airway spaces within the volume to allow for the visualization and measurement of the

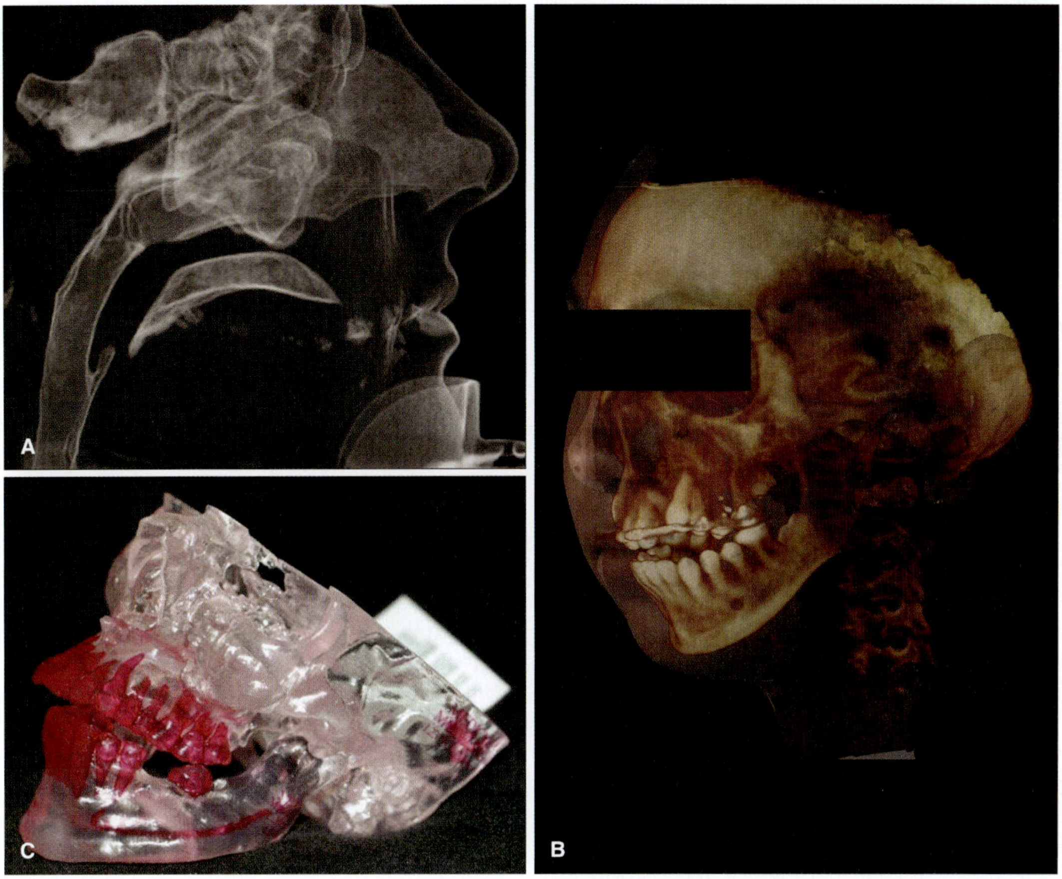

Figure 8.21 Some examples of advanced reconstruction techniques. *A*: Volume rendering of airway anatomy. *B*: 3D photos can be generated using stereophotogrammetry and then overlaid on a CBCT volume rendering to create a virtual patient. *C*: Physical analogues of a volume can be printed using a stereolithographic printer.

sinuses and airway (Figure 8.21A; see also Chapter 13). The volumes also can be merged with 3D photographs that were generated using stereophotogrammetry systems that use multiple cameras to capture an image simultaneously from multiple angles (Hatcher & Dial, 2009). The result is a marriage of the patient's soft tissue features and the hard tissue skeleton (Figure 8.21B). Some software also has the ability to export the segmented CBCT volume into a stereolithography (STL) file format. This reformatted volume then can be used by a stereolithographic printer to create a physical 3D model of the CBCT volume (Figure 8.21C). This technique can be useful particularly for patients with craniofacial deformities or a history of facial trauma.

THE ROLE OF THE ORAL AND MAXILLOFACIAL RADIOLOGIST

In addition to the region of interest, every CBCT scan taken should be evaluated in its entirety (Carter *et al.*, 2008). This is the same principle that has governed orthodontists and general dentists alike in their interpretation of 2D projectional radiographs. As discussed in Chapters 1, 6 and 7, the concept that the dental practitioner who ordered the radiograph is responsible for interpreting its contents is not new. Indeed, the diagnostician, whether a dentist, orthodontist, or oral maxillofacial radiologist, is legally responsible for identifying any pathology in the entire imaged volume and referring patients for follow-up when clinically significant findings are noted on the scan.

Dentists and orthodontists receive substantial training in dental school and orthodontic residency about how to interpret and diagnose pathology on conventional 2D radiographs. When it comes to interpreting CBCT scans, appropriate curriculae still are being developed and implemented within programs and schools, and the training is not yet ubiquitous. During this transition period, it is incumbent upon the prescribing clinician to become trained in interpreting CBCT scans. After attending continuing education courses and studying the available literature, the clinician then should identify his or her personal comfort level regarding the interpretation of CBCT scans. Some clinicians may feel confident diagnosing only the orthodontically relevant anatomy of the scan and will refer the scans to an oral and maxillofacial radiologist to evaluate the remainder of the volume. Other clinicians may feel confident in their ability to identify abnormalities in the scans, following which he or she may request further evaluation by an oral and maxillofacial radiologist. Ultimately, the responsibility to identify these personal boundaries of capabilities lies on the shoulders of the clinician who is prescribing the scan since he or she is responsible for the contents of the volume (Zinman *et al.*, 2010; see also Chapter 7). An appropriate protocol for CBCT image interpretation, reporting, and follow-up is presented in Chapter 1.

THE FUTURE OF CBCT AND ORTHODONTICS

The future of CBCT orthodontics lies in "integration." As the technology becomes more ubiquitous, orthodontists will begin to see more products and services being offered with CBCT integration. As prudent practitioners, it will be incumbent upon each orthodontist to evaluate the value of the service or product and the benefits to his or her patients versus the risks. As radiation doses decrease, these services and products will gain momentum and ultimately play an important role not only in how orthodontists diagnose their patients, but also in the choice of tools used to treat them.

Though intraoral scanners have allowed us to begin moving away from taking impressions, their inability to capture the anatomy and relationships of the roots has been their weakness (Stevens *et al.*, 2006). Unlike intraoral scanners, CBCT scans can capture and display the entire dentoalveolar structure, but currently lack the spatial resolution required for the fabrication of study models or appliances unless the scan duration, frame acquisition, and radiation output of the scan is increased. This dilemma places the responsibility back on the clinician to decide what is in the best interest of each individual. Every case should be evaluated individually to determine if traditional orthodontic imaging and its lower radiation dose are sufficient to facilitate an outcome that meets both the patient's and doctor's expectations. Conversely, the orthodontist should be trained sufficiently to identify patients for whom traditional imaging would be inadequate and who instead would benefit from the increased diagnostic information derived from a CBCT scan.

CONCLUSIONS

This chapter provides insights on the benefits of CBCT imaging in orthodontic diagnosis and treatment planning, as well as the protocols for reconstructing scans, interpreting images, and utilizing them in orthodontic practice. As hardware and software continue to evolve, CBCT scans and other emerging technologies likely will become increasingly integrated into the orthodontic practice. CBCT technology thus offers new horizons to the profession, and the need to learn how to utilize it is in the best interest of every orthodontist. The motto of Dr. G.V. Black, the father of modern dentistry, stated: "The professional man has no right to be other than a continuous student." As we strive to be continual students, we also should recognize that if we fail to do so, the profession will not wait for us, but quickly will pass us by. In the words of the Carnegie Commission on Higher Education

(1970): "Health professionals must remain students throughout their professional careers or face partial obsolescence."

References

Ackerman, J.L., Proffit, W.R., Sarver, D.M., *et al.* (2007) Pitch, roll, and yaw: describing the spatial orientation of dentofacial traits. *American Journal of Orthodontics and Dentofacial Orthopedics*, 131 (3), 305–310.

Athanasiou, A.E. & Van Der Meij, A.J.W. (1995) Posteroanterior (frontal) cephalometry. In Athanasiou, A.E. (ed.), *Orthodontic Cephalometry*. 1st ed. Mosby-Wolfe, London, pp. 141–161.

Ballrick, J.W., Palomo, J.M., Ruch, E., *et al.* (2008) Image distortion and spatial resolution of a commercially available cone-beam computed tomography machine. *American Journal of Orthodontics and Dentofacial Orthopedics*, 134 (4), 573–582.

Becker, A., Chaushu, S., & Casap-Caspi, N. (2010a) Cone-beam computed tomography and the orthosurgical management of impacted teeth. *Journal of the American Dental Association*, 141 (Suppl 3), 14S–18S.

Becker, A., Chaushu, G., & Chaushu, S. (2010b) Analysis of failure in the treatment of impacted maxillary canines. *American Journal of Orthodontics and Dentofacial Orthopedics*, 137 (6), 743–754.

Bjerklin, K. & Ericson, S. (2006) How a computerized tomography examination changed the treatment plans of 80 children with retained and ectopically positioned maxillary canines. *Angle Orthodontist*, 76 (1), 43–51.

Botticelli, S., Verna, C., & Cattaneo, P.M. (2011) Two-versus three-dimensional imaging in subjects with unerupted maxillary canines. *European Journal of Orthodontics*, 33 (4), 344–349.

Broadbent, B.H., Sr., Broadbent, B.H., Jr., & Golden, W.H. (1975) *Bolton Standards of Dentofacial Developmental Growth*. Mosby, St. Louis, MO.

Buzug, T.M. (2008) *Computed Tomography: From Photon Statistics to Modern Cone-Beam CT*. Springer, Berlin.

Carnegie Commission on Higher Education (1970) *Higher Education and the Nation's Health Policies for Medical and Dental Education*. McGraw-Hill, New York.

Carter, L., Farman, A., Geist, J., *et al.* (2008) American Academy of Oral and Maxillofacial Radiology executive opinion statement on performing and interpreting diagnostic cone beam computed tomography. *Oral Surgery, Oral Medicine, Oral Pathology, Oral Radiology, and Endodontics*, 106 (4), 561–562.

Cevidanes, L.H., Oliveira, A.E., Motta, A., *et al.* (2009) Head orientation in CBCT-generated cephalograms. *Angle Orthodontist*, 79 (5), 971–977.

Cevidanes, L.H., Alhadidi, A., Paniaqua, B., *et al.* (2011) Three-dimensional quantification of mandibular asymmetry through cone-beam computerized tomography. *Oral Surgery, Oral Medicine, Oral Pathology, Oral Radiology, and Endodontics*, 111 (6), 757–770.

Chakeres, D.W. (1984) Clinical significance of partial volume averaging of the temporal bone. *American Journal of Neuroradiology*, 5 (3), 297–302.

Cho, H.J. (2009) A three-dimensional cephalometric analysis. *Journal of Clinical Orthodontics*, 43 (4), 235–252.

Damstra, J., Oosterkamp, B.C., Jansma, J., *et al.* (2011) Combined 3-dimensional and mirror-image analysis for the diagnosis of asymmetry. *American Journal of Orthodontics and Dentofacial Orthopedics*, 140 (6), 886–894.

Endo, M., Tsunoo, T., Nakamori, N., *et al.* (2001) Effect of scattered radiation on image noise in cone beam CT. *Medical Physics*, 28 (4), 469–474.

Farronato, G., Garagiola, U., Dominici, A., *et al.* (2010) "Ten-point" 3D cephalometric analysis using low-dosage cone beam computed tomography. *Progress in Orthodontics*, 11 (1), 2–12.

Faure, J., Oueiss, A., Marchal-Sixou, C., *et al.* (2008) Three-dimensional cephalometry: applications in clinical practice and research. *L'Orthodontie Francaise*, 79 (1), 13–30.

Forsberg, C.T., Burstone, C.J., & Hanley, K.J. (1984) Diagnosis and treatment planning of skeletal asymmetry with the submental-vertical radiograph. *American Journal of Orthodontics*, 85 (3), 224–237.

Gribel, B.F., Griebel, M.N., Manzi, F.R., *et al.* (2011) From 2D to 3D: an algorithm to derive normal values for 3-dimensional computerized assessment. *Angle Orthodontist*, 81 (1), 3–10.

Grummons, D.C. & Kappeyne Van De Coppello, M.A. (1987) A frontal asymmetry analysis. *Journal of Clinical Orthodontics*, 21 (7), 448–465.

Halazonetis, D.J. (2012) Cone-beam computed tomography is not the imaging technique of choice for comprehensive orthodontic assessment. *American Journal of Orthodontics and Dentofacial Orthopedics*, 141 (4), 402–407.

Haney, E., Gansky, S.A., Lee, J.S., *et al.* (2010) Comparative analysis of traditional radiographs and cone-beam computed tomography volumetric images in the diagnosis and treatment planning of maxillary impacted canines. *American Journal of Orthodontics and Dentofacial Orthopedics*, 137 (5), 590–597.

Hans, M.G., Valiathan, M., & Palomo, J.M. (2011) Cone beam computed tomography: a link with the past, a promise for the future. *Seminars in Orthodontics*, 17 (1), 81–87.

Hatcher, D.C. & Aboudara, C.L. (2004) Diagnosis goes digital. *American Journal of Orthodontics and Dentofacial Orthopedics*, 125 (5), 512–515.

Hatcher, D.C. & Dial, C. (2009) Three-dimensional surface imaging of the face. *Journal of the California Dental Association*, 37 (3), 193–197.

Holberg, C., Steinhäuser, S., Geis, P., *et al.* (2005) Cone-beam computed tomography in orthodontics: benefits and limitations. *Journal of Orofacial Orthopedics*, 66 (6), 434–444.

Jacobson, R.L. (2006) Three-dimensional cephalometry. In Jacobson, A. & Jacobson, R.L. (eds.), *Radiographic Cephalometry: From Basics to 3-D Imaging*. 2nd ed. Quintessence, Chicago, IL, pp. 249–266.

Kim, S.J., Park, S.B., Kim, Y.I., *et al.* (2012) The reliability of cone-beam computed tomography (CBCT): generated frontal cephalograms. *Journal of Cranio-Maxillo-Facial Surgery*, 40 (8), e331–e336.

Kimpe, T. & Tuytschaever, T. (2007) Increasing the number of gray shades in medical display systems: how much is enough? *Journal of Digital Imaging*, 20 (4), 422–432.

Larson, B.E. (2012) Cone-beam computed tomography is the imaging technique of choice for comprehensive orthodontic assessment. *American Journal of Orthodontics and Dentofacial Orthopedics*, 141 (4), 402–410.

Mah, J.K., Enciso, R., & Jorgensen, M. (2003) Management of impacted cuspids using 3-D volumetric imaging. *Journal of the California Dental Association*, 31 (11), 835–841.

Mah, J.K., Huang, J.C., & Choo, H. (2010) Practical applications of cone-beam computed tomography in orthodontics. *Journal of the American Dental Association*, 141 (Suppl 3), S7–S13.

Molen, A.D. (2010) Considerations in the use of cone-beam computed tomography for buccal bone measurements. *American Journal of Orthodontics and Dentofacial Orthopedics*, 137 (Suppl 4), S130–S135.

Molen, A.D. (2011) Comparing cone beam computed tomography systems from an orthodontic perspective. *Seminars in Orthodontics*, 17 (1), 34–38.

Moshiri, M., Scarfe, W.C., Hilgers, M.L., *et al.* (2007) Accuracy of linear measurements from imaging plate and lateral cephalometric images derived from cone-beam computed tomography. *American Journal of Orthodontics and Dentofacial Orthopedics*, 132 (4), 550–560.

Motokawa, M., Sasamoto, T., Kaku, M., *et al.* (2011) Association between root resorption incident to orthodontic treatment and treatment factors. *European Journal of Orthodontics*, 34 (3), 350–356.

Park, J.U., Kook, Y.A., & Kim, Y. (2012) Assessment of asymmetry in a normal occlusion sample and asymmetric patients with three-dimensional cone beam computed tomography. *The Angle Orthodontist*, 82 (5), 860–867.

Peck, J.L., Sameshima, G.T., Miller, A., *et al.* (2007) Mesiodistal root angulation using panoramic and cone beam CT. *The Angle Orthodontist*, 77 (2), 206–213.

Ricketts, R.M., Bench, R.W., Hilgers, J.J., *et al.* (1972) An overview of computerized cephalometrics. *American Journal of Orthodontics*, 61 (1), 1–28.

Robinson, A.H. & Petchenik, B.B. (1976) *The Nature of Maps: Essays Toward Understanding Maps and Mapping*. University of Chicago Press, Chicago, IL.

Scarfe, W.C. & Farman, A.G. (2008) What is cone-beam CT and how does it work? *Dental Clinics of North America*, 52 (4), 707–730.

Sheats, R.D., McGorray, S.P., Musmar, Q., *et al.* (1998) Prevalence of orthodontic asymmetries. *Seminars in Orthodontics*, 4 (3), 138–145.

Stevens, D.R., Flores-Mir, C., Nebbe, B., *et al.* (2006) Validity, reliability, and reproducibility of plaster *vs* digital study models: comparison of peer assessment rating and Bolton analysis and their constituent measurements. *American Journal of Orthodontics and Dentofacial Orthopedics*, 129 (6), 794–803.

Swennen, G.R.J. (2005) 3-D cephalometric analysis. In Swennen, G.R.J., Schutyser, F., & Hausamen, J.E. (eds.), *Three-Dimensional Cephalometry: A Color Atlas and Manual*. 1st ed. Springer-Verlag, Berlin, Germany, pp. 241–288.

Tsiklakis, K., Donta, C., Gavala, S., *et al.* (2005) Dose reduction in maxillofacial imaging using low dose cone beam CT. *European Journal of Radiology*, 56 (3), 413–417.

Walker, L., Enciso, R., & Mah, J. (2005) Three-dimensional localization of maxillary canines with cone-beam computed tomography. *American Journal of Orthodontics and Dentofacial Orthopedics*, 128 (4), 418–423.

Zinman, E.J., White, S.C., & Tetradis, S. (2010) Legal considerations in the use of cone beam computer tomography imaging. *Journal of the California Dental Association*, 38 (1), 49–56.

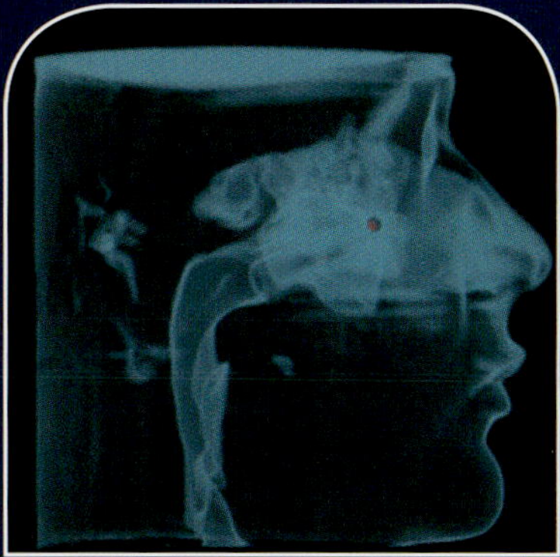

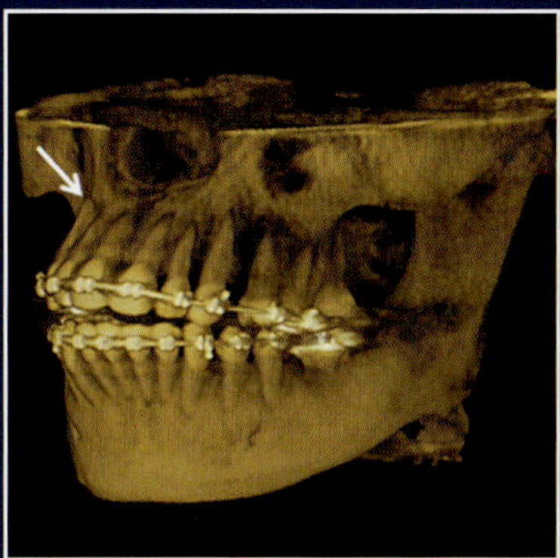

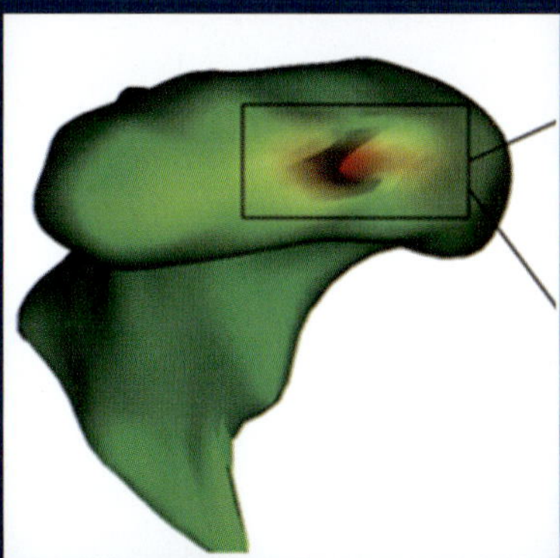

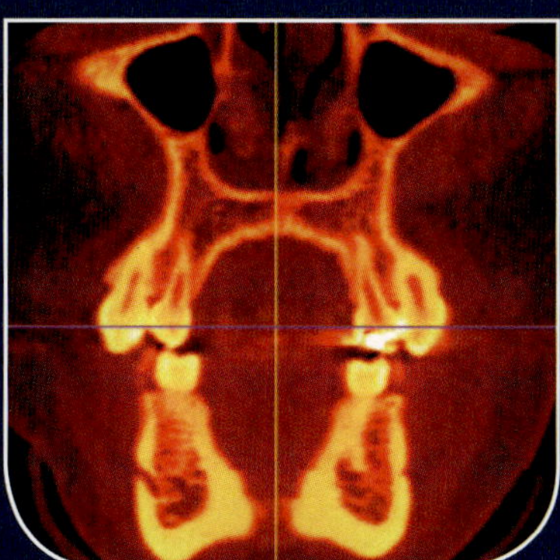

PART 3

Diagnosis and Treatment Planning

9 How to Interpret Cone Beam Computed Tomography Scans

Christos Angelopoulos, DDS, MS

INTRODUCTION

Cone beam computed tomography (CBCT) scans, as all diagnostic images, are prescribed mainly for three reasons: to assist in diagnosis, to assist in presurgical planning, and to assess the results of certain types of treatments or periodic evaluations (McDonald, 2011). The nature and progression of some diseases is such that diagnostic imaging ultimately could facilitate their identification and diagnosis. Diagnostic imaging is used most frequently in order to reveal pathology in areas of the human body that are not visible directly. In addition, diagnostic imaging is used to reveal features of a disease that may not be clear and may be crucial in its identification and progression.

Significant information about the disease in question may be revealed from its radiographic appearance. The analysis of a radiographic image (traditionally named radiographic interpretation) has a dual goal: the detailed review of the appearance of the diseased tissue in order to identify most or all of the features with which the pathological entity presents, and the review of the remainder of the tissues and structures included in the diagnostic image or the imaging volume in volumetric imaging, in order to rule out possible silent and, up to that point, incidental disease (Rege *et al.*, 2012). Although dental professionals strive to meet both goals in all dental diagnostic images, this becomes rather crucial in cone beam imaging due to the novelty of the modality and the overall lack of familiarity with multiplanar imaging in the profession (Angelopoulos, 2008).

The overall excitement in the dental profession about CBCT is illustrated by the numerous publications on this topic in dental literature. This has raised some concerns in the maxillofacial radiology community specifically regarding the ability of diagnosticians to recognize normal and abnormal

Cone Beam Computed Tomography in Orthodontics: Indications, Insights, and Innovations, First Edition. Sunil D. Kapila.

anatomy accurately and to identify incidental findings (Koong, 2010; Jacobs, 2011; Scarfe *et al.*, 2012). This chapter presents a sequential and logical approach to navigating three-dimensional (3D) volumes in order to distinguish normal from abnormal anatomy and to identify pathologies and incidental findings. Specifically, we provide general principles and protocols to follow in identifying, characterizing, and potentially arriving at differential diagnosis for any given lesion. A detailed site-specific presentation of lesions and pathologies are provided in Chapter 10.

PROTOCOLS FOR IMAGING, QUALITY ASSURANCE, AND IMAGE RECONSTRUCTION

Before we address CBCT image analysis, it is important to address some factors that may affect one or more of the steps of the analysis process and ultimately the diagnostic outcome.

Selection of the appropriate CBCT imaging protocol

A thorough clinical examination, either intraoral or extraoral or both depending on the diagnostic concern, will dictate the CBCT imaging protocol to be selected. The imaging protocol includes the field of view (FOV) and the voxel resolution of the scan to be acquired. Most of the CBCT scanners currently available in the market provide adjustable FOV that range from an area of exposure as small as 50 × 50 mm, which is adequate for examining two to three teeth and their surrounding structures, to 150 × 150 mm, which is large enough to examine more than two-thirds of the patient's head (see Chapter 2). Moreover, current CBCT scanners can acquire volumetric data with a voxel size between 0.08 and 0.4 mm, which provide images with an exceptional detail for hard tissue evaluation. The size of the pathological entity under investigation and the extent of the affected region will dictate the FOV to be selected (Scarfe & Farman, 2008). Facial asymmetries, large developmental defects, and facial trauma are some of the conditions that should steer the clinician toward the selection of an extended FOV (large imaging volume). On the contrary, implant site assessment, single tooth impactions, tooth defects, and periapical pathology are evaluated better using smaller FOV. Concomitantly, diagnostic tasks requiring high detail almost always mandate engaging a small voxel resolution to achieve the needed image resolution. Examples of such diagnostic tasks include periapical pathology, external and internal root resorption, ankylosis, and root fractures.

Scans acquired for surgical planning of pathologies or lesions should be limited to the areas of interest determined by the clinical examination and the extent of the affected region. Once more, the desired resolution is determined by the level of detail that is required to meet the objectives of the diagnostic task at hand.

CBCT scans as well as other radiographic procedures often are performed to assess the progression of disease or the outcome of a certain treatment or surgery (follow-up). The frequency of the follow-up examinations should be based on the suspected rate of the disease progression; certain pathological entities admittedly advance faster than others and no set rule exists as to the periodicity of these examinations. Once more, the follow-up clinical examination will determine how frequently these scans should be acquired. Post-surgical follow-up or post-treatment scans are prescribed to assess the progress of treatment or surgery or healing. Osseous tissue healing is slow and these scans may be acquired every 6–12 months; they also may be substituted with other simpler diagnostic images (panoramic or periapical radiographs) if the clinician is satisfied by the progress of the tissue healing. As always, the need for follow-up imaging and the selection of the appropriate type of imaging is determined after a clinical examination indicates that such an evaluation may be helpful. Progress of the treatment rendered is judged by comparing the follow-up radiographic examinations made at different time intervals after treatment or surgery with the initial radiographic examination performed before treatment or surgery.

While the above parameters provide some guidance on imaging procedures, a great deal of flexibility exists in the selection of the proper CBCT imaging protocol. The optimal protocol should be based ultimately on the clinician's judgment, knowledge, and professional responsibility, with the clinical examination as the deciding factor.

CBCT scan quality assurance

Poor image quality may obscure fine details in a scan, and, as a result, slight or early changes in the region of interest (ROI) may be missed; this, in turn, may compromise diagnosis. In fact, the link between the high image quality and the diagnostic efficiency is well established in the literature (White & Pharoah, 2004). The most common factors affecting image quality in a CBCT scan are patient motion during the scan acquisition and artifacts. Although current CBCT scanners acquire a scan rather fast (between 5 and 30 seconds), patient motion may occur during the scan and may have a detrimental effect in image quality. Strict adherence to the manufacturer's recommendations on patient positioning and stabilization in the scanner may reduce the likelihood of motion. A thorough review of the entire volumetric data after the scan is acquired—while the patient still is present—should be performed in order to identify signs of patient motion in the scan. If there is evidence of patient motion in the scan such as blurred images or double margins, the scan should be redone.

Artifacts are observed frequently in CBCT scans; they may deteriorate image quality and compromise diagnosis, sometimes rather significantly (Bechara *et al.*, 2012). Metallic restorations are the most frequent cause of artifacts. They present with alternating bright and dark bands or a "sunray" appearance and may make it impossible to evaluate any areas of the scan that may overlap with the pathology or lesion being investigated. In fact, the finer the diagnostic task at hand, the lower the diagnostic contribution of a CBCT scan will be in the presence of metallic artifacts, irrespective of the size or the resolution of the FOV selected. As a result, diagnoses regarding recurrent caries assessment, crown and root fractures, early periodontal defects, and other defects around or in contact with metallic restorations are difficult, if not impossible, to be made. Under such circumstances, the clinician's knowledge and experience will assist him or her to develop realistic expectations about the diagnostic efficiency of this exciting imaging modality.

Selection of proper reconstructions

Multiplanar imaging was introduced to dentistry with computed tomography (CT); however, the introduction of CBCT has spread its utilization to a large number of diagnostic tasks in dentistry. In simple words, multiplanar imaging or reformatting (MPR) is the ability of the clinician, or any user, to reconstruct any kind of image he or she wishes from an already acquired volumetric dataset or imaging volume. This admittedly was somewhat of a novelty for the dental profession. Dental professionals, with exception of maxillofacial radiologists and maxillofacial surgeons, rarely had any kind of exposure with the kind of diagnostic potential that MPR offers (Angelopoulos, 2008; Angelopoulos & Aghaloo, 2011). As a result, it is not uncommon for the most frequent reconstructions from an imaging volume to be panoramic images and sometimes cross-sectional images (sections perpendicular to a specific structure); these reconstructions target teeth and their surrounding structures almost exclusively. Although such standard reconstructions can contribute considerably to diagnosis, they may not be the answer to all diagnostic issues. Moreover, these select reconstructions may exclude a great deal of important data. Since some MPRs provide more diagnostic information for certain diagnostic tasks than others, it is the clinician's professional responsibility to be knowledgeable about these options in order to utilize them when needed. Therefore, when reviewing and preparing for image analysis and diagnosis, it is crucial to include all those reconstructions that may contribute to further our understanding of the specific diagnostic question and not to limit these views to some standard images (such as panoramic, cephalometric, or cross-sectional) or other images simply because they are familiar. Thus, for example, some specific indications of images for various purposes include the following: (1) 3D reconstructions are exceptional for the evaluation of gross asymmetry of the maxillofacial region and clefts and fractures in the maxilla mandible or mid-face; (2) paranasal sinuses and their draining sites are assessed best in coronal reconstructions; and (3) the best images to evaluate the airway are axial and sagittal reconstructions of the neck.

ANALYSIS OF CBCT IMAGES

Follow a system

The most important rule in reviewing a CBCT scan or other diagnostic images is to apply a systematic approach in order to ensure that no available diagnostic information is missed. An example of such an approach might be dividing the imaging volume in several smaller sections based on anatomical location such as the maxilla and maxillary teeth, mandible and mandibular teeth, nose and paranasal sinuses, temporomandibular joints (TMJs) and the neck, cervical spine, and skull base, and ensuring that all these sections will be reviewed and analyzed for possible clinically significant findings. This requires discipline, and it may take some time and practice to establish a pattern so as to make it almost "second nature" to follow this process, wherein steps of an algorithm are followed sequentially without any exceptions. If needed, a prepared template with these steps or anatomical locations to be reviewed can be used as a prompt and to record the findings. The same template also may be utilized even for limited field scans where no notes are included for the anatomical regions that have been omitted from the scan. In reviewing each of the anatomical regions mentioned above, special attention is paid to the "chief complaint" or the reason for the scan acquisition. Often the review may start from the region of concern, since it is natural to try to identify "what's wrong" first. This is a common practice in most, if not all, disciplines of medicine and dentistry. This is an acceptable approach, as are modifications to the algorithm described above to fit the clinician's needs better. However, the instant satisfaction of identifying "what's wrong" in the region of concern may contribute to omission of one or more steps of the algorithm, which, in turn, may result in overlooking significant diagnostic findings.

Collecting diagnostic information

The review of a CBCT scan is a step-by-step analysis of all abnormal radiographic findings or features with the goal of recognizing and collecting as much information as possible that is available in the various image reconstructions (White & Pharoah, 2004). Analysis of the collected information may lead the clinician to a diagnosis or, more frequently, to a short list of possible diagnoses.

As a first step, *the disease or the abnormality has to be identified*. For this purpose, the diagnostician should look for irregularities in the appearance of the region that the clinical examination and/or other findings have indicated as the area of concern, including changes in the shape and size or density affecting hard or soft tissue or both at the site. Alterations in the cortical or cancellous bone pattern (Figure 9.1 and Figure 9.2) are a frequent result of disease. Although dentists largely are familiar with normal and abnormal appearance of the osseous tissue in traditional dental diagnostic images, getting acquainted with irregular appearance of tissues in CBCT may require substantial exposure to and experience with these images (Ahmed *et al.*, 2012). With regard to soft tissues, CBCT images show minimal differences in density of various soft tissues (Figure 9.3); their changes in disease processes are almost impossible to identify unless the disease has caused either extensive destruction of the soft tissue involved or has induced the production of dystrophic calcifications (see Chapter 10).

The clinician also should look for asymmetry (Figure 9.4) and/or differences between the right and left side in gross anatomical structures such as the heads of the mandibular condyles, mandibular ramii, paranasal sinuses, and walls of the airway. Asymmetry often is a sign of unilateral growth or atrophy and may indicate disease. As opposed to developing diseases that tend to be unilateral, anatomical variations tend to be bilateral. Unfortunately, the anatomical variation between different individuals and sometimes even within the same individual adds a considerable amount of difficulty in diagnosis in some cases of asymmetric findings.

Noting the exact location of the abnormality or suspected disease is crucial in the diagnostic process.

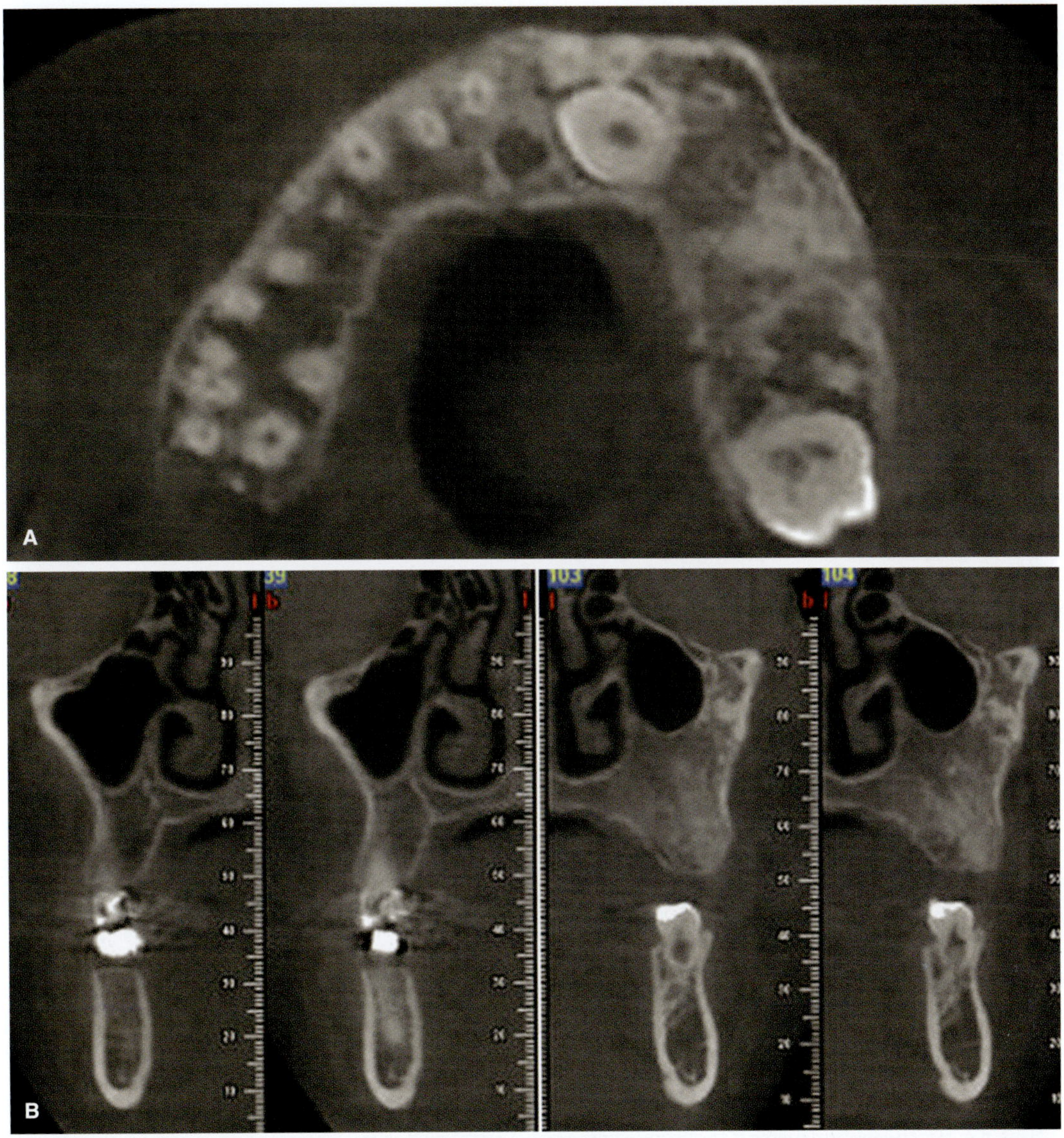

Figure 9.1 Axial (*A*) and cross-sectional (*B*) images of the maxilla depicting an asymmetry between the right and left side of the maxillary bone. Note the difference in the density of the alveolar bone between the left and right sides. This is the kind of information to be documented when reviewing the region of interest.

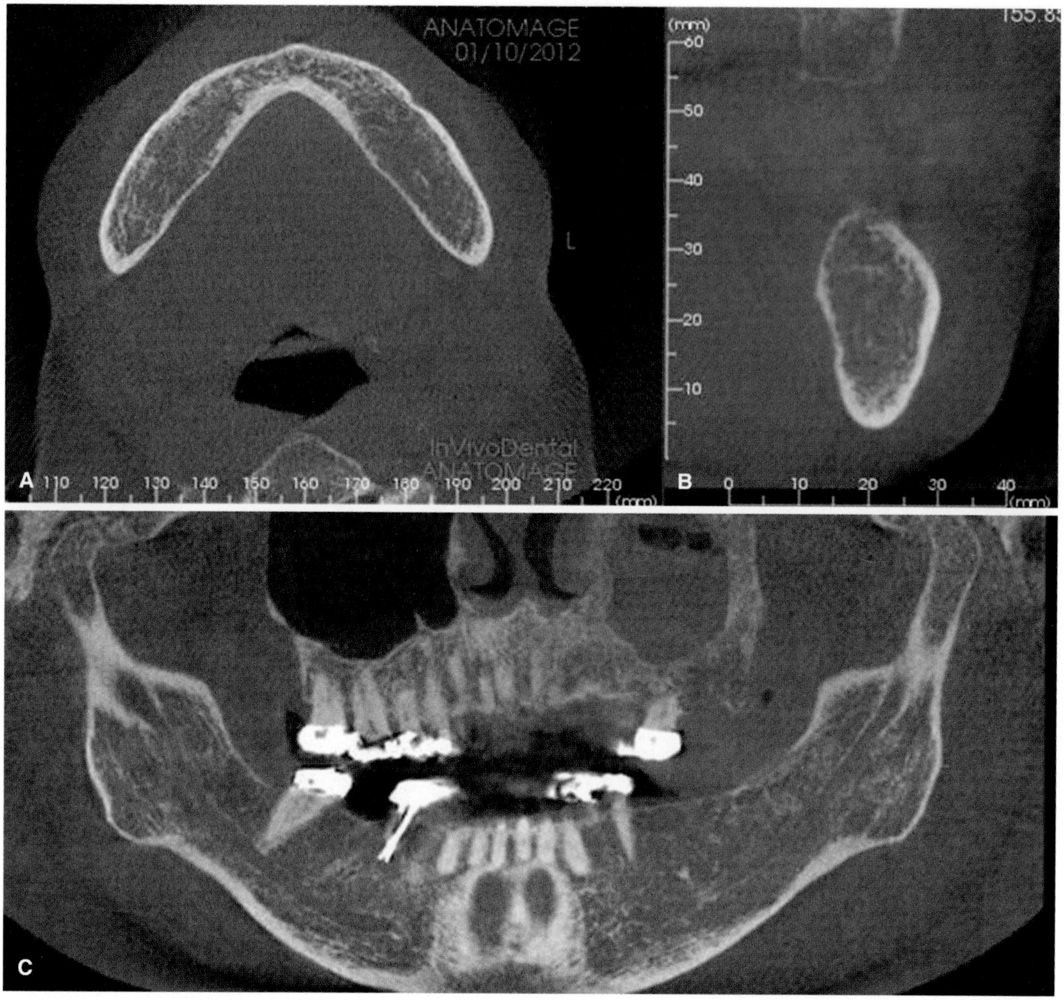

Figure 9.2 Axial (*A*), cross-sectional (*B*), and panoramic (*C*) reconstructions of the maxillofacial region of a 65-year-old female patient. Note the generalized rarefaction (low density) of the mandibular bone and the thinning of the mandibular cortex best depicted in the cross-sectional image. Such an observation should trigger the clinician to investigate for possible osteoporosis.

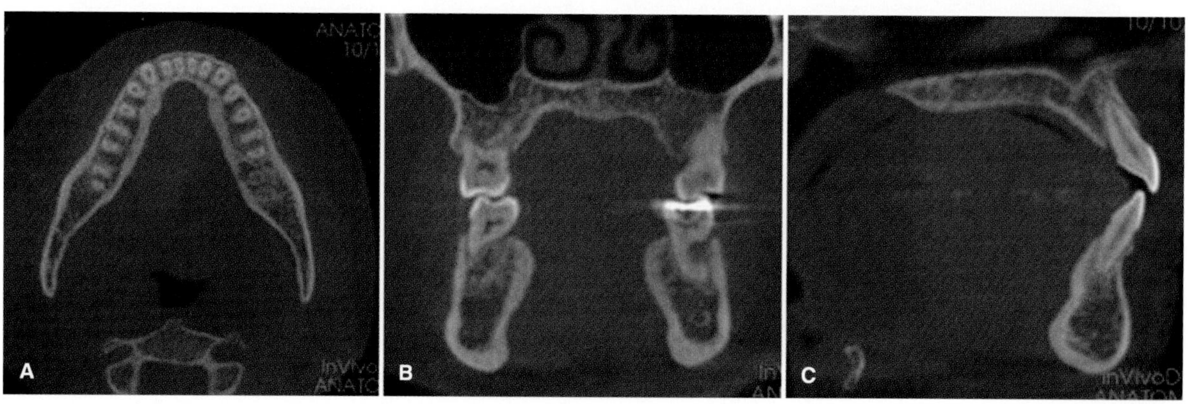

Figure 9.3 Axial (*A*), coronal (*B*), and sagittal (*C*) images of the floor of the mouth. Note the lack of distinction between the various soft tissue structures, namely, muscles, glands, and fat. The low soft tissue contrast on CBCT images makes it difficult to assess possible density differences between various soft tissues and changes that may result from disease.

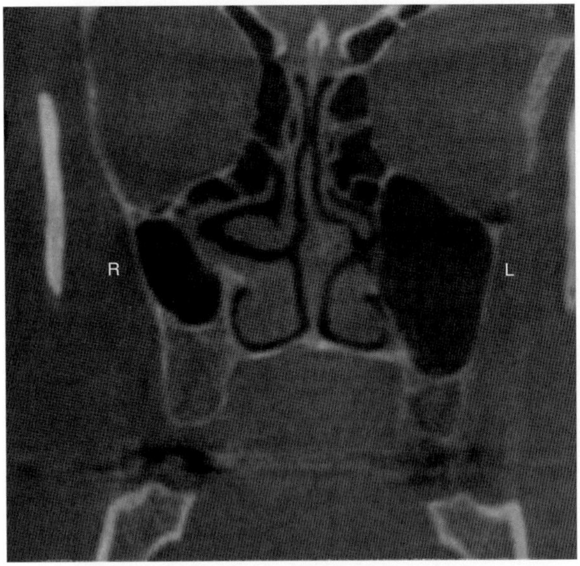

Figure 9.4 Coronal section of the maxillary sinuses showing a marked asymmetry between the right (R) and the left (L) maxillary sinus. This is consistent with right maxillary sinus hypoplasia and is a developmental defect that requires no further action.

Thus, it is important to identify all the anatomical structures in proximity to the area under examination, which will assist considerably in revealing the tissue of origin. Most of the pathological entities in the maxillofacial region follow a domestic pattern: they develop and grow within the tissue from which they have originated. The only exceptions are systemic conditions and metastatic disease. For example, if an intraosseous, suspected pathological entity under examination is identified in tooth-bearing areas of the jaws, the possibility that it is odontogenic in origin is fairly high (Figure 9.5). On the contrary, if it is located below the mandibular canal or in proximity to the floor of the maxillary sinuses (non-tooth-bearing areas), the chance of the tooth-related pathology is low (Figure 9.6). Similarly, if an unknown calcification is identified in the anatomical location of one of the major salivary glands, there is a strong possibility that it is a silalolith (Figure 9.7 and Figure 9.8). Thus, it is essential that the diagnostician be familiar with the anatomy of the maxillofacial region and its appearance in CBCT images. Admittedly, this is not easy to acquire since anatomical information of fine structures such as the maxillofacial structures, paranasal sinuses, skull base, and neck is scattered among multiple texts. In addition, certain anatomical structures, including those familiar to dental professionals in traditional imaging, become harder to identify in sectional imaging due to lack of training and experience. The ongoing utilization of MPR imaging by the dental profession, with appropriate experience or training or both, will provide the required comfort level in the identification of the various craniofacial anatomic structures and the variations in their presentation on images.

The next step is to *focus on the pathological entity and its appearance*. The various pathological entities that may be seen in the maxillofacial region differ in appearance. Different imaging characteristics often are a reflection of their nature, growth pattern, aggressiveness, and potential damage. These features have been studied in depth and are listed in several textbooks; however, most of these descriptions refer to traditional dental imaging, specifically intraoral and panoramic images. Although little has been written collectively until now on imaging characteristics of intraosseous maxillofacial diseases observed with advanced imaging modalities including CBCT, this deficiency in the literature had been overcome largely by the details provided in Chapter 10 of this book. With regard to the features of soft tissue pathological entities in CBCT imaging, there is no information available at all, probably because the poor soft tissue contrast of CBCT makes it impossible to distinguish and describe any pathological entity originating from soft tissue. Unless such soft tissue lesions affect the normal shape and size of known neighboring anatomical structures (airway, nasal cavity) or invade osseous structures, they likely will be unidentifiable in CBCT scans and will continue to grow silently unless diagnosed clinically or by other diagnostic methods.

The shape and borders of an unknown lesion will provide some hints about its nature and growth rate. Slow-growing pathological entities usually demonstrate a smooth border, whereas irregular borders often characterize more aggressive ones. Cystic lesions usually are round or ovoid in shape within the constraints of the shape of the jaw in the region they have developed. The border of a lesion

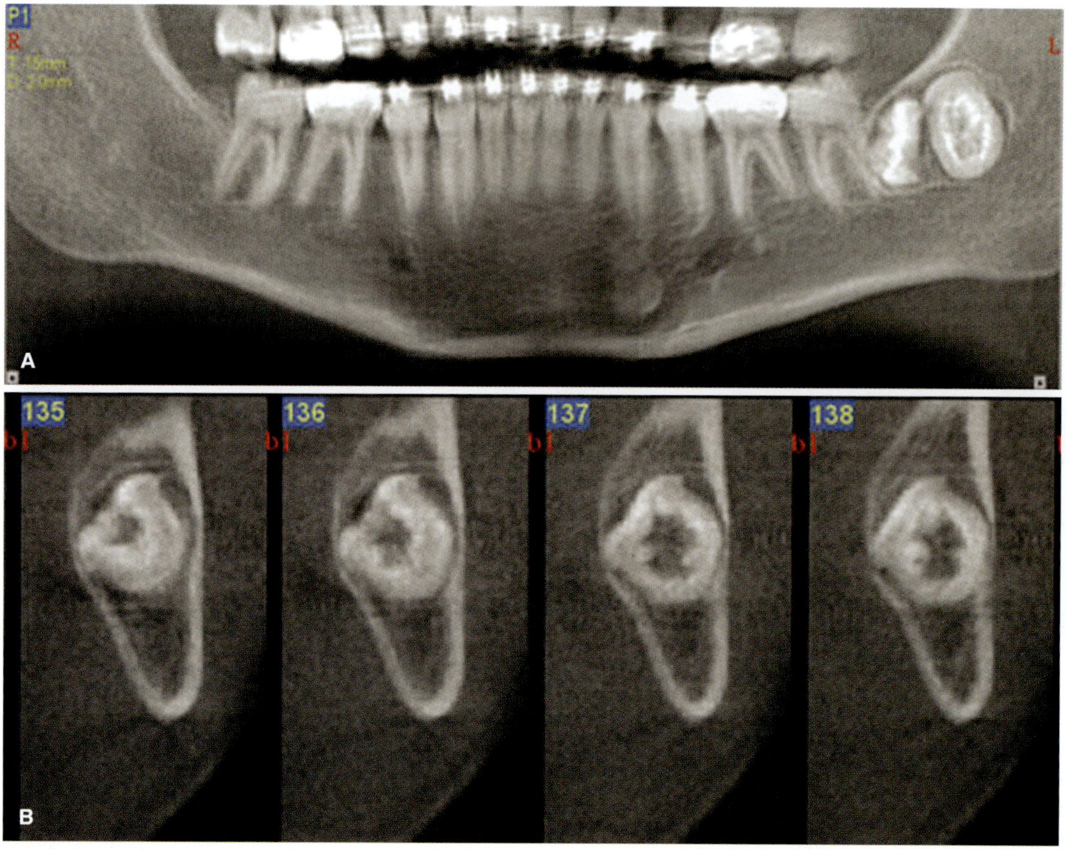

Figure 9.5 Panoramic (*A*) and cross-sectional images (*B*) depicting a large, well-defined, corticated lesion that contains a large radiopaque core. The density of the core is similar to that of teeth. The clearly delineated borders and the expansion of the bony cortices instead of erosion or destruction indicate a mass that is benign in nature. Note that the location of this mass (above the left mandibular canal) is a strong indicator that this mass is odontogenic in origin. In fact, this was a compound ondontoma. Odontomas are by far the most common odontogenic tumors.

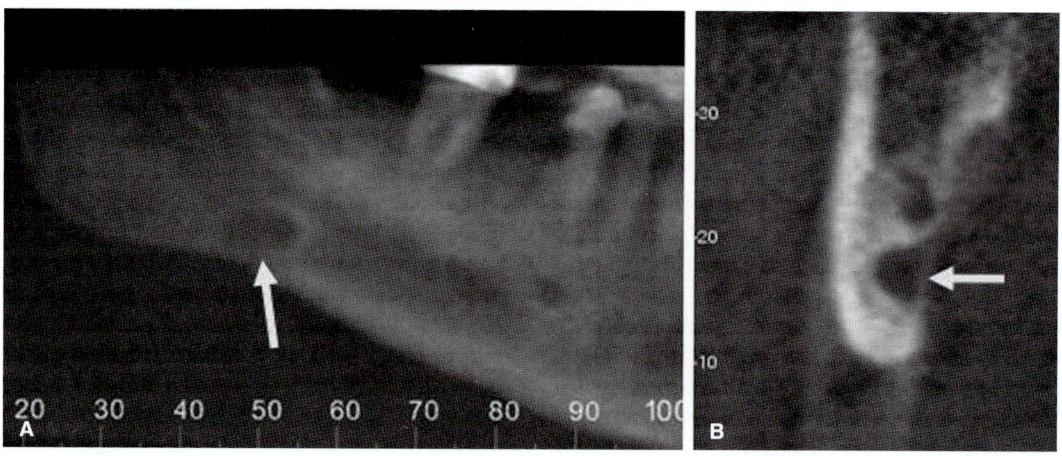

Figure 9.6 *A:* Cropped panoramic reconstruction depicting a well-defined, corticated low-density lesion below the right mandibular canal that has thinned the inferior mandibular cortex. The location of the lesion below the mandibular canal indicates that the origin of this entity is not odontogenic, because this is not a tooth-bearing region. *B:* The cross-sectional image of that region revealed that this was a concavity on the lingual aspect of the mandibular bone and not an intraosseous lesion. This appearance is almost pathognomonic for a submandibular gland depression or defect also known as Stafne's cyst.

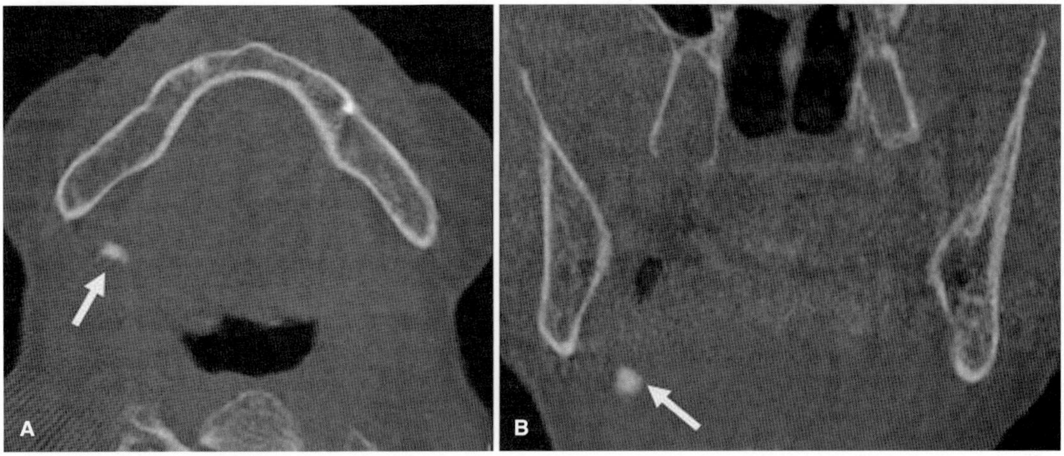

Figure 9.7 Axial (*A*) and coronal (*B*) sections at the level of the floor of the mouth depicting a well-defined, high-density structure (arrows) that is identified just medial and inferolingually to the right mandibular angle. Although the poor soft tissue contrast of CBCT prevents the delineation of the submandibular salivary glands—which blend with the rest of the soft tissue structures of the neck due to similar density—knowledge of the anatomical location of the gland assists in the characterization of the above high-density structure as a sialolith.

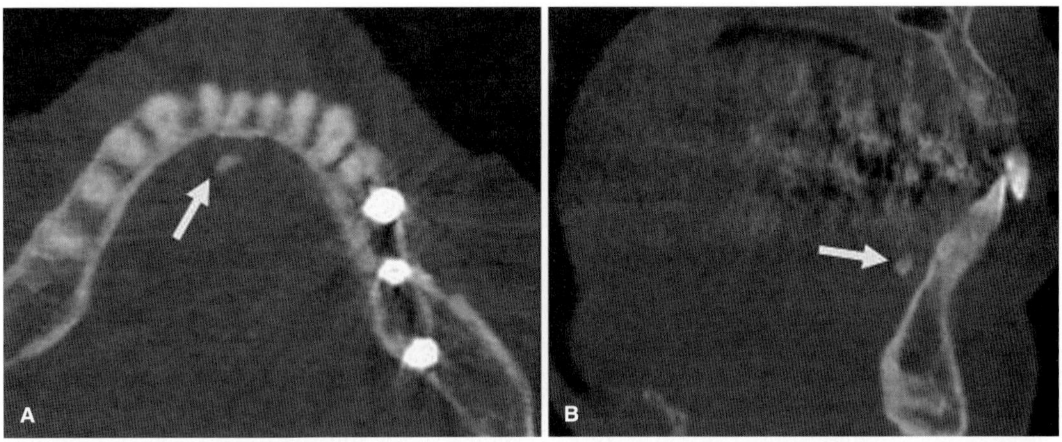

Figure 9.8 Axial (*A*) and sagittal (*B*) sections showing a small calcification just lingual to the incisors. The calcification is in proximity to the orifice of the right submandibular or sublingual salivary glands' ductal system. This is a common site for small stones. As a result, the characterization of such a calcification as a sialolith in the ductal system of either the right submandibular salivary gland or the sublingual salivary gland is valid.

is described as "well defined" or "poorly defined" based on how clear the distinction is between the diseased and healthy tissues. Presence of a well-defined, corticated border around an intraosseous lesion usually is a sign of a benign, slow-growing lesion (Figure 9.9). Larger cystic lesions may expand, contributing to the thinning of bony cortices, and, on some occasions, may perforate these cortices. In such cases, it is possible that the lesion may communicate with the oral cavity and become contaminated. Contaminated cystic lesions frequently behave like abscesses and may lose their

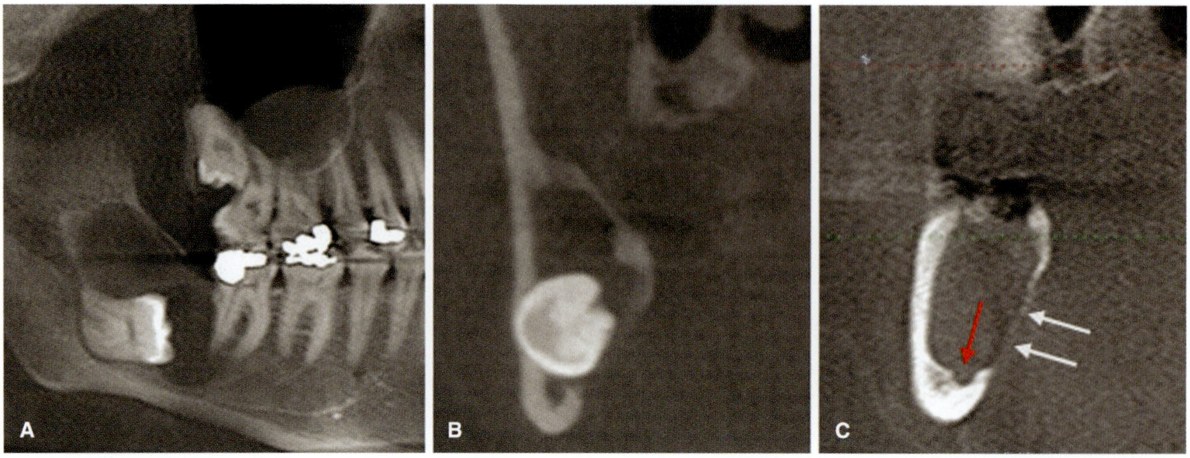

Figure 9.9 Panoramic (*A*) and cross-sectional (*B* and *C*) images of the right posterior mandible, which depict a well-defined lesion that is ovoid in shape and that is extended around an impacted right mandibular third molar. The lesion has expanded the buccal and lingual cortices and has thinned and possibly perforated the lingual cortex (white arrows). However, despite the expansion, it appears to be within the constraints of the mandibular bone. The above features all are characteristic of a benign lesion. The most likely diagnosis in this case is a dentigerous cyst. Note the displaced mandibular canal into the inferior cortex (red arrow) and the perforation of its superior wall.

clear delineation (Figure 9.10). In poorly defined lesions, the diseased tissue blends with the surrounding bone; this appearance is seen commonly in solid pathological entities that mostly are benign tumors (Figure 9.11). Lesions that demonstrate erosive or permeative borders are rather aggressive; another sign of aggressiveness is a "moth-eaten" destruction pattern or borders of the affected bone (Figure 9.12). The above most frequently characterize malignancies or osteomyelitis.

The internal architecture of the pathological entity under examination will contribute to the differentiation between a solid mass (tumor) and a cystic lesion. Lesions that demonstrate a uniform, low-density (radiolucent) content often are cystic lesions. The vault of a lesion that is cystic in appearance sometimes is divided into a number of smaller chambers; this number may vary from a few to several. These chambers are known as loculations and the internal structure of such a lesion is called multilocular. Some odontogenic cysts (odontogenic keratocyst, dentigerous cyst) and a number of benign odontogenic tumors (ameloblastoma, odontogenic myxoma) demonstrate a multilocular internal pattern (Figure 9.13). Lesions that demonstrate a high-density internal structure or radiopacity may be abnormal osseous tissue such as sclerotic bone formation (Figure 9.14) or solid masses such as tumors (Figure 9.15).

The effects of the lesion on the surrounding tissues vary and will provide information about the behavior of the developing pathology. Slow-growing lesions most frequently will displace teeth, cause root resorption, expand bony cortices, and generally displace anatomical structures in the vicinity as they try to find space to grow in order to form space-occupying masses. Such lesions may displace the floor of the maxillary sinuses and nasal cavities, sometimes considerably, if they are developing in the maxilla (Figure 9.16A,B), or the mandibular canal and mental foramen, if they are developing in the mandible. While this commonly is seen in sizable pathological entities, it may be seen even in smaller ones contributing to the commonly known "halo effect" (Figure 9.16C). When one recognizes the findings discussed above as effects of an unknown lesion, benign pathological entities such as cysts or benign neoplasms should be considered first as possible diagnoses.

In contrast, rapidly growing lesions most frequently erode bony cortices instead of expanding them, invade neighboring anatomical structures

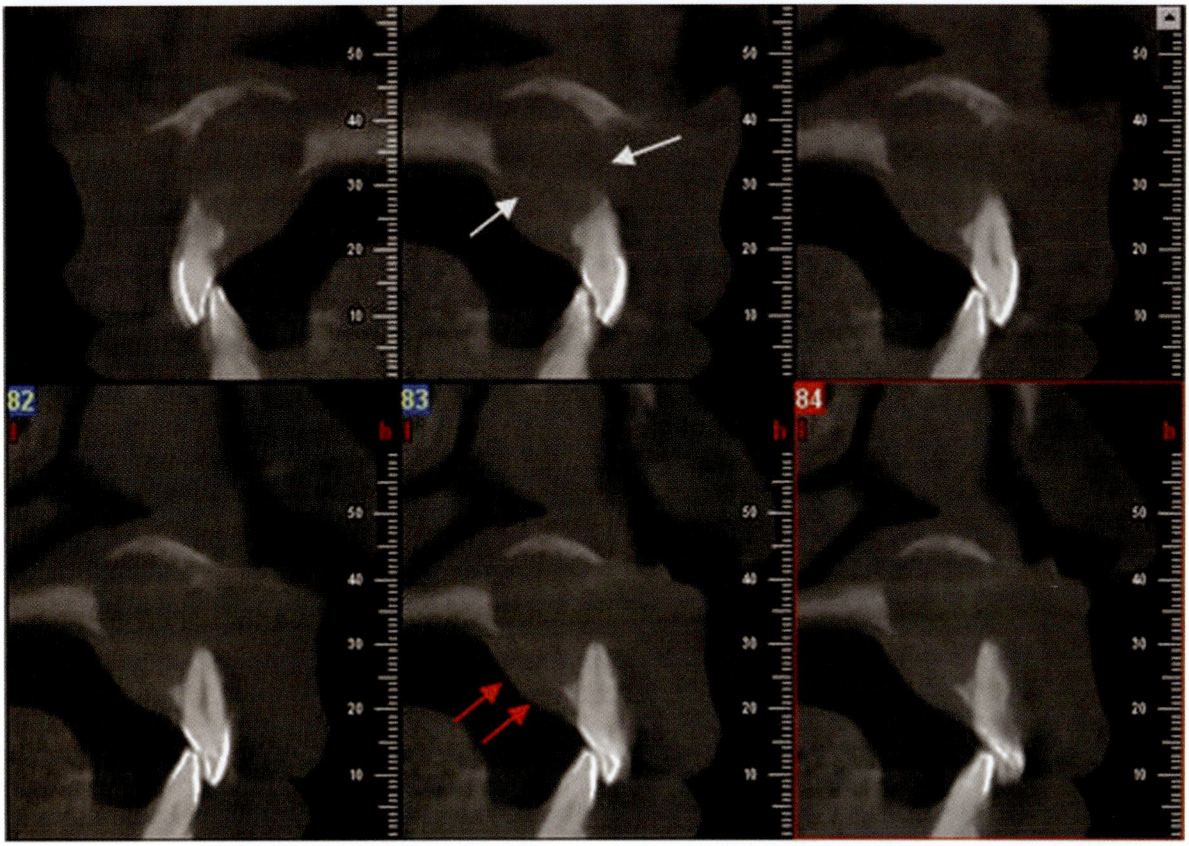

Figure 9.10 Sagittal sections showing a large, round, fairly well-defined lesion that is cystic in appearance in the central incisor location, along the maxillary midline, that has perforated the labial as well as the palatal cortex (white arrows). The lack of a corticated border most likely is an indication that the cystic lesion is contaminated through communication with the oral cavity. Note the projection of the lesion into the oral cavity due to the expansion of the palatal mucosa (red arrows). The cystic lesion was fluctuating on palpation of the labial and palatal aspect of the alveolar ridge.

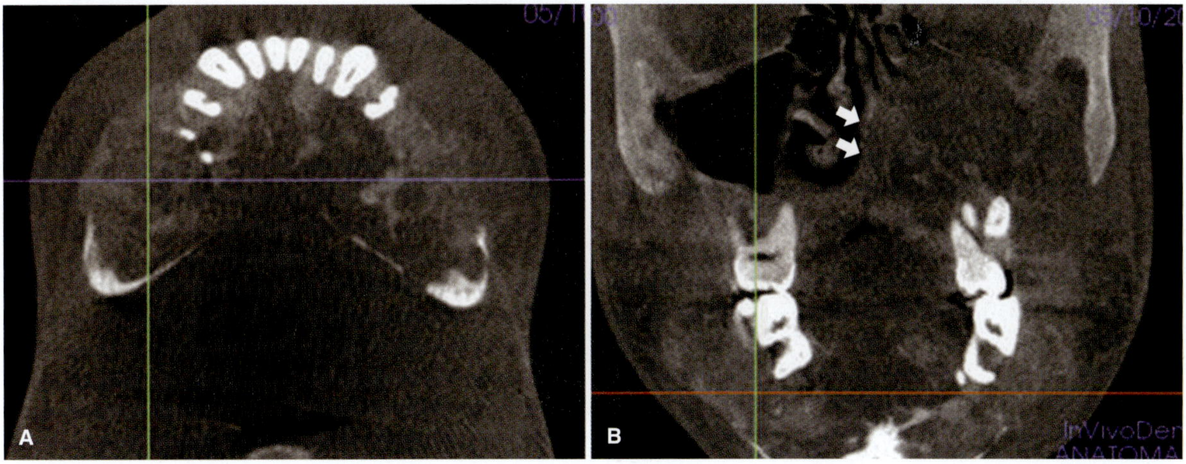

Figure 9.11 Axial (*A*) and coronal (*B*) sections showing multiple, mixed in appearance, expansile masses throughout the maxilla and the mandible. The lesions are blending with the healthy osseous tissues and their borders are impossible to distinguish. They occupy the entire mandible and a large portion of the maxilla and the nasal cavity. The arrows show that the lesions under investigation are in contact with the nasal septum and appear to be rather invasive. The patient's history of hyperparathyroidism and the above-mentioned radiographic findings suggest these lesions most likely are brown tumors.

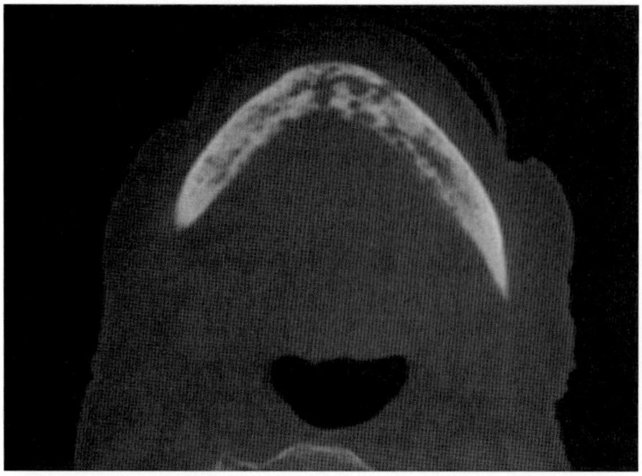

Figure 9.12 Axial section of the mandible showing a characteristic "moth-eaten" appearance of the inferior border of the mandible, extending approximately from the region of the left to right first molars. The lesion has eroded the lingual and the mandibular cortices and consists of multiple small, poorly defined radiolucencies. The above features are suggestive strongly of either a malignant lesion or osteomyelitis. In this case, the pathology was a metastatic lesion.

instead of displacing them, and grow fast around teeth instead of moving them. In other words, they generally cause significant destruction in the region they grow, irrespective of the tissue of origin. These features characterize rather aggressive pathological entities and, when they are recognized, one should include malignant neoplasms in formulating a list of possible diagnoses. As always, there are a few exceptions to this rule; osteomyelitis, an inflammatory disease of bone and bone marrow, is almost indistinguishable radiographically from malignant or metastatic disease (Figure 9.17).

Abnormalities originating from soft tissue may be observed when reviewing a CBCT, although a CBCT scan rarely will be prescribed for the assessment of a pathological entity that is identified within soft tissue and causes no effects in the neighboring hard tissues. The only exception might be airway restriction or obliteration. Consequently, most of these soft tissue abnormalities might be incidental findings on CBCT that otherwise typically are silent. The two main features of soft tissue abnormalities that may raise the diagnostician's

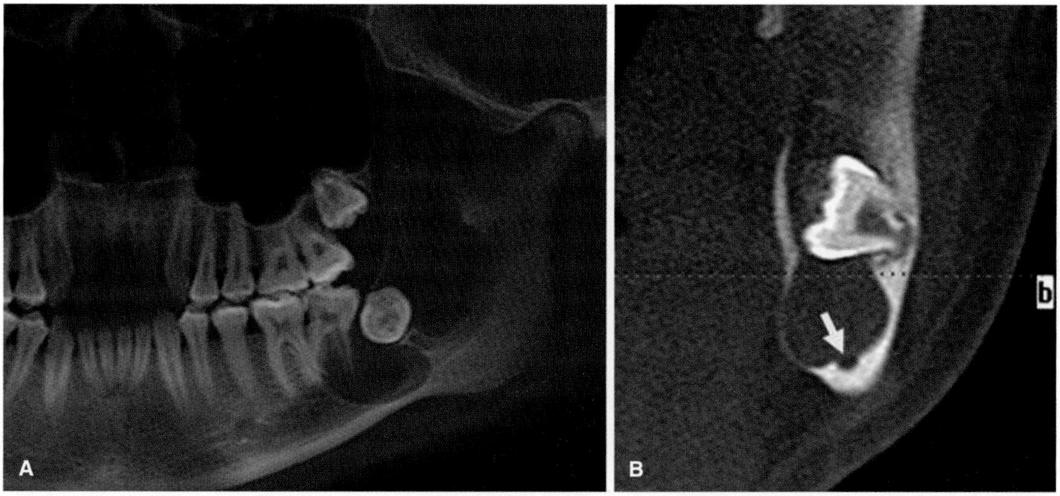

Figure 9.13 A panoramic view (*A*) and coronal section (*B*) of a lesion with a multilocular or multiple-chamber pattern involving an impacted third molar. This frequently is characteristic of more aggressive pathological entities such as odontogenic keratocystic tumor or ameloblastoma. In this case, the lesion has expanded and thinned both cortices of the left mandibular ramus and has displaced the second molar and the left mandibunar canal (arrow). The confirmed diagnosis in this case was odontogenic keratocystic tumor.

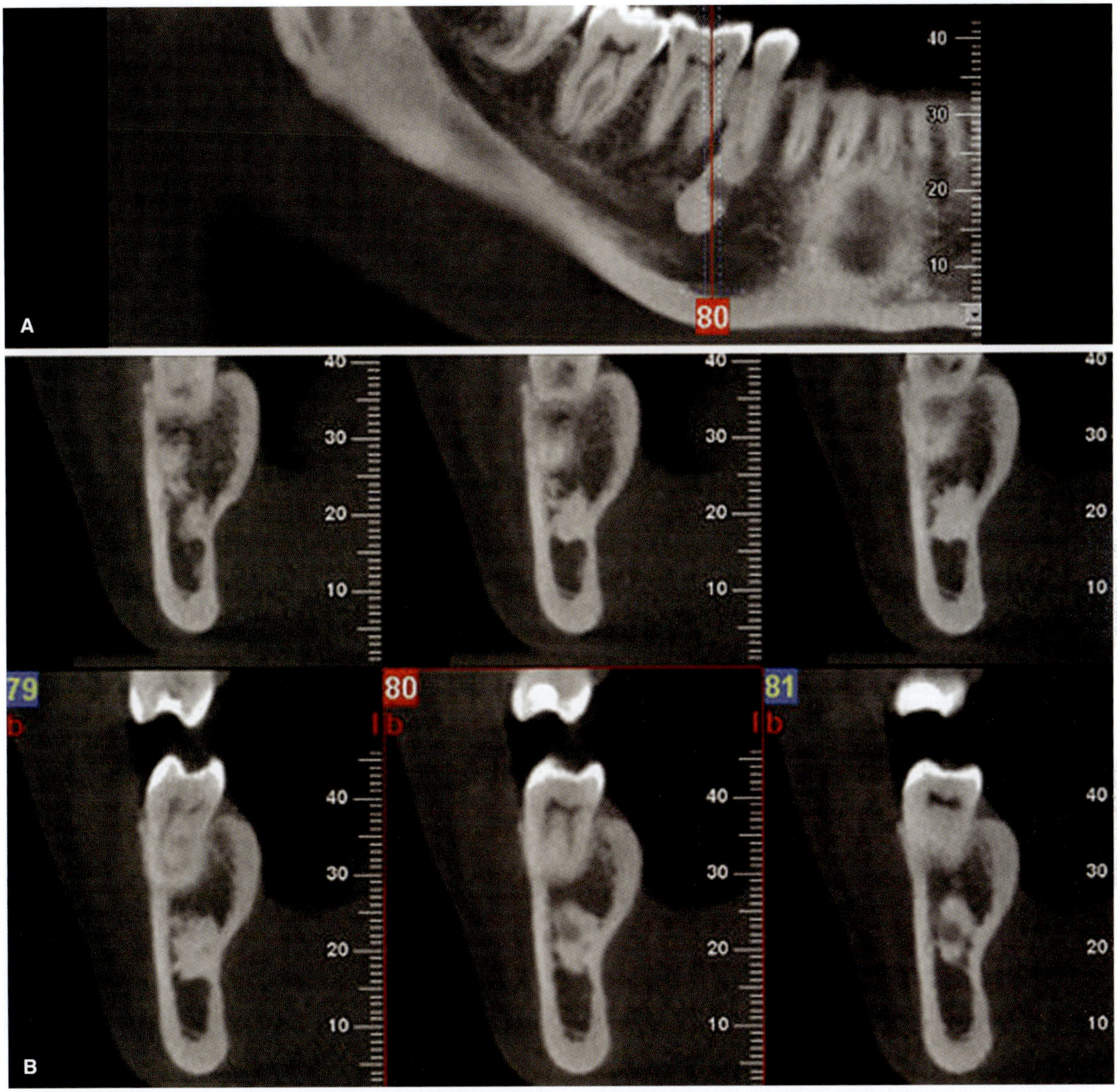

Figure 9.14 A panoramic view (*A*) and coronal sections (*B*) of a well-defined, homogenous, high-density lesion (similar in density to cortical bone) in contact with the apex of a premolar and just superior to the right mandibular canal. There is clear distinction between the lesion and the surrounding healthy osseous tissues. The most likely diagnosis is either idiopathic osteoscleoris or enostosis, both of which are benign pathological entities that are characterized by dense bone.

suspicions and steer him or her to investigate further for a possible disease include its effects on the neighboring tissues or anatomical structures and the presence of dystrophic calcifications, which are described below in greater detail.

A growing mass in the soft tissue may alter the contours of the anatomical structures in its vicinity, which might be identifiable even if the mass itself is not. This frequently may cause asymmetry between the ipsilateral and contralateral sides,

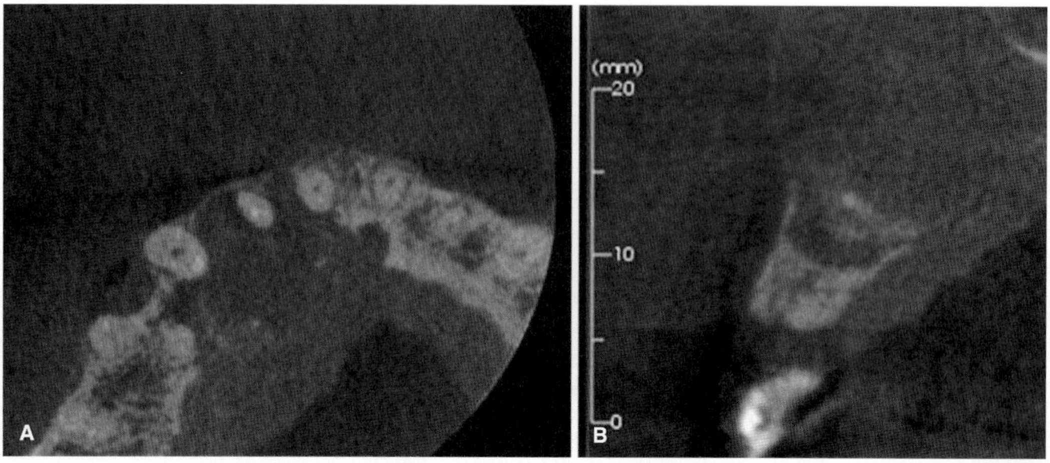

Figure 9.15 Axial (*A*) and sagittal (*B*) sections of an expansile, moderately defined lesion in the apical region of teeth maxillary right canine to central incisor in the anterior maxilla. The lesion has expanded and thinned the maxillary cortices significantly. Thick radiopaque flecks within the lesion most likely indicate a solid mass, typically a benign tumor.

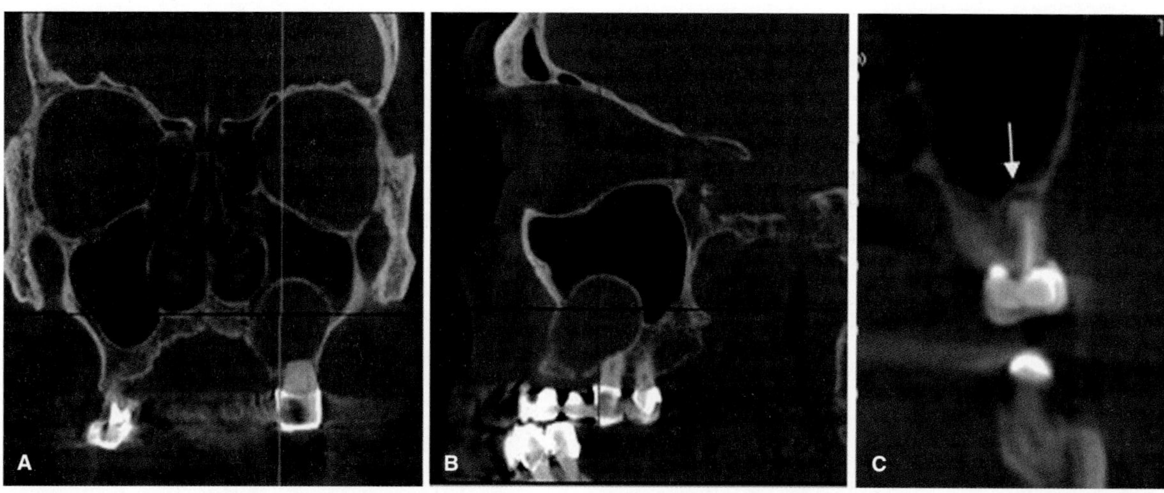

Figure 9.16 Coronal (*A*) and sagittal (*B*) sections showing considerable displacement of the floor of the left maxillary sinus caused by a well-delineated cystic lesion. There is no evidence of invasion of the maxillary sinus, however, since there is no interruption in the continuity of its floor. The lesion appears to have originated from a molar tooth and most likely is a radiocular cyst (inflammatory cyst). This is known as "halo effect." *C:* Even lesions that are smaller in size can cause a "halo effect." A small periapical lesion, most likely a periapical granuloma, has displaced the floor of the maxillary sinus superior without invading it (arrow).

which also may be identifiable and may indicate the growing abnormality indirectly. For example, an effect may be observed on the shape and size of the airway caused by soft tissue disease developing at its walls or even deeper, such that the growing lesion may cause some shifting of the airway walls that may be noticeable even if it is asymptomatic. This most frequently will present itself as asymmetry between the right and left sides of the airway at a certain level or throughout its

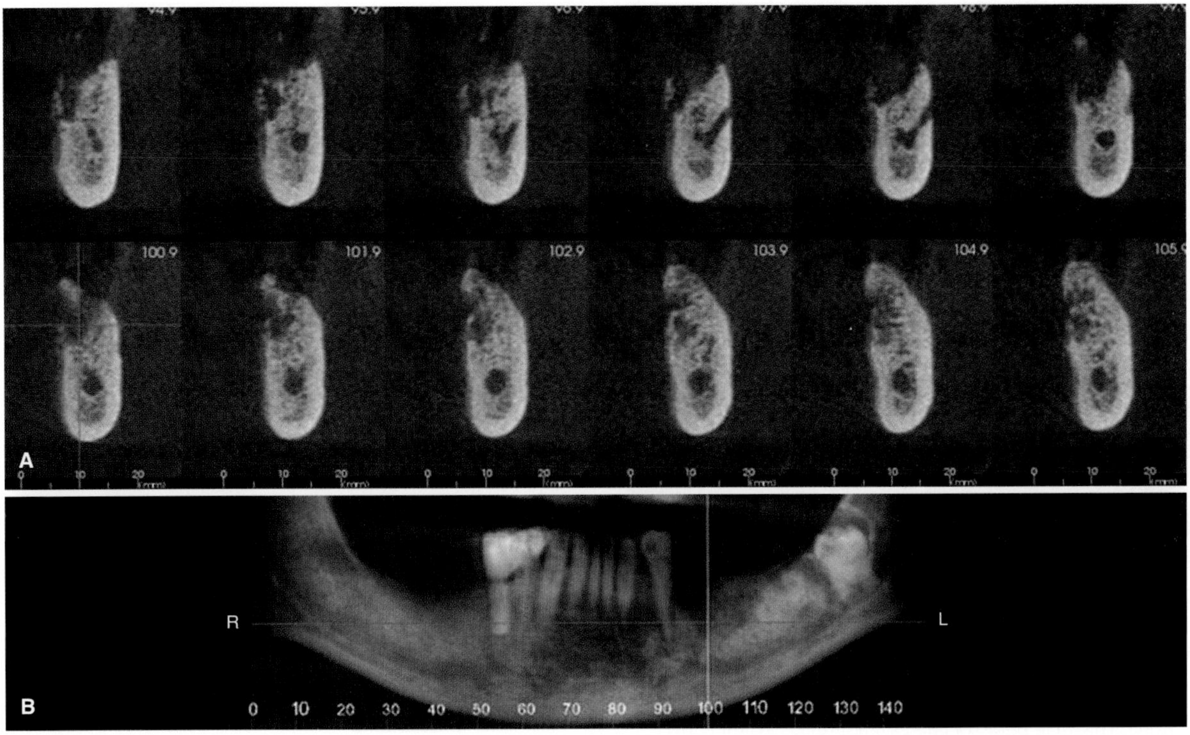

Figure 9.17 Coronal sections (*A*) and panoramic view (*B*) showing a permeative lesion on the lingual aspect of the mandibular bone in the left premolar region. The lesion is rather irregular in shape and demonstrates several small erosions. Loose fragments of bone, known as sequestrae (or sequestrations), are the result of destruction of the osseous tissue as the pathological entity progresses to deeper layers of bone. These features are suggestive of an aggressive and invasive lesion. Only malignant disease and osteomyelitis show this appearance. In fact, the two are indistinguishable if there is no clinical history that indicates chronic inflammation on the latter entity.

course (Figure 9.18). If the developing abnormality affects all walls of the airway, an overall narrowing of the airway diameter may result with the accompanying airway restriction, providing an explanation for clinical symptoms such as sleep apnea.

A growing soft tissue mass also may have an effect in osseous structures. This may be revealed in one of two possible ways: a slowly growing mass may alter the hard tissue contours such as bony cortices and the shape and size of foramina and canals through remodeling of bone. This most frequently reflects the behavior of a benign tumor that may have originated in the soft tissue. Although the tumor itself may not be identifiable due to inadequate soft tissue contrast, its effects on bone contours reveal its existence and location (Figure 9.19). More aggressive soft tissue pathological entities such as invasive tumors or malignant neoplasms may erode and invade the osseous structures in their vicinity, if these lie in the path of the growing tumor. An example of such an effect is the erosion of the lingual mandibular cortex toward the inferior border caused by a malignant neoplasm on the floor of the mouth (Figure 9.20).

A second indicator of an otherwise unidentifiable soft tissue condition is the presence of dystrophic calcifications, namely, calcifications that develop in areas where no calcified material is supposed to be present. Soft tissue abnormalities or pathologies sometimes are detected neither because of obvious changes in the soft tissue of origin nor because of effects on the neighboring structures,

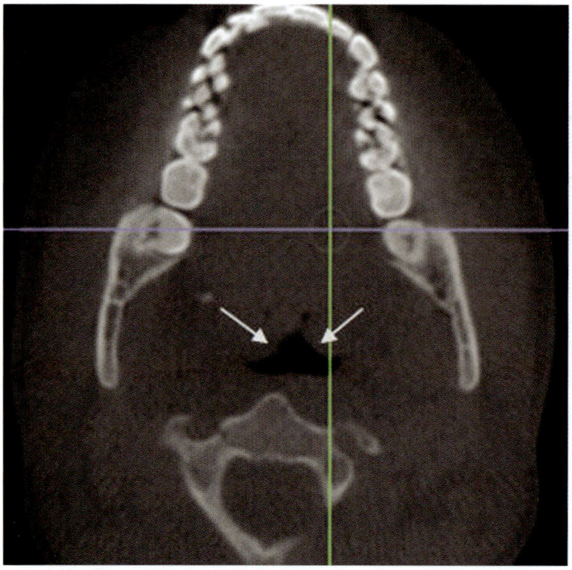

Figure 9.18 Axial section showing marked narrowing of the airway at the level of the floor of the mouth caused by soft tissue masses projecting into the lumen of the airway bilaterally (arrows). The narrowing in that region most likely is the cause of hypertrophic tonsillitis (inflammation of the tonsils). This may be associated with airway-obstructive phenomena such as sleep apnea.

but because of the tendency of the developing disease to produce calcifications. In other words, the presence of calcifications in areas of soft tissue structures points to the otherwise undetected disease. Carotid artery atheromatosis (Figure 9.21) and sialolithiasis (Figure 9.7 and Figure 9.8) are two characteristic examples of soft tissue diseases that frequently are found incidentally on CBCT scans.

CONCLUSIONS

All the approaches presented in this chapter are aimed toward helping the diagnostician collect all significant diagnostic information by means of reviewing CBCT images in a systematic fashion. In addition, noting detailed features of the findings often will steer the diagnostician toward a specific direction, further helping to narrow the pathology or finding. Toward achieving these goals, the clinician should address the following questions:

Is the suspected abnormality a true pathological entity or an anatomical variant? A sound

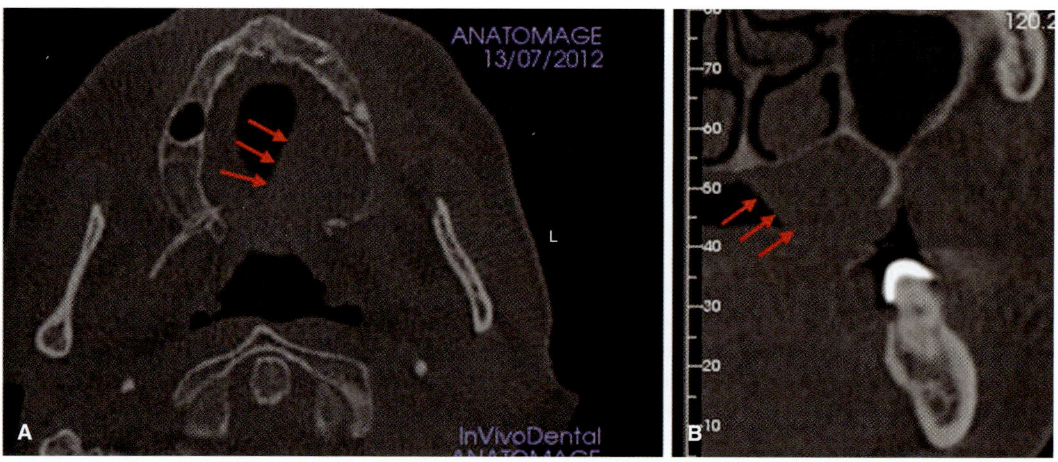

Figure 9.19 Axial (*A*) and coronal (*B*) sections of the left posterior maxilla, depicting a soft tissue mass in the palatal mucosa (arrows) that has caused marked thinning and scalloping of the alveolar ridge in the posterior maxilla and has shifted the floor of the nasal cavity superior. Soft tissue pathology often may be identified with CBCT by its effects on surrounding structures. In this case, the shifting of the floor of the nasal cavity and the scalloping of the alveolar ridge may be associated with a benign soft tissue mass (tumor).

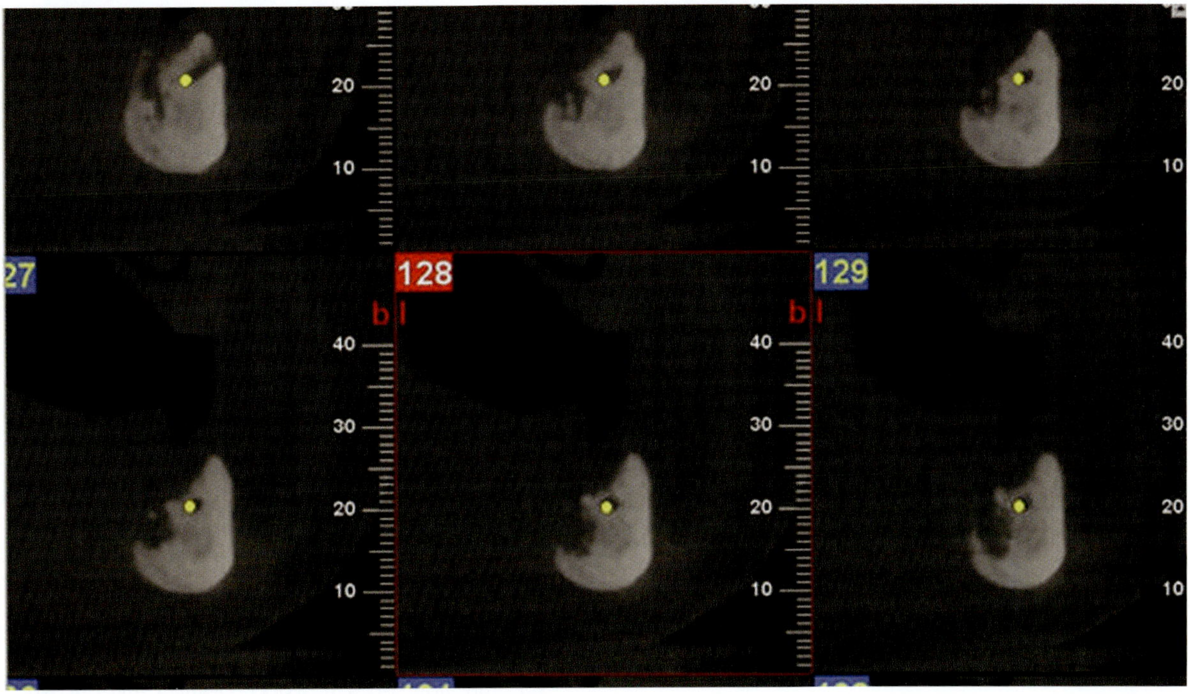

Figure 9.20 Coronal sections showing a permeative lesion invading the lingual aspect of the mandibular bone in the premolar region. The appearance of the lesion indicates an aggressive type of pathological entity, probably a malignant lesion. In fact, this was a squamous cell carcinoma of the floor of the mouth, which invaded the mandibular bone from the lingual aspect.

knowledge of the anatomy of the maxillofacial region and its variations will help provide an answer to this question. If one has the experience and the knowledge to exclude normal anatomy and its variants as a suspected abnormality, then, by extension, any other significant findings are likely to be disease. There is no doubt that anatomical variations are the main reasons that raise the suspicion of possible pathology.

From where did this lesion originate? Certain alterations in the appearance of the affected region, the tissues in the vicinity of the suspected pathological entity, and mostly indirect effects in the surrounding tissues will reveal whether the abnormality in question has a osseous tissue or soft tissue as its origin.

Is this a benign or a malignant lesion? Irregular shape, fast growth, and invasive and destructive behavior indicate a malignancy. In contrast, slow-growing round or ovoid-shaped lesions that displace and push the neighboring tissues instead of invading them usually point toward benign pathological entities such as cysts or benign tumors.

Is there anything else that I might be missing? Thorough review of the entire imaging volume available will ensure that no incidental disease is missed.

What's next? Few pathological entities can be diagnosed from their radiographic features exclusively. In most cases, the diagnostician may formulate a list of possible diagnoses. Keeping a record of all the findings and notes of each reviewed CBCT scan will be of great assistance as a patient record for future use as well as a legal record and will enhance communication with other clinicians.

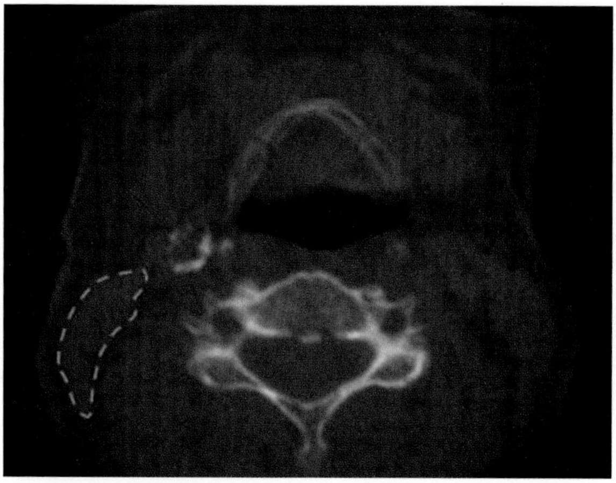

Figure 9.21 Coronal section of a circular high-density structure (red arrows: calcification) in the right common carotid artery (atheromatic plaque) just lateral to the airway and antromedially to the sterno-cleidomastoid muscle (dotted line). Although the blood vessel is not seen in the CBCT images, the knowledge of its anatomical location and its course may point to the diagnosis of atheromatic disease.

References

Ahmed, F., Brooks, S.L., & Kapila, S.D. (2012) Efficacy of identifying maxillofacial lesions in cone-beam computed tomographs by orthodontists and orthodontic residents with third-party software. *American Journal of Orthodontics and Dentofacial Orthopedics*, 141, 451–459.

Angelopoulos, C. (2008) Cone beam tomographic imaging anatomy of the maxillofacial region. *Dental Clinics of North America*, 52 (4), 731–752.

Angelopoulos, C. & Aghaloo, T. (2011) Imaging technology in implant diagnosis. *Dental Clinics of North America*, 55 (1), 141–158.

Bechara, B., McMahan, C.A., Geha, H., *et al.* (2012) Evaluation of a cone beam CT artefact reduction algorithm. *Dentomaxillofacial Radiology*, 41 (5), 422–428.

Jacobs, R. (2011) Dental cone beam CT and its justified use in oral health care. *JBR-BTR*, 94 (5), 254–265.

Koong, B. (2010) Cone beam imaging: is this the ultimate imaging modality? *Clinical Oral Implants Research*, 21 (11), 1201–1208.

McDonald, D. (2011) *Oral and Maxillofacial Radiology: A Diagnostic Approach*. Wiley-Blackwell, Chichester, UK.

Rege, I.C., Sousa, T.O., Leles, C.R., *et al.* (2012) Occurrence of maxillary sinus abnormalities detected by cone beam CT in asymptomatic patients. *BMC Oral Health*, 12 (1), 30.

Scarfe, W.C. & Farman, A.G. (2008) What is cone-beam CT and how does it work? *Dental Clinics of North America*, 52 (4), 707–730.

Scarfe, W.C., Li, Z., Aboelmaaty, W., *et al.* (2012) Maxillofacial cone beam computed tomography: essence, elements and steps to interpretation. *Australian Dental Journal*, 57 (Suppl 1), 46–60.

White, S. & Pharoah, M. (2004) *Oral Radiology: Principles and Interpretation*. 5th ed. Mosby, St. Louis, MO.

10 Detection of Incidental Findings in Cone Beam Computed Tomography Imaging and Their Clinical Implications

Erika Benavides, DDS, PhD, and Paul C. Edwards, MSc, DDS, FRCD(C)

INTRODUCTION

The introduction of cone beam computed tomography (CBCT) to dentistry in the late 1990s transformed the way the profession as a whole analyzes the oral and maxillofacial complex. Dental providers, who previously were limited to two-dimensional (2D) images of three-dimensional (3D) anatomical structures, now have the ability to visualize the hard tissues of the head and neck in all the desired planes as well as in 3D reconstructions. The principal limitation of CBCT is that the soft tissue resolution is limited to visualization of the soft tissue profile, the airway, and the relatively higher density muscles and major salivary glands.

Since the introduction of CBCT is relatively recent, many dentists have not been trained to identify the cross-sectional anatomy visualized in CBCT imaging; an overview is provided in Chapter 9. In addition, CBCT scans may reveal occult pathology and incidental findings of varying clinical significance located in structures outside a dentist's conventional area of expertise.

The frequency of incidental findings identified by CBCT has been reported to be as high as 3.2 findings per scan (Price *et al.*, 2012). Not surprisingly, individual studies have reported different frequencies of these incidental findings, depending on the field of view (FOV) employed, the average age of the population studied, and the method used to categorize these findings (Miles, 2006, 2010; Cha *et al.*, 2007; Rogers *et al.*, 2011). Price and colleagues (2012) reviewed 272 consecutive CBCT scans and found that the most prevalent incidental discoveries were airway-associated findings (35%), soft tissue calcifications (20%), lesions of bone (17.5%), temporomandibular joint (TMJ; 15.4%), endodontic etiology (11.3%), developmental dental lesions (0.7%), and pathologic lesions (0.1%). Of these findings, 16.1% required intervention/referral and 15.6% required monitoring; the remainder (68.3%) required no further treatment. Similarly, Caglayan & Tozoglu (2012) conducted a

Cone Beam Computed Tomography in Orthodontics: Indications, Insights, and Innovations, First Edition. Sunil D. Kapila.

review of 207 consecutive CBCT scans and reported that the highest number of incidental findings was noted within the airway structures (51.8%), followed by the presence of impacted teeth (21.7%), TMJ-associated lesions (11.1%), endodontic lesions (4.3%), condensing osteitis (1%), and miscellaneous other processes (2.9%). Lack of recognition of these incidental findings can have significant medicolegal implications (Zinman *et al.*, 2010; see also Chapter 7). On the other hand, the untrained clinician may have a higher likelihood of reporting false-positive findings, which could result in unnecessary healthcare costs and patient anxiety (Kapila *et al.*, 2011; Ahmed *et al.*, 2012).

In orthodontics, the use of extended or large FOV CBCT scans is relatively common since one of the principal applications of CBCT imaging is the evaluation of the craniofacial complex prior to orthognathic surgery or, in some instances, as an alternative to traditional 2D radiographic imaging even in nonsurgical cases. Using an extended FOV increases the likelihood of discovering incidental pathology since a larger volume of the head and neck is imaged.

A recent study demonstrated that orthodontists and orthodontic residents failed to detect approximately 67% of incidental lesions while having a 50% false-positive detection rate. These numbers decreased to 33% and 30%, respectively, after 3 hours of training by an oral and maxillofacial radiologist (Ahmed *et al.*, 2012). This highlights the importance of having an oral and maxillofacial or medical radiologist assist with the interpretation of CBCT scans.

The objective of this chapter is to provide information on the radiographic presentation and locations of incidental and pathological findings in CBCT scans, as well as their clinical implications. The overall goal of this chapter is to enhance the diagnostician's ability to identify these lesions and undertake appropriate steps where needed. More specifically, we review incidental findings under the categories of (1) intracranial soft tissue calcifications and lesions, (2) extracranial soft tissue calcifications, (3) airway lesions, (4) lesions of the paranasal sinuses and nasal cavity, (5) tooth-related findings and developmental defects of the jaws, (6) TMJ-associated processes, (7) lesions of the cervical spine, and (8) other miscellaneous findings. Within each of these sections, we provide tables summarizing the CBCT presentation, age and sex distribution, and clinical implications, including the recommended follow-up for each CBCT lesion or finding.

INTRACRANIAL SOFT TISSUE CALCIFICATIONS AND LESIONS

Internal carotid calcifications

Internal carotid calcifications represent deposits of fat, cholesterol, and associated inflammatory cells that contribute to the formation of a plaque within the artery. Progressive narrowing of the internal diameter of the arterial lumen reduces the maximum volume of blood flow. This process ultimately may result in decreased vessel elasticity and erosion of the vessel walls. Plaque deposits also can become dislodged and transported to other structures, resulting in pulmonary emboli or deep vein thrombosis, or may lead to a myocardial infarction or stroke. On CBCT imaging, internal carotid calcifications are seen as high-density, well-defined, single or ring-like opacities commonly located on either side of the sella turcica or the sphenoid sinus (Figure 10.1; Table 10.1). They tend

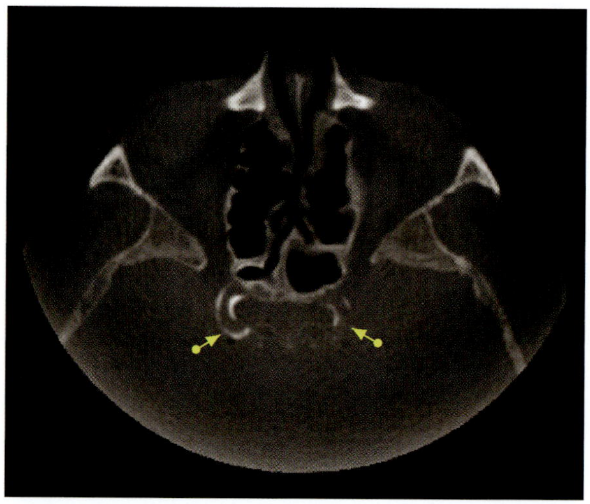

Figure 10.1 Internal carotid calcifications. Axial CBCT section reveals bilateral, well-defined, high-density ring-shaped opacity (arrows) lateral to the sphenoid sinus.

Table 10.1 Summary of CBCT presentation, age and sex distribution, additional diagnostic features, and recommended follow-up of intracranial soft tissue calcifications and lesions.

Condition or incidental finding	Radiographic location	CBCT presentation	Typical age range	Sex distribution	Frequency in CBCT scans	Clinical and other diagnostic features	Follow-up
Internal carotid calcification	Lateral to sella turcica or spenoid sinus	High-density, well-defined, single, or ring-like	Older adults	M > F	0.5% (Price *et al.*, 2012)	Possible medical history of cardiovascular disease	Refer to MD: CT and/or MRA
Pineal gland calcification	Midline of brain in pineal gland area	High-density, well-defined, single or cluster, irregularly shaped	Adults, rare in children	Unknown	Unknown	Possible history of sleep disorders and/or schizophrenia	Refer to MD: CT and/or MRI
Pituitary gland tumors	Within sella turcica	Thinning or sloping of the floor of sella turcica	Adults (20–50 years old)	M = F	Unknown	Endocrine disorders	Refer to MD: CT and/or MRI

CT, computed tomography; MRI, magnetic resonance imaging; MRA, magnetic resonance angiogram.

to be bilateral and are more common in older male patients. The prevalence of identifiable intracranial carotid calcifications in CBCT scans has been reported to be as high as 0.5% (Price *et al.*, 2012). Overall, intracranial calcifications have been reported to occur in greater than 80% of older Caucasian individuals (Bos *et al.*, 2012). The presence of intracranial carotid calcifications has been linked to smoking, hypercholesterolemia, and a history of cardiac disease (deWeert *et al.*, 2009). These calcifications are an indicator of arterial stenosis, which is associated with an increased risk of stroke. Therefore, identification of internal carotid calcification by CBCT imaging mandates referral for further medical evaluation.

Pineal gland calcifications

The pineal gland is a small endocrine gland located between the two hemispheres of the brain, approximating the center. It is larger in children, with a decrease in size noted after the onset of puberty. It produces the serotonin derivative melatonin, a hormone that affects the modulation of wake/sleep patterns and seasonal functions and plays an important role in sexual development and metabolism. In CBCT scans, calcifications of the pineal gland area can be seen as a single lesion or a cluster of multiple small high-density, well-defined, irregularly shaped opacities, typically 3–5 mm or smaller (Figure 10.2; Table 10.1). Pineal gland calcifications have been linked to sleep disorders and schizophrenia (Bersani *et al.*, 1999; Kunz *et al.*, 1999); these are rare in children younger than 6 years of age. When found in this age group or when greater than 1 cm in diameter, the possibility of a pineal gland tumor should be considered.

Pituitary gland tumors

The possibility of a pituitary adenoma, the most common neoplasm arising within the substance of the pituitary gland, should be suspected when the pituitary gland measures greater than 9 mm in the superior to inferior dimension. These occur with equal frequency in males and females, typically in individuals between the ages of 20 and 50 years. On CBCT imaging, thinning and sloping of the floor of the sella turcica may be noted. On occasion, extension into the sphenoid sinus also may be evident (Figure 10.3A; Table 10.1). Although relatively uncommon, calcifications within the pituitary gland can be seen in association with certain secretory pituitary tumors (Figure 10.3B). Therefore, the presence of any of these radiographic findings requires further evaluation by medical computed tomography (CT) or magnetic resonance imaging (MRI).

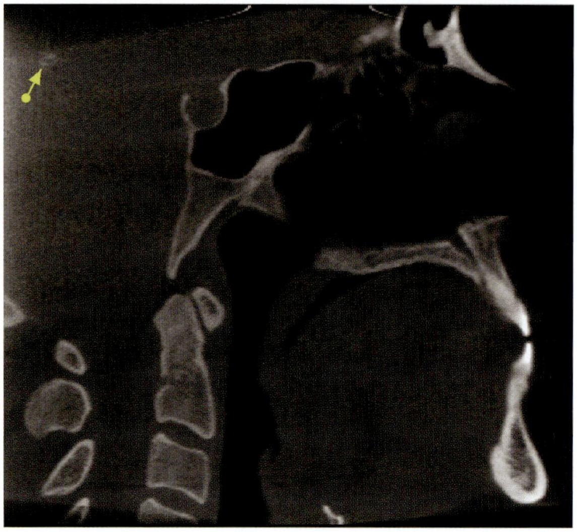

Figure 10.2 Pineal gland calcification. Sagittal CBCT section reveals a single, high-density, well-defined calcification in the midline in the area of the pineal gland (arrow).

EXTRACRANIAL SOFT TISSUE CALCIFICATIONS

Carotid space calcifications

The most common location for carotid artery calcifications is at the bifurcation of the common carotid artery into the internal and external branches of the carotid artery, which is located at the level of the C3-C4 vertebrae. The incidence of carotid calcifications in a general dental population has been reported to be as high as 5% in older patients (Lewis & Brooks, 1999). On CBCT scans, Price and associates (2012) reported an incidence of 1.5%. In axial CBCT imaging, these calcifications are seen within the carotid space, located medial and anterior to the sternocleidomastoid muscle (Figure 10.4A,B; Table 10.2) as single,

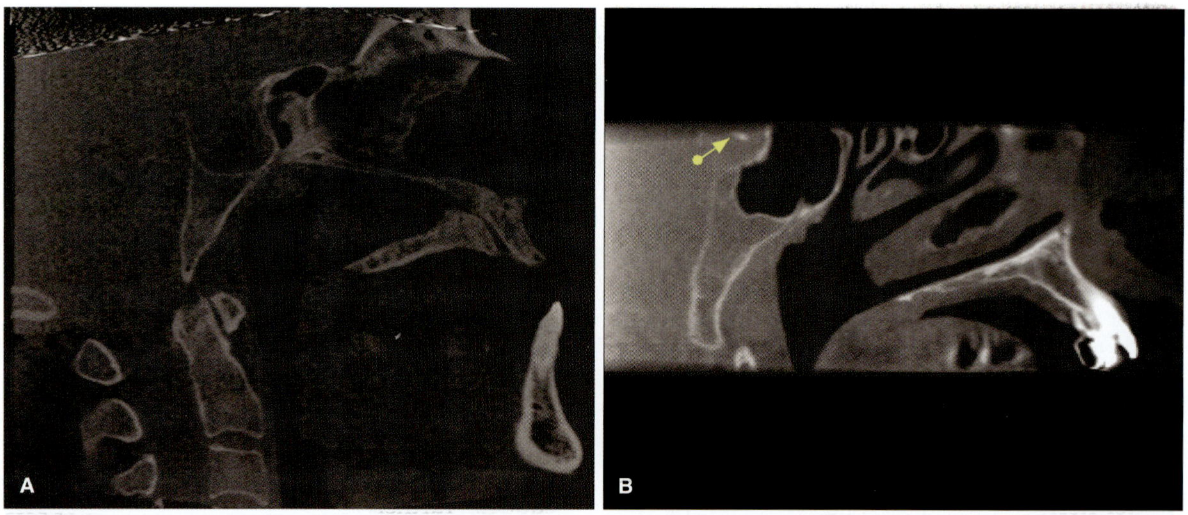

Figure 10.3 *A*: Pituitary adenoma. Sagittal CBCT section reveals an enlarged sella turcica (21 mm diameter) with thinning of the floor. *B*: Pituitary gland calcification. Sagittal CBCT section reveals an irregular, high-density calcification (arrow) within the sella turcica.

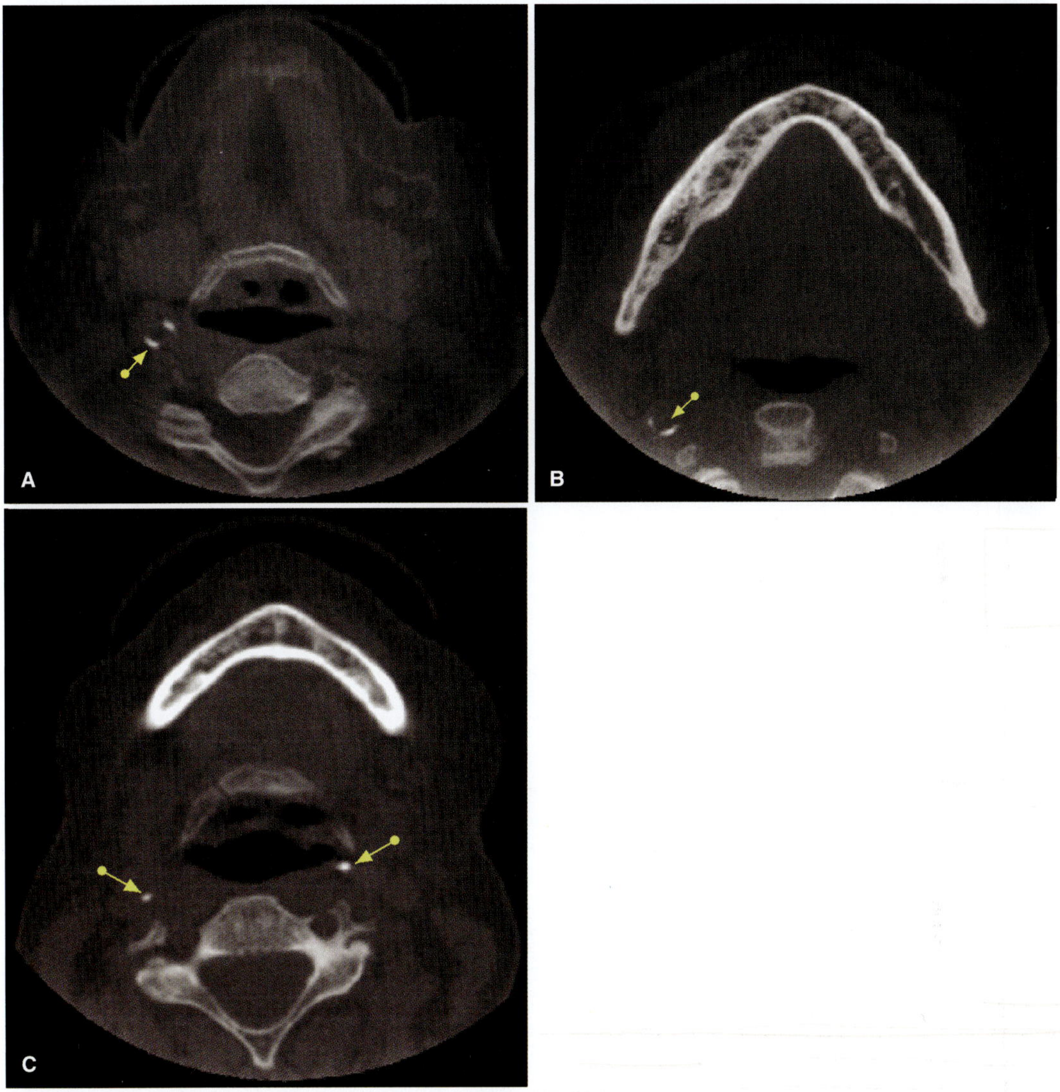

Figure 10.4 Carotid calcifications. *A*: Axial CBCT section at the level of C2-C3 reveals a well-defined, high-density, ring-shaped calcification (arrow). *B*: Axial CBCT section at the level of C3-C4 reveals two well-defined, high-density, ring-shaped calcifications (arrow) within the carotid space, medial and anterior to the sternocleidomastoid muscle. *C*: Axial CBCT section at the level of C4 reveals a small, well-defined, high-density carotid space calcification on the right side (arrow) and calcification of the stylohyoid ligament in proximity to the greater horn of the hyoid bone on the left side (arrow).

multiple, or ring-like well-defined high-density opacities. It is important to note that the tip of the greater horn of the hyoid bone is located in close proximity to the carotid space and may be mistaken for a single carotid calcification, particularly when this "calcification" is located toward the inferior edge of the FOV (Figure 10.4C). The presence of calcifications within the carotid space requires further medical evaluation. Doppler ultrasound has been found to be useful in determining the exact location and degree of arterial stenosis (Ravon *et al.*, 2003).

Table 10.2 Summary of CBCT presentation, age and sex distribution, additional diagnostic features, and recommended follow-up of extracranial soft tissue calcifications.

Condition or incidental finding	Radiographic location	CBCT presentation	Typical age range	Sex distribution	Frequency in CBCT scans	Clinical and other diagnostic features	Follow-up
Carotid space calcifications	Medial and anterior to the SCM on axial plane, between C3-C4 on sagittal plane	High-density, well-defined, single, multiple, or ring-like	Older adults	M > F	1.5% (Price *et al.*, 2012)	Possible medical history of cardiovascular disease	Refer to MD: US
Sialoliths	Within the three major glands or their ducts	High-density, well-defined, single or multiple, uni- or bilateral	Adults	M = F	Unknown	Possible gland swelling and/or pain at meal times	Correlate with clinical exam and manage accordingly
Tonsilloliths	Within palatine, lingual, or pharyngeal tonsils	High-density, well-defined, single or multiple, uni- or bilateral	Young adults	M = F	16% (Aspestrand & Kolbenstvedt, 1987)	Possible history of chronic inflammation or infection, possible halitosis	Correlate with clinical exam and manage accordingly
Calcified sylohyoid or stylomandibular ligaments	Extending from styloid process and/or close to hyoid bone	High-density, well-defined, enlongated calcifications	Adults	Unknown	Unknown	Possible facial or neck pain, dysphagia, or taste disturbances	Correlate with clinical exam to rule out possible Eagle's Syndrome and manage accordingly
Calcified lymphnodes	Any of the head and neck lymph nodes	High-density, well-defined, irregularly shaped, cauliflower-like appearance, usually multiple	Adults	Unknown	Unknown	May indicate presence of metastatic disease	Refer to MD: US, CT, and/or MRI
Phleboliths	Within a vein, venule, or hemangioma that is not contained within bone	High-density, multiple, laminated, may have an onion skin-like appearance	Adults	Unknown	Unknown	Highly suggestive of a hemangioma or venous malformation, predisposition to thrombus formation	Refer to MD: CT, MRI, MRA, US
Intradermal calcifications	Within skin	High-density, well-defined, single to multiple	Adults	Unknown	Unknown	Possible history of acne, surgery, trauma, or systemic disease involving altered calcium metabolism	Correlate with clinical exam and medical history

US, ultrasound; CT, computed tomography; MRI, magnetic resonance imaging; MRA, magnetic resonance angiogram; SCM, sternocleidomastoid muscle; C3, third cervical vertebra; C4, fourth cervical vertebra.

Sialoliths

Sialoliths are crystallized minerals that can be found in the parenchyma or the ductal system of the parotid, submandibular, or sublingual salivary glands, with approximately 80% of the cases involving the submandibular gland. Submandibular gland sialoliths are located near the hilum of the gland or in the proximal portion of Wharton's duct. Sialoliths may cause pain and swelling of the affected gland, particularly at meal times, and may be associated with decreased salivary flow. On CBCT imaging, they present as single to multiple, unilateral, or bilateral high-density calcifications within the salivary gland or their ductal system (Figure 10.5; Table 10.2). Correlation with clinical examination for the presence of associated signs and symptoms helps to determine the need for additional imaging (sialogram with plain film radiography, CT, or ultrasound) and/or the appropriate treatment.

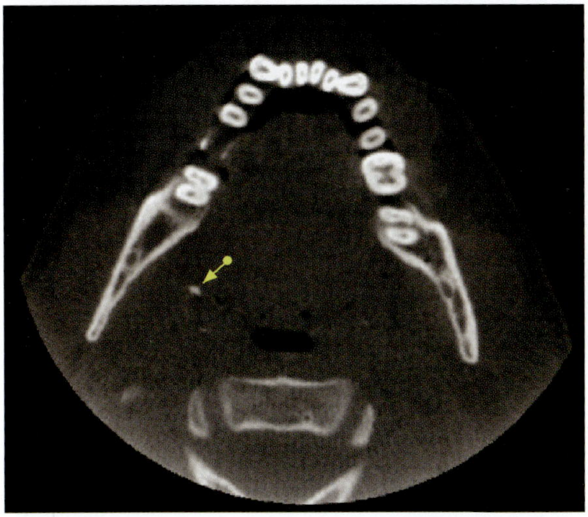

Figure 10.5 Submandibular gland sialolith. Axial CBCT section demonstrates a sialolith (arrow) in the area of the submandibular gland.

Tonsilloliths

Tonsilloliths represent clusters of calcified material that form in the crevices of the palatine tonsils and rarely within the lingual or pharyngeal tonsils (Figure 10.6; Table 10.2). On CBCT imaging, tonsilloliths are seen as single to multiple small high-density calcifications that may be unilateral or bilateral (Figure 10.7; Table 10.2). Tonsilloliths are a common incidental imaging finding, identified in up to 16% of patients (Aspestrand & Kolbenstvedt, 1987). Their presence may indicate a history of

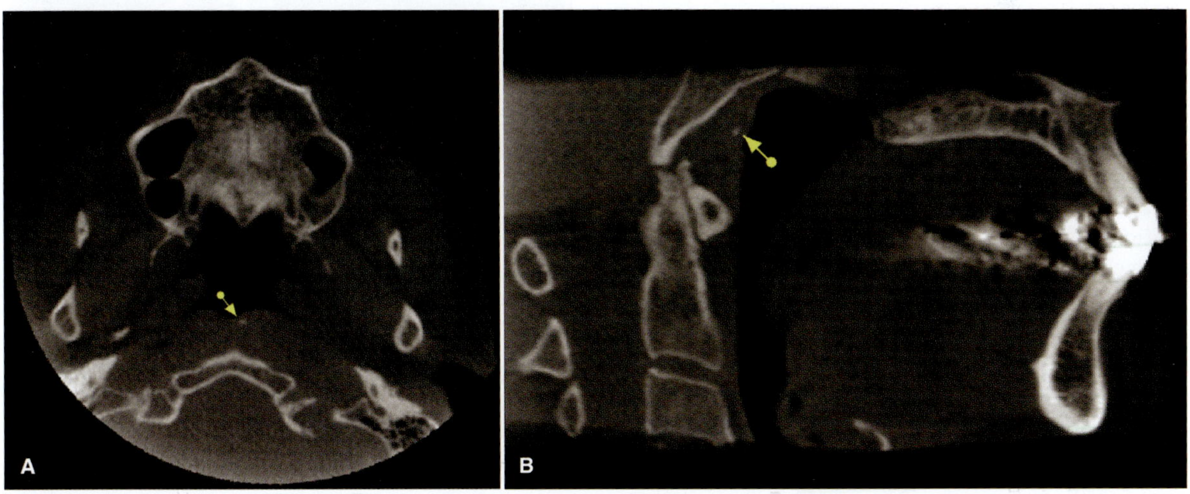

Figure 10.6 Pharyngeal tonsilloliths. Images reveal a small pharyngeal tonsillolith in axial (*A*) and sagittal (*B*) sections (arrows).

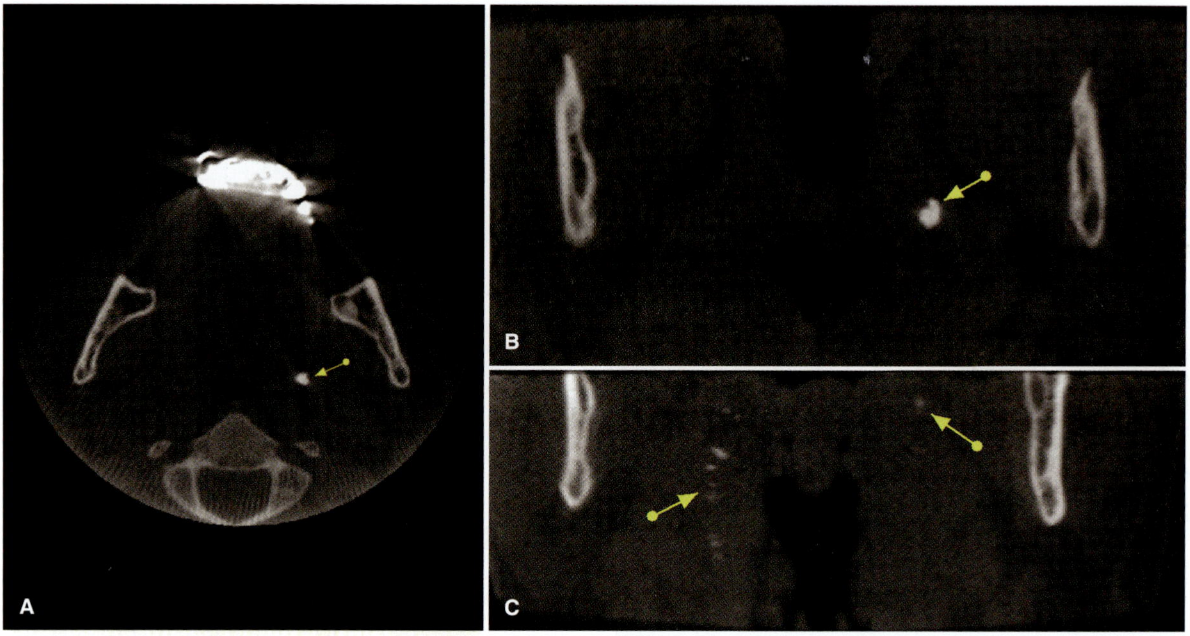

Figure 10.7 Palatine tonsilloliths. *A*: Single, relatively large tonsillolith visualized in the axial plane (arrow). *B*: The same tonsillolith visualized in the coronal plane (arrow). *C*: Multiple bilateral tonsilloliths of a different patient seen in coronal CBCT section (arrows).

chronic inflammation or infection; they have been found to be associated with halitosis.

Calcified ligaments

Unilateral or bilateral calcification of the stylohyoid or stylomandibular ligament (Figure 10.8; Table 10.2) is a frequently noted incidental finding on panoramic radiography and CBCT imaging (Radfar *et al.*, 2008). Approximately 4% of the general population has an elongated styloid process and a partially calcified stylohyoid ligament. However, only 4% of this group is symptomatic. The etiology of this process is unknown, although congenital factors, trauma, or an inflammatory process that leads to the proliferation of granulation tissue that eventually becomes calcified have been implicated. This calcification can cause compression of adjacent structures, including the glossopharyngeal nerve, trigeminal nerve, chorda tympani, and sympathetic nerves within the carotid sheath, resulting

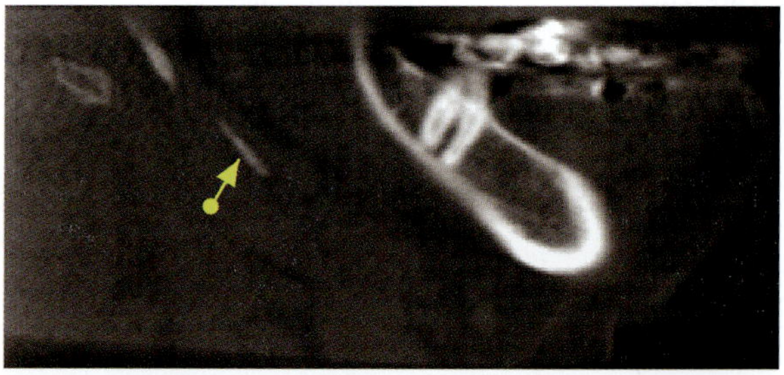

Figure 10.8 Calcified stylomandibular ligament. Sagittal CBCT section reveals a well-defined, high-density linear opacity (arrow) inferior to the styloid process and extending toward the angle of the mandible. The styloid process has attachments to two ligaments: the stylohyoid ligament, which extends from the tip of the styloid process to the lesser cornu of the hyoid bone, and the stylomandibular ligament, which extends from the styloid process to the angle of the mandible. It is necessary to trace the path on successive CBCT sections to differentiate between calcifications of these two ligaments.

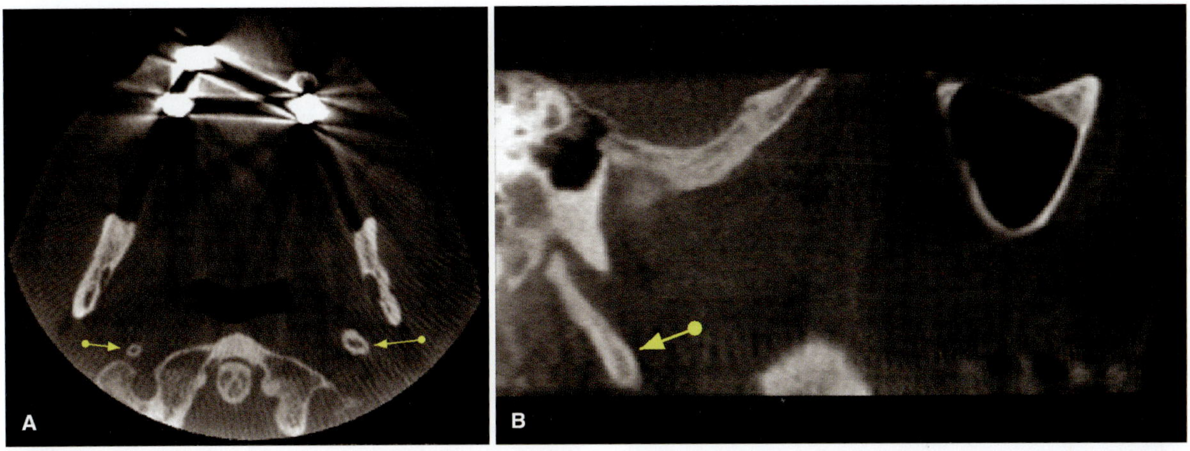

Figure 10.9 Enlarged styloid process. *A*: Axial CBCT section reveals significant asymmetry in the diameter of the right and left styloid processes (arrows). *B*: Sagittal CBCT section confirms the enlargement of the left styloid process (arrow).

in facial and neck pain, particularly when turning the head laterally. These also may be associated with a foreign-body sensation within the throat, dysphagia, or taste disturbances. When these symptoms are present, Eagle's Syndrome should be suspected. Eagle's Syndrome commonly is found in adults between the ages of 30 to 50 years, with women being affected more often than men. Treatment of symptomatic patients may require surgical removal of the calcified ligament.

On CBCT imaging, a styloid process greater than 30 mm in length is considered "elongated" and partial calcification of the stylohyoid or stylomandibular ligaments should be suspected (Figure 10.9A,B; Table 10.2). Correlation with clinical examination is important to determine the need for further evaluation and/or treatment.

Calcified lymph nodes

Of the approximately 800 lymph nodes in the human body, about 300 are located in the head and neck region. CBCT will identify the presence of calcifications within lymph nodes, which may indicate the presence of chronic inflammation or infection. These usually present as well-defined, irregularly shaped calcifications that may have a cauliflower-like appearance (Figure 10.10; Table 10.2). Occasionally, the presence of calcified lymph nodes may be associated with metastatic disease.

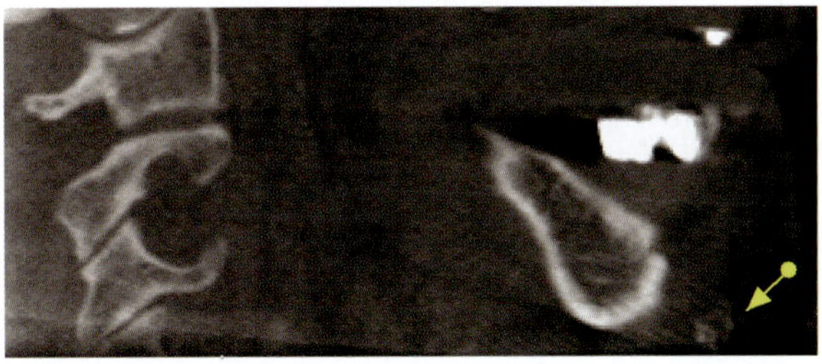

Figure 10.10 Submental lymph node calcification. Sagittal CBCT section reveals a well-defined, irregularly shaped calcification in the submental area, consistent with a calcified lymph node (arrow).

The presence of cervical metastatic nodal disease is a major prognostic determinant for patients with head and neck cancer, associated with a significantly reduced patient survival. Traditionally, contrast-enhanced CT and/or MRI are used to identify and classify the extent and distribution of lymph node involvement in patients with head and neck cancer. Since CBCT presents limited soft tissue visualization, medical CT or ultrasound is recommended if the presence of cervical lymphadenopathy is suspected (Jank *et al.*, 2003).

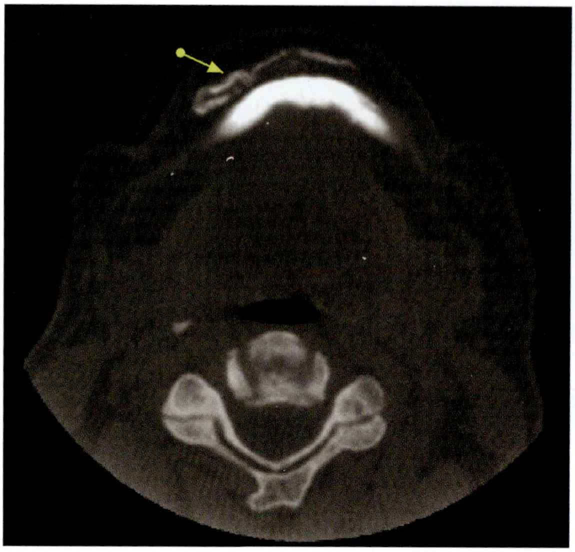

Figure 10.11 Intradermal post-surgical changes. Axial CBCT section showing intradermal calcifications and scar tissue in the chin area after plastic surgery (arrow).

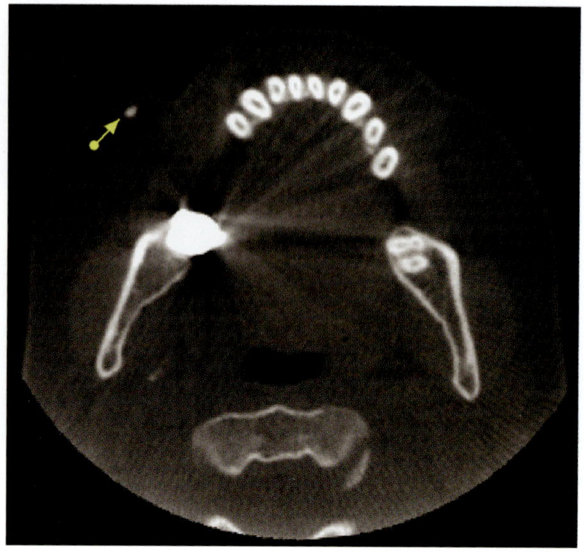

Figure 10.12 Subdermal calcification. This axial CBCT section shows a small, round, well-defined subcutaneous calcification (arrow).

Phleboliths

A phlebolith represents a calcified vascular thrombus within a vein, venule, or hemangioma that is not contained within bone (Scarfe & Farman, 2010). The formation of a phlebolith appears to be related to the presence of a vascular anomaly, which predisposes the patient to the formation of a thrombus, which ultimately may calcify. On CBCT imaging, these usually are multiple laminated high-density calcifications that may have an onion skin-like appearance. The presence of a phlebolith is highly suggestive of the presence of an underlying hemangioma or the presence of venous malformations (Eivazi *et al.*, 2012). Medical consultation is therefore recommended.

Intradermal calcifications

CBCT images can reveal small calcium deposits that may form under the skin as a result of an injury or at the site of a previous surgical incision (Figure 10.11; Table 10.2). Multiple skin calcifications also may indicate the presence of systemic disease involving alterations in calcium metabolism. Based on underlying etiology, skin calcifications may be classified as metastatic, dystrophic, iatrogenic, or idiopathic (Walsh & Fairley, 1995). In contrast to dystrophic calcifications, metastatic cutaneous calcifications usually are associated with elevated serum calcium or phosphate levels.

Cutaneous ossification (osteoma cutis) is another intradermal radiopacity that may be observed within the skin and underlying soft tissues. Cutaneous ossification can be divided into primary (15%) and secondary (85%) forms. Secondary osteoma cutis develops within pre-existing neoplastic or inflammatory skin lesions (Cottoni *et al.*, 1993; Fazeli *et al.*, 1999). On CBCT imaging, intradermal calcifications are noted as small, well-defined, single to multiple, high-density areas within the skin or subcutaneous structures (Figure 10.12; Table 10.2).

AIRWAY

Airway narrowing and asymmetry

Narrowing or asymmetry of the pharyngeal space noted in CBCT imaging may be artifacts caused by

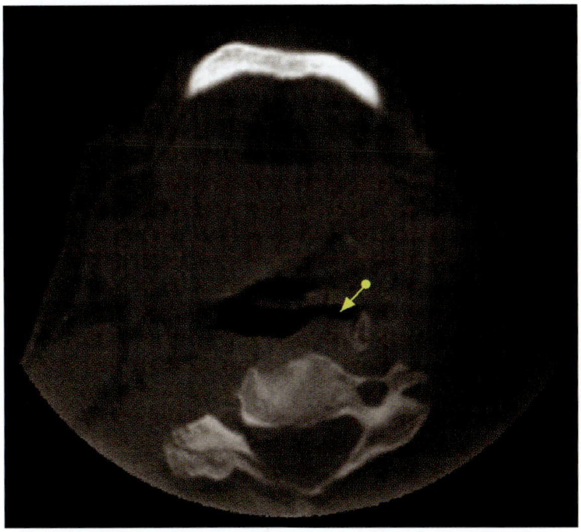

Figure 10.13 Airway asymmetry caused by papillary thyroid cancer. Axial CBCT section reveals anterior displacement of the left aspect of the posterior pharyngeal wall (arrow). On further investigation, it was determined that the patient had stage II papillary thyroid carcinoma.

breathing or swallowing during imaging or by the presence of hypertrophic tonsils. This imaging finding also may be associated with the presence of sleep apnea (see also Chapter 13) or benign or malignant tumors originating in any of the adjacent head and neck spaces (Figure 10.13; Table 10.3). A systematic and thorough review of the shape and width of the oropharyngeal and nasopharyngeal spaces of CBCT images in the axial, coronal, and sagittal planes should help to identify the presence and potential cause of airway asymmetry based on the location and direction of displacement. However, the exact cause of airway narrowing or asymmetry cannot be established based on the CBCT appearance alone (Figure 10.14). Clinical correlation and review of the patient's medical history are essential in order to determine the need for medical consultation or further imaging studies.

Obstruction of the lateral pharyngeal recess

The lateral pharyngeal recess (fossa of Rosenmuller) of the pharyngeal mucosal space may be asymmetric due to the presence of inflammatory debris and asymmetries in the volume of lymphoid tissue (Harnsberger, 1995). This asymmetric appearance can lead to the impression of a mass in the pharyngeal mucosal space (Figure 10.15; Table 10.3). To rule out this possibility, the adjacent deep spaces (parapharyngeal and retrophraryngeal spaces) must be evaluated. If the soft-tissue planes are maintained, the "mass" probably is not real. However, since the soft tissue contrast resolution of CBCT is limited, depending on the age of the patient and the presence or absence of a history of a recent upper respiratory illness, correlation with clinical evaluation of the mucosa and referral for otorhinolaryngological (ENT) consultation is recommended.

LESIONS OF THE PARANASAL SINUSES AND NASAL CAVITY

The nasal cavity, paranasal sinuses, and nasopharynx comprise functionally interrelated anatomic structures. While divided into separate structures based on defined anatomic landmarks, for all practical purposes, pathological processes in one of these structures predictably affect adjacent structures.

The paranasal sinuses include the bilateral maxillary, frontal, ethmoid, and sphenoid sinuses. Pathology of the paranasal sinuses is a common incidental finding on CBCT scans. In one retrospective review of 166 consecutive CBCT scans of the maxillofacial region taken for the primary purpose of implant treatment planning or for evaluation of TMJ disease, impacted teeth, or jaw pathology, 152 separate and potentially clinically significant findings involving the sinonasal complex were noted (Edwards *et al.*, 2007). In this study, incidental findings that would have been visible readily on a full mouth series of intraoral radiographs or on panoramic views (e.g., antral pseudocysts) were excluded, as were any findings that were related to the primary indication for ordering the scan (e.g., evaluation for maxillary sinusitis in the presence of an oro-antral fistula). Ritter and associates (2012) identified the presence of maxillary sinus pathologies in 56% of CBCTs evaluated, with a trend to higher occurrence in older (>60 years of age) and

Table 10.3 Summary of CBCT presentation, age and sex distribution, additional diagnostic features, and recommended follow-up of airway findings.

Condition or incidental finding	Radiographic location	CBCT presentation	Typical age range	Sex distribution	Frequency in CBCT scans	Clinical and other diagnostic features	Follow-up
Airway narrowing and asymmetry	Along airway; at any level	Displacement of pharyngeal walls	Any age	Unknown	18.8% (Cha *et al.*, 2007)	May indicate presence of hypertrophic tonsils in younger patients, sleep apnea, or presence of underlying tumor; also may be caused by breathing or swallowing artifacts	Correlation with clinical exam and medical history to determine need for otorhinolaryngological (ENT) consultation
Obstruction of lateral pharyngeal recess	Lateral pharyngeal recess	Asymmetry in size or shape	Adults	Unknown	Unknown	May indicate variation of normal anatomy, an underlying tumor, or breathing artifact	Refer for ENT consultation

ENT, ear, nose and throat.

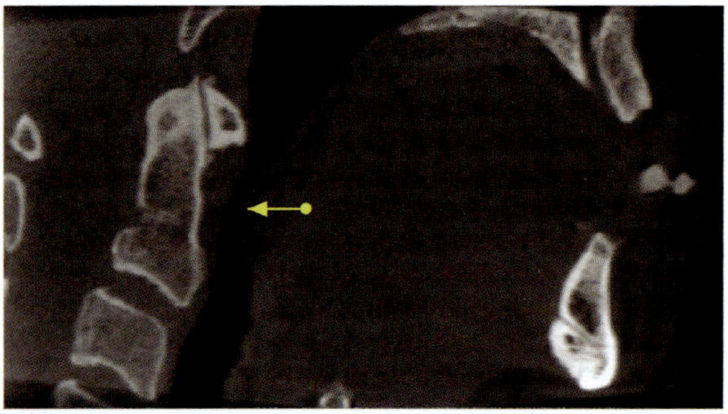

Figure 10.14 Airway narrowing. Sagittal CBCT section reveals significant narrowing of the airway (arrow). This incidental finding can be caused by swallowing artifacts or can be associated with sleep apnea.

male patients. Although pathology is identified most commonly in the maxillary sinuses, the remaining paranasal sinuses also are imaged when using large FOV CBCT scans as in orthodontic treatment planning. In another retrospective study, sphenoid sinus pathosis was observed in 11.9% of 227 consecutive dental patients who had undergone CBCT imaging (Bourek *et al.*, 2008).

The most common pathologies associated with the paranasal sinuses are inflammatory in origin, specifically sinusitis and sinonasal polyposis. One study reported that such inflammatory changes of the paranasal sinuses are found incidentally in 33% of dental CBCT scans reviewed (Scanlon *et al.*, 2007).

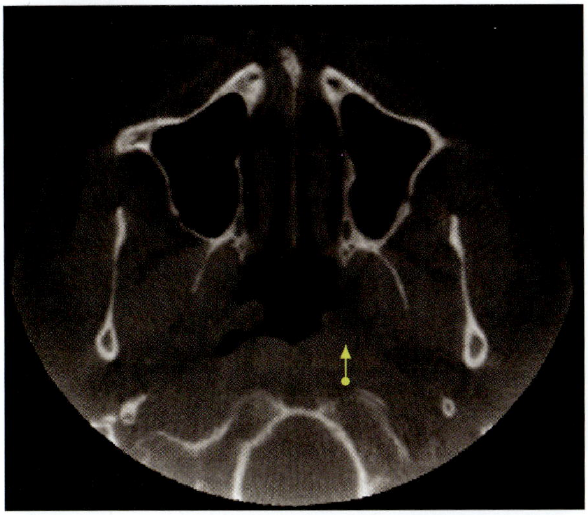

Figure 10.15 Obstruction of left lateral pharyngeal recess. Axial CBCT section reveals asymmetry at the level of the lateral pharyngeal recess (fossa of Rosenmuller; arrow). This asymmetry could be caused by inflammatory or neoplastic changes in the pharyngeal, parapharyngeal, or pharyngeal mucosal neck spaces.

Sinusitis and rhinosinusitis

Sinusitis is defined best as inflammation of the mucosa that lines the paranasal sinuses. When the nasal cavity also is involved, which occurs relatively frequently, it is termed rhinosinusitis. The most common causes of acute rhinosinusitis include viral (e.g., following an upper respiratory tract infection), bacterial, and fungal infections (Figure 10.16; Table 10.4). Rhinosinusitis is classified as chronic when both the characteristic symptoms (nasal congestion and/or discharge, facial pain, and dysosmia) and objective evidence of sinus disease confirmed by endoscopic or radiographic examination are present for longer than 12 weeks. Obstruction of the openings between the paranasal sinuses and the nasal cavity (the ostiomeatal complex), by interfering with proper drainage, plays a fundamental role in the pathogenesis of most cases of chronic mucosal inflammation. Factors that may predispose to the development of chronic sinusitis include atopy, acquired or developmental structural abnormalities (e.g., deviated septum, concha bullosa, small sinus ostia), and the presence of nasal polyps (Hamilos, 2011). Inflammation of dental origin (e.g., pulpal- or periodontal-induced inflammation) is estimated to account for approximately 10% of cases of chronic maxillary sinusitis (Figure 10.17; Table 10.4; Mehra & Jeong, 2009).

Chronic sinusitis is evidenced on CBCT as mucosal thickening, opacification of air cells, and reactive osseous thickening of the sinus cavity walls (Figure 10.18; Table 10.4). These findings, however, while suggestive of chronic sinusitis, are not pathognomonic. In contrast, identification of sinus opacification, air-fluid levels, and localized thickening of the antral mucosa in CBCT images is suggestive of acute sinusitis.

Using stringent radiographic criteria that included partial or complete opacification of the sphenoid sinus with concomitant reactive osseous sclerosis, Edwards and coworkers (2007) found that chronic maxillary sinusitis was evident in 16 of 166 patient CBCT scans, while combined ethmoid and sphenoid sinusitis was noted in an additional 13 patients. Sphenoid sinusitis was noted in 3.1% of the scans reviewed, with the majority of these patients showing no involvement of other sinuses.

Severe complications of acute and chronic rhinosinusitis are rare in adults, but are noted more commonly in association with frontal sinus involvement. Bone erosion may be seen but is uncommon. Serious complications include osteomyelitis, orbital and periorbital cellulitis, intracranial meningitis, intracranial abscesses, and cavernous sinus thrombosis (Rosenfeld *et al.*, 2007).

Nasal and sinonasal (sinus) polyps

Nasal polyps, relatively common inflammatory lesions presenting as smooth surfaced nodular soft tissue prominences of the nasal mucosa, represent the end product of a number of underlying sinonasal conditions, the most common being recurrent acute or chronic rhinosinusitis and allergic rhinitis. The most common site of involvement is the middle meatus. Although less common, polyps also may develop within the paranasal sinuses ("sinus polyps"). In the previously noted study (Edwards *et al.*, 2007), radiographic findings suggestive of

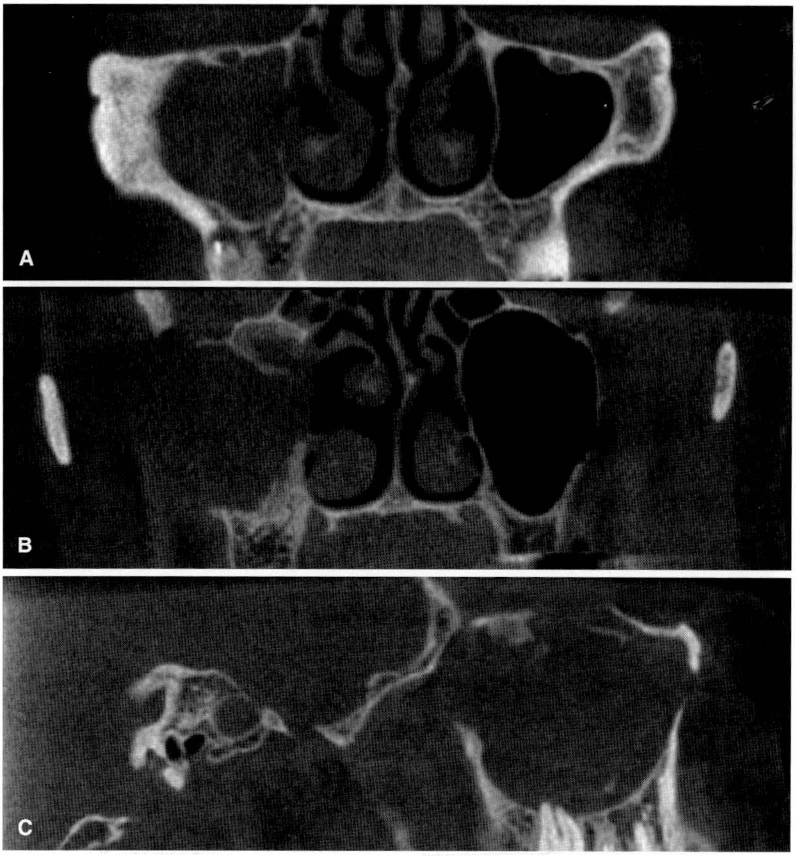

Figure 10.16 Fungal sinusitis. Coronal (*A* and *B*) and sagittal (*C*) CBCT sections reveal complete opacification of the right maxillary sinus with thickening and destruction of the sinus walls.

maxillary polyps were evident on CBCT in 23 of 166 scans, and combined ethmoid and sphenoid sinusitis polyps were noted in an additional 17 scans. Sphenoid sinus polyps, noted in 7.9% of scans reviewed, were associated with pathologies of the other sinuses, namely maxillary, ethmoid, or both in two thirds of affected patients.

Polyps appear on CBCT scans as noncorticated dome-shaped nodular soft tissue density lesions (Figure 10.19A; Table 10.4). Bony remodeling, although uncommon, typically is subtle if present (Figure 10.19B,C).

Sinonasal polyposis is a relatively benign process. Symptoms, where present, are similar to those of chronic rhinosinusitis and may include nasal obstruction, post-nasal drainage, facial and maxillary dental pain, sinus pressure, and anosmia. Sinonasal polyps predispose to obstruction of the ostiomeatal complex, leading to impaired drainage, secondary infection, and a persistence of the chronic inflammatory process within the paranasal sinuses and nasal cavity (Table 10.4). In children with multiple polyps, cystic fibrosis should be ruled out. Treatment involves systemic or topically applied (nasal spray) therapy. For larger polyps, especially those causing structural changes, or polyps unresponsive to conservative therapy, endoscopic sinus surgery, typically combined with enlargement of the ostea (functional endoscopic sinus surgery), should be considered.

Table 10.4 Summary of CBCT presentation, age and sex distribution, additional diagnostic features, and recommended follow-up of lesions of paranasal sinuses and nasal cavity.

Condition or incidental finding	Radiographic location	CBCT presentation	Typical age range	Sex distribution	Frequency in CBCT scans	Clinical and other diagnostic features	Follow-up
Sinusitis (acute)	Sinuses	Sinus opacification, air-fluid levels, localized thickening of antral mucosa	Adults, occasionally children	M = F	Unknown (somewhat common)	Serious complications rare but are more common with frontal sinus involvement	Refer for ENT consultation
Sinusitis (chronic)	Sinuses	Mucosal thickening, opacification of air cells, osseous thickening of sinus cavity walls	Adults	M = F	15 to 20% (Edwards *et al.*, 2007)	Serious complications rare but are more common with frontal sinus involvement (e.g., osteomyelitis, orbital and periorbital cellulitis, intracranial meningitis, intracranial abscesses, cavernous sinus thrombosis)	Refer for ENT consultation
Sinonasal polyps	Middle meatus and paranasal sinuses	Noncorticated dome-shaped nodular soft tissue density	Adults	M = F	10 to 20% (Edwards *et al.*, 2007)	Predisposes to obstruction of ostiomeatal complex, leading to impaired drainage, secondary infection	Refer for ENT consultation
Mucous retention pseudocyst	Maxillary sinus floor	Dome-shaped, soft tissue density	Adults, occasionally children	M = F	Common	No significance	No treatment
Oral-antral fistulae	Maxillary sinus floor	Defect of osseous floor of maxillary antrum with associated soft tissue hyperplasia	Adults	M = F	Unknown (somewhat common)	May be associated with unilateral chronic maxillary sinusitis	Refer to OMFS

(Continued)

Table 10.4 *(Continued)*

Condition or incidental finding	Radiographic location	CBCT presentation	Typical age range	Sex distribution	Frequency in CBCT scans	Clinical and other diagnostic features	Follow-up
Antroliths and foreign material	Maxillary sinus	Well-circumscribed density; density varies depending on etiology	Adults	M = F	Unknown (somewhat common)	Typically no significance; occasionally associated with maxillary sinus inflammation	No treatment unless signs/ symptoms of associated inflammation
Post-surgical changes	Maxillary sinus (most common site)	Varies depending on prior surgical procedure (well-defined defect of osseous structures at surgical site)	Adults, rarely children	M = F	Unknown (somewhat common)	Typically no significance; differentiate from pathologic process	No treatment
Schneiderian papillomas	Sinuses and nasal cavities	Destructive lesion +/− associated irregular soft tissue density	Adults	Unknown	Unknown (rare)	Extensive morbidity; possibility of carcinomatous change	Refer for ENT consultation
Malignant sinonasal neoplasms	Sinuses and nasal cavities	Destructive lesion	Older adults	Unknown	Unknown (rare)	Extensive morbidity; death	Refer for ENT consultation
Anatomic variations of nasal cavity: nasal septum deviations and concha bullosa	Nasal cavity (septum and middle concha)	Asymmetry of nasal turbinates/nasal conchae	Adults, occasionally children	M = F	20% deviated septum, 60% concha bullosa (Smith *et al.* 2010a)	No significance (unclear if surgical intervention alters risk of developing chronic rhinosinusitis in patients with deviated nasal septum or concha bullosa)	No treatment (informed consent prior to surgical/ orthodontic intervention)

ENT, ear, nose and throat; OMFS, oral and maxillofacial surgeon.

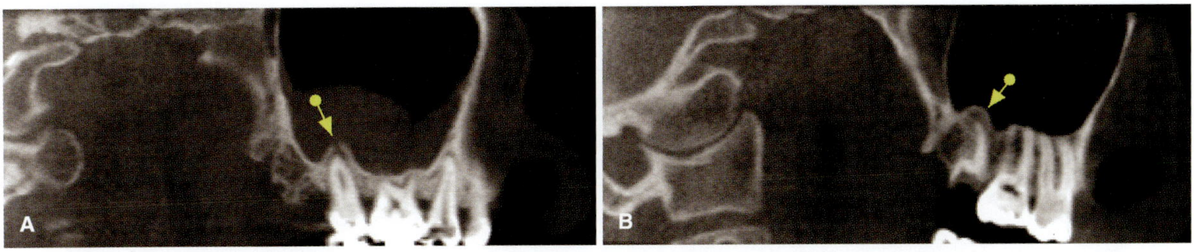

Figure 10.17 Mucosal thickening of odontogenic origin. *A*: Sagittal CBCT section reveals odontogenic maxillary sinus mucositis (arrow). *B*: Sagittal CBCT section showing odontogenic maxillary sinusitis with periostitis (arrow).

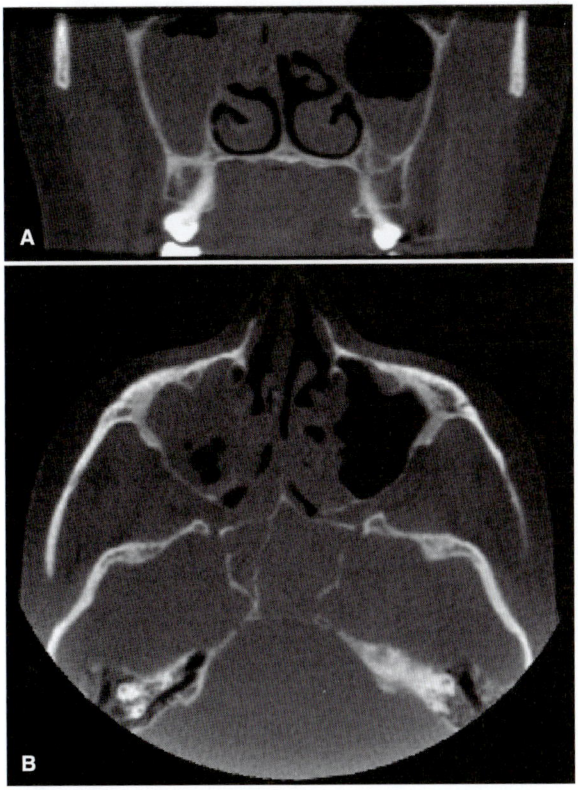

Figure 10.18 Mucosal thickening associated with pansinusitis. *A*: Coronal CBCT section reveals partial opacification of the right maxillary sinus. *B*: Axial CBCT section reveals additional involvement of the ethmoid air cells and sphenoid sinus in the same patient.

Mucous retention pseudocysts

The mucous retention pseudocyst represents a nondestructive reactive accumulation of fluid between the bony floor of the sinus (typically, the maxillary antrum, where it is termed an "antral pseudocyst") and the antral mucosa that lines the sinus (Table 10.4). Antral pseudocysts are relatively common, presenting in upward of 10% of the population (Carter *et al.*, 1998). Their exact underlying etiology has not been determined definitively but is believed to be multifaceted, involving inflammation of sinus of odontogenic origin and a probable allergic component.

Antral pseudocysts are identified readily on routine panoramic radiographs as single, noncorticated, dome-shaped radiopacities overlying the floor of the maxillary sinus, characteristically centered at its greatest concavity (Figure 10.20; Table 10.4). CBCT typically does not contribute to the identification of these lesions, except in atypical presentations. These may need to be distinguished from true sinus mucoceles most commonly involving the frontal sinuses, which are destructive, expansile epithelial-lined cysts caused by obstruction of the sinus ostia, and from mucous retention cysts, which represent small mucous-filled cysts that develop secondary to overproduction of mucinous material by obstructed minor seromucinous glands often found in association with sinus polyps. Early antral pseudocysts may be indistinguishable radiographically from a single sinus polyp of the maxillary sinus floor, although the latter tends to be more polypoid in appearance and often multiple in number.

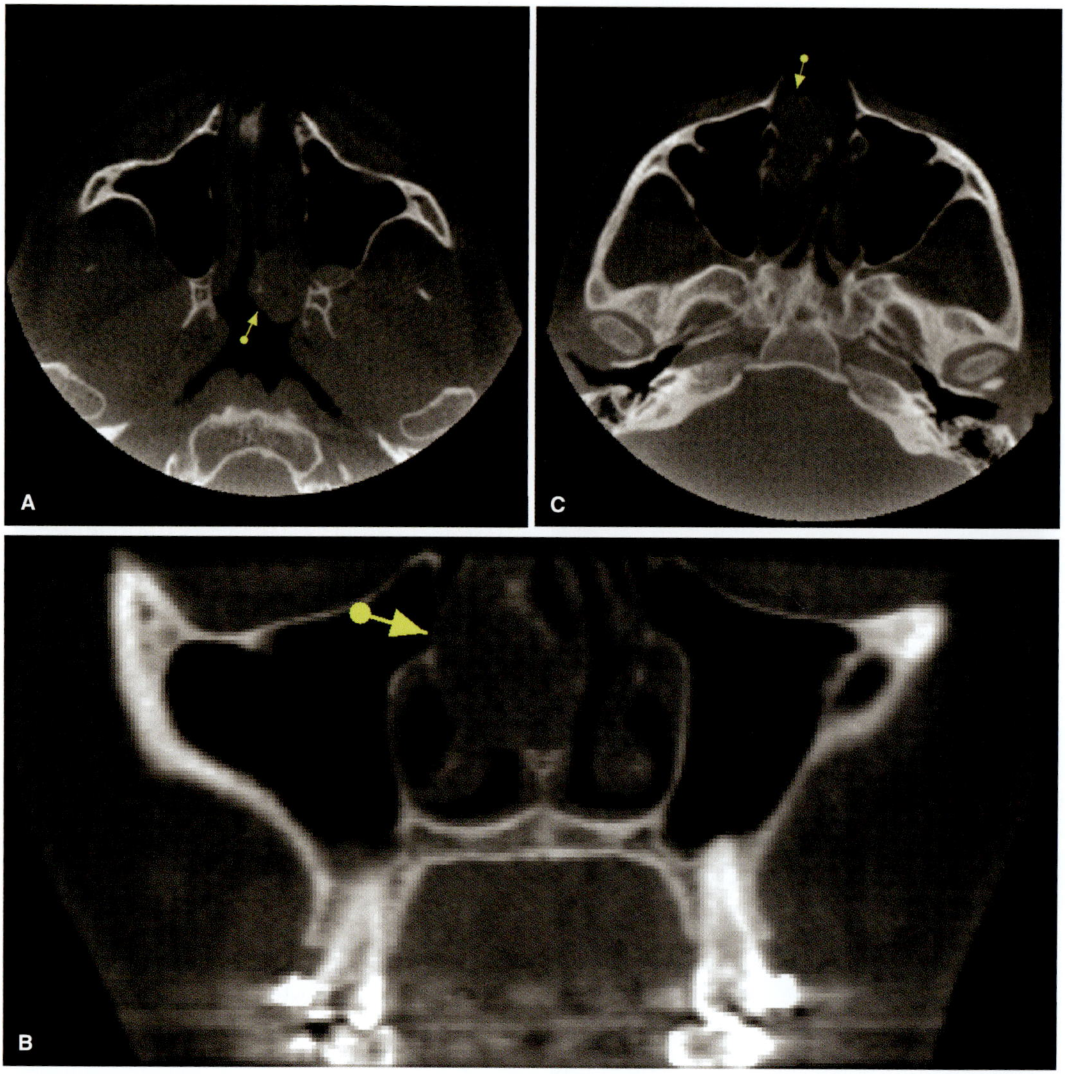

Figure 10.19 Nasal polyp. *A*: Axial CBCT section showing nasal polyp in the posterior aspect of the left inferior nasal turbinate (arrow). *B*: Coronal section demonstrating nasal polyp in the anterior aspect of the right middle nasal turbinate (arrow), causing thinning of the nasal cavity walls and displacement of the nasal septum. *C*: Nasal polyp seen in axial CBCT section of the same patient (arrow).

Once a convincing presumptive diagnosis has been rendered, treatment is not required. The diagnosis of antral pseudocyst appears to be of minimal clinical consequence. For example, it has been demonstrated that the presence of a maxillary antral pseudocyst is associated with a low frequency of sinus membrane perforation and post-surgical maxillary sinusitis following sinus augmentation surgery (Mardinger *et al.*, 2007).

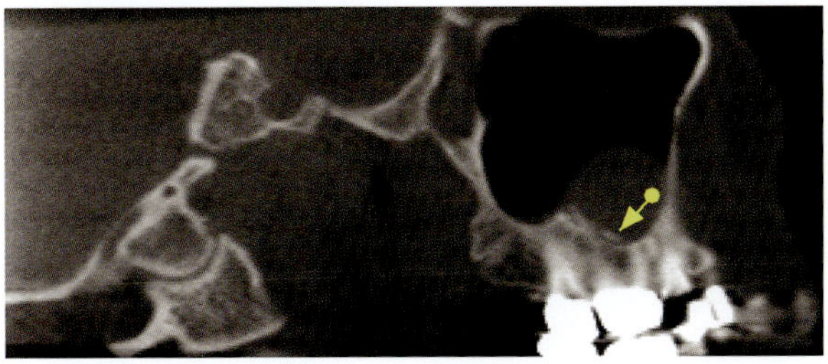

Figure 10.20 Maxillary antral pseudocyst. Sagittal CBCT section reveals a dome-shaped, soft-tissue density on the floor of the maxillary sinus. Incidentally noted is a linear high-density opacity immediately above the floor of the maxillary sinus (arrow), consistent with an antrolith.

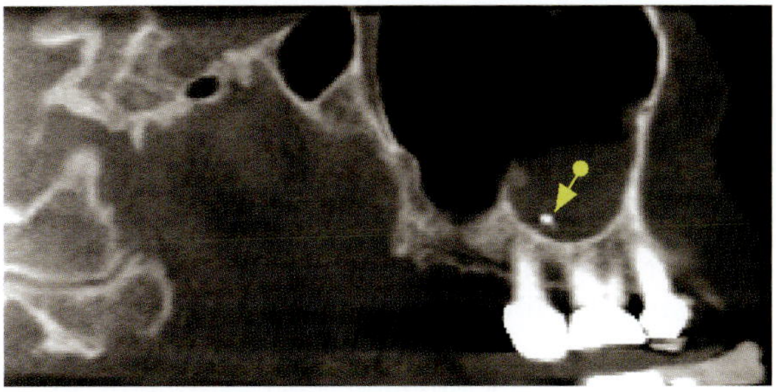

Figure 10.22 Metal-density foreign body. Sagittal CBCT section reveals a well-circumscribed, high-density spherical opacity (arrow) within the maxillary sinus adjacent to the roots of the second molar. Note the low-density opacity within the maxillary sinus, consistent with maxillary sinus inflammation, surrounding the foreign material.

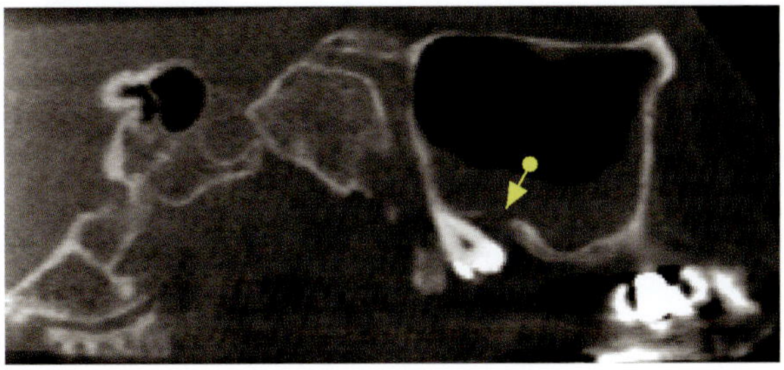

Figure 10.21 Sagittal CBCT section showing an oro-antral communication (arrow).

Oral-antral fistulae

Oral-antral fistulae (Mehra & Murad, 2004) represent pathologic communications between the oral cavity and maxillary sinus that commonly develop as a consequence of maxillary molar tooth extraction or other surgical procedures involving the posterior maxillary alveolar process and/or sinus. These are associated with a small percentage of cases of unilateral chronic maxillary sinusitis and are identifiable readily on CBCT imaging as a defect in the osseous floor of the maxillary antrum with associated soft tissue hyperplasia in the antral floor (Figure 10.21; Table 10.4). Treatment involves surgical repair of the defect, either through endoscopic surgery or a modified Caldwell-Luc procedure.

Antroliths and foreign material

While calcified masses within the maxillary sinus, termed antroliths, generally are identifiable readily on panoramic imaging, their presence may be obscured on occasion by superimposition of adjacent hard tissue in conventional 2D radiography (Figure 10.20). The development of antroliths appears to be related to the presence of endogenous (e.g., mucous, erythrocytes) or exogenous material, such as gutta percha or endodontic sealer (Figure 10.22; Table 10.4), or the presence of organisms (e.g., fungal) that act as a nidus for calcification and growth (Güneri *et al.*, 2005).

Post-surgical changes

Surgical interventions in the sinonasal complex can result in post-surgical changes that may be noted on CBCT imaging. Caldwell-Luc procedures involving osteotomy of the anterior sinus wall and creation of an artificial opening of the sinus into the inferior nasal meatus have been superseded largely by functional endoscopic sinonasal surgery for treatment of chronic rhinosinusitis in which appropriate nonsurgical intervention has failed (Table 10.4). Despite these evolutions, post-surgical changes to the sinonasal complex, predominantly bony defects on the lateral maxillary wall post-Caldwell-Luc procedure, were identified in nine of 166 scans reviewed by Edwards and colleagues (2007).

The surgical ciliated cyst represents an epithelial-lined cystic cavity that develops following traumatic or surgical implantation of a portion of the sinus antral lining involving the maxillary bone. Radiographically, these may resemble a routine developmental odontogenic cyst, although most patients will report a prior history of a Caldwell-Luc procedure to the area (Chindasombatjaroen *et al.*, 2009).

Schneiderian papillomas

Three pathologically distinct papillomatous lesions develop from the respiratory mucosa that lines the sinonasal structures: the exophytic, inverted, and oncocytic Schneiderian ("cylindrical cell") papillomas. These are locally destructive lesions with unlimited growth potential that can result in significant morbidity if not excised surgically and completely (Figure 10.23; Table 10.4). A variable percentage of Schneiderian papillomas, in particular the inverted and oncocytic types, are associated with synchronous or metachronous carcinomatous change (Barnes, 2002).

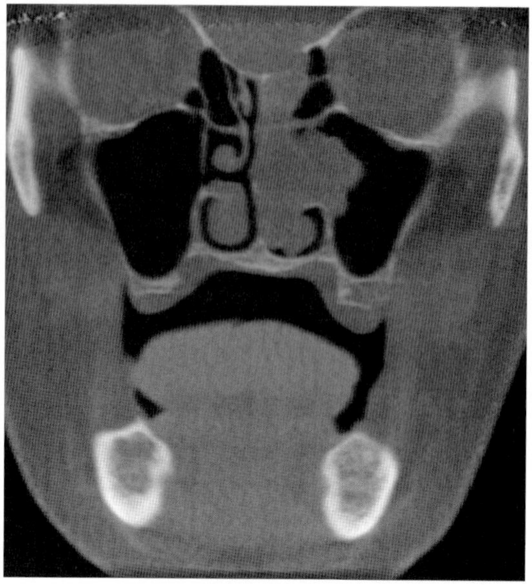

Figure 10.23 Inverted sinonasal papilloma. Coronal CBCT section suggests the papilloma most likely originates within the left nasal cavity and extends into the left maxillary sinus, causing destruction of the medial sinus/lateral nasal cavity wall.

Malignant sinonasal neoplasms

Sinonasal malignancies range from non-Schneiderian-derived tumors such as squamous cell carcinoma, small cell neuroendocrine carcinoma, olfactory neuroblastoma, lymphoepithelial carcinoma, and mucosal melanomas to more site-specific respiratory mucosa-derived neoplasms including nonkeratinizing carcinoma, sinonasal undifferentiated carcinoma, nasopharyngeal carcinoma, and intestinal-type adenocarcinoma (Franchi *et al.*, 2011). Fortunately, malignant neoplasms of the paranasal sinuses and nasal cavity are infrequent, with carcinomas of the nasal cavity and paranasal sinuses accounting for less than 1% of all malignancies. Approximately 60% of these carcinomas originate in the maxillary sinus, 30% in the nasal cavity, and 10% in the ethmoid sinuses. Malignant neoplasms of the sphenoid and frontal sinuses are exceedingly rare.

Sinonasal malignancies, particularly early stage lesions, may be indistinguishable from sinonasal polyps and Schneiderian papillomas on CBCT imaging (Table 10.4). Large destructive lesions such as the true sinus mucocele or the Schneiderian papilloma may simulate malignant sinonasal neoplasms radiographically. Clinically, malignant processes in the maxillary sinus often are misdiagnosed as discomfort and/or swelling of inflammatory odontogenic origin, especially when the characteristic warning signs of dysesthesia or paresthesia are overlooked (Edwards *et al.*, 2006).

Anatomic variations of the nasal cavity: nasal septum deviations and concha bullosa

The nasal cavity is located between the hard palate and the skull base, separated into bilateral structures by the nasal septum, which, in turn, is

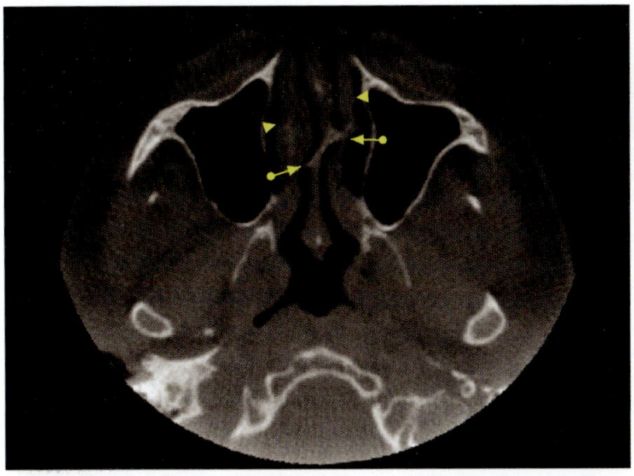

Figure 10.24 Nasal septum deviation. Axial CBCT section reveals nasal septum deviation (arrows) as well as asymmetry of the nasal turbinates (arrowheads).

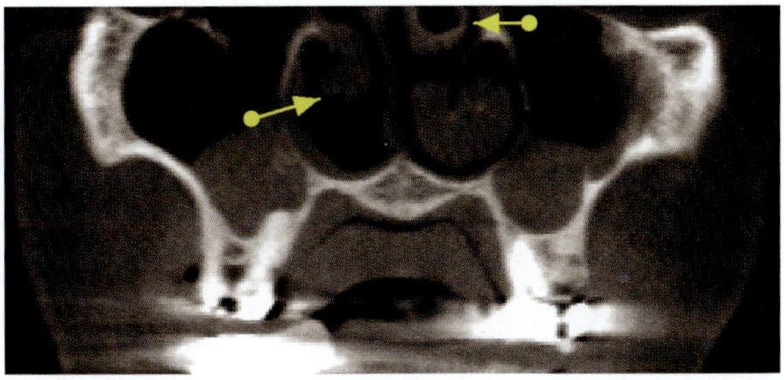

Figure 10.25 Concha bullosa on the left middle turbinate (left arrow) and asymmetry of the nasal conchae. Coronal CBCT section reveals significant atrophy of the right inferior nasal turbinate (right arrow).

composed of an anterior cartilaginous component and a posterior osseous component formed by the ethmoid bone, vomer, and maxillary bones (Norton, 2011; see also Chapter 9). Deviation of the nasal septum is a common, typically developmentally acquired finding characterized by displacement of the nasal septum from the midline (Figure 10.24; Table 10.4; Maples *et al.*, 2008).

The lateral nasal walls include three projections: the superior, middle, and inferior turbinates, overlying openings to the sphenoid and posterior ethmoid sinuses (superior turbinates); the frontal, maxillary, and anterior ethmoid sinuses (middle turbinates); and the nasolacrimal ducts (inferior turbinates). Pneumatization of the middle turbinate (middle nasal "concha") is a common anatomic variant termed "concha bullosa" (Figure 10.25; Zinreich *et al.*, 1988; Smith *et al.*, 2010b).

It is widely accepted that obstructions of the ostiomeatal complex, by interfering with ventilation and mucociliary clearance from the sinuses, may predispose affected patients to chronic sinus disease. Less understood is the role of a deviated nasal septum or enlargement of the middle turbinates in the pathogenesis of sinonasal sinusitis. Studies exploring potential associations between nasal septal deviations and/or the presence of concha bullosa and chronic sinus disease have produced contradictory findings (Bolger *et al.*, 1991; Collet *et al.*, 2001; Stallman *et al.*, 2004; Subramanian *et al.*, 2005). In a review of 883 CBCT scans, pneumatization of at least one concha was noted in 67.5%, a deviated septum (defined as a deviation of >4 mm from the midline) in 19.4%, and mucosal thickening consistent with maxillary sinusitis in 50.0% of the patients (Smith *et al.*, 2010a). No statistically significant relationship was evident between the presence of concha bullosa and/or nasal septal deviation and the incidence of maxillary sinusitis.

Despite these findings, it remains unclear what effect surgical or nonsurgical orthodontic intervention may have on the risk of developing chronic rhinosinusitis in patients with concha bullosa or deviated nasal septum. Until more definitive data are available, it may be prudent to advise patients in whom these anatomic variants are noted on CBCT that the risk of developing chronic rhinosinusits following orthodontic or orthognathic surgery remains to be determined, but is likely to be minimal.

TOOTH-RELATED FINDINGS AND DEVELOPMENTAL DEFECTS OF THE JAWS

Periradicular and pericoronal lesions

The common inflammatory periradicular lesions (e.g., periapical granuloma, periapical cyst, external and internal root resorption, condensing osteitis) and lesions of developmental origin involving

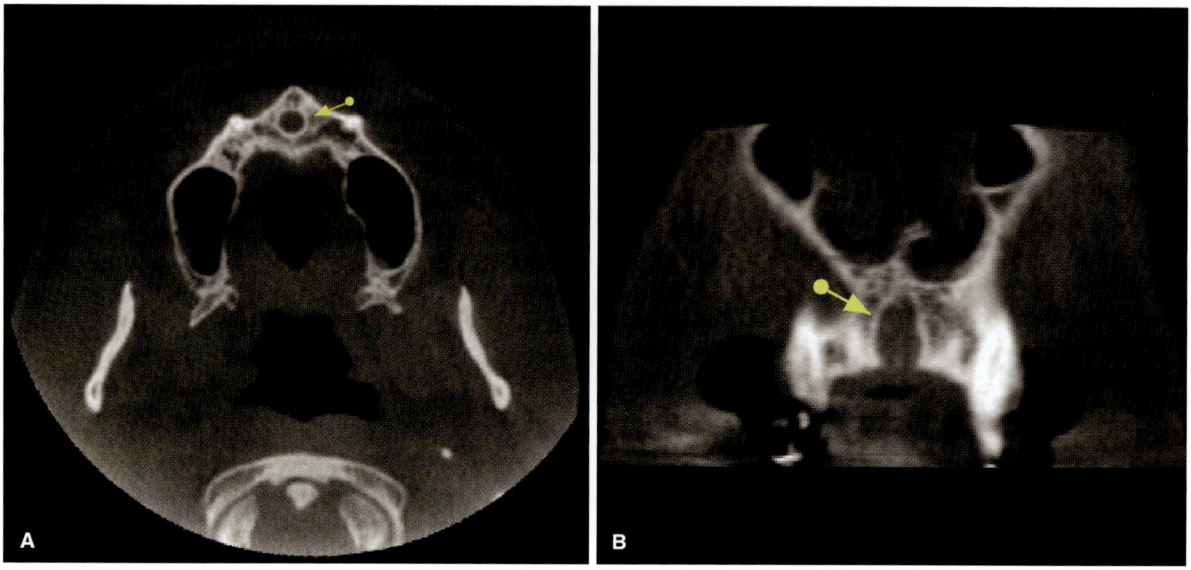

Figure 10.26 Prominent nasopalatine canal. *A*: Axial CBCT section reveals an enlarged nasopalatine canal that measures approximately 6 mm in diameter (arrow). Correlation with the clinical exam will help determine the need for biopsy in this borderline case. *B*: Coronal CBCT section of the same patient displaying the enlarged nasopalatine canal (arrow).

the jaws (e.g., dentigerous cyst, idiopathic osteosclerosis, odontogenic keratocyst or "keratocystic odontogenic tumor," nasopalatine duct cyst, benign fibro-osseous lesions) are visualized readily on conventional panoramic and plain film radiographs (Edwards, 2009). While CBCT can provide valuable information as to the nature of the lesion, with the routine availability of high quality plain films, it is infrequent for these lesions to be noted first on CBCT (Figure 10.26). On occasion, however, CBCT can identify small lesions before they have caused sufficient demineralization to be visible on plain films and may provide more definitive information when visualization on plain films is complicated by the superimposition of adjacent structures (Figure 10.27; Table 10.5).

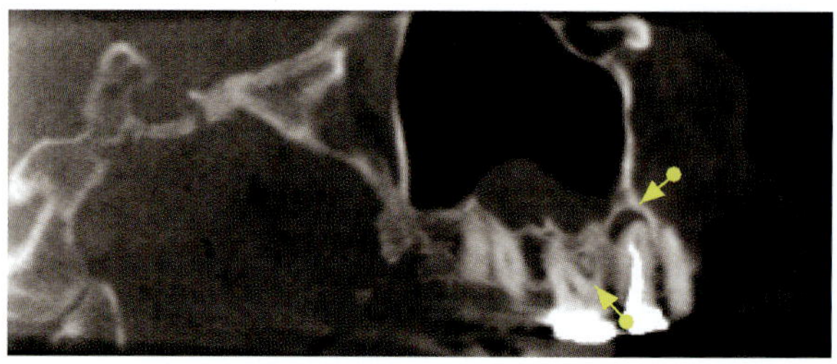

Figure 10.27 Periapical pathology in endodontically treated maxillary right second premolar (arrow pointing down) and furcation involvement in maxillary right first molar (arrow pointing up).

Developmental cortical defects of the mandible

The most common and best recognized of these variants is the developmental mandibular lingual salivary gland depression, also known by the eponym "Stafne bone cyst" or "Stafne defect" (Philipsen *et al.*, 2002). Other synonyms include static bone cyst and posterior lingual cortical defect. The Stafne defect represents a solitary, relatively static, lingual cortical depression located between the angle of the mandible and the first molar, below the inferior alveolar canal, attributed to resorptive pressure from the adjacent normal submandibular gland or other associated connective tissue (e.g., adipose tissue; Figure 10.28; Table

Table 10.5 Summary of CBCT presentation, age and sex distribution, additional diagnostic features, and recommended follow-up of tooth-related findings and developmental defects of the jaws.

Condition or incidental finding	Radiographic location	CBCT presentation	Typical age range	Sex distribution	Frequency in CBCT scans	Clinical and other diagnostic features	Follow-up
Periradicular and pericoronal lesions	Mandible, maxilla and (less commonly) maxillary sinuses	Varies depending on underlying process	Adults, occasionally children	M = F	Unknown (somewhat common)	Identification and management of underlying process required	Correlate with clinical exam and manage accordingly
Developmental cortical defects of mandible	Lingual of posterior mandible, below inferior alveolar canal	Well-defined concavity of lingual cortical plate; cortex intact	Adults (>40 years of age)	M > F	Unknown (somewhat common)	No significance	No treatment

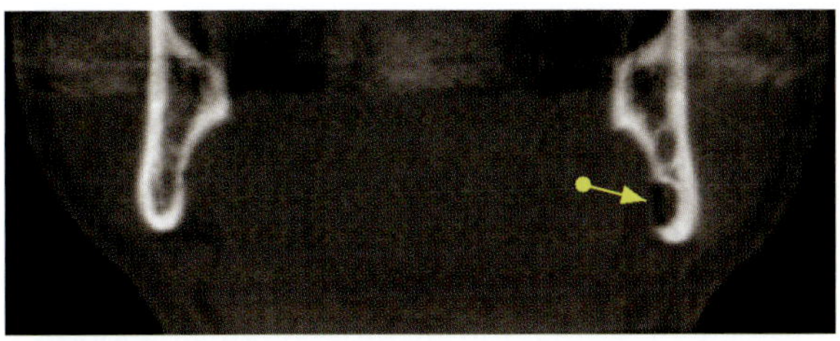

Figure 10.28 Stafne bone defect. This CBCT coronal section reveals a well-defined depression on the lingual aspect of the mandible displaying an intact lingual cortex (arrow).

10.5). These are identified readily as incidental findings on panoramic radiographs.

The anterior lingual cortical defect is similar to the Stafne defect in that it is characterized by a concavity involving the cortical mandibular plate (Philipsen *et al.*, 2002). The anterior lingual variant, like the Stafne defect, is more common in middle-aged and older males and, like its more posterior counterpart, consists histologically of normal salivary gland and/or adipose tissue.

Radiographically, the location of the "lesion" and the demonstration of an intact lingual cortical plate usually are pathognomonic. These entities have no diagnostic or pathologic significance other than the potential for misdiagnosis. With the more widespread use of CBCT in the dental field, it is expected that smaller lesions of clinically nonconsequential nature that otherwise may be difficult to discern by conventional radiography are likely to be identified more frequently.

TEMPOROMANDIBULAR JOINT (TMJ)

There are a number of common conditions affecting the TMJ space that may be noted incidentally on CBCT scans, ranging from inflammatory and degenerative conditions to neoplastic processes. While more details of these observations and their implications are provided elsewhere in this textbook (see Chapter 12), the most common clinicpathologic and radiographic TMJ findings are summarized below.

Degenerative joint disease: articular flattening, subcondral osteosclerosis, articular erosion, osteophytosis, and subchondral cyst formation

Degenerative joint disease of the TMJ complex, commonly referred to as osteoarthritis or osteoarthrosis, occurs in response to supraphysiologic activity on the joint, which can range from normal forces on a structurally altered joint (e.g., mechanical instability secondary to loss of posterior support) to parafunctional activity (e.g., bruxism). Altered forces on the joint may result in bony and soft tissue remodeling, ranging from subchondral sclerosis and flattening of the articular curvature of the joint (Figure 10.29A; Table 10.6) to thinning of the articular cartilaginous surface. Eventually, this may progress to erosion of the articular surface of the condyle, irregular cortical outlines, reduced joint space, loose bodies within the joint space (Figure 10.29B), osteophyte formation (Figure 10.29C), subchondral cyst formation (Figure 10.29D), and resorption of the condylar head.

These changes can be visualized on CBCT imaging, particularly in the more advanced stages of the disease. In a proof of concept cadaveric study where histologic features were compared with CBCT radiographic findings, it was demonstrated that identification of specific radiographic changes (increased condylar head bone density, subchondral sclerosis, and/or osteophyte formation) were of diagnostic value in identifying late stage osteoarthritic changes, but not early or intermediate stage changes (Wasserburger *et al.*, 2007a).

While the anatomy of the articular disc is assessed best by MRI studies, it has been demonstrated that condyles with associated perforations of the articular disc have statistically significant increases in mean bone density of the medial, central, and lateral zones of the condyle relative to unaffected condyles (Wasserburger *et al.*, 2007b).

It is important to note that while one or more imaging techniques commonly are employed in the assessment of patients with classical signs and symptoms of temporomandibular joint disease (TMJD), there is limited available evidence to support their routine use for this purpose. As concluded in a recent systematic review, there are a limited number of studies, all with low to moderate levels of evidence, to support the efficacy of routine MRI in the evaluation of inflammatory and degenerative TMJD (Limchaichana *et al.*, 2006). Similarly, another systematic review concluded that "the scarcity of studies on the therapeutic efficacy of MRI in TMJD and the absence of such studies for CT do not support the concept that these exams are indicated in the diagnosis of TMJD when a symptomatic patient seeks treatment" (Ribeiro-Rotta *et al.*, 2011).

Inflammatory conditions of the TMJ

The radiographic changes described above as degenerative joint disease are nonspecific. Similar radiographic changes including erosion of the condylar head, fibrosis, and mandibular and subchondral cysts of the condyle can be seen in the spectrum of inflammatory TMJDs that include rheumatoid arthritis, infectious arthritis (e.g., late stage Lyme disease), gout (chronic deposition of monosodium urate crystals), and calcium pyrophosphate crystal deposition disease (pseudogout, chondrocalcinosis).

Reactive, cystic, and neoplastic lesions of the TMJ

Other conditions with a propensity to involve the TMJ space that may be noted incidentally on routine CBCT imaging include synovial chondromatosis, a reactive process involving the proliferation of synovial-like tissue that characteristically results in the formation of numerous loose cartilaginous bodies within the joint space, and pigmented villonodular synovitis, an idiopathic, locally aggressive, and destructive process of uncertain potential or origin (Table 10.6). Ganglion cysts, pseudocysts derived from degeneration of the joint capsule, and true synovial cysts of bone are rare entities that typically represent late findings in a myriad of conditions characterized by degeneration of the articular surface (Sano *et al.*, 2004). Malignant neoplasms of the TMJ are rare, with metastatic lesions being more common than primary malignancies (Dos Santos & Cavalcanti, 2002). Clinically, these initially often mimic the more common degenerative or inflammatory TMJ conditions. More advanced disease will present on CBCT as unilateral destructive lesions with irregular margins.

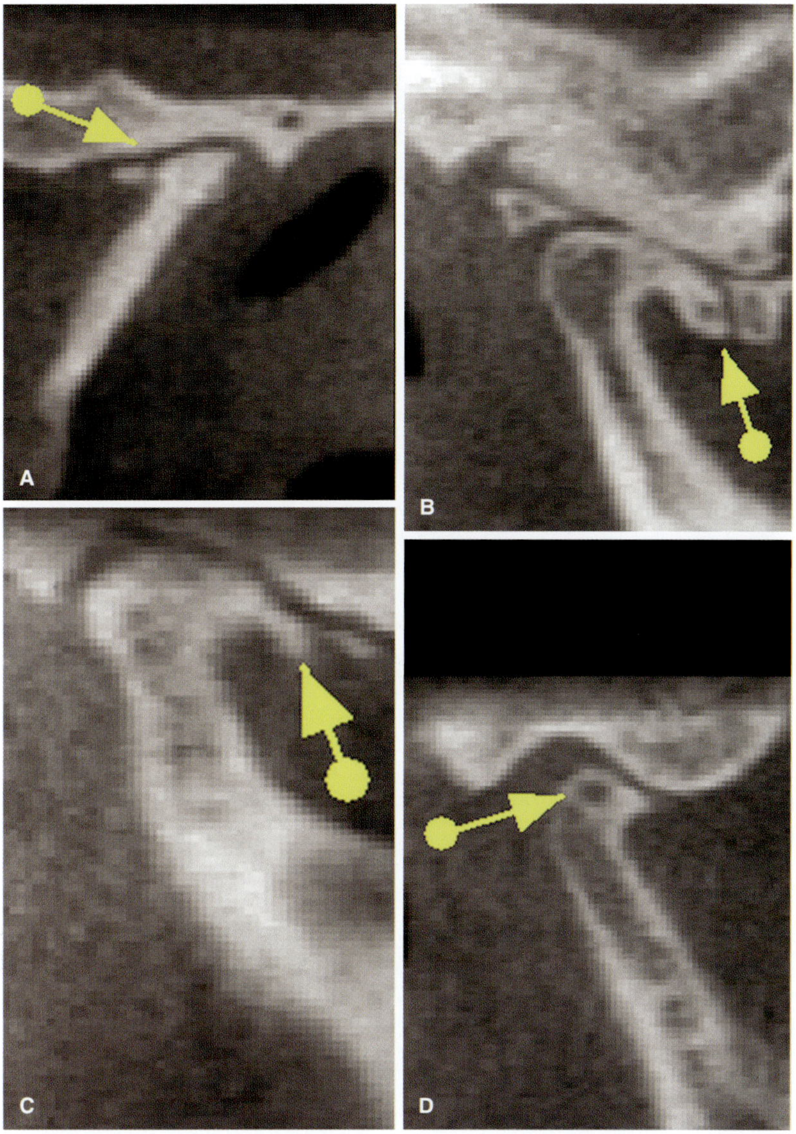

Figure 10.29 Degenerative changes of the TMJ. *A*: Severe flattening and subchondral sclerosis of the condyle and glenoid fossa (arrow). *B*: Severe flattening, osteophytosis and loose bodies in the TMJ (arrow). *C*: Osteophytosis (arrow). *D*: Subchondral cyst formation (arrow).

As these conditions typically involve a significant soft tissue and/or fluid component, MRI or conventional CT with contrast typically will offer better detail and a stronger presumptive radiographic diagnosis compared with CBCT.

Developmental and traumatically acquired anomalies in TMJ size and/or shape

CBCT studies readily can identify developmental osseous disorders including morphological

Table 10.6 Summary of CBCT presentation, age and sex distribution, additional diagnostic features, and recommended follow-up for temporomandibular joint (TMJ) findings.

Condition or incidental finding	Radiographic location	CBCT presentation	Typical age range	Sex distribution	Frequency in CBCT scans	Clinical and other diagnostic features	Follow-up
Degenerative joint disease and inflammatory conditions of TMJ	Condyle and glenoid fossa	Subchondral sclerosis, flattening of articular curvature, increased condylar head bone density, osteophyte formation	Adults (>40 years of age)	M = F	Unknown (somewhat common)	Varies from no signs/ symptoms to TMJ pain, restricted opening	No treatment unless accompanied by signs/ symptoms of TMJ dysfunction (informed consent prior to orthodontic intervention)
Reactive, cystic and neoplastic lesions of TMJ	Condyle and/or glenoid fossa	Varies depending on underlying process	Adults (>40 years of age)	Unknown	Unknown (rare)	Varies from no signs/ symptoms to TMJ pain, restricted opening	Depends on specific entity
Developmental and traumatically acquired anomalies in TMJ size and/ or shape	Varies	Varies	Varies	Varies	Unknown (rare)	Depends on specific entity	Depends on specific entity
Degenerative changes of TMJ	Condyle and/or glenoid fossa	Subchondral sclerosis, flattening, osteophytosis, cyst, erosion	Older adults	M = F	17.6% (Miles, 2006)	Patient may or may not have signs and symptoms	Correlate with the clinical exam to determine need for referral to TMJ specialist

changes, condylar hypoplasia (Figure 10.30; Table 10.6), condylar hyperplasia, coronoid hyperplasia, bifid condyles, and previous condylar fractures with residual joint deformities (Figure 10.31). These findings are of substantial relevance to orthodontic assessment and treatment planning particularly when obvious facial asymmetry (see also Chapter 21) or limited mandibular range of movement is present.

CERVICAL SPINE

Surface and bone density changes of the cervical spine: remodeling, flattening, exostoses, osteophytosis, osteosclerosis, and osteopenia

The analysis of the cervical vertebral maturation (CVM) from lateral cephalometric radiographs is

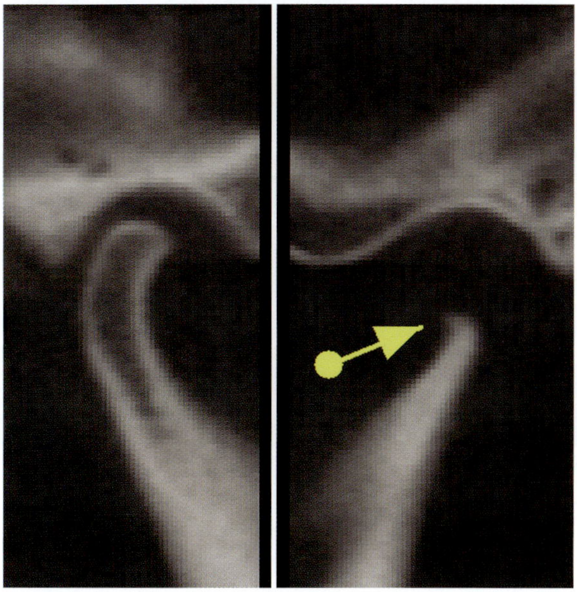

Figure 10.30 Condylar hypoplasia. Corrected sagittal CBCT section of the right and left TMJs show significant left condylar hypoplasia in a 17-year-old male patient.

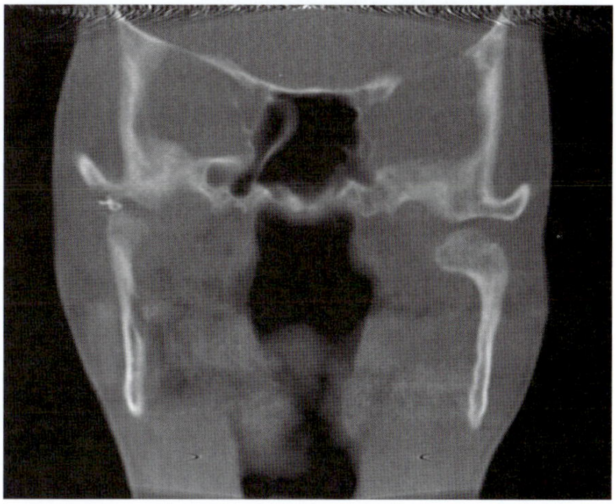

Figure 10.31 Old malpositioned TMJ fracture. Coronal CBCT section reveals significant condylar asymmetry as a result of medially displaced healed left condylar neck fracture.

an important method to identify the peak stage of mandibular growth in orthodontic patients (Baccetti *et al.*, 2002). Although cervical vertebrae C1 through C4 typically are visualized on extended FOV CBCT scans, and are likely to be helpful in assessing peak mandibular growth from their 2D reconstructions, the potential for enhanced assessment of growth stages from the entire 3D CBCT data has not been elucidated yet.

Degenerative changes of the cervical spine are a relatively common incidental CBCT finding, particularly in older patients. These changes include remodeling of the surface of the vertebrae, including flattening, exostosis formation (Figure 10.32A,B; Table 10.7), and osteopytosis (Figure 10.32C), as well as changes in bone density, including osteopenia (Figure 10.32D) and osteosclerosis (Figure 10.32C). The significance of these findings should be determined by correlating them with the medical history and the presence of clinical signs and symptoms. In some cases, multiple areas of decreased bone density found in the cervical spine may indicate the presence of systemic osteometabolic diseases such as osteomalacia, which can occur in young adults (Cakur *et al.*, 2012). It also is important to keep in mind that the spine is the third most common site for cancer metastasis, following the lung and the liver. Ten percent of metastatic lesions are found in the cervical spine; therefore, correlation with medical history of primary cancer is of particular importance when determining the nature of bone density changes in the cervical vertebrae (Jenis *et al.*, 1999).

Calcified ligaments of the cervical spine

Of the multiple cervical spine ligaments, the alar, transverse ligament of atlas, and nuchal ligaments most commonly present internal calcifications that can be detected on CBCT imaging. The alar ligament connects the sides of the dens process of C2 vertebra to the tubercles on the medial side of the occipital condyle. The transverse ligament of atlas is a thick, band-like ligament that is located posterior to the dens process of C2 vertebra and encircles it as an extension of the anterior arch of C1 vertebra (Figure 10.33A,B; Table 10.7). The nuchal ligament extends from the external occipital protuberance and the median nuchal line to the spinous process of the seventh cervical vertebra (Figure 10.33C,D).

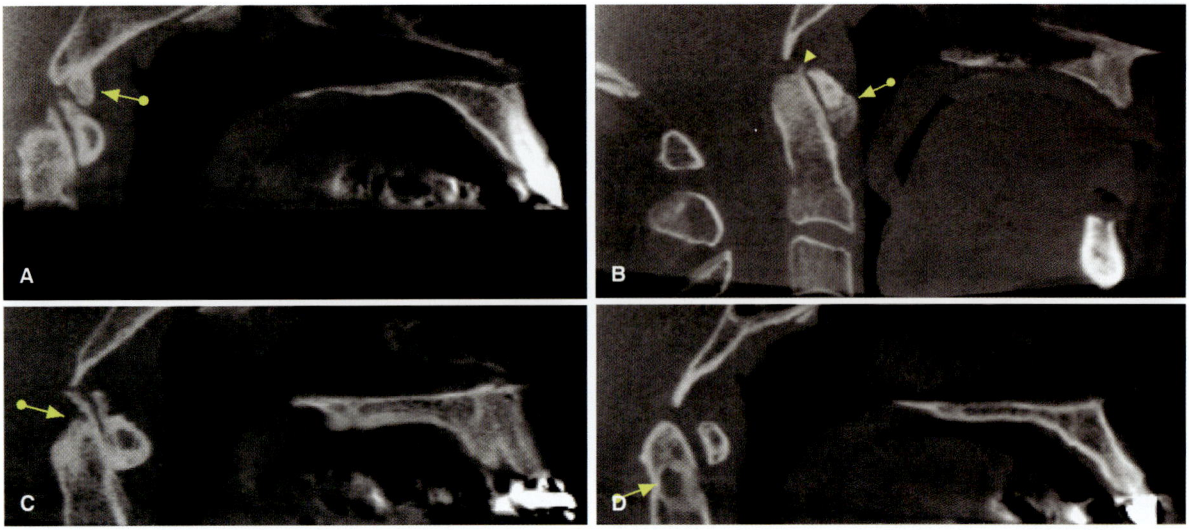

Figure 10.32 Degenerative changes of the cervical spine including exostosis, ostesclerosis, osteopenia, and intraosseous cyst. *A*: Sagittal CBCT section reveals well-defined exostosis (arrow) on the inferior aspect of the clivus. *B*: Sagittal CBCT section reveals an irregular high-density osseous mass or exostosis in the anterior-inferior aspect of the anterior arch of C1 vertebra (arrow). *C*: Osteosclerosis (arrow) and osteophytosis (arrowhead) are noted in the superior aspect of the dens process of C2 and the anterior arch of C1, respectively, on this sagittal CBCT section at the midline level. *D*: Sagittal CBCT section reveals multiple areas of decreased bone density (osteopenia) and a well-defined intraosseous cyst (arrow).

Table 10.7 Summary of CBCT presentation, age and sex distribution, additional diagnostic features, and recommended follow-up of findings in the cervical spine.

Condition or incidental finding	Radiographic location	CBCT presentation	Typical age range	Sex distribution	Frequency in CBCT scans	Clinical and other diagnostic features	Follow-up
Degenerative changes of cervical spine	Anterior arch of C1, dens process of C2 (most common), and/or body of cervical vertebrae included in the scan	Deformation, subchondral sclerosis, oseophytosis, intraosseous cyst formation, erosion	Older adults	M = F	8.4% (Miles, 2006)	Patient may or may not have signs and symptoms	Correlate with medical history and clinical exam to determine need for medical consultation
Calcified ligaments of cervical spine	Alar, transverse ligament of atlas, and nuchal ligaments	High-density, well-defined calcifications along the ligament, partial or complete	Older adults	M = F	Unknown	May indicate history of trauma	No treatment unless there is spinal cord compression

C1, first cervical vertebra (atlas); C2, second cervical vertebra (axis).

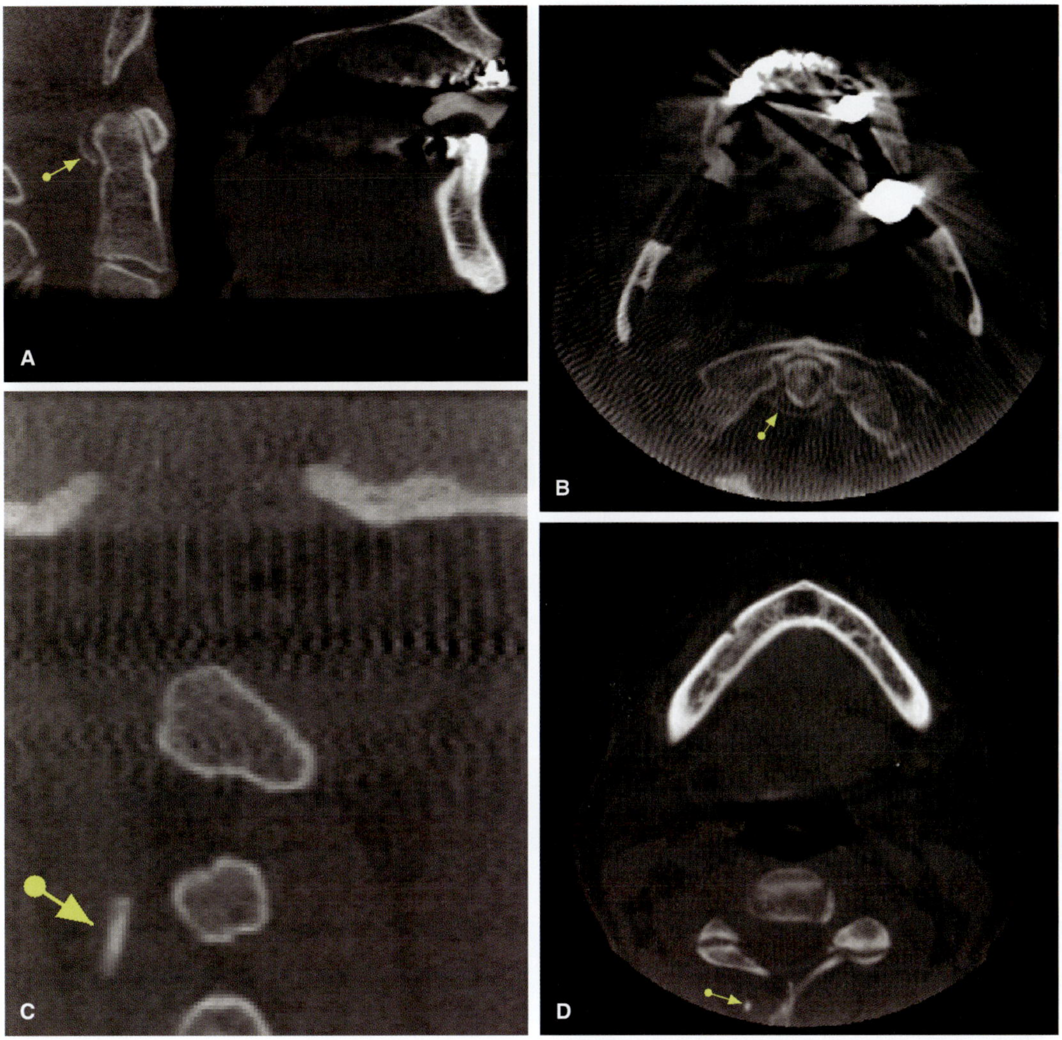

Figure 10.33 Calcified cervical spine ligaments. Sagittal (*A*) and axial (*B*) CBCT sections showing calcified transverse ligament of atlas (arrows). Coronal (*C*) and axial (*D*) CBCT sections depicting calcified nuchal ligament at the C3-C4 level (arrows).

Calcification of these ligaments is found more commonly in older, male patients or as a result of excessive stress, strain, or trauma applied to the neck as seen in violinists and weight lifters. This type of incidental finding usually carries low clinical significance unless the calcified ligament appears to be compressing the spinal cord (Figure 10.34A,B), in which case referral for further medical evaluation is recommended.

MISCELLANEOUS FINDINGS

Cosmetic surgery, soft tissue implants, post-surgical changes, and foreign bodies

Accessories such as nose rings and studs (Figure 10.35; Table 10.8), as well as cosmetic surgery including chin, cheek, and other soft tissue implants (Figure 10.36A,B; Table 10.8) can be seen in CBCT

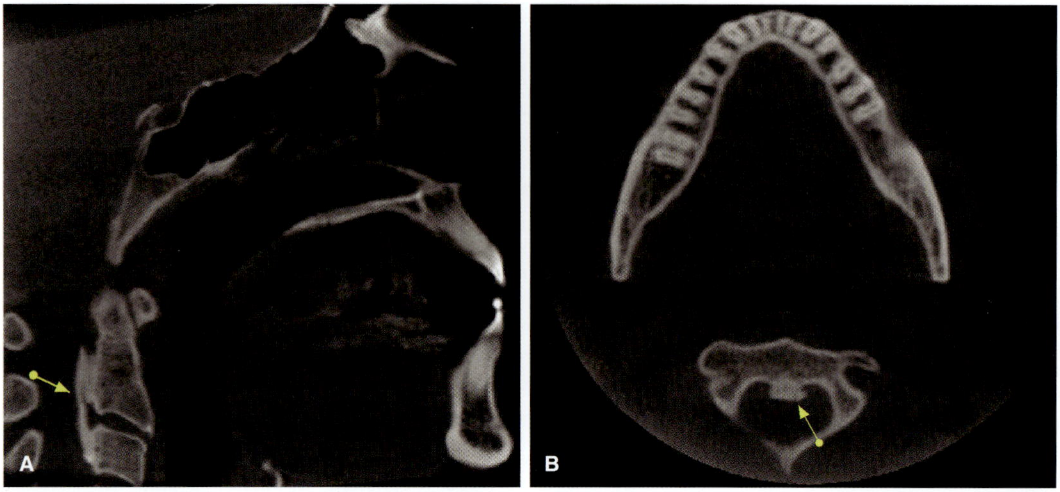

Figure 10.34 Calcified ligament causing possible spinal cord compression. *A*: Sagittal CBCT section reveals a linear, well-defined, high-density calcification in the posterior aspect of the dens process of C2 and the body of C3 vertebrae (arrow) that appears to occupy the spinal cord space partially in a 36-year-old female patient. *B*: Axial CBCT section of the same patient displaying the calcified ligament (arrow).

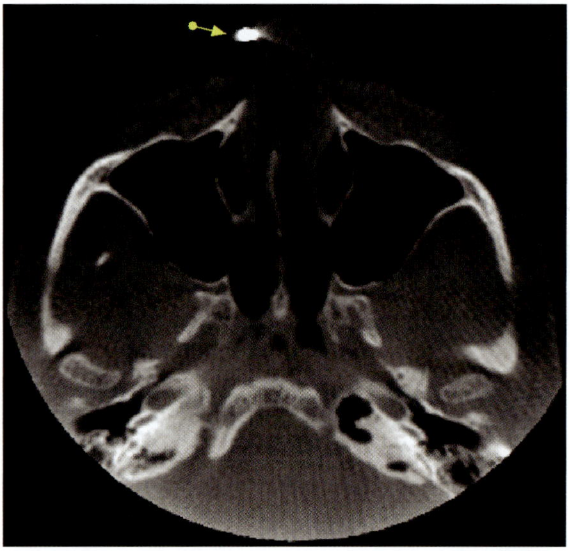

Figure 10.35 Axial CBCT section showing nose ring contributing to a metal streaking artifact (arrow).

scans as foreign bodies of varying size, shape, and density depending on the material used. In the latter cases, determination of previous surgical history can help facilitate the assessment of any alterations in the anatomical structures in proximity to the implants. Similarly, in patients who have undergone therapy for head and neck cancer and are likely to reveal soft and hard tissue changes on post-surgical CBCT scans, correlating the CBCT findings with medical history will aid in the accurate interpretation of the images (Figure 10.37).

Soft tissue lesions within the external acoustic meatus

Lesions within the external acoustic meatus can range from the simple impaction of cerumen to neoplasias of the temporal bone. Since the external acoustic meatus is a dermal-lined canal, dermatologic disorders affecting other areas of the skin also can affect the epithelium of the external auditory canal. Approximately 80–90% of the soft tissue masses found within this canal are benign. Of these benign lesions, cholesteatomas and keratosis obturans are the most common (Table 10.8). A cholesteatoma represents a cystic collection of squamous epithelium that may cause pain, purulent otorrhea, erosion of the canal walls, and periostitis in an older age group. Keratosis obturans is an accumulation of squamous debris in the external acoustic canal that often is bilateral and frequently

Table 10.8 Summary of CBCT presentation, age and sex distribution, additional diagnostic features, and recommended follow-up of miscellaneous CBCT findings.

Condition or incidental finding	Radiographic location	CBCT presentation	Typical age range	Sex distribution	Frequency in CBCT scans	Clinical and other diagnostic features	Follow-up
Soft tissue implants and other foreign bodies	Chin, cheek, other	Varying size, shape, and density depending on material; usually denser than soft tissue	Adults	M = F	Unknown	History of surgery	Correlate with medical history and manage accordingly
Soft tissue lesions within external acoustic meatus	Within external acoustic meatus	Soft-tissue density, well defined, oval in shape	Depends on lesion (cholesteatoma, older adults; keratosis obturans, adolescents and young adults)	Unknown	Unknown	May indicate the presence of cerumen or lesion	Correlate with possible clinical signs and symptoms to determine need for ENT consultation

ENT, ear, nose and throat.

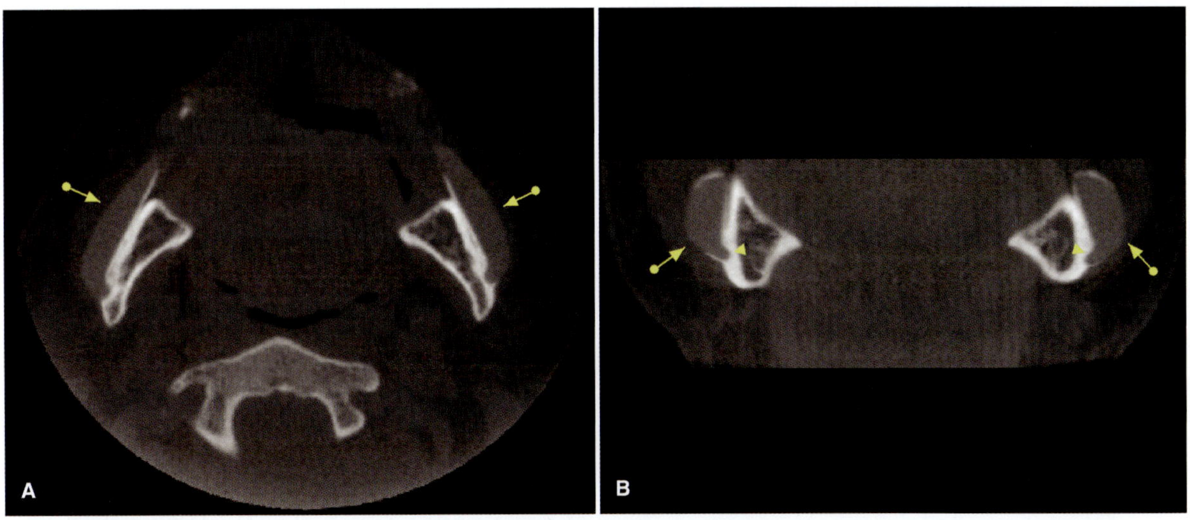

Figure 10.36 Bilateral cheek implants. Axial (*A*) and coronal (*B*) CBCT sections reveal symmetric cheek implants (arrows) of higher density compared with the adjacent soft tissue structures and possible small osteotomy sites (arrowheads) at the posterior-inferior aspect of the buccal mandibular cortex used to create the implant bed. The coronal CBCT section (*B*) also reveals a high-density superior border of cheek implants.

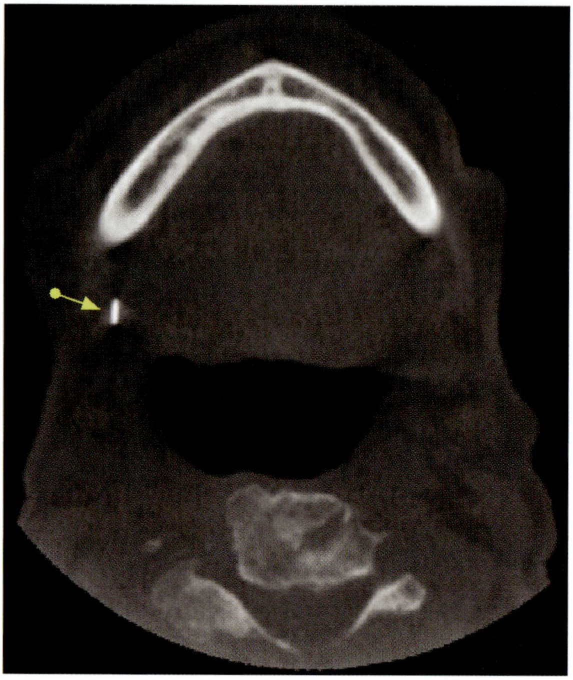

Figure 10.37 Post-surgical changes in a patient with history of carcinoma of the right submandibular gland. Axial CBCT section reveals surgical stent (arrow) and increased airway space after surgical resection of the submandibular gland followed by chemo-radiation therapy.

is found in a younger age group. It also may cause pain, canal hyperemia, and the formation of granulation tissue that occasionally is associated with hearing loss (Wenig, 1993; Selesnick, 1996; Tran *et al.*, 1996). Therefore, when soft-tissue density foreign bodies or suspected lesions are found within the external auditory meatus, careful evaluation of the canal walls for possible signs of erosion and referral for otorhinolaryngological evaluation is recommended (Figure 10.38).

CONCLUSIONS

In this chapter, we have reviewed several representative findings of potential clinical significance that may be noted incidentally not only in large, but also in smaller FOV CBCT scans of the craniofacial complex. As discussed elsewhere in this textbook (see Chapter 7), the diagnostician bears legal and ethical responsibilities for identifying all anomalies in the prescribed FOV that potentially may affect the patient's health and, where appropriate, to refer the patient for follow-up. Because of these ramifications and a multitude of incidental findings that can be present in CBCT scans, some of which occur frequently, it is imperative that diagnosticians have the skill set to identify these

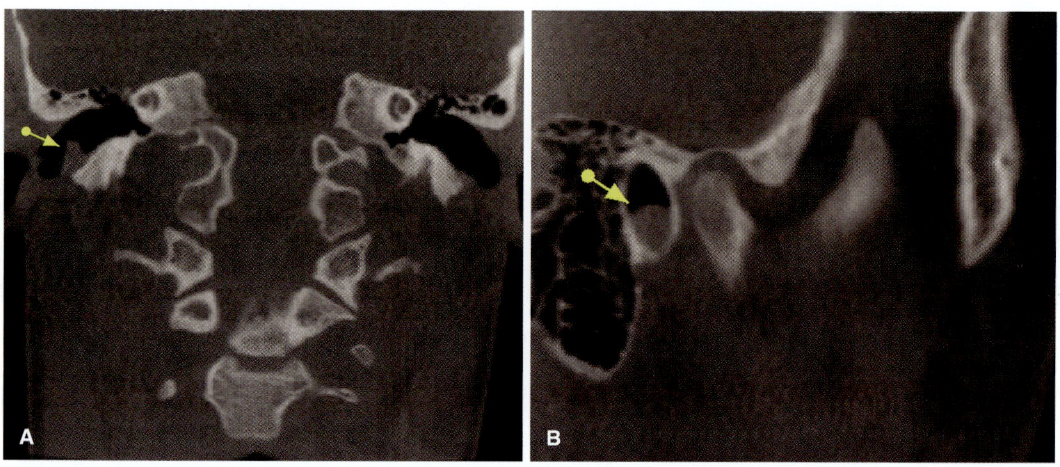

Figure 10.38 Soft tissue lesion (arrow) in the external auditory meatus. *A*: Coronal CBCT section reveals a well-defined, soft-tissue density lesion along the floor of the right external acoustic meatus. *B*: Sagittal CBCT section confirms the absence of erosion of the canal walls.

lesions anywhere within the scan. Finally, it is stressed that, absent relevant signs or symptoms or other appropriate justifications for performing the CBCT study (see Chapters 1 and 6 for indications and protocols for CBCT imaging), because of radiation considerations, routine CBCT imaging cannot be justified solely for screening for potential pathologic findings.

ACKNOWLEDGMENTS

We sincerely thank Dr. Neil Norton, Associate Dean for Student Affairs (Creighton University, Omaha, NE) and Dr. Tarnjit Saini, Lt. Colonel (U.S. Army) for their critical contribution to the many studies referenced in this chapter.

References

Ahmed, F., Brooks, S.L., & Kapila, S.D. (2012) Efficacy of identifying maxillofacial lesions in cone-beam computed tomographs by orthodontists and orthodontic residents with third-party software. *American Journal of Orthodontics and Dentofacial Orthopedics*, 141, 451–459.

Aspestrand, F. & Kolbenstvedt, A. (1987) Calcifications of the palatine tonsillary region: CT demonstration. *Radiology*, 165, 479–480.

Baccetti, T., Franchi, L., & McNamara, J.A., Jr. (2002) An improved version of the cervical vertebral maturation (CVM) method for the assessment of mandibular growth. *Angle Orthodontist*, 72, 316–323.

Barnes, L. (2002) Schneiderian papillomas and nonsalivary glandular neoplasms of the head and neck. *Modern Pathology*, 15, 279–297.

Bersani, G., Garavini, A., Taddei, I., *et al.* (1999) Computed tomography study of pineal calcification in schizophrenia. *European Psychiatry*, 14, 163–166.

Bolger, W.E., Butzin, C.A., & Parsons, D.S. (1991) Paranasal sinus bony anatomic variations and mucosal abnormalities: CT analysis for endoscopic sinus surgery. *Laryngoscope*, 101, 56–64.

Bos, D., Van Der Rijk, M.J., Geeraedts, T.E., *et al.* (2012) Intracranial carotid artery atherosclerosis: prevalence and risk factors in the general population. *Stroke*, 43 (7), 1878–1884.

Bourek, H., Saini, T.S., Edwards, P.C., *et al.* (2008) Incidental recognition of sphenoid sinus pathosis during routine cone beam computed tomography of dental patients. *Journal of Dental Research*, 87 (Spec Issue A), 240.

Caglayan, F. & Tozoglu, U. (2012) Incidental findings in the maxillofacial region detected by cone beam CT. *Diagnostic and Interventional Radiology*, 18, 159–163.

Cakur, B., Sumbullu, M.A., Dagistan, S., *et al.* (2012) The importance of cone beam CT in the radiological detection of osteomalacia. *Dentomaxillofacial Radiology*, 41, 84–88.

Carter, L.C., Calamel, A., Haller, A., *et al.* (1998) Seasonal variation in maxillary antral pseudocysts in a general clinic population. *Dentomaxillofacial Radiology*, 27, 22–24.

Cha, J.Y., Mah, J., & Sinclair, P. (2007) Incidental findings in the maxillofacial area with 3-dimensional cone-beam imaging. *American Journal of Orthodontics and Dentofacial Orthopedics*, 132, 7–14.

Chindasombatjaroen, J., Uchiyama, Y., Kakimoto, N., *et al.* (2009) Postoperative maxillary cysts: magnetic resonance imaging compared with computerized tomography. *Oral Surgery, Oral Medicine, Oral Pathology, Oral Radiology, and Endodontics*, 107, e38–e44.

Collet, S., Bertrand, B., Cornu, S., *et al.* (2001) Is septal deviation a risk factor for chronic sinusitis? Review of literature. *Acta Oto-Rhino-Laryngologica Belgica*, 55, 299–304.

Cottoni, F., Dell'Orbo, C., Quacci, D., *et al.* (1993) Primary osteoma cutis: clinical, morphological, and ultrastructural study. *American Journal of Dermatopathology*, 15, 77–81.

Deweert, T.T., Cakir, H., Rozie, S., *et al.* (2009) Intracranial internal carotid artery calcifications: association with vascular risk factors and ischemic cerebrovascular disease. *American Journal of Neuroradiology*, 30, 177–184.

Dos Santos, D.T. & Cavalcanti, M.G. (2002) Osteosarcoma of the temporomandibular joint: report of two cases. *Oral Surgery, Oral Medicine, Oral Pathology, Oral Radiology, and Endodontics*, 94, 641–647.

Edwards, P.C. (2009) Pathology of the hard tissues of the jaws. In Rosen, C.L. (ed.), *Primer on the Metabolic Bone Diseases and Disorders of Mineral Metabolism*. 7th ed. American Society for Bone and Mineral Research, Washington, DC, pp. 501–505.

Edwards, P.C., Hess, S., & Saini, T. (2006) Sinonasal undifferentiated carcinoma of the maxillary sinus. *Journal of the Canadian Dental Association*, 72, 161–165.

Edwards, P.C., Scanlon, C., III, Norton, N., *et al.* (2007) Review of extragnathic pathology noted during routine volumetric computed tomography. *Oral Surgery, Oral Medicine, Oral Pathology, Oral Radiology, and Endodontics*, (Abstract, AAOMP annual meeting), Suppl. 1.

Eivazi, B., Fasunla, A.J., Guldner, C., *et al.* (2012) Phleboliths from venous malformations of the head and neck. *Phlebology*, Feb 1 (Epub ahead of print).

Fazeli, P., Harvell, J., & Jacobs, M.B. (1999) Osteoma cutis (cutaneous ossification). *Western Journal of Medicine*, 171, 243–245.

Franchi, A., Miligi, L., Palomba, A., *et al.* (2011) Sinonasal carcinomas: recent advances in molecular and phenotypic characterization and their clinical implications. *Critical Reviews in Oncology/Hematology*, 79, 265–277.

Güneri, P., Kaya, A., & Kaliskan, M.K. (2005) Antroliths: survey of the literature and report of a case. *Oral Surgery, Oral Medicine, Oral Pathology, Oral Radiology, and Endodontics*, 99, 517–521.

Hamilos, D.L. (2011) Chronic rhinosinusitis: epidemiology and medical management. *Journal of Allergy and Clinical Immunology*, 128, 693–707.

Harnsberger, H.R. (1995) *Handbook of Head and Neck Imaging*. 2nd ed. Mosby, St. Louis, MO.

Jank, S., Robatscher, P., Emshoff, R., *et al.* (2003) The diagnostic value of ultrasonography to detect occult lymph node involvement at different levels in patients with squamous cell carcinoma in the maxillofacial region. *International Journal of Oral and Maxillofacial Surgery*, 32, 39–42.

Jenis, L.G., Dunn, E.J., & An, H.S. (1999) Metastatic disease of the cervical spine: a review. *Clinical Orthopaedics and Related Research*, 359, 89–103.

Kapila, S., Conley, R.S., & Harrell, W.E., Jr. (2011) The current status of cone beam computed tomography imaging in orthodontics. *Dentomaxillofacial Radiology*, 40, 24–34.

Kunz, D., Schmitz, S., Mahlberg, R., *et al.* (1999) A new concept for melatonin deficit: on pineal calcification and melatonin excretion. *Neuropsychopharmacology*, 21, 765–772.

Lewis, D.A. & Brooks, S.L. (1999) Cartoid artery calcification in a general dental population: a retrospective study of panoramic radiographs. *General Dentistry*, 47, 98–103.

Limchaichana, N., Petersson, A., & Rohlin, M. (2006) The efficacy of magnetic resonance imaging in the diagnosis of degenerative and inflammatory temporomandibular joint disorders: a systematic literature review. *Oral Surgery, Oral Medicine, Oral Pathology, Oral Radiology, and Endodontics*, 102, 521–536.

Maples, A.D., Saini, T.S., Bourek, H., *et al.* (2008) Prevalence of nasal septal aberrations using cone beam computed tomography. *Journal of Dental Research*, 87 (Spec Issue A), 243.

Mardinger, O., Manor, I., Mijiritsky, E., *et al.* (2007) Maxillary sinus augmentation in the presence of antral pseudocyst: a clinical approach. *Oral Surgery, Oral Medicine, Oral Pathology, Oral Radiology, and Endodontics*, 103, 180–184.

Mehra, P. & Jeong, D. (2009) Maxillary sinusitis of odontogenic origin. *Current Allergy and Asthma Reports*, 9, 238–243.

Mehra, P. & Murad, H. (2004) Maxillary sinus disease of odontogenic origin. *Otolaryngologic Clinics of North America*, 37 (2), 347–364.

Miles, D.A. (2006) Clinical experience with cone-beam volumetic imaging: report of findings in 381 cases. *US Dentistry*, 2–7.

Miles, D.A. (2010) Occult pathology detected in cone beam data volumes. *Alpha Omegan*, 103, 146–150.

Norton, N.S. (2011) *Netter's Head and Neck Anatomy for Dentistry*. 2nd ed. Saunders-Elsevier, Philadelphia.

Philipsen, H.P., Takata, T., Reichart, P.A., *et al.* (2002) Lingual and buccal mandibular bone depressions: a review based on 583 cases from a world-wide literature survey, including 69 new cases from Japan. *Dentomaxillofacial Radiology*, 31, 281–290.

Price, J.B., Thaw, K.L., Tyndall, D.A., *et al.* (2012) Incidental findings from cone beam computed tomography of the maxillofacial region: a descriptive retrospective study. *Clinical Oral Implants Research*, 23 (11), 1261–1268.

Radfar, L., Amjadi, N., Aslani, N., *et al.* (2008) Prevalence and clinical significance of elongated calcified styloid processes in panoramic radiographs. *General Dentistry*, 56, e29–e32.

Ravon, N.A., Hollender, L.G., McDonald, V., *et al.* (2003) Signs of carotid calcification from dental panoramic radiographs are in agreement with Doppler sonography results. *Journal of Clinical Periodontology*, 30, 1084–1090.

Ribeiro-Rotta, R.F., Marques, K.D., Pacheco, M.J., *et al.* (2011) Do computed tomography and magnetic resonance imaging add to temporomandibular joint disorder treatment? A systematic review of diagnostic efficacy. *Journal of Oral Rehabilitation*, 38, 120–135.

Ritter, L., Lutz, J., Neugebauer, J., *et al.* (2012) Prevalence of pathologic findings in the maxillary sinus in cone-beam computerized tomography. *Oral Surgery, Oral Medicine, Oral Pathology, Oral Radiology, and Endodontics*, 111, 634–640.

Rogers, S.A., Drage, N., & Durning, P. (2011) Incidental findings arising with cone beam computed tomography imaging of the orthodontic patient. *Angle Orthodontist*, 81, 350–355.

Rosenfeld, R.M., Andes, D., Bhattacharrya, N., *et al.* (2007) Clinical practice guidelines: adult sinusitis. *Otolaryngology—Head and Neck Surgery*, 137, S1–S31.

Sano, T., Yamamoto, M., Okano, T., *et al.* (2004) Common abnormalities in temporomandibular joint imaging. *Current Problems in Diagnostic Radiology*, 33, 16–24.

Scanlon, C., III, Saini, T.S., Norton, N., *et al.* (2007) Systematic protocol for cone beam computed tomography interpretation. *Journal of Dental Research*, 86 (Spec Issue A), 466.

Scarfe, W.C. & Farman, A.G. (2010) Soft tissue calcifications in the neck: maxillofacial CBCT presentation and significant. *American Association of Dental Maxillofacial Radiographic Technicians Newsletter*, 2 (2), 3–15.

Selesnick, S.H. (1996) Diseases of the external auditory canal. In *Otolaryngologic Clinics of North America*, 29 (5), 725–886.

Smith, K.D., Edwards, P.C., Saini, T.S., *et al.* (2010a) The prevalence of concha bullosa and nasal septal deviation and their relationship to maxillary sinusitis by volumetric tomography. *International Journal of Dentistry*, 2010, pii 404982.

Smith, K.D., Lanphier, T.F., Edwards, P.C., *et al.* (2010b) Using cone beam computed tomography (CBCT) imaging to study the incidence of concha bullosa in the nasal cavity. *Clinical Anatomy*, 23, 490.

Stallman, J.S., Lobo, J.N., & Som, P.M. (2004) The incidence of concha bullosa and its relationship to nasal septal deviation and paranasal sinus disease. *American Journal of Neuroradiology*, 25, 1613–1618.

Subramanian, S., Rampal, G.R., Wong, E.F., *et al.* (2005) Concha bullosa in chronic sinusitis. *Medical Journal of Malaysia*, 60, 535–539.

Tran, L.P., Grundfast, K.M., & Selesnick, S.H. (1996) Benign lesions of the external auditory canal. *Otolaryngologic Clinics of North America*, 29 (5), 807–825.

Walsh, J.S. & Fairley, J.A. (1995) Calcifying disorders of the skin. *Journal of the American Academy of Dermatology*, 33, 693–706.

Wasserburger, M., Dendinger, E.J., Edwards, P.C., *et al.* (2007a) Assessing bone density changes in condyles using cone beam CT. *Journal of Dental Research*, 86 (Spec Issue A), 461.

Wasserburger, M., Edwards, P.C., Saini, T., *et al.* (2007b) A comparison of dental iCAT scans and routine histological slides in observing osteoarthritic changes in the mandibular condyles of cadavers. *Federation of American Societies for Experimental Biology Journal*, 21, 623–624.

Wenig, B.M. (1993) Non-neoplastic diseases of the ear and neoplasms of the ear. In Wenig, B.M., *Atlas of Head and Neck Pathology*. W.B. Saunders, Philadelphia, pp. 24–25.

Zinman, E.J., White, S.C., & Tetradis, S. (2010) Legal considerations in the use of cone beam computer tomography imaging. *Journal of the California Dental Association*, 38, 49–56.

Zinreich, S.J., Mattox, D.E., Kennedy, D.W., *et al.* (1988) Concha bullosa: CT evaluation. *Journal of Computer Assisted Tomography*, 12, 778–784.

11 3D Orthodontic Diagnosis and Treatment Planning

Juan Martin Palomo, DDS, MSD, Manish Valiathan, DDS, MSD, and Mark G. Hans, DDS, MSD

INTRODUCTION

In the 20th century, the cephalogram was a pioneering advance that led to many fundamental insights into the changes in the neurocranium and face during growth and with treatment. This imaging approach also became a standard part of orthodontic records for confirming diagnosis and treatment plans, as well as evaluating treatment outcomes (Broadbent, 1931). However, cephalograms provide only a compressed two-dimensional (2D) view of the complex three-dimensional (3D) craniofacial structures. The need for 3D information for orthodontic purposes has been evident for decades, and several attempts have been made to achieve this goal (Savara, 1965; Solow, 1970; Baumrind & Frantz, 1971; Hixon, 1972; Ricketts, 1972; Goldberg, 1973; Maganzini, 1974; Thurow, 1981; Bookstein, 1982; Vig, 1982; Baumrind *et al.*, 1983a, 1983b; Grayson *et al.*, 1988; Bookstein *et al.*, 1991; Altobelli *et al.*, 1993). More recently, the introduction of relatively low cost, high resolution, cone beam computed tomography (CBCT) has provided researchers and clinicians with the tool needed to acquire those images in 3D (Kau *et al.*, 2005; Palomo *et al.*, 2005; Kapila *et al.*, 2011). Given its attributes, CBCT imaging may become the 21st century's equivalent of what the cephalometer was for orthodontics in the 20th century.

CBCT provides more diagnostic information, unobstructed views of anatomy, relative density information, and an easy-to-understand complete radiographic view of the orthodontic patient. With regard to image quality, completeness, and versatility, CBCT has clear advantages over the cephalometer; however, its higher ionizing radiation results in a benefit/risk ratio that is not always weighted positively toward CBCT. In keeping with the "as low as reasonably achievable" (ALARA) principle, if ionizing radiation were reduced below that of current orthodontic radiographic series, it is possible that orthodontists would take CBCT

Cone Beam Computed Tomography in Orthodontics: Indications, Insights, and Innovations, First Edition. Sunil D. Kapila.

scans on most if not all of their patients, and the cephalometer would become obsolete.

The radiation received by the patient from a CBCT scanner for a large field of view (FOV), which often is preferred for orthodontic imaging, can be different depending on the scanner used (see Chapters 2 and 3). Although these are low doses relative to medical radiographic imaging, there are substantial differences in radiation doses between different CBCT scanners even when used for the same purpose (Pauwels *et al.*, 2012; see Chapters 2 and 3). The current ionizing radiation dose of CBCTs could be lowered further by technique standardization, the use of optimized and customized imaging protocols, and improvements of CBCT scanners as discussed elsewhere in this book (see Chapters 2 and 5). Thus, just as there are specific computed tomography (CT) protocols for different radiographic exams in medicine, rather than using a standardized CBCT protocol for every orthodontic patient, specific protocols that provide the desired images and may help lower the radiation can be developed for each patient or procedure. CBCT scanner optimization, which could be achieved by modifications to the hardware and/or software also could help to lower ionizing radiation doses. These modifications include utilization of pulsed mode radiation and the optimization of radiation arc, post-scan adjustments, scanning time, receptor sensitivity, numbers of rotations, collimators, and filters (see Chapters 2 and 5).

The utility of CBCT in orthodontic diagnosis is constrained partially due to the lack of universally acceptable protocols and availability of reproducible and quantifiable analyses. The purpose of this chapter is to provide insights into the protocols that we have developed at Case Western Reserve University (CWRU) for CBCT imaging of orthodontic patients and approaches for qualitative and quantitative analyses of these images to extract important diagnostic information. This chapter, therefore, provides one example, but not the only approach, of utilizing CBCT in the evaluation of craniofacial structures that could be useful in orthodontic diagnosis and treatment planning. Variations of these protocols and approaches and their customization to complex cases also are presented elsewhere in this book (see Chapters 1, 8, and 23).

CBCT'S ROLE IN ORTHODONTIC DIAGNOSIS AND TREATMENT PLANNING

The primary purpose of imaging is to answer questions that otherwise cannot be addressed clinically or to confirm or rule out what was found during a clinical exam. Thus CBCT, like other radiographic examinations, offers another important tool in our armamentarium that, depending on the information required, may or may not be useful. In order to decide which tool to use, it is essential to understand what this approach has to offer and to know how to use it. CBCT technology offers a range of options. Current scanners offer a multitude of image sizes and several options for mA, kVp and even voxel size (see Chapter 2). We have evolved from the time that a radiograph was just a radiograph; now the image can be customized to fit our needs. More important, with all these tools at our disposal, the clinician needs to know which imaging protocol would enhance the understanding of the patient's clinical findings best. Despite these advantages of CBCT, the initial clinical exam remains the most important step in orthodontic diagnosis. Such direct evaluation allows the clinician to use three senses: listening to the patient's description of his or her condition and main goals for treatment outcome, assessing the face and dentition along with facial animation, and analyzing function including the movements of the temporomandibular joints (TMJs) and the intra- and extraoral musculature. This evaluation, together with a complete review of the medical and dental history and assessment of treatment needs and wants, will determine which additional diagnostic information may be required, including which if any imaging modality is necessary to confirm the findings, help in treatment planning, and rule out any current or potential problems during treatment. Thus, even though radiographs, whether 2D or 3D, may be used to refine diagnosis and help corroborate treatment plans, no imaging modality is a substitute for the clinical examination of the patient.

A skilled clinician will use diagnostic tests such as cephalometric analysis to confirm the diagnoses. It is common to use quantitative methods to supplement subjective evaluation because this leads to more consistent diagnoses and, subsequently, to more consistent treatments. For example, the lateral cephalometric technique enables the clinician to characterize skeletal and dentoalveolar morphology of patients in the midline. This information improves our understanding of the underlying basis of malocclusions with reference to midline structures in both the sagittal and vertical planes. All of the standard lateral cephalometric analyses answer five basic questions about the patient's midline skeletal and dentoalveolar relationships, namely:

(1) What is the position of the maxilla with respect to the cranial base?
(2) What is the position of the mandible with respect to the cranial base?
(3) What is the position of the maxillary teeth with respect to the maxilla?
(4) What is the position of the mandibular teeth with respect to the mandible?
(5) What are the vertical proportions of the facial thirds?

Norms have been developed for each of these five anatomic relationships that, with some exceptions, aid the clinician to characterize the malocclusion and to arrive at the most appropriate strategies for correction of the discrepancies. Although normative information for CBCT analysis may be useful, the need for CBCT norms may not be as critical as that for the cephalogram because a CBCT image is more akin to the patient than the cephalogram: unlike in the case of a cephalogram, the anatomy viewed in a CBCT is unobstructed, accurate, and distortion-free while also being able to provide all the information available from cephalometry. For example, the precise position of impacted teeth, their contact with other teeth and position, and alignment of roots do not require the determination of distances or angles in order to be helpful (see Chapters 15 and 16). The 3D and/or multiplanar visualization in such clinical situations may be adequate for the experienced clinician to derive an optimal treatment plan. The availability of information from these additional views represents some of the many situations in which CBCT can contribute to modification to an orthodontic treatment plan by providing information not accessible by any other available means. While these clinical scenarios may not require CBCT norms for extracting important diagnostic information, several other situations exist in which CBCT norms may be useful for treatment decision.

Enlow & Hans (2008) noted that lateral cephalograms often reveal dental compensations that mask underlying skeletal discrepancies. In fact, anatomic compensations, which include dental compensations, are the primary reason why more than 95% of all first molars fit within 6mm (the distance between Angle Class II and Class III molar relationships) in human populations, even though there clearly is more than 6mm of anatomic variation in mandibular size among humans. As revealed by cephalometrics and widely accepted in the field, dental compensations such as mandibular dental protrusion often accompany mandibular skeletal retrognathia. Not surprisingly, similar dental compensations exist in the transverse dimension. This chapter uses newly derived CBCT norms to illustrate how these compensations can be identified and then used to help plan treatment in the transverse dimension. Interestingly, while mandibular length has not been easy to modify clinically, transverse maxillary skeletal and dental width, as well as mandibular dental width, can be altered by the orthodontist. This makes the identification of transverse compensation especially relevant to the modern clinician.

THE CWRU COMPREHENSIVE CBCT ANALYSIS

At CWRU, we currently have two different CBCT scanners that, in addition to having true 2D cephalometric and panoramic radiographic capabilities, provide up to 10 possible FOVs. Our CBCT scanners have been optimized with decreased radiological settings in combination with image quality optimization, which substantially reduces the amount of ionizing radiation exposure (Kwong *et al.*, 2008; Palomo *et al.*, 2008). However, the approaches to analyzing a CBCT and making the best possible use of the information it provides has not been standardized yet. For educational purposes and to facilitate the transition from 2D to 3D imaging, we have partially standardized approaches to managing and using 3D CBCT volumes.

In the past, the orthodontic electronic records for our patients included the standard three extraoral photos, five intraoral photos, a panoramic radiograph, and a cephalogram. With the inclusion of the CBCT volume, there are additional images to include in the records and review on the computer. The volume can be viewed in both 3D and multiplanar modes. The multiplanar reconstructs (MPRs) incorporate axial, coronal, and sagittal views with slices that can be as thin as the voxel size. The 3D view can be visualized from every direction by rotating it; however, this rendering is not truly a 3D image since it is displayed on a computer screen instead of as a holographic representation. The 3D displays also can appear different when using different software packages. Software image filters can be applied to create a smoother image, and several operator-controlled features allow the display of different density ranges that, depending on the settings, can show the same areas either covered or uncovered by bone. Due to display inaccuracies and inconsistencies in image filters, the most reliable and consistent method for analyzing a CBCT image uses the multiplanar mode.

Image management protocol and obtaining standardized views

The CWRU imaging protocol starts with importing the CBCT volume into the patient's electronic chart. This is important because it allows quick access of the complete 3D volume during appointments. Even though the complete 3D volume is imported into the patient's file, there still is value in creating standardized views that represent different areas of the craniofacial complex and can be used to track progress or outcome assessment.

In order to create different views in a standardized way, the first step is the CBCT volume orientation within the software. Unlike cephalograms, a CBCT volume does not have rigid orientation hardware such as ear rods and nasion rests available during imaging. Also unlike cephalograms, a 3D image needs to be oriented in all three planes of space. Precise orientation of the volume is necessary in order to assess asymmetries and deviations accurately from normality while going through the MPR images.

Landmarks and plane

Although other volume orientation methods are available (see Chapter 8 for an example), the CWRU orientation method uses five biologically relevant anatomical structures and one plane (Wu *et al.*, 2012). The structures, used together with a brief rationale on their selection, are as follows and are depicted in Figure 11.1.

(1) **The optic foramina** are bilateral structures located in the sphenoid bone. The optic nerve along with the ophthalmic artery passes through these structures. The center of this and the other two foramina (listed below) are found by visual inspection as they enter the sphenoid bone and the x, y, and z coordinates of these points are recorded.
(2) **The foramina ovale** also are bilateral structures located in the posterior and lateral portion of the sphenoid bone.
(3) **The foramen cecum** is a midline structure located where the frontal bone articulates with the ethmoid bone.
(4) **The McRae's plane** is located in sagittal view and is defined as a line drawn from the anterior margin of the foramen magnum (basion) to the posterior border (opisthion). The McRae's plane commonly is used in neurosurgery as a stable reference for orienting the head in the sagittal plane. It also illustrates the degree of deformity and aids in surgical decision making with regard to fixation and stabilization (Goel, 2004). Aligning the McRae's plane prevents superior and inferior tilting of the head at the time of surgery.

Method for orienting the head in three planes of space

The coronal view is used to align the centers of the left and right optic foramina to correct any left or right tilt of the volume (Figure 11.1A). The axial view is used to align the centers of the left and right foramina ovale to correct any rotation of the volume (Figure 11.1B). The sagittal view is used to correct for superior and inferior tilting of head by aligning the axial plane to overlap with the McRae's plane (Figure 11.1C).

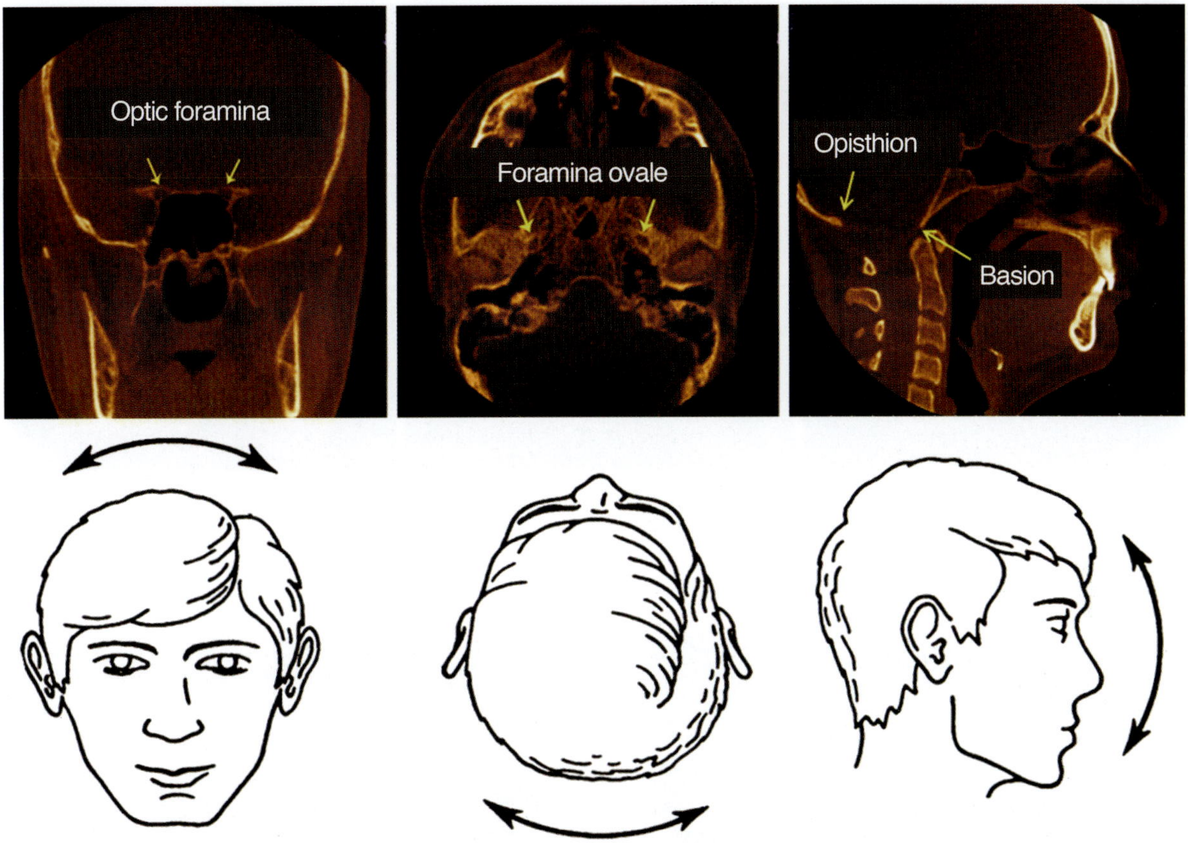

Figure 11.1 CBCT volume orientation using all three planes of space. (Based on Wu *et al.* (2012); drawings courtesy of Robert W. Patricy.)

Capturing the views

The next step is to create different cuts or views of the volume necessary to synthesize our findings. Instead of two images (cephalogram and panorex), we now create 30 different views from a CBCT as listed below.

Right, frontal, and left solid views

These three views mimic the extraoral photographs, but show skeletal tissue instead (Figure 11.2). The display settings used do not permit transparency and, therefore, aid in the visualization of root coverage and bone anatomy. The soft tissue outline is not viewed often in these images.

Right, frontal, and left side transparency views

These three views are similar to the ones depicted in Figure 11.3, but show transparency of skeletal tissue and the soft tissue outline (Figure 11.3). The lateral images are taken in a half-skull mode to eliminate superimposition of bilateral structures. Thus, when creating the right side view, the left side is cropped off so as not to interfere with the final image, and vice versa.

Cephalogram and Bolton analysis

During the 2D to 3D transition, it still is important to utilize the knowledge base provided by cephalometry. Therefore, we generate a good quality cephalogram from the CBCT volume and use the

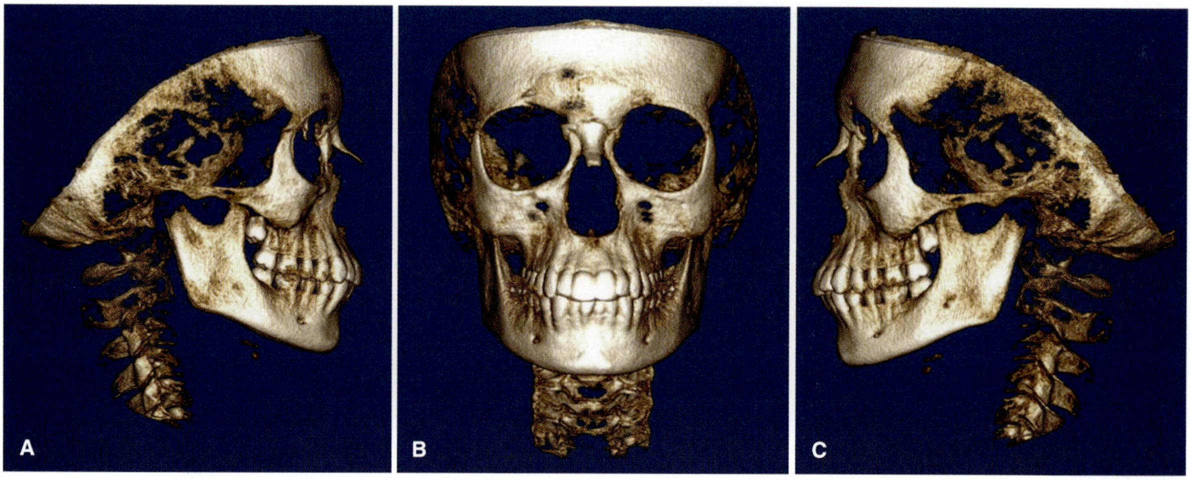

Figure 11.2 *A*: Right side solid view. *B*: Frontal solid view. *C*: Left side solid view.

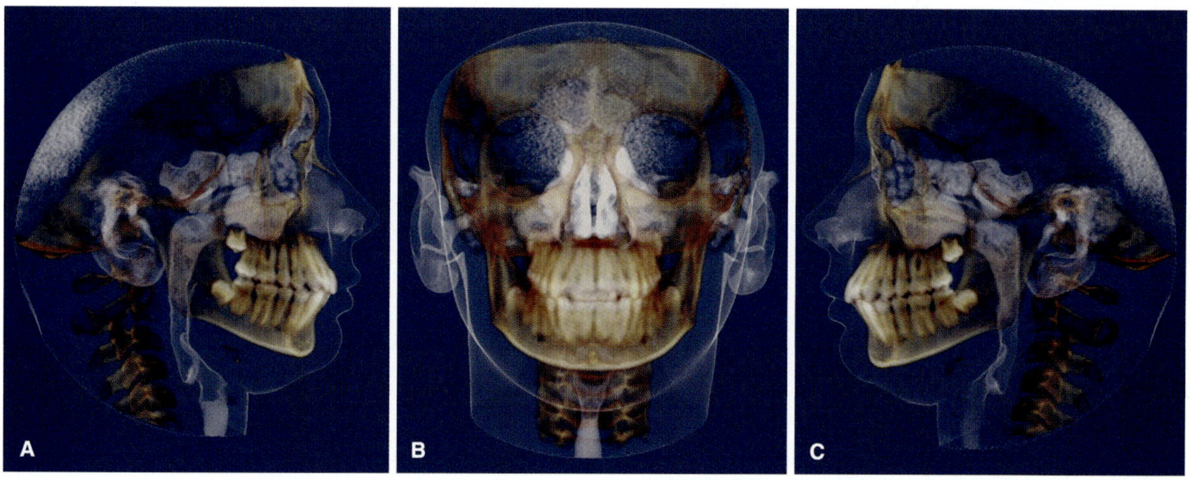

Figure 11.3 *A*: Right side transparency view. *B*: Frontal transparency view. *C*: Left side transparency view.

traditional cephalometric analyses (Figure 11.4A). We also superimpose specific age templates of the Bolton Standards on the cephalogram to assess sagittal dental and skeletal positions, as well as vertical dimension. This approach complements the goals of other cephalometric analyses and provides a cross-referencing check between cephalometrics and the Bolton Standards (Figure 11.4B).

Panoramic radiograph

As with the cephalogram, the panoramic radiograph, even though inherently distorted, continues to be utilized during the transition from 2D to 3D imaging because it provides a general view of the dentition. A panoramic radiograph can be created from a CBCT scan by identifying the arch curve to

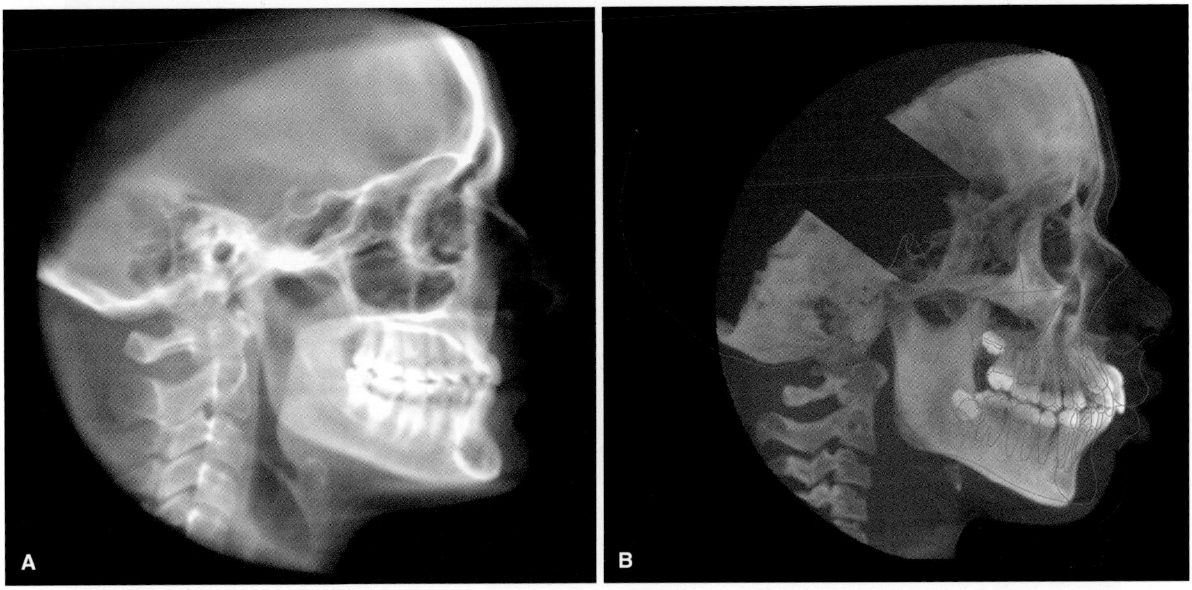

Figure 11.4 *A*: A CBCT-generated cephalogram. *B*: Reconstructed cephalogram superimposed with age- and sex-specific Bolton standard tracing.

be reconstructed as a tomographic view. If the curve is not identified properly and needed compensations are not incorporated into it, the resultant panoramic image can misrepresent some areas due to distortions, shortening, or elongation of the anatomy. Since the reconstructed panoramic image leaves room for operator error, it is important to confirm the panoramic radiographic findings on root parallelism, position, and presentation of other anatomic structures with 3D views of the volume (Figure 11.5).

Temporomandibular joint tomogram

Visualization of the TMJs is done more efficiently through reconstructed tomograms, which can be created easily out of a CBCT volume. Checks for symmetry, shape, size, and condylar position provide insights into normal or abnormal anatomy and relationships of the condyle to the fossa (Figure 11.6).

Airway volume and area of maximum constriction

The airway can be segmented automatically, but to standardize the method and allow comparisons at different time points, anatomical limits should be used. The superior and inferior limits used at CWRU were modified slightly from the limits used by Ogawa and colleagues (2007). The airway volume is defined as the volume of pharynx that is between the palatal plane (anterior nasal spine–posterior nasal spine [ANS-PNS]) and extends to the posterior wall of the pharynx and a plane constructed from the most antero-inferior point of the second cervical vertebrae parallel to the palatal plane (Figure 11.7 and Figure 11.8; El & Palomo, 2010, 2011, 2013; El *et al.*, 2011).

Since the airway volume shows much variation between individuals and with growth, it is important also to collect the area of maximum constriction. This measure represents the area where air probably will find the greatest resistance of passage.

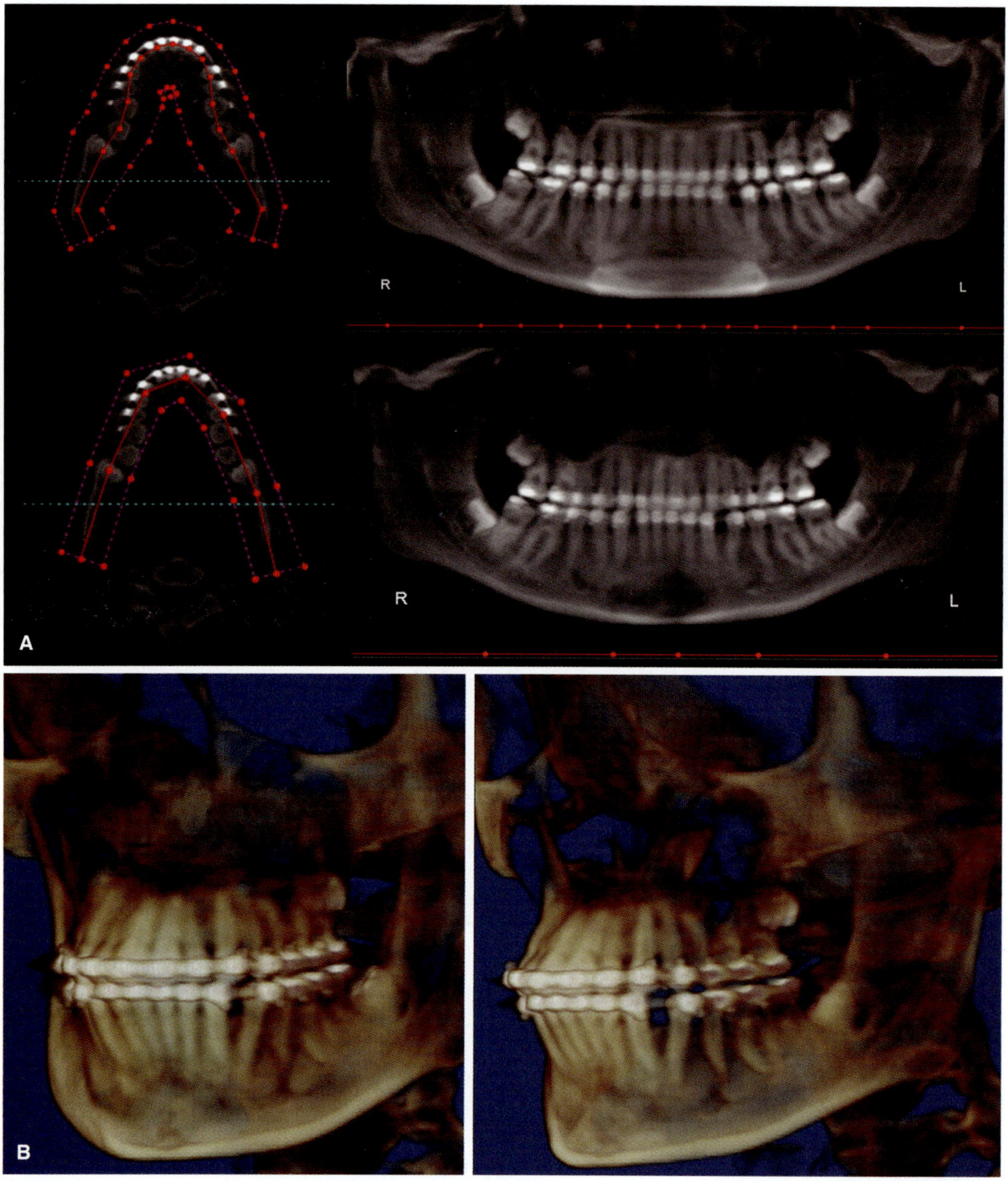

Figure 11.5 *A*: Panoramic radiograph generated from a CBCT volume is under greater operator control than traditional panoramic radiographs. The resulting image is dependent on the points and lines chosen for the tomographic reconstruction by the operator. A thick tomographic section with lines following contours of the arch results in a panoramic radiograph (upper panel) that shows substantial differences from one constructed by a thinner tomographic section and an arch contour that is created with fewer points and angles (lower panel). *B*: Confirmation of findings from the constructed panoramic radiograph with 3D reconstructions is recommended.

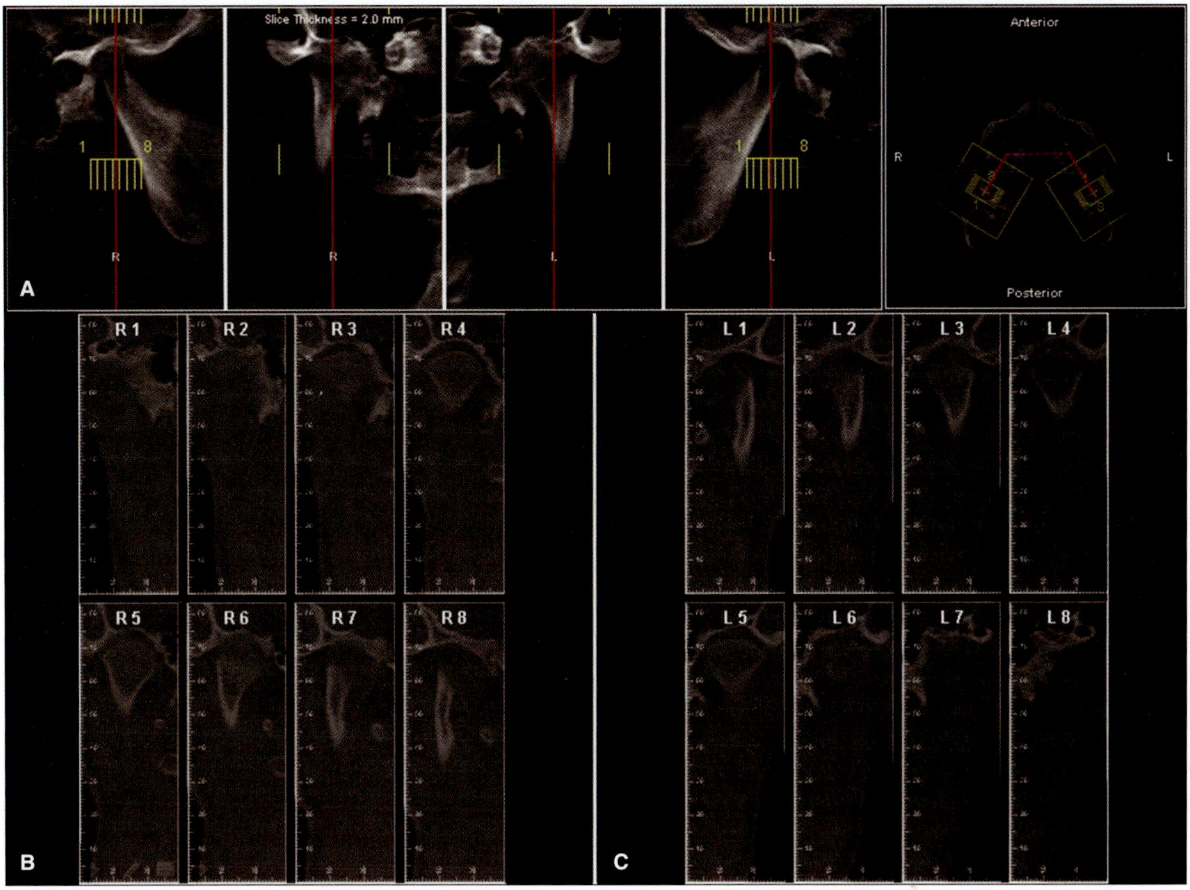

Figure 11.6 TMJ study can be generated out of a CBCT volume. *A*: Sites of tomographic cuts. *B* and *C*: Coronal tomograms of right and left TMJs, respectively.

The maximum constricted area as well as its position within the segmented volume also is determined automatically. One lateral and one frontal view of the segmented airway, together with the volume and maximum constricted area values, are stored in the patient's electronic chart.

Maxillary and mandibular intercanine and intermolar widths

In order to assess skeletal widths, both maxillary and mandibular intercanine and inter-first molar distances at the cemento-enamel junction level are measured and captured on the image (Figure 11.9).

Maxillary and mandibular root apices position

Maxillary and mandibular anterior crowding are some of the most common reasons for orthodontic treatment and for relapse. A single axial slice of the region close to the root apices can be useful to the orthodontist for determining torque needs and to check if an apparent clinical alignment also has translated to the apical area. These views can be compared during treatment by using a standardized method of orientation. Even though a view such as this has not been available to orthodontists prior to the introduction of CBCT, its applications to treatment are relatively self-evident (Figure 11.10).

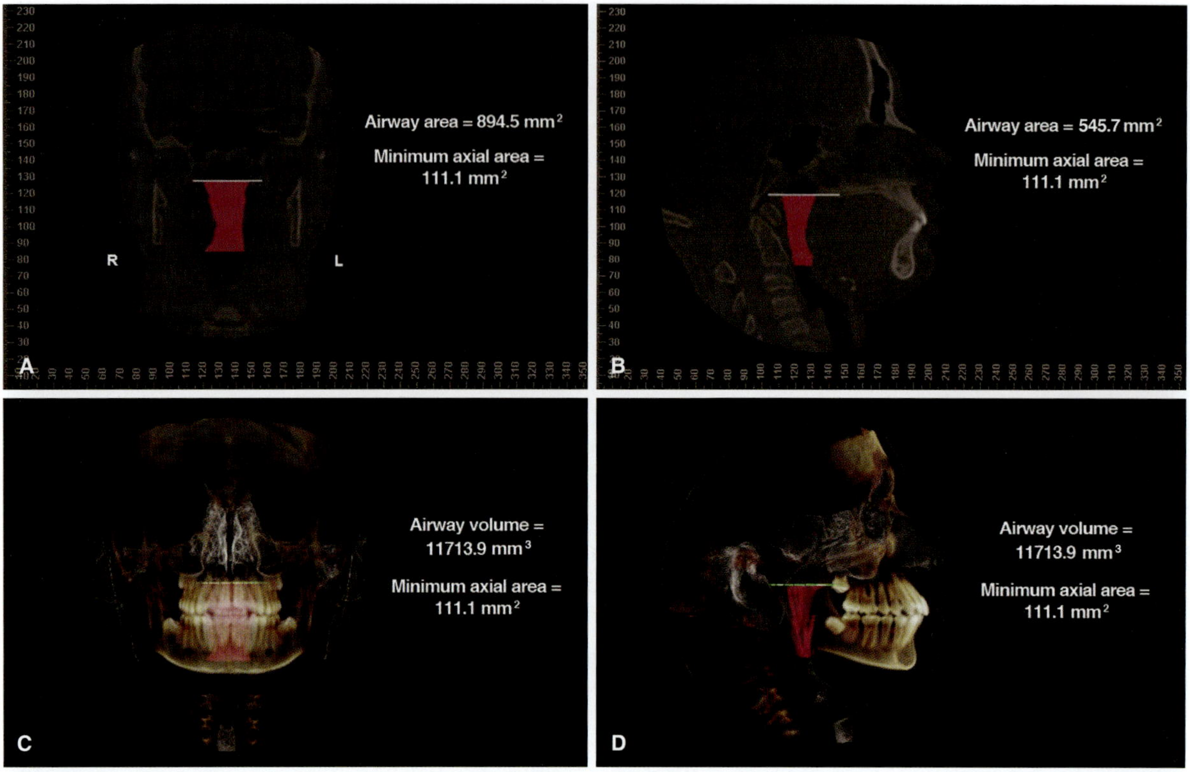

Figure 11.7 Total airway area and area of maximum constriction in frontal (*A*) and lateral (*B*) sections. Total airway volume and area of maximum constriction in frontal (*C*) and lateral (*D*) 3D volumetric renderings.

The CWRU transverse analysis

A transverse analysis has been developed similar to other cephalometric techniques consisting of twelve bilateral angular measurements. These measurements, derived from coronal slices, help to diagnose the transverse dimension and aid in treatment decisions (e.g., the use of skeletal or dental expansion). These measurements are depicted in Figure 11.11 and can be described as follows:

(1) Maxillary and mandibular right and left canine buccolingual inclination (degrees).
(2) Maxillary and mandibular right and left first molar buccolingual inclination (degrees).
(3) Right and left intercanine angulation (degrees).
(4) Right and left intermolar angulation (degrees).

THE CWRU TRANSVERSE ANALYSIS

The diagnosis of maxillary transverse deficiency has been inconsistent within the orthodontic community. Some clinicians make this diagnosis on the basis of the presence of a unilateral or bilateral posterior dental crossbite. Others make the diagnosis based on the shape of the maxillary dental arch. Still others prefer to use the height and width of the palatal vault. In addition, the concept of a relative maxillary transverse deficiency in Class II patients has been proposed. In this instance, the dental casts of a Class II patient are occluded in the Class I molar position, thus "revealing" a maxillary transverse deficiency. This last diagnostic maneuver is flawed, especially since the tapering nature of all dental arches necessarily results in a "relative" maxillary transverse deficiency in all Class II cases, except those with a Brodie bite. This lack of

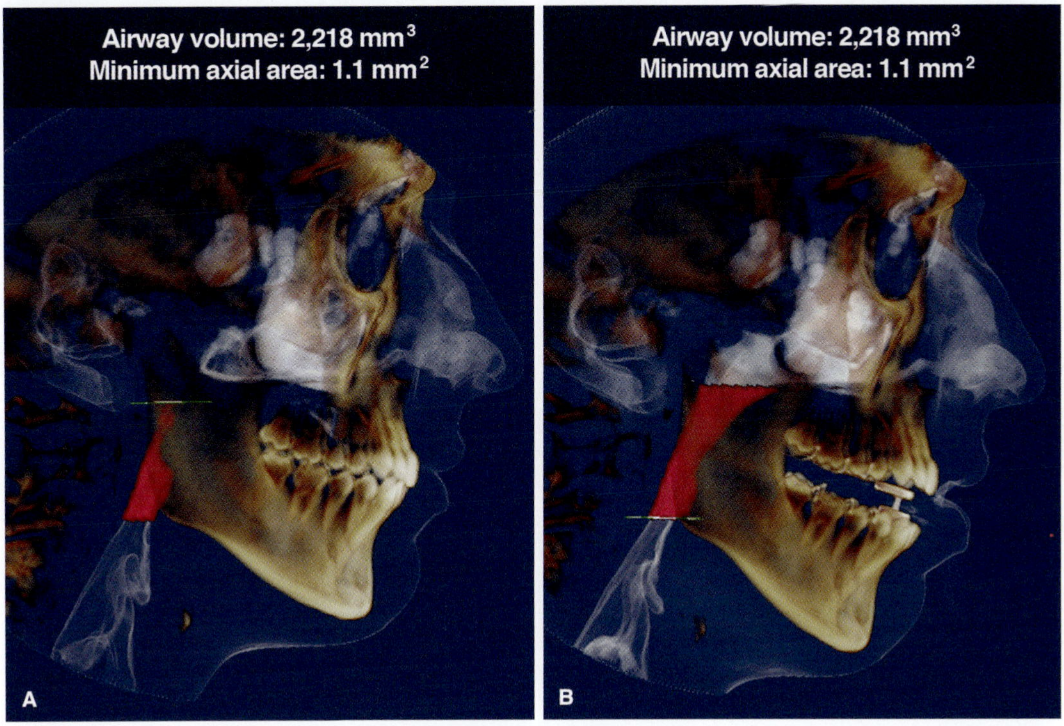

Figure 11.8 Change in airway volume and area of maximum constriction shown above the images of a patient with obstructive sleep apnea without (*A*) and with (*B*) an intraoral appliance that advances and opens the bite.

criteria for the diagnosis of what is expected to be a relatively common condition has led to a variety of treatment plans based on empiric rather than biologic evidence.

The buccolingual inclination of teeth can change significantly during treatment. By using lateral cephalometrics, the orthodontist monitors changes that occur sagittally and vertically in both maxillary and mandibular incisors. Such changes can occur with the use of large rectangular archwires or with increase in arch perimeter needed to resolve crowding. But orthodontic treatment changes are not limited to the incisors. When looking retrospectively at orthodontically treated cases, it is evident that significant changes occur in canines and first molars during treatment (Table 11.1 and Table 11.2; Evangelinakis *et al.*, 2010; Karamitsou *et al.*, 2011; Shewinvanakitkul *et al.*, 2011; Miyamoto *et al.*, 2012). These changes may happen unnoticed and may play a role in the stability of the resulting occlusion.

In addition to helping to provide guidelines to manage changes in the buccolingual inclination of teeth, a set of norms also can aid in decisions regarding transverse dimensions, providing valuable diagnostic information needed for treatment decisions such as whether to undertake dental versus skeletal expansion (rapid maxillary expansion [RME]). With this goal in mind, we developed norms for "The CWRU Transverse Analysis" by averaging the buccolingual inclinations of canines and first molars in individuals showing ideal posterior occlusion and intermaxillary relationships (Figure 11.12). The CWRU method allows treatment plans to be developed to address specific elements of the patient's malocclusion. It is hoped

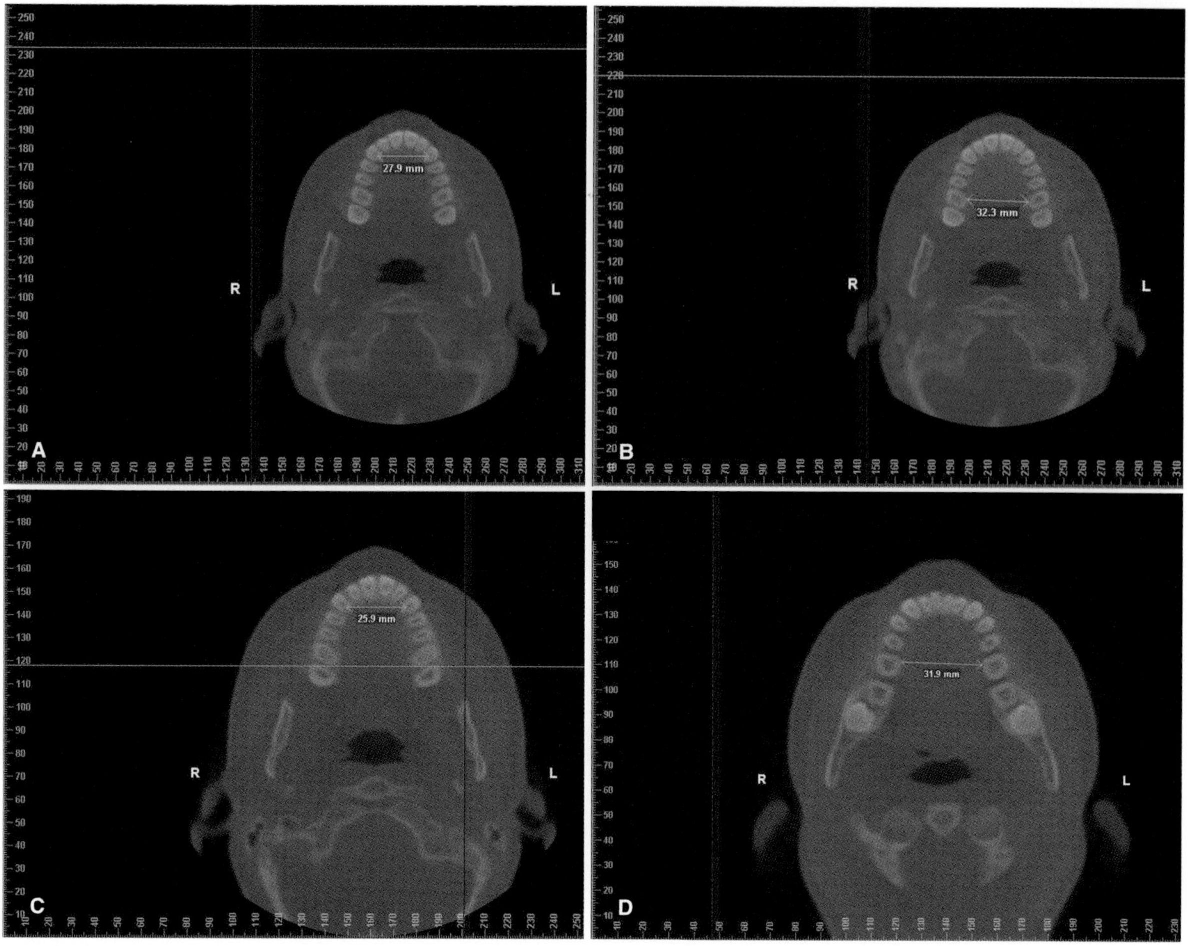

Figure 11.9 Axial slices at the tooth cemento-enamel junction used to measure and document maxillary and mandibular intercanine and intermolar widths. *A*: Maxillary intercanine width. *B*: Maxillary intermolar width. *C*: Mandibular intercanine width. *D*: Mandibular intermolar width.

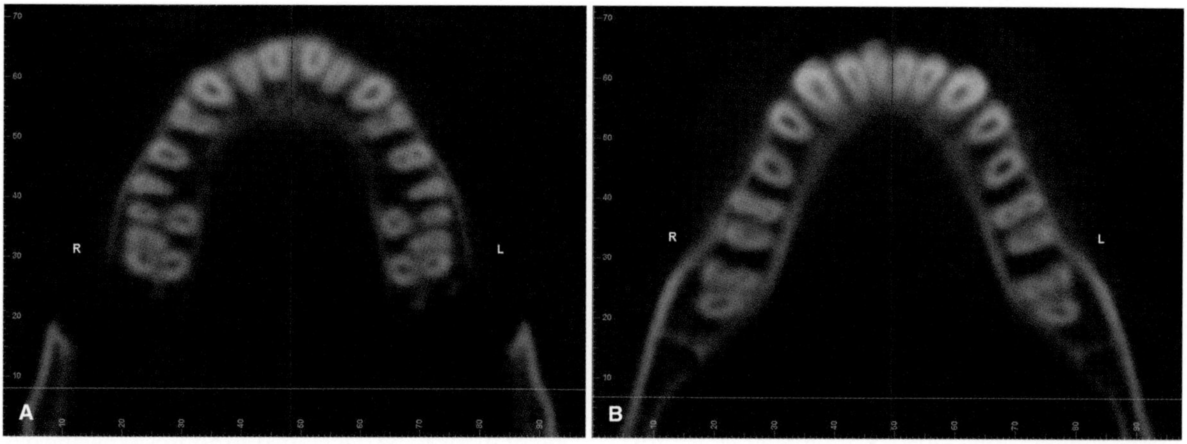

Figure 11.10 Axial plane images to visualize regions near the root apices of maxillary (*A*) and mandibular (*B*) teeth.

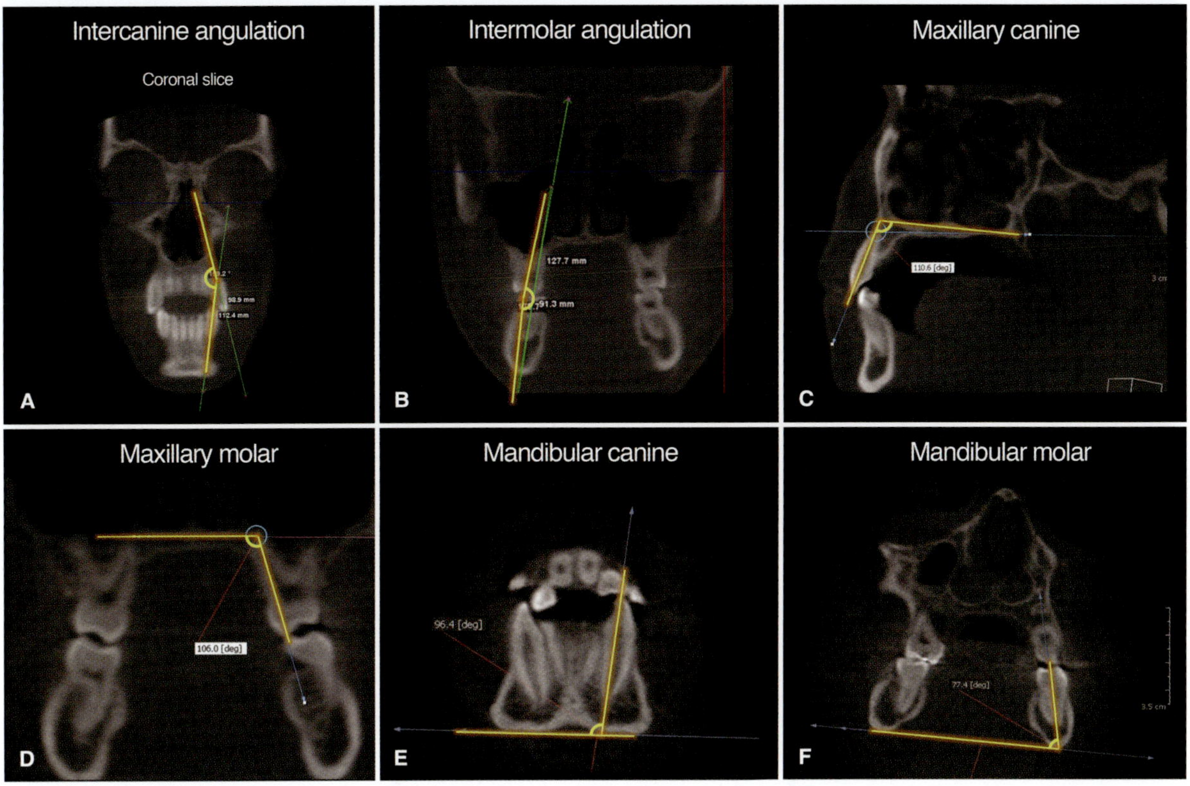

Figure 11.11 Coronal sections depicting buccolingual inclinations of canines and molars to their respective counterparts (*A* and *B*) and to maxillary (*C* and *D*) and mandibular (*E* and *F*) reference planes using the CWRU transverse analysis. The maxillary measurements are made from the tooth's long axis to the line traced on the lower border of the nasal cavity; the mandibular measurements are made for the long axis to a line representing the mandibular plane.

Table 11.1 Means (±SD) and ranges of initial, final, and change in buccolingual inclination and distances of maxillary canines and molar in orthodontically treated cases.

Variable (N = 70)	Initial		Final		Change	
	Mean ± SD	Range	Mean ± SD	Range	Mean ± SD	Range
Right canine (°)	106.1 ± 4.8	97.0 to 119.3	104.7 ± 5.7	88.6 to 115.8	−1.4 ± 4.8	−17.2 to 8.7
Left canine (°)	105.9 ± 5.6	90.8 to 119.6	105.0 ± 5.7	88.8 to 121.1	−0.9 ± 4.4	−12.4 to 8.3
Intercanine (mm)	33.9 ± 2.7	27.5 to 39.8	34.9 ± 2.1	30.3 to 39.1	1.0 ± 1.8*	−3.7 to 5.1
Right molar (°)	101.9 ± 4.9	85.7 to 112.5	103.2 ± 4.4	95.6 to 115.6	1.3 ± 4.2	−6.0 to 14.4
Left molar (°)	102.1 ± 4.9	89.7 to 112.7	102.5 ± 5.1	84.4 to 112.5	0.4 ± 3.9	−9.6 to 7.7
Intermolar (mm)	45.3 ± 2.6	38.1 to 50.6	46.5 ± 2.6	39.9 to 52.9	1.2 ± 1.4*	−3.1 to 4.3

* $p < 0.05$.

Table 11.2 Means (±SD) and ranges of initial, final, and change in buccolingual inclination and distances of mandibular canines and molar in orthodontically treated cases.

Variable (N = 70)	Initial		Final		Change	
	Mean ± SD	Range	Mean ± SD	Range	Mean ± SD	Range
Right canine (°)	96.8 ± 3.9	88.6 to 108.6	93.9 ± 4.1	85.3 to 103.8	−2.9 ± 3.9	−13.4 to 5.5
Left canine (°)	97.8 ± 4.6	88.5 to 111.1	94.7 ± 4.8	81.7 to 106.5	−3.1 ± 4.6	−13.4 to 5.5
Intercanine (mm)	25.8 ± 2.2	21.0 to 31.6	27.0 ± 1.8	22.6 to 31.5	1.2 ± 1.7	−4.2 to 6.9
Right molar (°)	76.4 ± 4.5	67.4 to 86.0	77.4 ± 5.0	65.6 to 90.6	1.1 ± 4.0	−7.9 to 11.0
Left molar (°)	74.7 ± 5.1	61.9 to 86.7	77.0 ± 4.9	66.4 to 91.9	2.2 ± 5.0	−13.4 to 13.2
Intermolar (mm)	41.23 ± 2.6	33.5 to 46.2	41.5 ± 2.4	35.5 to 48.0	0.3 ± 1.6	−4.0 to 3.8

Note: The data presented here are from a sample different from the one in Table 11.1, even though the sample size is the same.

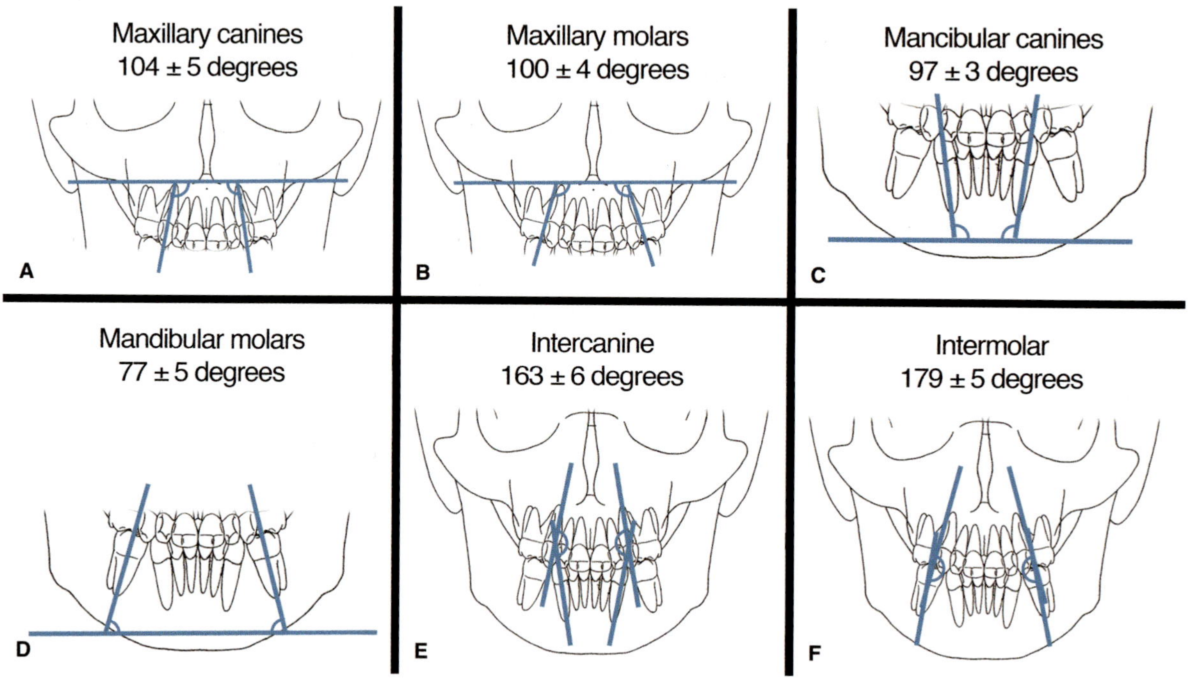

Figure 11.12 *A–F*: Norms for maxillary and mandibular canine and molar inclinations used in the CWRU transverse analysis.

that the use of objective data to develop treatment plans will eliminate some of the guesswork and variability in treatment decisions for these common conditions.

Rationale

For the CWRU method, angular norms rather than linear norms were chosen. This decision is based on two factors. First, the lateral limits of the dental arches are not known; therefore, a linear measure showing either excess or deficient length would be impossible to determine. Second, the idea of a single measurement of maxillary or mandibular width that could be applied to all individuals is an unlikely scenario due to biologic variability in size and shape of the human face. We assume that because teeth are anchored in the alveolar bone, they must necessarily be good markers of the lateral limits of the skeletal base. This is true especially in the mandible where there is no possibility for skeletal expansion of arch width. For these reasons, the CWRU analysis uses six angular measures to answer the following clinical questions, responses for which include "normal," "excessive," or "deficient": (1) What is the transverse dimension of the maxilla? and (2) What are the buccolingual inclinations of the maxillary and mandibular first molars and canines?

DEVELOPING NORMS FOR THE CWRU TRANSVERSE ANALYSIS

Population norms versus selected normals

Two approaches can be used to establish normative data for use in diagnosis and treatment planning. The first is to use population norms. This technique relies on the mathematical property called regression to the mean. As the number of subjects increases in the sample, the value for any given measurement in that sample tends toward the mean value of the sample. Of course, this mean value is influenced by both normal and abnormal individual values. The second approach is to derive norms from a select sample that satisfies specific criteria. Using a well-known example from cephalometrics, the population norm for the angulation of the lower incisor to the mandibular plane (IMPA) is 95°, while the Tweed norm based on a selected sample is 90°. In both these instances, not only is the mean value of importance, but so is the standard deviation or sample variability, particularly when used for treatment planning. In general, we are interested most in identifying individuals who differ from the mean value by greater than one standard deviation because it is likely that this level of variation from the norm is of clinical importance. For most of the transverse measurements in our analysis, the standard deviation is on the order of 5° (Streit *et al.*, 2012).

How to do the analysis?

The measurement of the buccolingual inclination of transverse dental angulations is relatively simple and can be performed using any software package that permits the CBCT volume to be opened and has a tool for measuring angles. Prior to measuring the buccolingual tooth inclinations, the CBCT volume should be oriented properly. In the case of maxillary measurements, the volume should be oriented on the palatal plane in the sagittal view and on the bizygomatic arches in the coronal view. To have the greatest possible accuracy and reliability, the angular measurements should be performed using the slice view.

The CWRU analysis evaluates the long axis buccolingual inclinations of all canines and first molars in slice views. The long axis of these teeth is measured relative to a line representing the mandibular plane for mandibular measurements and a line traced on the lower border of the nasal cavity for maxillary measurements (Figure 11.11 and Figure 11.12). The long axis for the maxillary molar is constructed from the mesiopalatal cusp tip to the palatal root apex, while that for mandibular molar is constructed from the root apex of the mesial root to the central groove on the crown. The long axis of the canine is constructed by joining the root apex to the tip of the cusp. These measurements can be performed with any commercially available DICOM viewer.

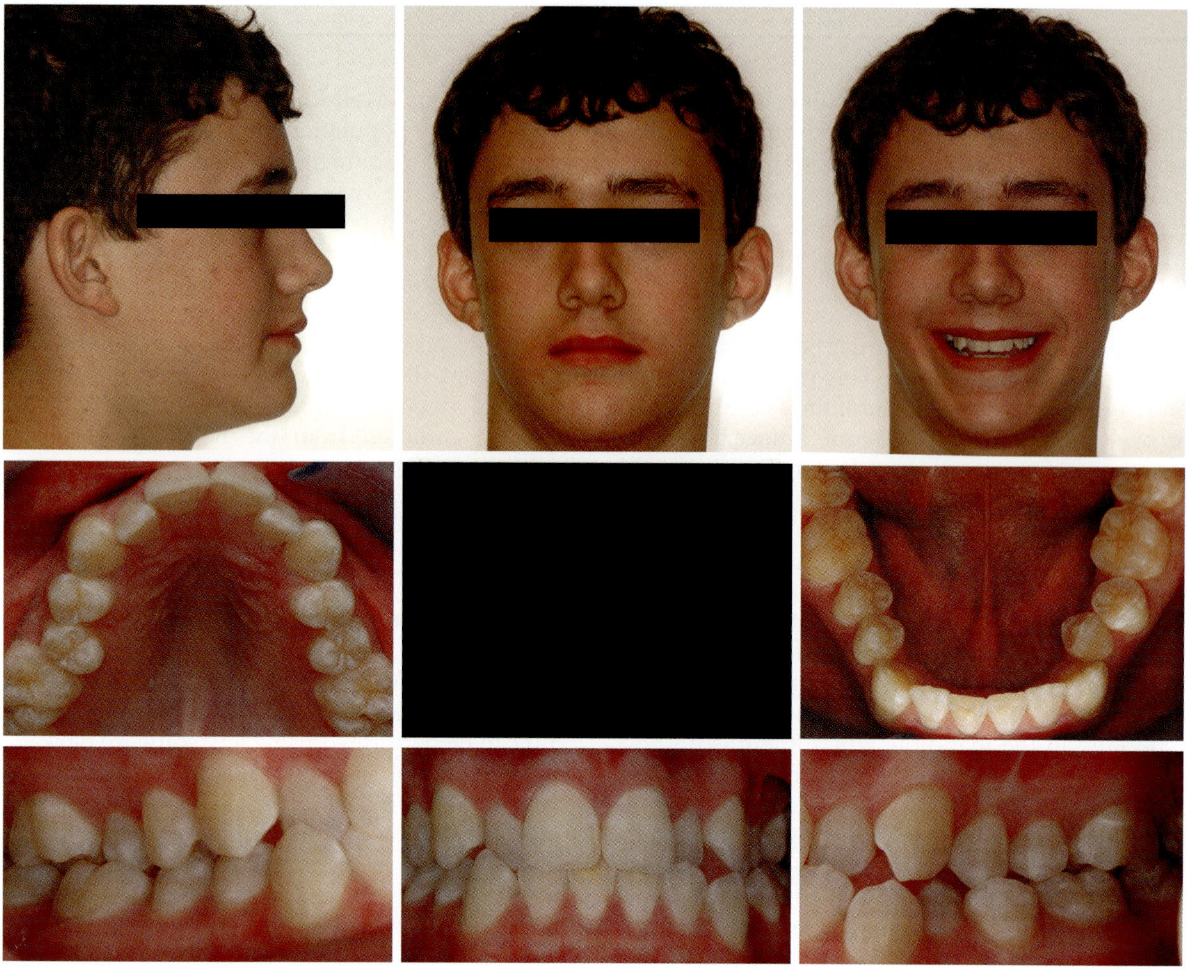

Figure 11.13 Pre-treatment photographs of Case I showing 13-year-old male with bilateral posterior crossbite not involving the molars. A dental expansion treatment approach was utilized in this case.

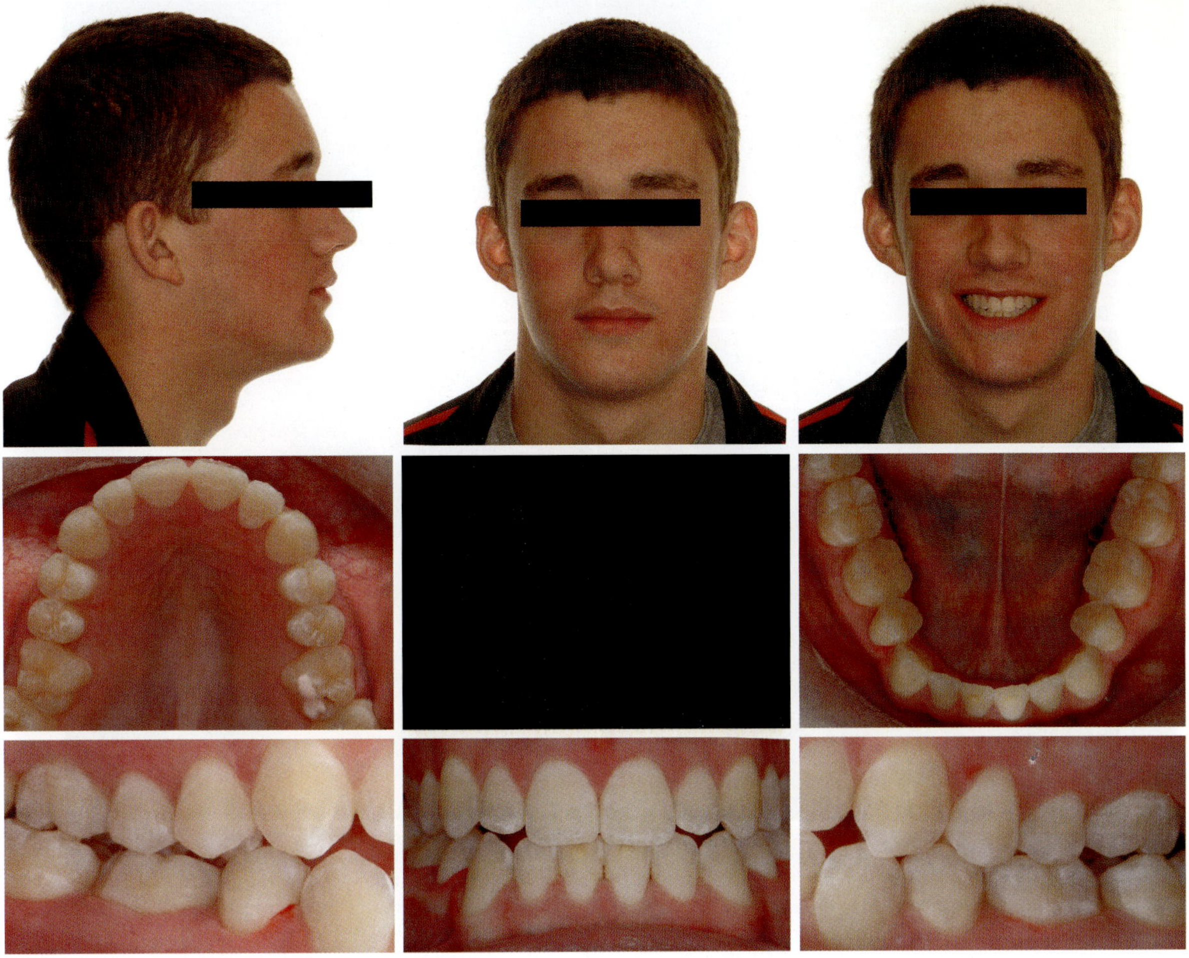

Figure 11.14 Case I. Post-treatment records showing inadequate correction of the posterior crossbite.

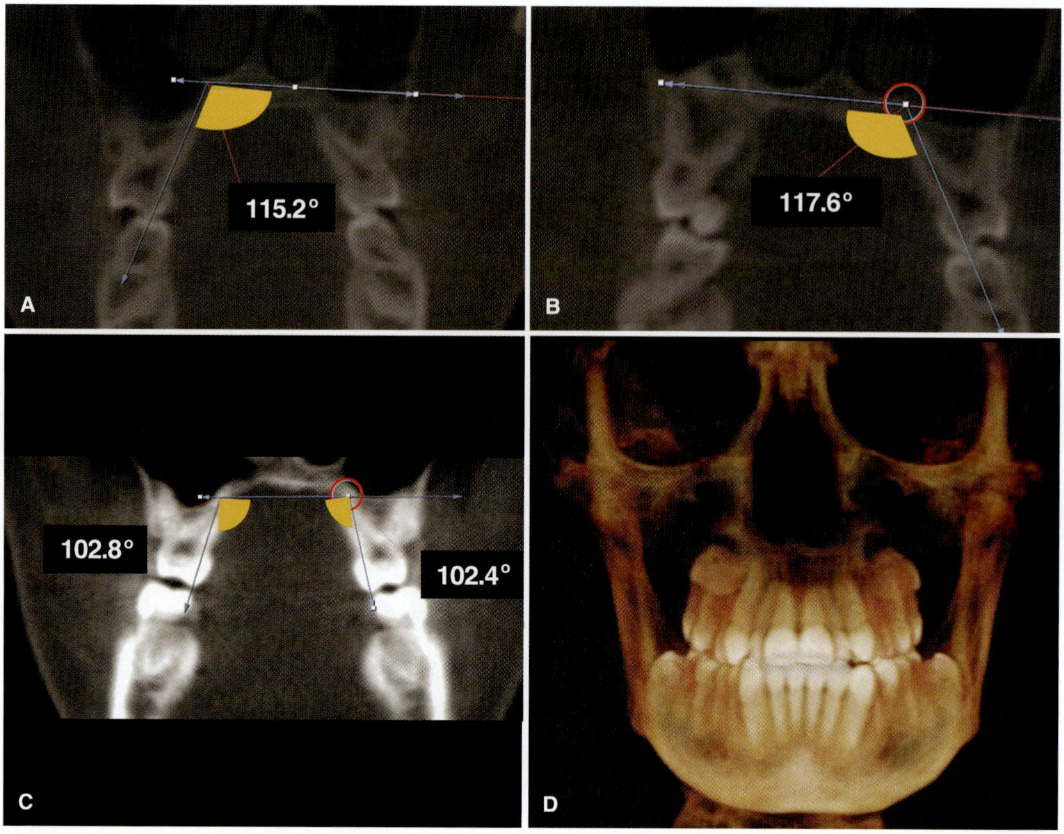

Figure 11.15 Case I. Pre-treatment transverse analysis reveals right (*A*) and left (*B*) molars at 115° and 117° inclination, respectively. This is greater than the molar angulation norm of 100° and suggests that the increased molar buccal inclination likely is due to a compensation for transverse skeletal deficiency. *C*: The final result shows that the maxillary molar angulations were changed to approximate the buccolingual norm, making the intermolar and skeletal transverse discrepancy more evident. *D*: Volumetric rendering of pre-treatment CBCT depicting buccolingual inclinations of the posterior teeth in 3D.

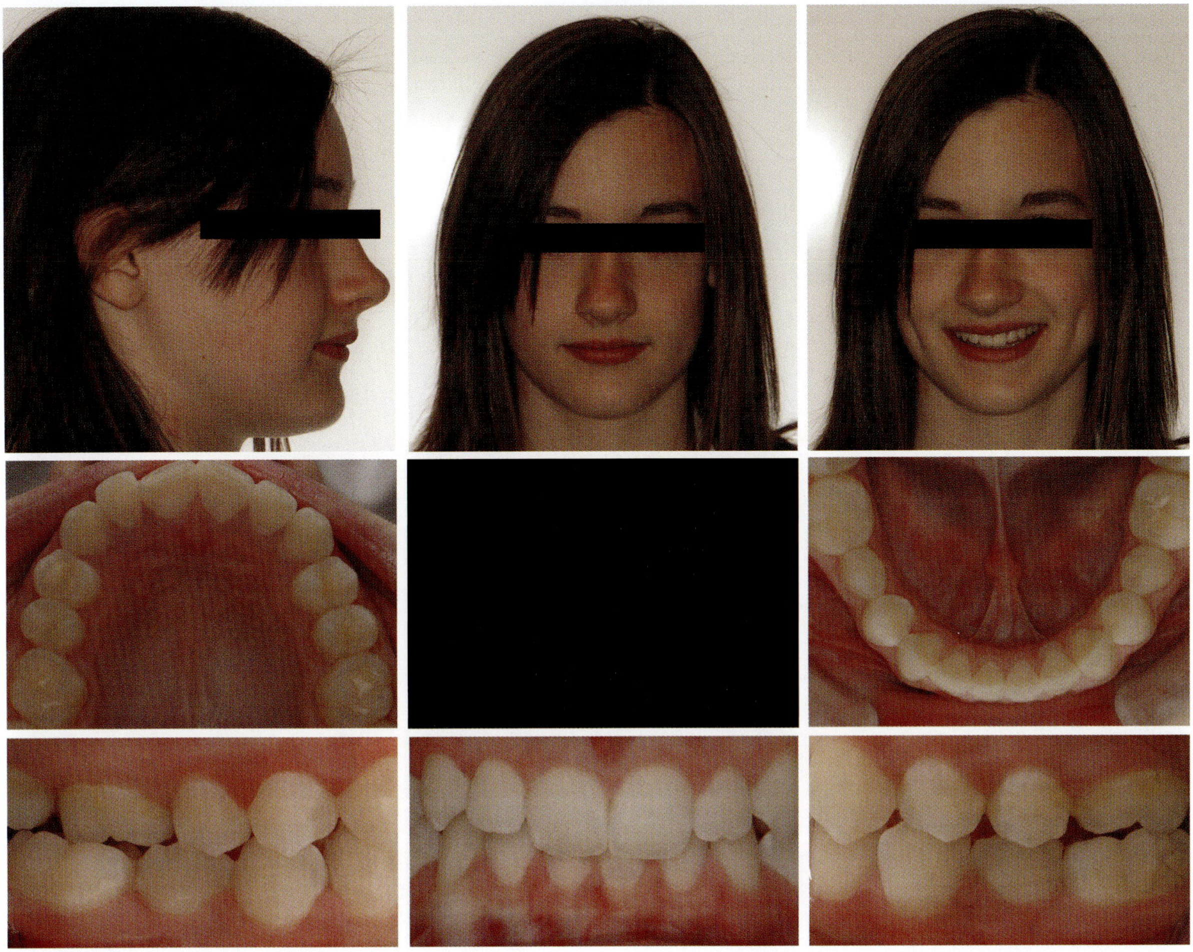

Figure 11.16 Case II. Pre-treatment records of a 12-year, 7-month-old female with posterior crossbite in the molar region with upright maxillary posterior teeth seen on 3D CBCT image. A dental expansion treatment approach was used in this case.

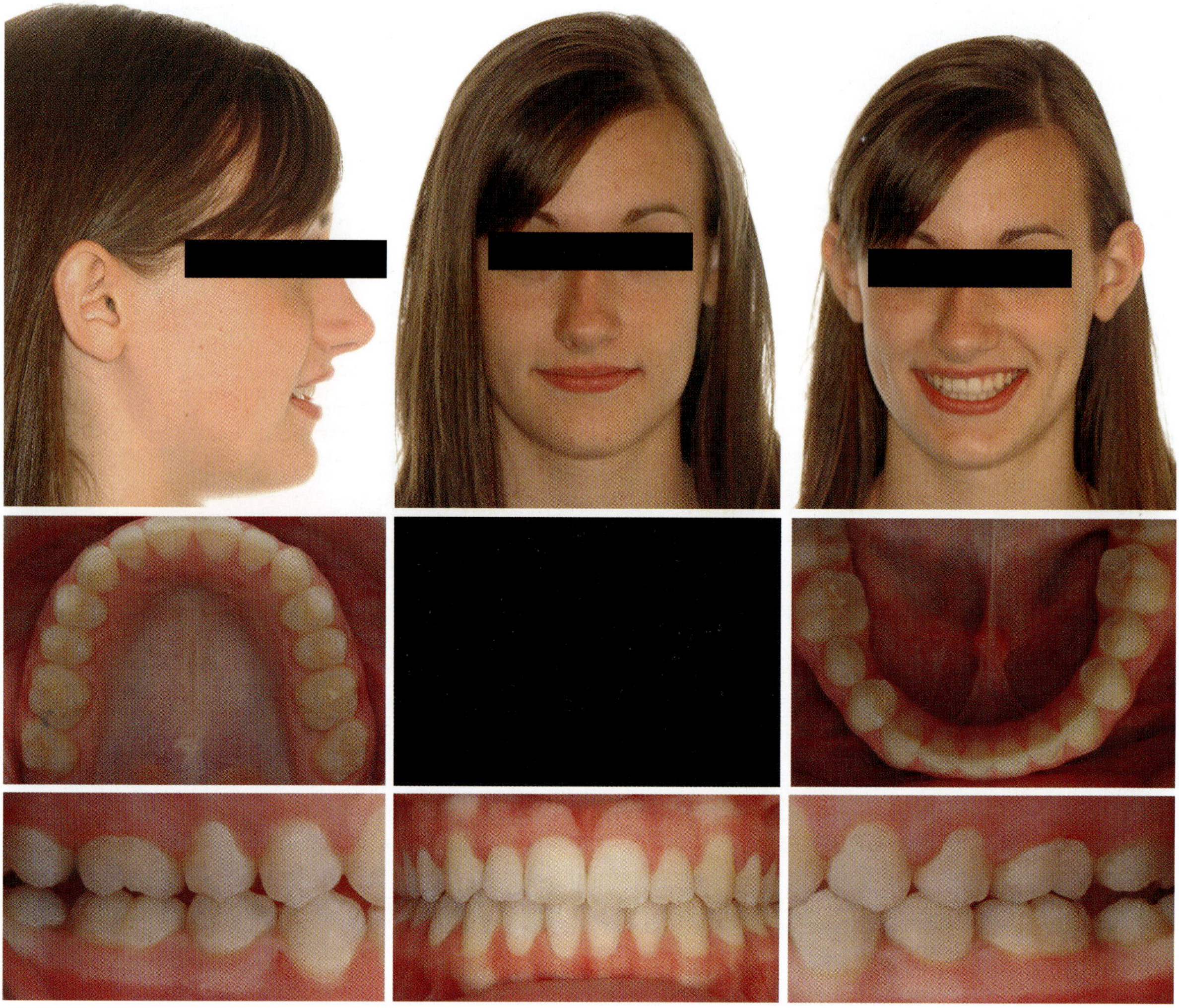

Figure 11.17 Case II. Post-treatment photos of patient showing correction of crossbite.

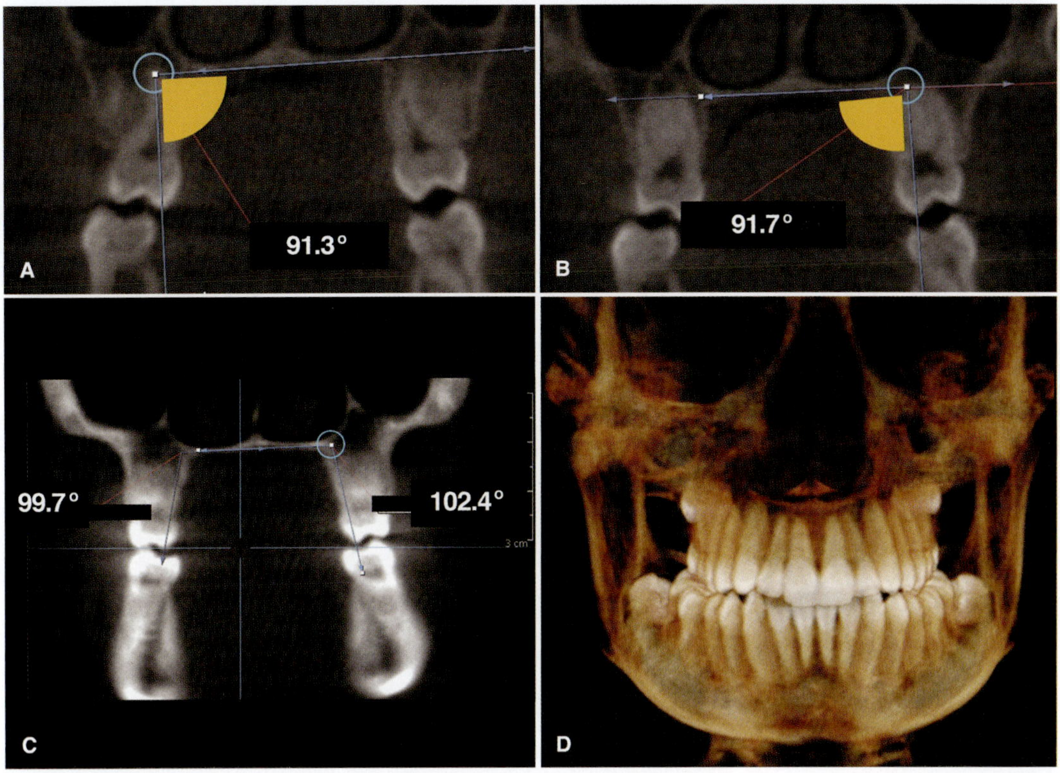

Figure 11.18 Case II. Pre-treatment transverse analysis reveals right (*A*) and left (*B*) molars at 91°, which is lower than the molar angulation norm of 100°. This suggests that the crossbite likely is due to dental inclination and that increasing the molar buccal inclination will correct the transverse deficiency. *C*: The final result shows that the maxillary molar angulations were increased close to the norm of 100° to help alleviate the crossbite. *D*: Volumetric rendering of pre-treatment CBCT depicting upright buccolingual inclinations of the posterior teeth in 3D.

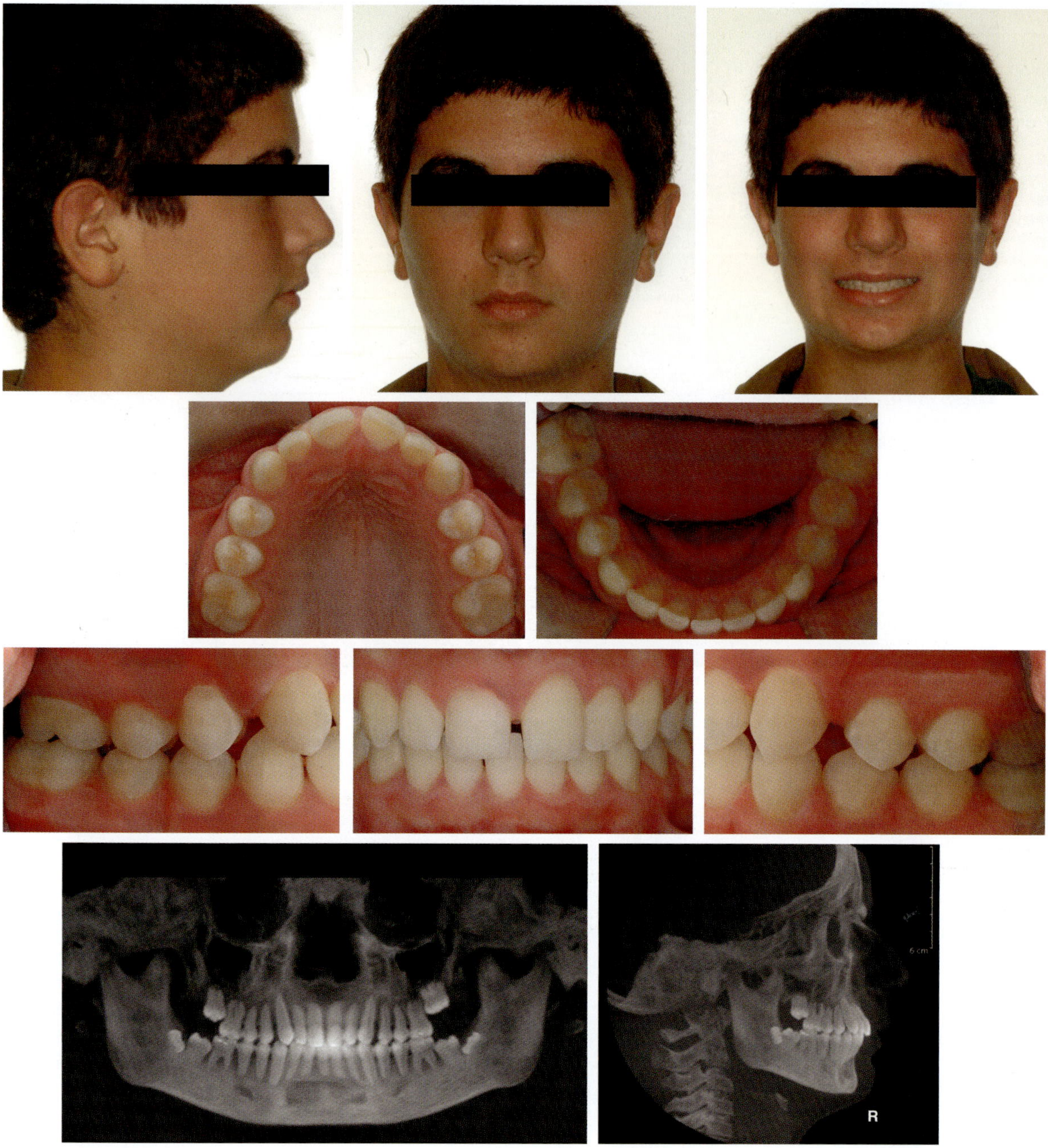

Figure 11.19 Case III. Pre-treatment photographs and radiographs of a teenage male with missing lower incisors and some upper anterior spacing.

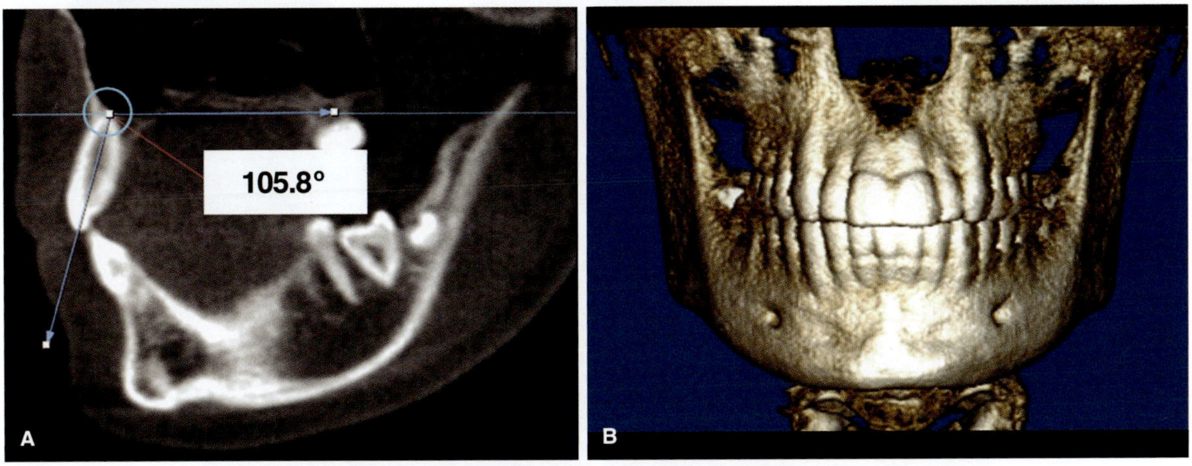

Figure 11.20 Case III. *A*: The pre-treatment bucco-lingual inclination of the maxillary right canine of 105.8° is close to the norm of 104°. *B*: Volumetric rendering shows sound bone support around all roots.

INTERPRETING THE ANALYSIS RESULTS: CASE REPORTS

The use of the norm of 100° for the buccolingual inclination of maxillary molars has been tested retrospectively in several cases. This norm shows strong diagnostic capabilities for the maxillary transverse dimension, detecting dental compensations and objectively showing when dental expansion is possible or when orthopedic expansion is indicated.

Such measures in combination with the buccolingual inclination of mandibular molars to the mandibular plane also can show whether compensations are present in the mandibular teeth. This information allows better control of orthodontic treatment, especially when preadjusted fixed appliances are used. In our retrospective inspection, there were cases in which dental compensations were not detected at the initial diagnosis; when such inclinations were decompensated by the pretorqued brackets, a crossbite that was not present at the beginning appeared or a mild crossbite worsened during treatment (Figure 11.13, Figure 11.14, and Figure 11.15). In contrast, cases that were treated successfully with the increase of the buccolingual inclination, also known as dental expansion, showed that the initial inclinations often were below the norm of 100° (Figure 11.16, Figure 11.17, and Figure 11.18), while cases where such an approach was not successful showed that dental compensations for transverse deficiency already were present at the start of treatment. Finally, the case depicted in Figure 11.19, Figure 11.20, Figure 11.21, and Figure 11.22 demonstrates a situation in which the normal pre-treatment buccolingual canine inclination was decreased to below norms during orthodontic treatment with potential adverse consequences on bone support.

CONCLUSIONS

This chapter outlines how information can be extracted from a CBCT volume in a standardized method, incorporated into the patient's records for clinical use, and quantified in the transverse plane to further aid in the diagnosis and treatment planning of the orthodontic patient.

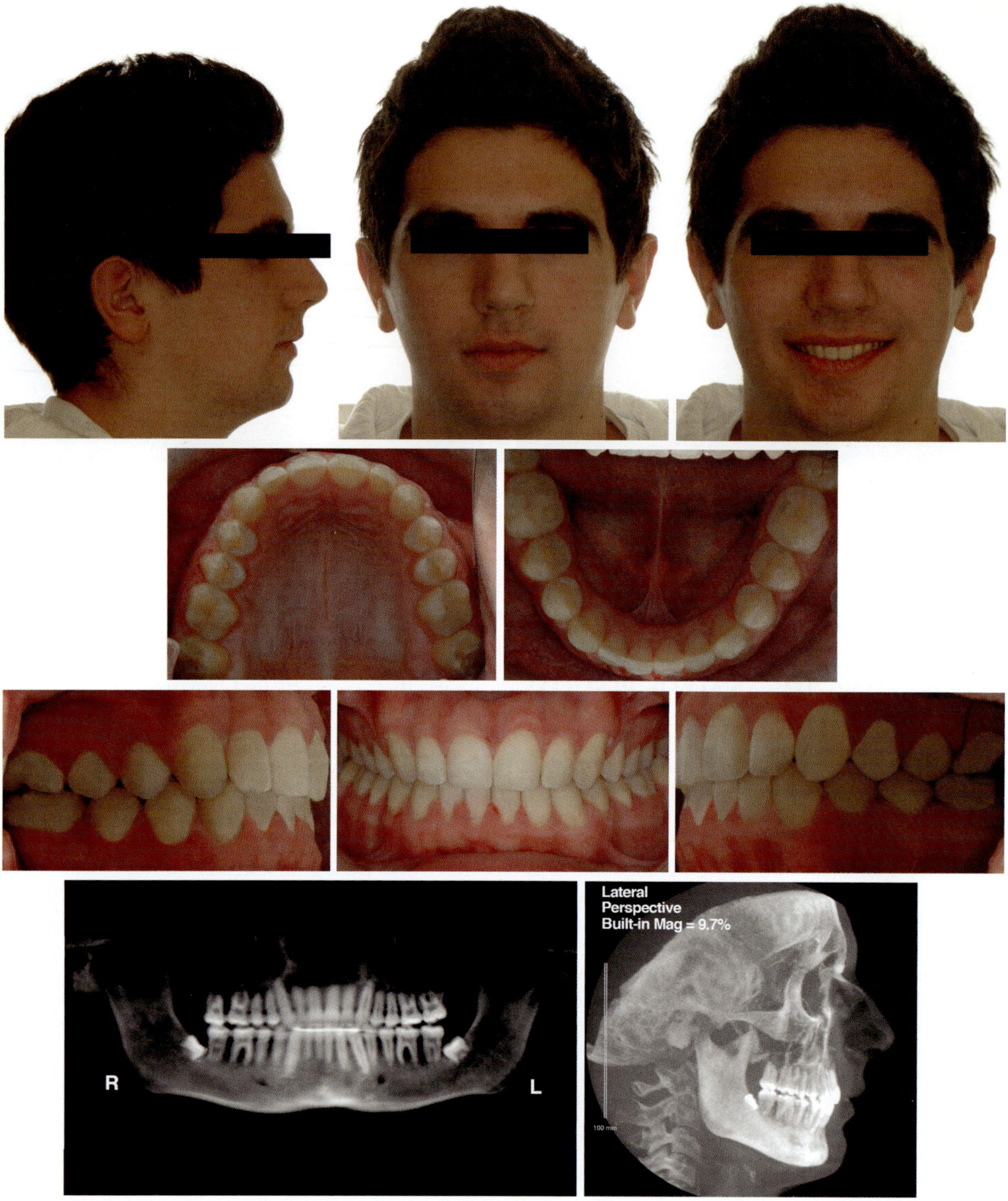

Figure 11.21 Case III. Post-treatment photographs and radiographs showing good orthodontic treatment results.

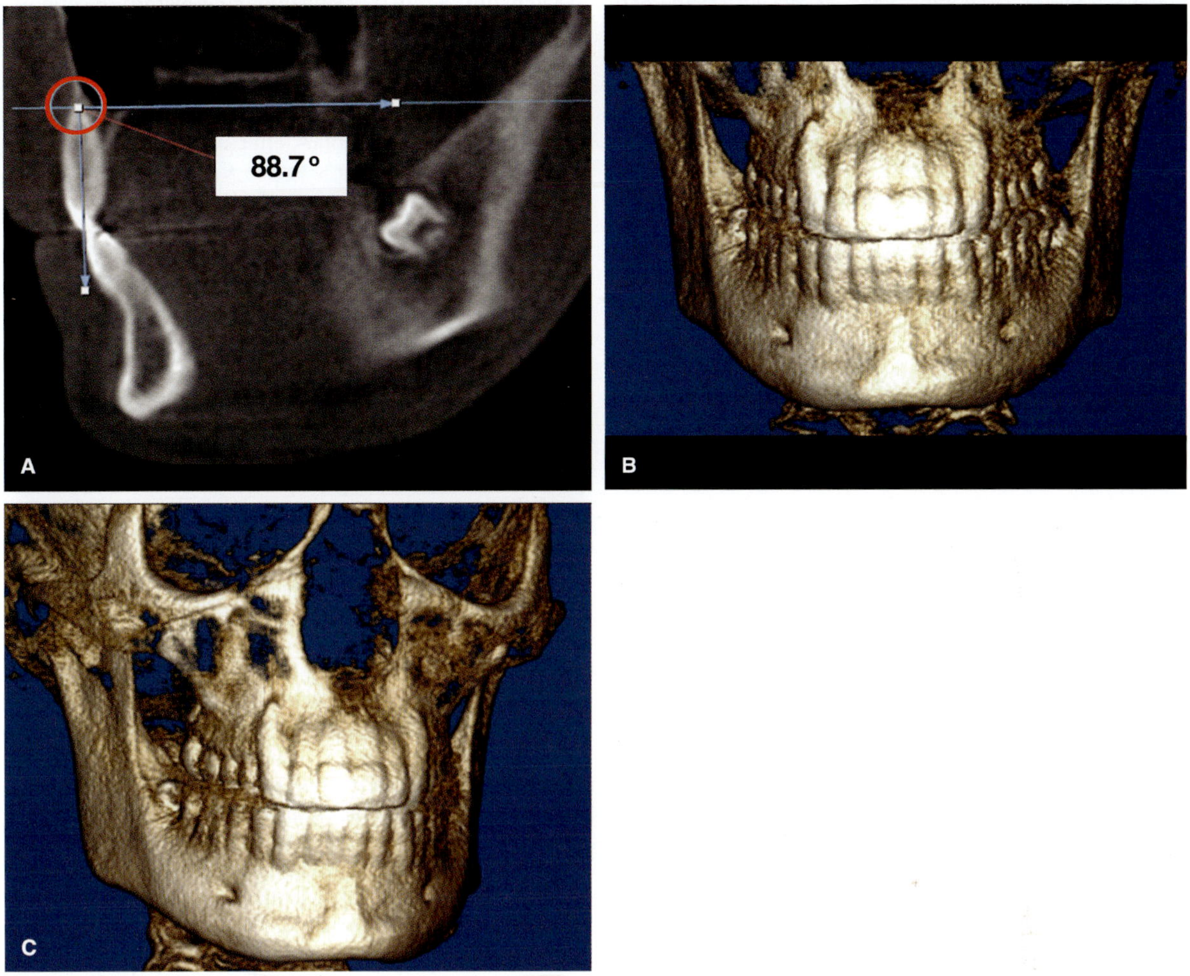

Figure 11.22 Case III. *A*: The post-treatment bucco-lingual inclination of the maxillary right canine has been decreased to 88.7°, which is substantially lower than the norm of 104°. *B* and *C*: Volumetric renderings show a potential concern for recession, attachment loss, or dehiscence around the root of the right canine.

References

Altobelli, D.E., Kikinis, R., Mulliken, J.B., *et al.* (1993) Computer assisted three-dimensional planning in craniofacial surgery. *Plastic and Reconstructive Surgery*, 92 (4), 576–585.

Baumrind, S. & Frantz, R. (1971) The reliability of head film measurements. 1: landmark identification. *American Journal of Orthodontics*, 60 (2), 111–127.

Baumrind, S., Moffit, F., & Curry, S. (1983a) The geometry of three dimensional measurements from paired coplanar X-ray images: a progress report. *American Journal of Orthodontics*, 84 (4), 313–322.

Baumrind, S., Moffit, F., & Curry, S. (1983b) Three-dimension X-ray stereometry from paired coplanar images: a progress report. *American Journal of Orthodontics*, 84 (4), 292–312.

Bookstein, F.L. (1982) On the cephalometrics of skeletal change. *American Journal of Orthodontics*, 82 (3), 177–198.

Bookstein, F.L., Grayson, B., Cutting, C.B., *et al.* (1991) Landmarks in three dimensions: reconstruction from cephalograms versus direct observation. *American Journal of Orthodontics and Dentofacial Orthopedics*, 100 (2), 133–140.

Broadbent, B.H. (1931) A new X-ray technique and its application to orthodontia. *Angle Orthodontist*, 1 (2), 45–66.

El, A.S., El, H., Palomo, J.M., *et al.* (2011) A 3D airway analysis of an obstructive sleep apnea surgical correction with cone beam computed tomography. *Journal of Oral and Maxillofacial Surgery*, 69 (9), 2424–2436.

El, H. & Palomo, J.M. (2010) Measuring the airway in 3D: a reliability and accuracy study. *American Journal of Orthodontics and Dentofacial Orthopedics*, 137 (Suppl 4), S50.e1–S50.e2.

El, H. & Palomo, J.M. (2011) Airway volume for different dentofacial skeletal patterns. *American Journal of Orthodontics and Dentofacial Orthopedics*, 139 (6), e511–e521.

El, H. & Palomo, J.M. (2013) An airway study of different maxillary and mandibular sagittal positions. *European Journal of Orthodontics*, 35, 262–270.

Enlow, D.H. & Hans, M.G. (2008) *Essentials of Facial Growth*. 2nd ed. Needham Press, Ann Arbor, MI.

Evangelinakis, N., Palomo, J.M., Narendran, S., *et al.* (2010) Changes in buccolingual inclination of mandibular canines and first molars after orthodontic treatment using CBCT. Master's thesis, Case Western Reserve University.

Goel, A. (2004) Treatment of basilar invagination by atlantoaxial joint distraction and direct lateral mass fixation. *Journal of Neurosurgery. Spine*, 1 (3), 281–286.

Goldberg, M. (1973) Cephalometrics. *International Journal of Orthodontics*, 11 (4), 111–129.

Grayson, B.H., Cutting, F.L., Bookstein, F.L., *et al.* (1988) The three dimensional cephalogram: theory, technique and clinical application. *American Journal of Orthodontics and Dentofacial Orthopedics*, 94 (4), 237–337.

Hixon, E.H. (1972) Cephalometrics: a perspective. *Angle Orthodontist*, 42 (3), 200–211.

Kapila, S., Conley, R.S., & Harrel, W.E. (2011) Current status of CBCT imaging in orthodontics. *Dentomaxillofacial Radiology*, 40 (1), 24–34.

Karamitsou, E., Palomo, J.M., Ntragatakis, M., *et al.* (2011) Pretreatment buccolingual inclination of maxillary canines and first molars. Master's thesis, Case Western Reserve University.

Kau, C.H., Richmond, S., Palomo, J.M., *et al.* (2005) Current products and practice: three-dimensional cone beam computerized tomography in orthodontics. *Journal of Orthodontics*, 32 (4), 282–293.

Kwong, J.C., Palomo, J.M., Landers, M.A., *et al.* (2008) Image quality produced by different cone-beam computed tomography settings. *American Journal of Orthodontics and Dentofacial Orthopedics*, 133 (2), 317–327.

Maganzini, A. (1974) Developmental history of cephalometrics: a review. *International Journal of Orthodontics*, 12 (1), 5–24.

Miyamoto, M., Palomo, J.M., Narendran, S., *et al.* (2012) Changes in buccolingual inclination of maxillary canines and first molars after orthodontic treatment using CBCT. Master's thesis, Case Western Reserve University.

Ogawa, T., Enciso, R., Shintaku, W.H., *et al.* (2007) Evaluation of cross-section airway configuration of obstructive sleep apnea. *Oral Surgery, Oral Medicine, Oral Pathology, Oral Radiology, and Endodontics*, 103 (1), 102–108.

Palomo, J.M., Yang, C.Y., & Hans, M.G. (2005) Clinical application of three-dimensional craniofacial imaging in orthodontics. *Journal of Medical Sciences*, 25 (6), 269–278.

Palomo, J.M., Rao, P.S., & Hans, M.G. (2008) Influence of CBCT exposure conditions on radation dose. *Oral Surgery, Oral Medicine, Oral Pathology, Oral Radiology, and Endodontics*, 105 (6), 773–782.

Pauwels, R., Beinsberger, J., Collaert, B., *et al.* (2012) SEDENTEXCT Project Consortium. Effective dose range for dental cone beam computed tomography scanners. *European Journal of Radiology*, 81 (2), 267–271.

Ricketts, R.M. (1972) The value of cephalometrics and computerized technology. *Angle Orthodontist*, 42 (3), 179–199.

Savara, B.S. (1965) A method for measuring facial growth in three dimensions. *Human Biology*, 37 (3), 245–255.

Shewinvanakitkul, W., Hans, M.G., Narendran, S., *et al.* (2011) Measuring buccolingual inclination of mandibular canines and first molars using CBCT. *Orthodontics & Craniofacial Research*, 14 (3), 168–174.

Solow, B. (1970) Computers in cephalometric research. *Computers in Biology and Medicine*, 1 (1), 41–49.

Streit, L., Palomo, J.M., Narendran, S., *et al.* (2012) The CWRU transverse analysis: developing norms. Master's thesis, Case Western Reserve University.

Thurow, R.C. (1981) Fifty years of cephalometric radiography. *Angle Orthodontist*, 51 (2), 89–91.

Vig, P.S. (1982) An orthodontist's view of some recent mathematical studies in cephalometrics. *American Journal of Orthodontics*, 81 (4), 341–342.

Wu, R., Palomo, J.M., Landers, M., *et al.* (2012) Anatomically based cranial landmarks for three-dimensional superimposition. Master's thesis, Case Western Reserve University.

12 Application of 3D TMJ Imaging to TMJDs, TMJ Functional Analyses, and Orthodontic Treatment Outcomes

Anna-Kari Hajati, DDS, PhD, Lucia H.S. Cevidanes, DDS, MS, PhD, Laura Iwasaki, DDS, MSc, PhD, Jeffrey C. Nickel, DMD, MSc, PhD, MRCD (C), Dipl ABO, and Sunil D. Kapila, BDS, MS, PhD

INTRODUCTION

The temporomandibular joint (TMJ) is a structure of substantial importance in clinical orthodontics. During growth, the joint components influence the development of the relationships between the upper and lower jaws, the occlusion, and the functioning masticatory system. In adults, the health of the TMJ and masticatory system depends on the capacity of these joint components to adapt to normal or abnormal function. TMJ pathologies that result in alterations to the size, form, and spatial and functional relationships of the joint components can lead to progressive changes and compensations that ultimately may affect jaw and tooth positions and occlusion. Such pathological TMJ conditions include temporomandibular joint disorders (TMJDs; also referred to as temoporomandibular disorders or TMD) and developmental disorders such as condylar hyperplasia, hypoplasia, or aplasia. TMJDs in turn include internal derangement or disc displacement, arthralgia, osteoarthritis (OA), and osteoarthrosis. Occlusal and functional changes associated with these pathological conditions include progressive anterior openbite and limitation or deviation of jaw movements (Helenius *et al.*, 2005; Koyama *et al.*, 2007; Alexiou *et al.*, 2009; Yura *et al.*, 2010).

The current diagnoses of TMJDs are based largely on signs and symptoms of the disease. However, it is acknowledged widely that an ideal diagnostic classification system for any disease or disorder including TMJDs should be based on etiology (National Institues of Health Technology Assessment Conference Statement on the Diagnosis and Management of TMDs, 1996). The first step toward an etiology-based system was introduced in 1992 (Dworkin & LeResche, 1992) and was known as the Research Diagnostic Criteria for temporomandibular disorders (RDC/TMD). The RDC/TMD index includes two axes: Axis I is related to physical diagnoses, primarily based on

Cone Beam Computed Tomography in Orthodontics: Indications, Insights, and Innovations, First Edition. Sunil D. Kapila.

clinical signs and symptoms; Axis II incorporates the psychological status of the patient and pain-related disability. This system has been used in many studies to date and is the basis of ongoing large-scale multisite epidemiological studies (Maixner *et al.*, 2011). The results of projects that validate the RDC/TMD have been reported recently (Anderson *et al.*, 2010; Ohrbach *et al.*, 2010; Truelove *et al.*, 2010; Look *et al.*, 2010a; Schiffman *et al.*, 2010a, 2010b) and the scientific evidence for clinical treatment of TMJDs has been reviewed (Cairns, 2010; List & Axelsson, 2010; Michelotti & Iodice, 2010; Ohrbach, 2010), setting the stage for improved approaches for diagnosing (Zhao *et al.*, 2011; Gonzalez *et al.*, 2011b) and treatment of TMJDs (Greene, 2010).

Imaging data currently are recommended to help differentiate the diagnosis of disc displacement diagnoses and arthralgia, OA, and osteoarthrosis (Look *et al.*, 2010b). Indeed, the RDC/TMD validation project supports the use of imaging to enhance the Axis I physical diagnoses protocol. Hence, the recommended TMJ imaging has evolved to include computed tomography (CT) and cone beam CT (CBCT) for diagnosis of osseous degenerative changes, and magnetic resonance imaging (MRI) for detecting disc displacements and effusion (Ahmad *et al.*, 2009). Comprehensive imaging criteria for TMJ diagnoses have been validated for image acquisition and analysis using CT (and by extension CBCT), MRI, and panoramic radiographs (Ahmad *et al.*, 2009). Furthermore, the validated combination of multidimensional imaging with computer-aided numerical modeling has produced novel insights and enhanced our understanding of the normal function and pathomechanics of the human masticatory apparatus. The increased use of CBCT, MRI, and joint kinematics methods allow us to understand better TMJ tissue dynamics during growth and aging that include adaptive and therapeutic remodeling as well as pathologic degradation and proliferation. However, despite the importance of TMJ morphologic assessment derived from imaging, treatment evaluations and risk assessments of TMJDs also must take into consideration function, pain and biological perspectives for the full clinical value of diagnostics to be realized. For this reason, in addition to providing an in-depth background on the applications of three-dimensional (3D) imaging to TMJD diagnostics and therapeutics, this chapter highlights clinical and biological data that are essential to attain comprehensive insights on the causes and pathogenesis of these disorders. A discussion on the known changes within the TMJ in response to growth modification orthodontic therapies also is included. Finally, since the applications of CBCT in the clinical assessment of the TMJs are still under study and development, we also have incorporated an overview of recent advances in methodologies and technologies that eventually will help in moving the diagnostic uses of 3D imaging into the clinical arena.

IMAGING OF THE TMJ

TMJDs include developmental and acquired disorders of the TMJ. Acquired disorders of the TMJ comprise arthralgia and inflammatory disorders such as rheumatoid arthritis (RA) and OA, disc dislocation or internal derangement, ankylosis, and fracture (Leeuw, 2008). While these diagnostic classifications are based primarily on clinical signs and symptoms, clinical examination alone is insufficient to describe fully the disease status and aid in the development of protocols for the management of hard tissue pathologies of the TMJ. Imaging is a necessary element in the diagnostic process (Petersson, 2010), but also is insufficient on its own for the management of disease (Wiese *et al.*, 2011).

Conventional radiographic imaging of the TMJ using panoramic radiographs and cephalograms results in disorted images with superimposed structures. Given that imaging with panoramic radiographs is unreliable and has a low sensitivity, analysis for structural changes using this imaging modality generally has been limited to evaluating gross changes in joint anatomy (Ahmad *et al.*, 2009; Shintaku *et al.*, 2009). Advancements in CT technologies and the introduction of CBCT with reduced radiation doses and costs relative to CTs have resulted in its increased utilization as the primary diagnostic imaging method for assessing TMJ bone morphology. CBCT is at least as reliable as conventional CT in detection of TMJ bone tissue changes and has superior reliability and greater accuracy than conventional tomograms in

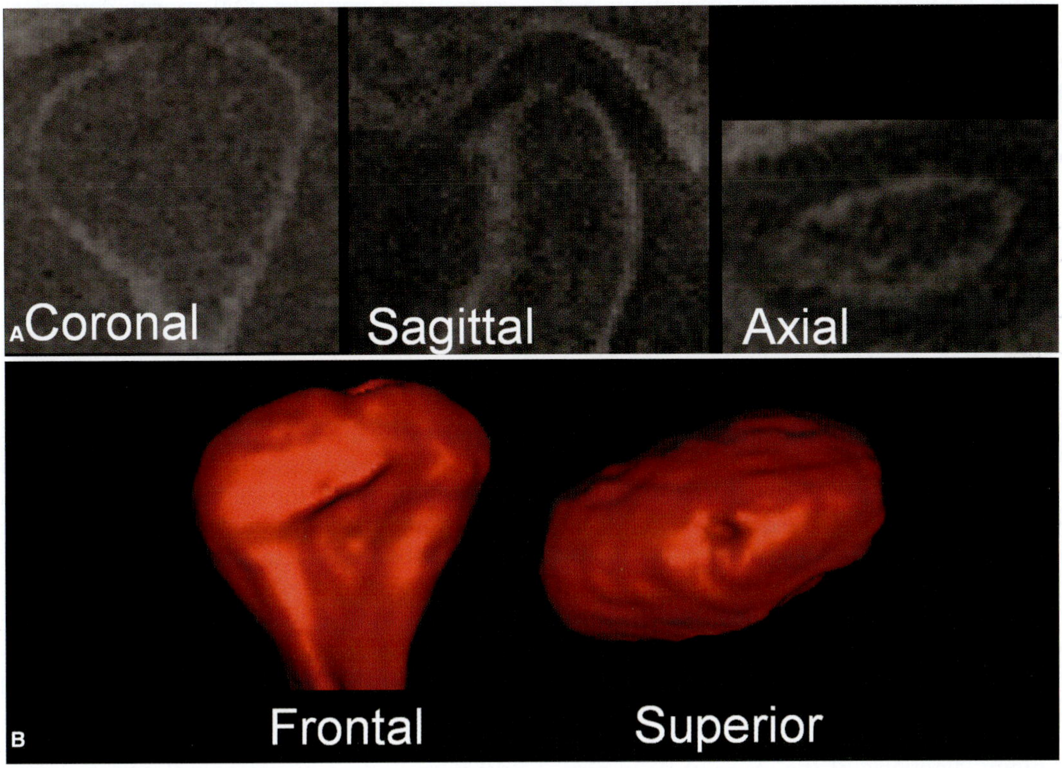

Figure 12.1 CBCT cross-sections in the three planes of space (*A*) that are utilized for construction of condylar 3D virtual surface model (*B*).

detecting TMJ erosions (Honda *et al.*, 2006; Honey *et al.*, 2007).

CBCT allows evaluation of TMJ hard tissue morphology and enables visualization of a wide spectrum of minor to overt osseous changes resulting from pathology, growth, and adaptive processes. A radiographic examination of the TMJ is an essential part in the diagnosis and management of TMJ diseases involving the bone that supports the articulating tissues. CBCT also allows for accurate detection and evaluation of pathological changes (Honda *et al.*, 2006; Honey *et al.*, 2007). Relative to conventional 2D radiography, the precise rendering of virtual 3D surface models of the TMJ bone anatomy enables practitioners to provide earlier and accurate identification of aberrations in the bone morphology (Figure 12.1) and in the congruency of bone surfaces that define the joint space (Crow *et al.*, 2005) in 3D. The following sections describe how CBCT can be utilized for (1) the diagnosis of different types of TMJ arthritides, (2) better understanding of TMJ bone remodeling, (3) specific applications of TMJ evaluations in orthodontic patients, and (4) 3D superimpositions for evaluating four-dimensional (4D) changes in TMJ bone architecture.

Arthritides and degenerative joint diseases

3D imaging of the TMJ provides essential information for detecting inflammatory and degenerative conditions of the TMJ bony tissues and to determine accurate intervention by longitudinally monitoring progression and responses to treatment (Okeson, 1996). The utility of 3D imaging applies to conditions such as OA, RA, juvenile idiopathic arthritis, psoriatic arthritis, gout, ankylosing spondylitis, idiopathic condylar resorption, and other less common diseases. Radiographic features of arthritides in the TMJ are similar regardless of whether the condition is local, such as for OA, or systemic, as in RA. Progression of OA, however, can be slower than that of RA, making radiographic signs less evident in OA compared with RA. Radiographic signs of bony changes associated with TMJ arthritides include irregular and possibly thickened cortical outlines (sclerosis), erosions, osteophyte formation, subchondral cysts, and flattening and narrowing of the joint space (Gynther *et al.*, 1996; Ahmad *et al.*, 2009; Alexiou *et al.*, 2009). In RA, when erosions are detected early, they also may predict progression and severity (van der Heijde *et al.*, 1992; van der Heijde, 1995; Forslind *et al.*, 2009).

CBCT images allow reliable detection and localization of hard tissue structural changes. The efficacy of CBCT for detecting osseous changes is superior to that of plane tomography and MRI (Honey *et al.*, 2007; Alkhader *et al.*, 2010). Possible indications for imaging of the TMJs with CBCTs include detection of bone abnormalities, characterization of the condylar and articular fossa bone morphology, diagnosis of the stage of bone morphologic changes, assessment of the progression of bony changes over time, or the response to a specific treatment (Ahmad *et al.*, 2009; De Vos *et al.*, 2009). The use of CBCT for orthodontic reasons also may increase the possibility for early detection of TMJ degenerative processes in an otherwise asymptomatic patient.

Upon diagnosis of initial signs of active TMJ destruction in a CBCT scan, it is essential to monitor active disease, either localized to the TMJ or systemic, before loading the joints with orthodontic/orthopedic forces or undertaking jaw surgery. Interpretation of CBCT findings, therefore, should be part of a complete analysis of the dental and medical history, as well as charting of the TMJ clinical signs and symptoms prior to the start of the orthodontic treatment. If a systemic inflammatory condition is suspected at the clinical examination, the patient should be referred for a medical evaluation, including necessary serological evaluation. It is important to keep in mind that structural bony changes of the TMJ alone do not reveal whether or not the disease is active, since there is no direct correlation between TMJ morphological changes and clinical findings in OA or RA (Celiker *et al.*, 1995; Hajati *et al.*, 2009). Early diagnosis and treatment of destructive inflammatory conditions is important to further control bone destruction successfully (Allaart *et al.*, 2006). As demonstrated in Figure 12.2 and as validated by studies regarding other joints, controlling the inflammation in patients with RA leads to repair of bone through formation of new bone at the base of deep erosions (Finzel *et al.*, 2011). Control of local inflammation, therefore, should be an important clinical goal for these patients.

Besides the radiographic signs of joint destruction in RA, there are several common risk factors for disease progression including systemic inflammatory markers, the shared epitope (SE) allele for the human leukocyte antigen (HLA), the presence of rheumatoid factor (RF), estrogen deficiency, and being female. A promising marker with high diagnostic specificity for RA is an antibody to cyclic citrullinated peptides (anti-CCP; Pfeilschifter *et al.*, 2002; van Venrooij *et al.*, 2003; Vittecoq *et al.*, 2004; Sanmartí *et al.*, 2007; Syversen *et al.*, 2008). Anti-CCP has been shown to predict RA more than 10 years before disease onset and to be a strong predictor of progression of joint destruction (Aho *et al.*, 1991, 1993; Rantapää-Dahlqvist *et al.*, 2003; Forslind *et al.*, 2004). It still is unknown whether appropriate markers or predictors may be detectable in other arthritides, such as idiopathic condylar resorption, in otherwise clinically and radiographically healthy individuals.

3D quantification of bony changes in TMJ condylar surface models constructed from CBCT volumes has been performed recently using shape correspondence analysis (Cevidanes *et al.*, 2010). Condylar resorption and apposition was localized and quantified in patients with TMJ OA, and the morphology was compared with a group of healthy controls. This method measures defects within 0.5 mm of the true defect size in simulation studies and in longitudinal follow-up of disease progression (Paniagua *et al.*, 2011). Software tools for comparing TMJ structural abnormalities across patients that will aid in developing a 3D diagnostic index of morphological variability currently are under development. The biggest challenge toward achieving this goal is deriving a dataset of a 3D

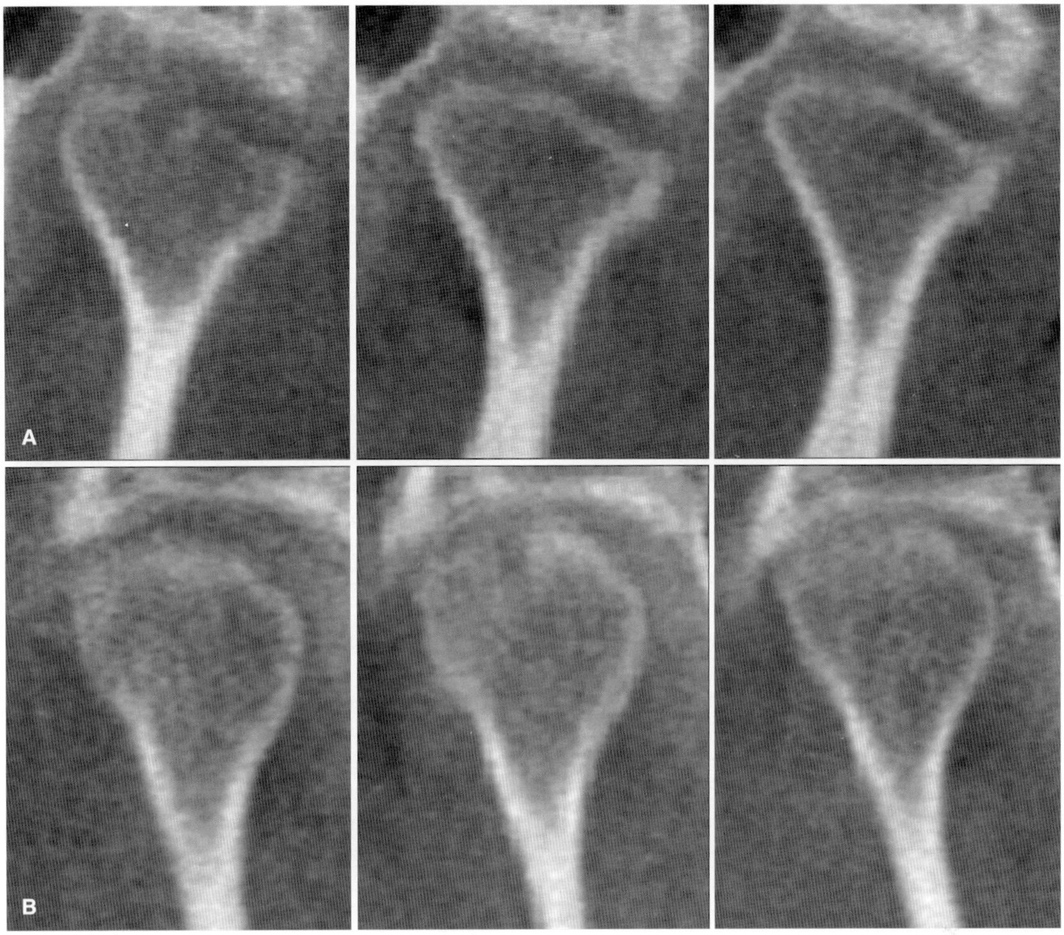

Figure 12.2 Longitudinal bone remodeling of the TMJ. Coronal cross-sectional views of the TMJ show the changes over a 2-year follow-up of the TMJ morphology in two patients with TMJ erosions. *A*: Patient showed marked TMJ erosion at first visit (left) and received intra-articular injection of glucocorticoids. At the 1-year follow-up (middle), the erosion had been repaired and the repair was stable at the 2-year follow-up (right), with possible mild surface flattening in that area. *B*: In the left panel at RA diagnosis, even though some loss of signal can be noted in the subchondral bone, no erosions were evident. The patient developed TMJ erosion during the 1-year follow-up and at that time was treated with intra-articular glucocorticoid injection (middle). New bone formation was observed at the 2-year follow-up, with some likely mild surface irregularity or flattening (right). Although the visualization and localization of bone formation and resorption can be noted in cross-sectional radiographic images, the quantification of longitudinal changes of 3D bone defects is not possible in cross-sectional slices.

population reference standard of normal TMJ morphologies when considerable individual variability exists in TMJ form and size among individuals and age groups.

As with CBCT, MRI is a noninvasive tomographic imaging technique that can produce cross-sectional images in any plane without morphologic distortion or magnification. In addition, MRI enables visualization of joint abnormalities not seen with any other imaging method and, thus, is considered to be the best method for diagnostic assessment of the TMJ status (Larheim, 2005). MRI is the only technique that allows simultaneous examination of all components of the TMJ, including soft tissues, articular cartilage, and bone, without ionizing radiation and its adverse effects.

The value of MRI for the detection of TMJ osseous abnormalities, however, is considered to be limited in comparison to CBCT (Alkhader *et al.*, 2010). Changes in TMJ bone marrow signals can be demonstrated with MRI revealing edema and osteonecrosis (Lieberman *et al.*, 1996; Larheim *et al.*, 1999). Since bone marrow changes on MRIs from hands and feet in early RA are an indicator for development of joint destruction (Conaghan *et al.*, 2003; McQueen *et al.*, 2003), similar findings for the TMJ may offer early indicators of future destructive changes.

Internal derangements of the TMJ

Ultrasound and MRI have been used to monitor synovitis and cartilage degradation in the knee (Peterfy *et al.*, 2008) and the TMJ (van Dijke *et al.*, 1997). Unlike the knee joint in which the bone is covered with hyaline cartilage, the mandibular condyle and eminence of the TMJ are lined by a thin layer of fibrocartilage. In addition, the TMJ disc that normally lies between the bony components also is comprised of fibrocartilage. The normal TMJ, as seen by MRI, is characterized differently in each cross-sectional view and jaw position. In the sagittal plane closed-mouth view, the disc clearly is depicted as a low-signal intensity band of biconcave-lens-like configuration. The posterior band lies approximately at the 12 o'clock position relative to the condylar head (Figure 12.3A). In the sagittal plane open-mouth view, the disc has a "bow tie" configuration and maintains its position between the condyle and the articular eminence (Figure 12.3B). The posterior disc attachment has a bright signal relative to the posterior band of the disc due to its rich network of fatty tissue. In the coronal plane, the disc has an arc-shaped configuration with the medial margin of the disc attaching to the medial pole of the condyle and with the lateral margin attaching to the lateral pole of the condyle.

Because of its ability to visualize the nonmineralized "soft tissues" of the disc and articular fibrocartilage in the TMJ, MRI is a preferable and proven method for the assessment of changes in morphology and/or spatial relationships that these tissues undergo during internal derangements of the TMJ, including joint effusion and disc displacements (Katzberg, 1990). Articular disc derangements may involve disc displacements and deformation. Displacements from the normal disc position may be partial or complete displacements of the disc away from the condylar head (Figure 12.3C). In open-mouth position, the disc may or may not be recaptured over the condylar head (Figure 12.3D). Coronal cross-sections can reveal medio-lateral disc displacements. Disc displacement is found in approximately 80% of patients with TMJ symptoms (Tasaki *et al.*, 1996). Additionally, Larheim and colleagues (2001) have reported that asymptomatic volunteers also may present early-stage disc displacement. More specifically, they found that while complete disc displacement is present in 40% of symptomatic joints compared with 2.4% of asymptomatic joints, partial disc displacement occurred in 22.6% and 21.8% of symptomatic and asymptomatic joints, respectively.

Large accumulations of joint fluid are seen only in symptomatic patients (Larheim *et al.*, 2001). Joint effusion is defined as the presence of increased intra-articular fluid and is seen best in T2-weighted closed-mouth MRI as an increased signal area (hyperintense signal) in the joint space. On opening the mouth, the accumulation is displaced within the joint space.

TMJ bone tissue remodeling

Continuous remodeling of the TMJ bony structures is a physiologic process aimed at adapting the articular surfaces to mechanical forces applied to the joint. This process continues during growth through late adulthood and is an essential biological response to normal functional demands, thereby ensuring homeostasis of joint form and function and maintenance of occlusal relationships (Smartt *et al.*, 2005). Bone tissue remodeling is accomplished by coordinated intercellular signals between the bone-forming osteoblasts and bone-resorbing osteoclasts, which, in turn, are thought to be induced by mechanical loading and controlled by locally produced cytokines, growth factors, hormones, and neuroregulators (Abe *et al.*, 1988; Lacey *et al.*, 1998; Shevde *et al.*, 2000; Michael *et al.*, 2005; Lerner, 2006a; Galal *et al.*, 2008). The

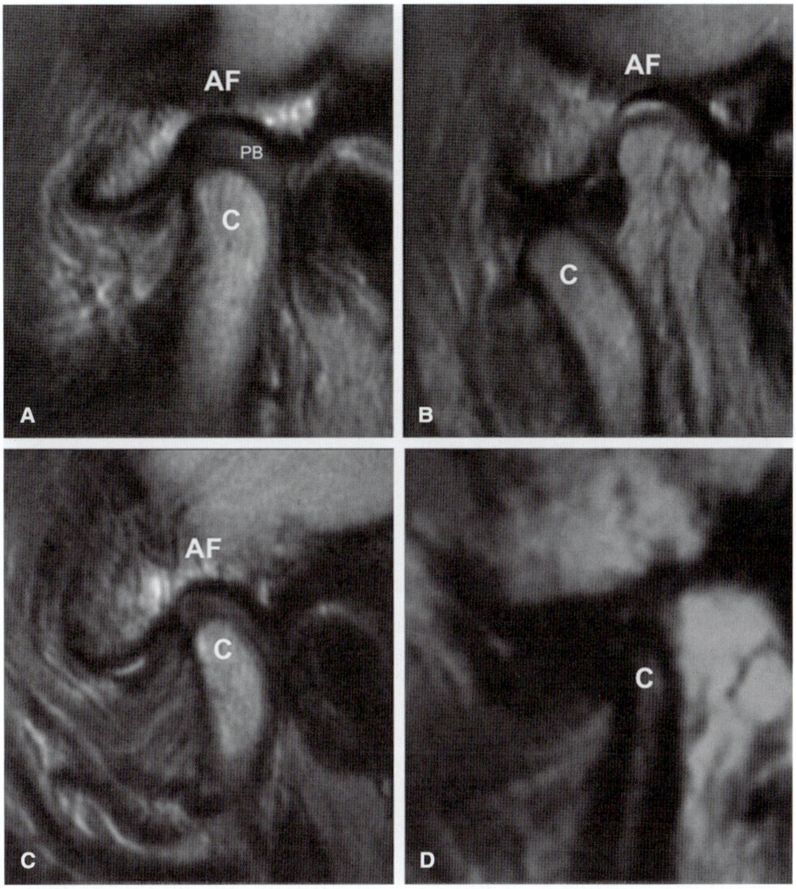

Figure 12.3 Articular disc appearance in sagittal sections from MRIs. *A*: Normal articular disc position in closed-mouth position where the posterior band is interposed between the condylar head and the articular fossa. *B*: In the open-mouth view, the normal disc has a "bow tie" configuration and maintains its position between the condyle and the articular eminence. The posterior disc attachment has a bright signal relative to the posterior band of the disk due to its rich network of fatty tissue. *C*: Partial disc displacement anteriorly to the condylar head in closed-mouth position. *D*: In open mouth, the displaced disc is pushed further anteriorly and cannot be recaptured over the condylar head. PB, posterior band; C, condylar head; AF, articular fossa.

pathogenic mechanisms that cause a predominance of bone tissue resorption under these circumstances might share several pathways in common with RA and periodontitis, two distinct conditions that are characterized with an overreactive inflammatory response (Lerner, 2006b).

The TMJ is subject to mechanical loading by normal- and para-function and orthopedic interventions; therefore, mechanical loading is a risk factor for articular bone resorption in individuals who have enhanced inflammatory response (i.e., Juvenile Idiopathic Arthritis [JIA] and RA). Interestingly, idiopathic articular bone tissue resorption may occur spontaneously without any diagnosis of general inflammatory disease or clinical signs and symptoms (Figure 12.4).

IMAGE-ASSISTED EVALUATION OF THE TMJ IN ORTHODONTIC TREATMENT

CBCT scans are indicated as part of the diagnostic records for specific clinical situations and may provide information regarding the TMJ's adaptive

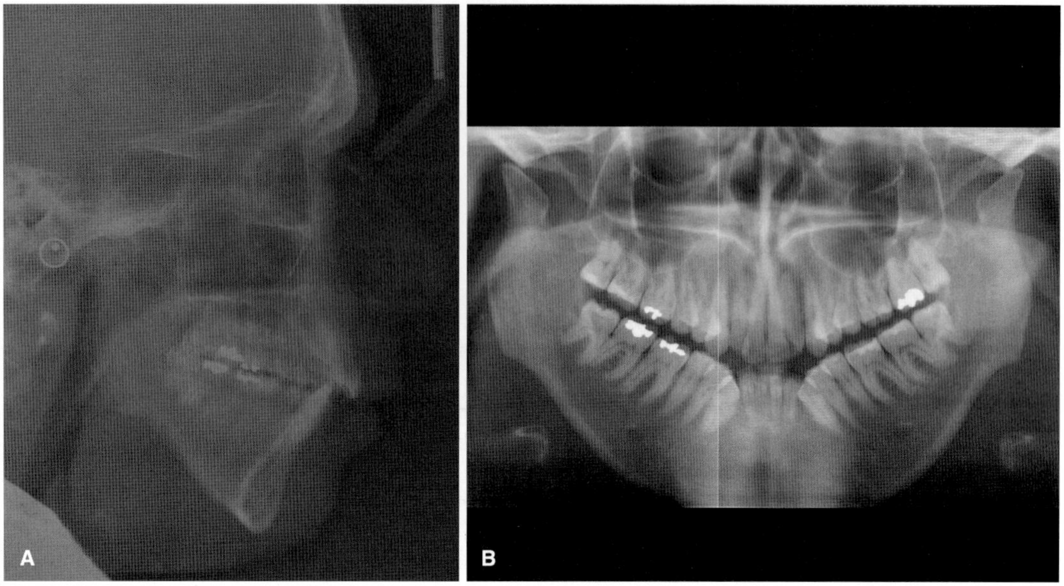

Figure 12.4 Pre-treatment cephalogram (*A*) and orthopantomogram (*B*) of an adult patient who sought orthodontic treatment for correction of bimaxillary crowding. The patient had no clinical signs or symptoms of TMJD nor a history of systemic arthritis. However, the cephalogram and orthopantogram demonstrate gross changes in the mandible, including a steep mandibular plane and condylar flattening, respectively.

capacity in response to orthodontic treatment. One important example of the latter includes the longitudinal assessment of TMJ bone tissue adaptation to mandibular advancement strategies. Earlier studies using CT have shown that orthopedic mandibular advancements with Herbst appliance result in condylar bone apposition and remodeling of the glenoid fossa in children and adolescents. Further studies using MRI have demonstrated that even nongrowing individuals can respond to orthopedic loading of the TMJ with resultant condylar bone apposition (Ruf & Pancherz, 1998, 1999). Finally, 3D CBCT imaging has been used to visualize successful treatment effects of distraction splint therapy during growth on mandibular asymmetry in unilateral manifestation of JIA (Stoustrup *et al.*, 2011).

Although previous work has assessed morphologic changes qualitatively in response to growth modification appliances, newer methodologies are becoming available that might provide better insights into these changes. Thus, the assessment of responses of the TMJ during therapies aimed at growth adaptation or therapeutic remodeling is an area in which 3D data acquisition from CBCT may be a valuable tool in enhancing our understanding and knowledge of the precise localization of treatment effects as well as the quantity of the changes achieved. Careful registration of 3D images is required to improve our current knowledge of TMJ bone tissue remodeling and displacements, evaluation of progress of orthodontic therapies or arthritis treatments, as well as risk assessments for disease. Additionally, CBCT scans and 3D models may enable the localization and quantification of previously unidentified bone tissue growth, remodeling, and degenerative patterns. However, in addition to using contemporary quantitative TMJ imaging approaches, it is essential to have a deeper understanding of its biological and functional attributes to better comprehend TMJ 3D morphology and the dynamics of its changes with orthodontic treatment and disease.

3D SUPERIMPOSITIONS FOR EVALUATION OF 4D CHANGES IN THE TMJ BONE

CBCT has been utilized to assess condylar remodeling longitudinally in treatment outcomes of surgery for almost a decade and, more recently, for determining changes during TMJ arthritides. The use of validated surface modeling and shape analysis quantification techniques for quantifying and localizing bone defects during progression and treatment of arthritis is illustrated in Figure 12.5 (Paniagua *et al.*, 2011). These models demonstrate the longitudinal development and partial repair of TMJ erosion. The patient was diagnosed with RA shortly before the first CBCT acquisition and a 3D model was processed (Figure 12.5B, left). There were no signs or symptoms in the TMJ disease at the time of the initial records or at the follow-ups. When active TMJ bone tissue resorption was discovered at the 1-year follow-up (Figure 12.5B, middle), local corticosteroid treatment was administered to suppress the pathologic inflammation. At the 2-year follow-up, the resorbed bone was rebuilt partially (Figure 12.5B, right). The magnitude and location of changes in bone contours between any two pairs of time points are depicted in Figure 12.5C.

Currently, superimposition of 3D surface models and shape analysis still is too time-consuming and computing-intensive to apply to routine clinical use. Several barriers including radiation doses (see Chapters 2 and 3), construction of CBCT surface models, image registration, and optimal methods for quantitation of the changes need to be overcome prior to more widespread use of CBCT for diagnostic or therapeutic imaging for longitudinal quantitative assessment of changes in the TMJ being performed routinely. Several of these challenges and their potential solutions toward a wider use of TMJ CBCT imaging are detailed below.

Construction of 3D surface models and image registration

Longitudinal quantitative assessment of bony changes requires construction of 3D surface models. Segmentation—the process of constructing 3D models by examining cross-sections of a volumetric data set to outline the shape of structures—remains a challenge (Adams & Bischof, 1994; Lie, 1995; Ma & Manjunath, 2000; Moon *et al.*, 2002), particularly when applied to physiologic or pathologic bone resorption and apposition of thin cortical bone areas in the TMJ condyles. The methods described by Gerig and coworkers (2003) addressing these technical difficulties, have been adapted by Cevidanes and associates (2005) to construct 3D craniofacial models, and more recently, have been applied to the TMJ.

Image registration is a core technology for many imaging tasks. The two most commonly used approaches for CBCT image registration applicable to the TMJ include cranial base superimpositions and regional superimpositions. Such superimpositions can be based on landmarks of reference or surfaces or the gray-level voxels of the CBCT volume. The methodology of choice for cranial base superimpositions has been developed into a sequence of fully automated volume-based registration (Figure 12.6). The major strength of these methods is that registration does not depend on the precision of the 3D surface models. The cranial base models are used only to mask anatomic structures that change with growth and treatment. The registration procedures actually compare the gray-level CBCT images containing only the cranial base voxel-by-voxel to calculate rotation and translation parameters between the two images and to register them on stable anatomic sites in 3D. As with 2D cephalometrics, cranial base superimpositions of 3D CBCT images assess longitudinal displacements of the condyle relative to the cranial fossa (Carvalho Fde *et al.*, 2010; Motta *et al.*, 2011), but do not separate these displacements from bone remodeling. Such an analysis to determine longitudinal changes in condylar remodeling (Figure 12.7A) and comparisons of condylar morphology across subjects requires regional superimpositions using surface-to-surface rigid registration on areas of the condylar neck and ramus (Figure 12.7B; Cevidanes *et al.*, 2010).

Quantitative measurements

Precise quantitative measurements are required for characterization of TMJ arthritides and longitudinal assessments of individual responses to diverse

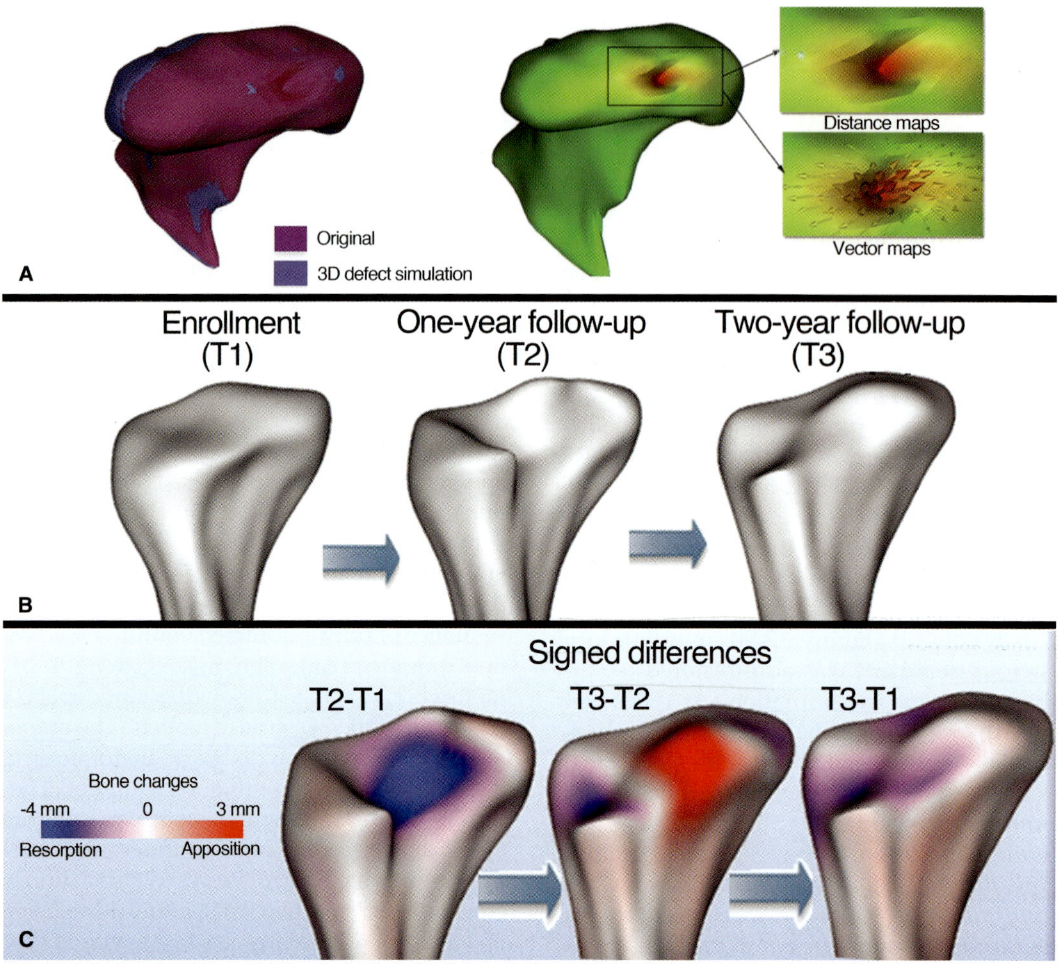

Figure 12.5 Construction of 3D virtual surface models from CBCT cross-sectional views. *A*: Shape analysis quantification of virtually simulated bone defects was validated compared with known values of simulated defects and allow quantification of corresponding 3D surface distances (Paniagua *et al.*, 2011). *B*: 3D surface models of a right TMJ condyle constructed from CBCT scans at the time of RA diagnosis (Timepoint 1 = T1), at 1-year (Timepoint 2 = T2) and 2-year follow-up (Timepoint 3 = T3). *C*: Quantification of changes using corresponding signed distances, where bone formation is shown in red and bone resorption in blue. In this condyle, bone resorption occurred as shown by subtracting the baseline model (T1) from the 1-year follow-up (T2) model. A partial repair of the erosion was visualized in the right image where the 1-year follow-up (T2) was subtracted from the 2-year follow-up (T3). Over the entire 2-year period (T3-T1), there was a net flattening of lateral pole of the condyle. The bar at the left of panel *C* represents the color scale of the magnitude of changes in surface contours between any two time points.

clinical protocols in order to support clinical decisions and to translate this knowledge to the needs of individual patients. Current quantification methods include volume measurements, landmark-based measurements, and analysis of surface models, as detailed below.

Volume measurements reflect an overall increase or decrease in size of an anatomic structure (Saccucci *et al.*, 2012). Structural changes at specific locations, however, are not reflected sufficiently in volume measurements. Volume assessment also does not reveal location and direction of

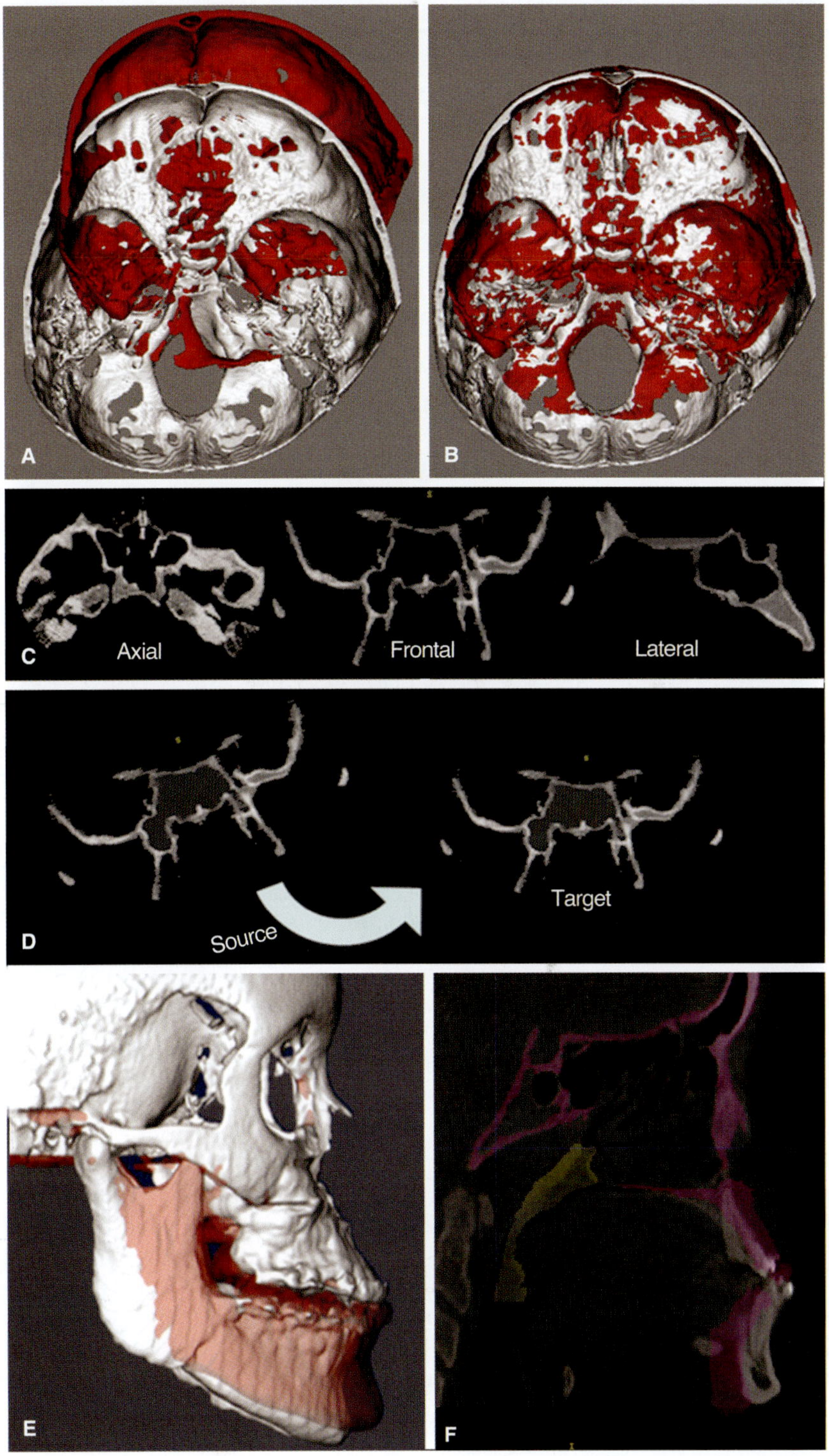

Figure 12.6 Cranial base registration of a patient who underwent jaw surgery. *A*: Pre-treatment cranial base model in white and post-surgery cranial base model in red. *B*: Matching of the pre- and post-treatment images on the cranial base is performed by voxel-based registration, shown in *C* and *D*. *C*: The post-surgery cranial base model (red in *A*), was used to mask all anatomic structures that changed with treatment to generate a gray-level intensity image containing only the cranial fossa for calculation of registration parameters. *D*: Fully automated calculation of rotational and translational parameters is performed to register the pre- and post-treatment images. *E*: Lateral view of the surface models overlayed in the cranial base showing the surgical displacements relative to the cranial base. *F*: CBCT gray-level sagittal cross-section with registered surface labels of post-treament models, showing the precision of cranial base fit using voxel-based registration.

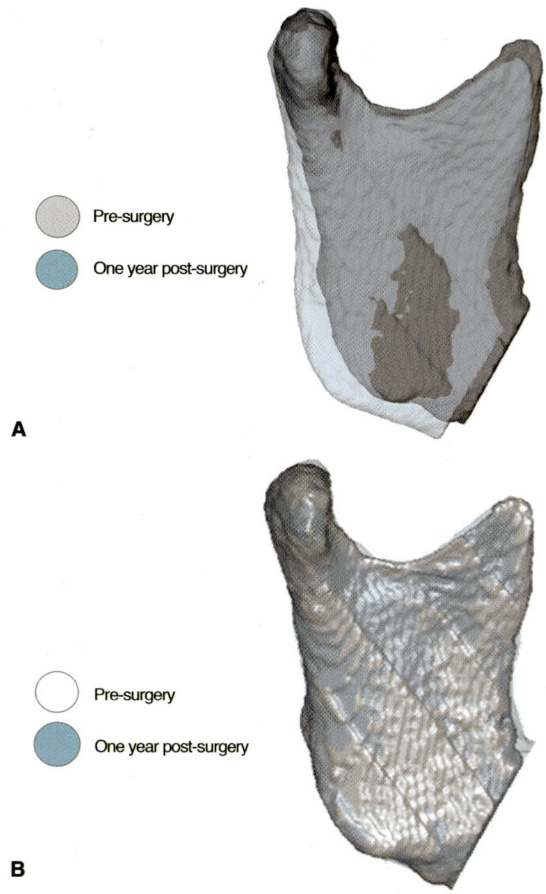

Figure 12.7 Comparison of mandibular ramus changes relative to (*A*) the cranial base to assess displacements and (*B*) the regional best fit to localize and assess bone remodeling.

proliferative or resorptive changes, which are relevant for assessment of clinical results or disease progression in the TMJ.

Another method for determining quantitative changes involves landmark-based measurements (Rohr, 2001). Because locating 3D landmarks on complex curving structures to represent components of craniofacial form is not a trivial problem (Dean *et al.*, 2000), this approach presents with limitations of errors related to landmark identification. As Bookstein (1991) noted, a lack of literature about suitable operational definitions exists for the landmarks in the three planes of space (coronal, sagittal, and axial). Although Gunz and coworkers (2004) and Andresen and associates (2000) proposed the use of semi-landmarks (i.e., landmarks plus vectors and tangent planes that define their location), it also is important to include information from whole curves and surfaces. The studies of Subsol and associates (1998) and Andresen and colleagues (2000) provided clear advances toward studies of curves or surfaces in 3D by referring to tens of thousands of 3D points in order to define geometry.

Finally, quantitative changes in the TMJ can be determined by the analysis of thousands of distances between registered surface models. Two common approaches for surface model analyses include measurements of the Closest Points between two surfaces and Shape Correspondence. Closest Point (CP) measurements between the surfaces at two time points can display changes with color maps, as proposed by Gerig and coworkers (2001). However, the CP method measures closest distances, not corresponding distances, between anatomical points on two or more longitudinally obtained images (Figure 12.8). For this reason, CP measurements completely fail to quantify large changes in bone during disease progression in a given patient and the differences in morphology between individuals.

In contrast to using thousands of arbitrary points in the surface meshes that often are not homologous points when using CP measurements between two registered surface models, Shape Correspondence computes corresponding or homologous point-based models in all registered models (Styner *et al.*, 2006). This method utilizes spherical harmonics-point distributed models (SHARM-PDM software) to determine anatomical correspondence or homology between thousands of points on different surfaces. The SPHARM-PDM software was developed as part of the National Alliance of Medical Image Computing (NA-MIC; NIH Roadmap for Medical Research) and has been adapted for the purpose of imaging of the hard tissues in the craniofacial complex (Paniagua *et al.*, 2010, 2011). The 3D virtual surface models are converted into a corresponding spherical harmonic description (SPHARM), which then is sampled into triangulated surface meshes (SPHARM-PDM). This work represents an improvement in outcome

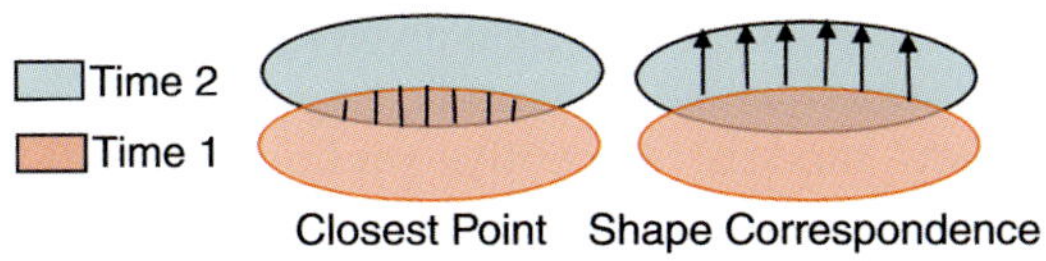

Figure 12.8 Diagram of two different methods, Closest Point surface measurements and Shape Correspondence measurements, to compute surface distances for quantifying longitudinal changes in condylar displacement. Note that the closest surface points fail to quantify the displacement when large translational changes occur. The Closest Points are linear distances (shown as lines), while the Shape Correspondence measurements are vectors (shown as lines with direction represented by arrows).

measurement as compared to CP correspondence-based analysis. CP still is the standard analysis used by most commercial and academic software, but it does not map corresponding surfaces based in anatomical geometry and usually underestimates rotational and large translational movements. For example, in the assessment of surgical outcomes, CP color maps measure surgical jaw displacement as the smallest separation between boundaries of the same structure, which may not be the correct anatomically corresponding boundaries on anatomical structures pre- and post-surgery (Figure 12.9).

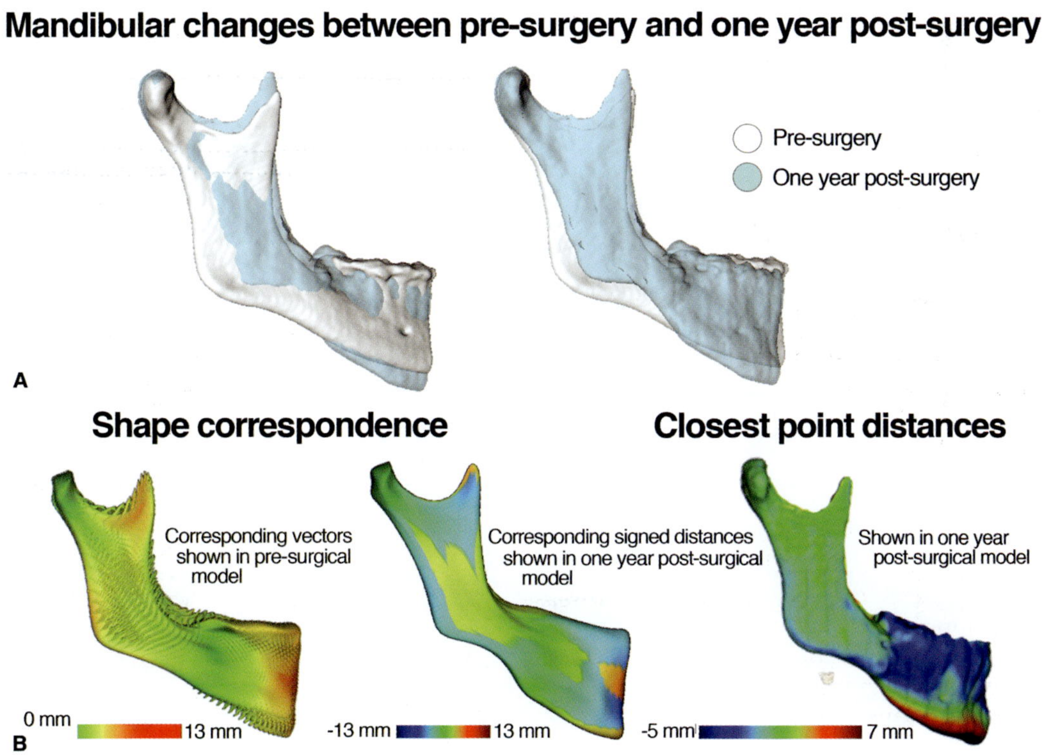

Figure 12.9 Mandibular 3D virtual surface models constructed from CBTCs of a patient where marked mandibular ramus bone resorption occurred after jaw surgery showing that Closest Point surface distances fail to quantify marked bone remodeling changes compared with Shape Correspondence. *A*: Two different versions of semi-transparent overlays of pre-surgery and 1-year post-surgery mandibular models to allow visualization of changes over time. *B*: Color maps using Shape Correspondence versus Closest Point surface distances demonstrate differences in measurements derived from the two methods for quantifying changes. The bars at the bottom represent the color scale of the magnitude of changes in surface contours determined through Shape Correspondence or Closest Point anlyses.

Statistical modeling of clinical and biological factors: integrated shape analysis

Statistical shape analyses can be carried out to test cross-patient group differences and to assess the correlation of morphologic variables with clinical and/or biological variables. The core of the ability to compute group mean and group variability (either parametric or nonparametric) is the correspondence procedure. This allows the association of any location on the condyle of Subject A with the correct location on the condyle of Subject B. Considerable intersubject variability also is accounted for in the model that captures the mean condylar morphology and variability around that mean morphology. A multivariate analysis of covariance is performed to estimate and compare group morphology models. Recently, preliminary studies have suggested that 3D virtual surface models can be used to detect and quantify even small bone changes in arthritic TMJ conditions (Cevidanes *et al.*, 2010; Paniagua *et al.*, 2010, 2011). Shape analysis of TMJ morphology potentially may enable the localization and quantification of previously unidentified bone tissue remodeling patterns and may reveal important relationships of morphologic variance to clinical signs and symptoms such as pain (Figure 12.10) as well as to biologic features (Helenius *et al.*, 2005; Wiese *et al.*, 2008a, 2008b; Hajati *et al.*, 2009, 2010).

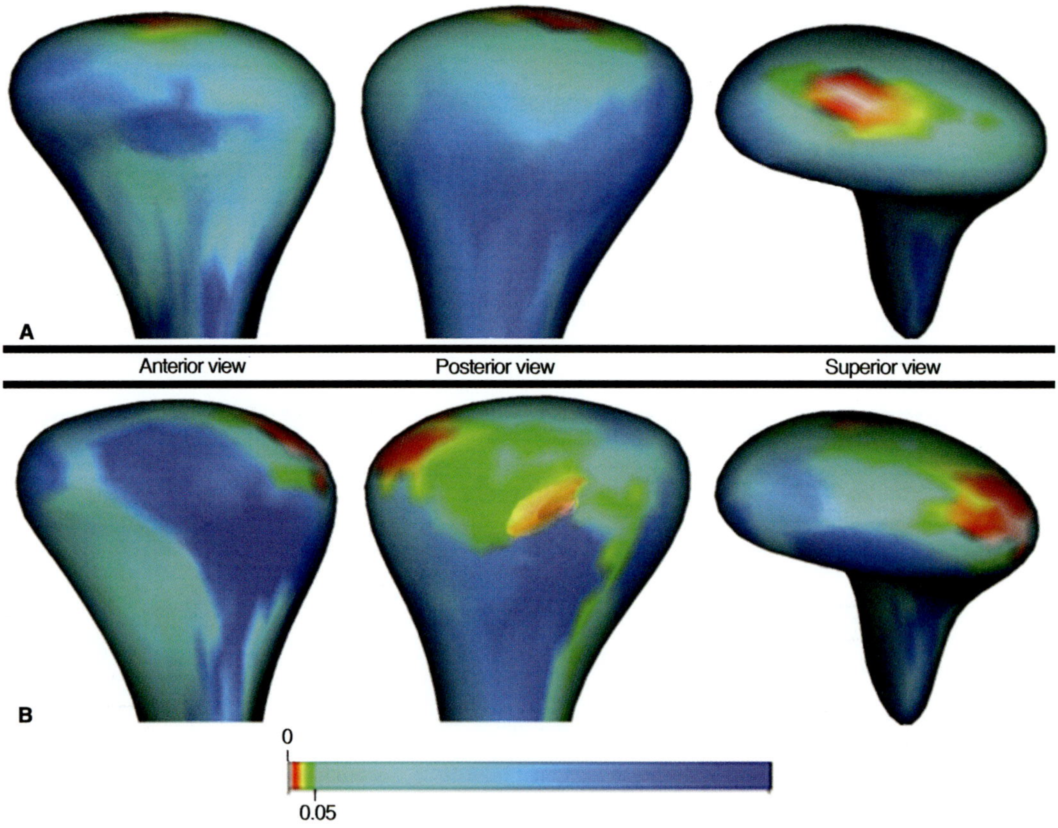

Figure 12.10 Statistical significance maps of correlations between local morphological differences in condylar shape and pain intensity. Significance maps show statistically significant correlations between pain intensity and morphologic differences in the superior surface of the condyle (*A*) and the lateral and posterior surfaces of the condyle (*B*). The color scale at the bottom represents correlation *p* values between pain and morphologic variance in the condyle relative to an average condyle.

Analysis of subchondral bone changes

Cross-sectional slices of CBCT or CT allow identification of subchondral cysts and diagnosis of subcortical sclerosis. Additionally, new image analysis applications for bone texture assessments now can elucidate the role of subchondral bone changes during the initiation, acceleration, and progression of arthritis. The bone beneath the fibrocartilage in the TMJ is the site of numerous dynamic morphological transformations, which are an integral part of the initiation of TMJ arthritis and not merely secondary manifestations of cartilage degradation. Altered bone morphology and associated mechanical properties are believed to influence articular cartilage integrity by distorting joint mechanics, leading to or enhancing joint degeneration.

MULTIDIMENSIONAL IMAGING AND NUMERICAL MODELING OF JAW BIOMECHANICS

Besides its utility visualizing the TMJ for disease diagnostics and responses to therapies, 3D imaging, combined with functional input of the muscles of mastication and central nervous system (CNS) increasingly is seen as key to understanding the pathogenesis of TMJD. This is because the functional and organizational adaptatio
and CNS may explain how the di
and symptoms progress and how p
logic processes could be mitigate... goal, the application of multidimensional imaging, in combination with computer-aided numerical modeling, has produced new insights and understanding of the normal function and pathomechanics of the human masticatory apparatus. The application of technologies to produce 3D and 4D data in human studies ranging from the CNS organization of the masticatory muscles to *in situ* TMJ disc mechanics and their likely clinical implications is summarized below.

3D geometry and CNS control of muscle activities

For static biting at a given position and in a given direction, the relationship between jaw muscle activity measured via electromyography (EMG) and bite force is predictable for nonfatiguing effort without feedback (Uchida *et al.*, 2002, 2008). The slope of this linear relationship varies as a function of the magnitude and sign (direction) of the 3D tooth-tipping moments produced by the bite forces (Figure 12.11). This relationship also is repeatable and reliable for a given bite-force position and

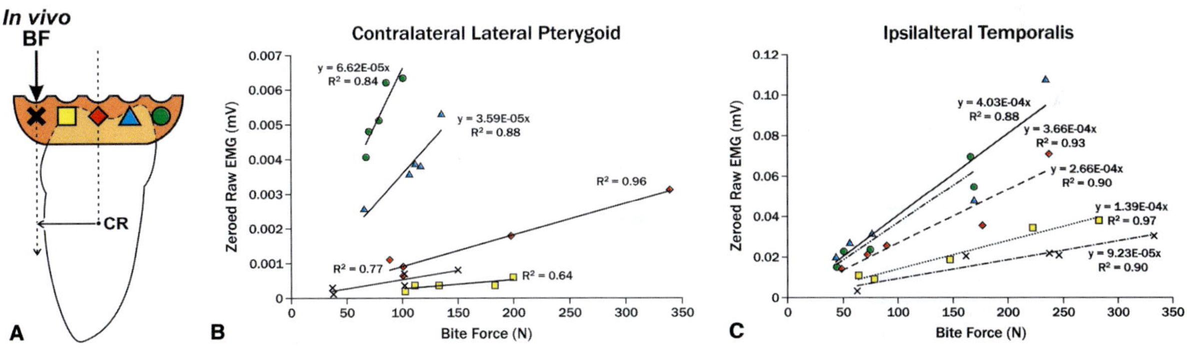

Figure 12.11 Biting tasks on the right molar (mesial view). *A*: To simulate the tooth tipping moments of modeled angular biting forces, progressive *in situ* biting at positions X, □, ◇, △, and ○ result in a progression from large + to − tipping moments due to the horizontal distance of biting force relative to the center of resistance (CR). Raw muscle activity (mV) versus biting force (N) plotted for the (*B*) contralateral lateral pterygoid and (*C*) ipsilateral temporalis muscles of one subject. Linear regression relations and slopes are shown for the five biting positions. Note that muscle activities per Newton of biting force for the contralateral lateral pterygoid muscle are highest during biting at the ○ position, which produces a lingual tipping moment. In contrast, this tipping moment is associated with the least amounts of ipsilateral temporalis muscle activities per Newton of bite force.

direction (Gonzalez *et al.*, 2011a). The distinct EMG bite-force relationship likely is due to CNS processing of periodontal mechanoreceptor information regarding the direction of load on the dentition and organizing of muscle outputs to support the applied load so that the jaw is steady. Data suggest that a complex relationship exists between direction of loading on the mandible and the CNS's regulation of muscle activities. This relationship is influenced by the 3D geometry of the anatomical components important to biting and the objective function employed by the CNS for control of the jaw musculature (Trainor *et al.*, 1995). Currently, objectives such as minimization of joint loads and minimization of muscle effort appear to fit the observed CNS organization of the muscles of mastication best during loading of the mandible. These and other objectives have been tested by comparing individual-specific numerical model predictions with individual-specific *in vivo* measurements (Nickel *et al.*, 2012). To date, these models have shown accuracies of 85–100% and have demonstrated that muscle responses to loads on the mandible are not obvious intuitively nor based on simple anatomical relationships such as the lines of action of the jaw muscles. These findings imply that muscles of mastication and their CNS control may regulate joint loads. A next step is to apply these validated models to explore and test clinical therapies with the potential to preserve and improve the health and longevity of the jaw muscles and TMJ tissues.

Symmetry and asymmetry of muscle organization

Computer-assisted numerical models using 3D geometries have been used primarily to study muscle forces and joint loads in healthy individuals (Nickel *et al.*, 2002, 2003; Iwasaki *et al.*, 2003a, 2003b), where it has been assumed that there is bilateral symmetry of CNS organization of the muscles of mastication. More recent studies have determined the accuracy of model-predicted muscle activation patterns in individuals with TMJD (Nickel *et al.*, 2012). During incisor biting, right-left symmetry of CNS organization of masticatory muscle output was more common in healthy individuals compared with TMJD subjects (Figure 12.12). The

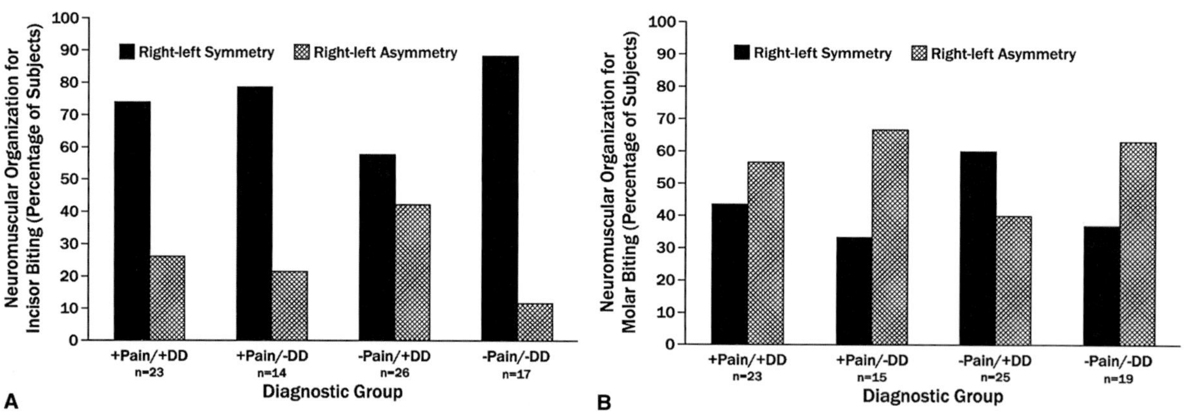

Figure 12.12 CNS organization of masticatory muscles. Ninety-one subjects participated in this study, which tested numerical model predicted muscle activities in healthy subjects and individuals with TMJD symptoms. The figures show the percentage of subjects in each diagnostic group showing symmetry (black columns) and asymmetry (striped columns) of neuromuscular organization during (*A*) incisor and (*B*) molar biting, based on matching of best-fit model type for right and left biting. Total numbers of subjects per group with bilateral data are indicated by "n." The diagnostic groups are designated with or without pain (+P or −P, respectively) and with or without disc displacement (+DD or −DD, respectively). Average model error in predicting muscle activities for all groups was ≤15% (Nickel *et al.*, 2012). Right-left symmetry in muscle organization was more common during incisor biting where nearly 90% of healthy individuals were symmetrical, while approximately 50–80% of sympotmatic subjects were symmetrical. In contrast, during molar biting, it was frequent to find within an individual muscle organization differing depending on biting side, which may reflect a preferred chewing side.

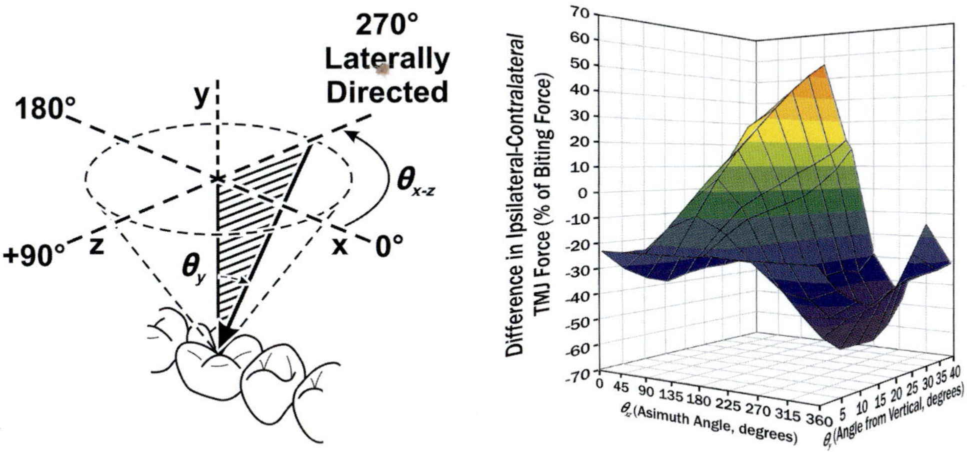

Figure 12.13 Difference in ipsilateral and contralateral TMJ forces averaged for seven subjects. Bite force (BF) angle (θ_y, θ_{xz}) where θ_y is the direction of the BF relative to the vertical axis, perpendicular to the occlusal plane, and varies between 0° and 40°; θ_{xz} (also known as the azimuth angle) is the direction of the BF in the occlusal plane and varies between 0° and 359°. Differences in TMJ forces are expressed as a percentage of a 100-unit bite force. Positive values (brighter colors) indicate that, on average, ipsilateral TMJ forces were larger than contralateral TMJ forces. Average differences in ipsilateral versus contralateral TMJ forces varied between +60% and −60% of the applied 3D bite force. A positive (+) value indicated that the ipsilateral TMJ force was relatively larger, and a negative (−) value, shown by darker colors, indicated that the contralateral TMJ force was relatively larger.

finding that TMJD subjects were more likely to have asymmetry in muscle organization during incisor biting may support the Pain Adaptation Model of muscle recruitment (Peck *et al.*, 2008), whereby the presence of pain contributes to a new recruitment strategy of motor units. The general consequences of asymmetry of neuromuscular objectives are that whenever minimization of muscle effort is invoked, loads increase on at least one TMJ (Iwasaki *et al.*, 2009b). Conversely, higher muscle forces are used to achieve minimization and equalization of TMJ loads when minimization of joint loads is desired (Trainor *et al.*, 1995).

CNS organization of muscle activation and TMJ loads

CNS control of the muscles of mastication affects the magnitude and direction of ipsilateral and contralateral TMJ loads (Iwasaki *et al.*, 2009b). Although it has been assumed that during unilateral biting the contralateral condyle is loaded more heavily, this is sometimes the case, but not always. In fact, validated numerical modeling indicates that differences in ipsilateral versus contralateral TMJ forces vary according to 3D bite-force direction (θ_y and θ_{xz}; Figure 12.13). Published data from seven healthy subjects showed ipsilateral versus contralateral joint load differences of +60% to −60% of the bite force, where a positive (+) value indicates that the ipsilateral TMJ force is relatively larger than contralateral TMJ force (Figure 12.13).

Validated numerical modeling was applied in another study of 17 healthy subjects and 17 individuals with TMJ disc displacement (Iwasaki *et al.*, 2009a). The objective was to explore between-group differences in mean ipsilateral and contralateral TMJ loads over various 3D biting angles. On average, subjects with TMJ disc displacement had higher relative predicted joint loads, especially during canine biting (Figure 12.14). These data support the hypothesis that TMJ disc failure is due to mechanical fatigue. Of course, magnitudes of load and consequent mechanical stresses are only one component in the fatigue of articulating tissues. Other potential contributing variables are frequency of load application and heritable traits

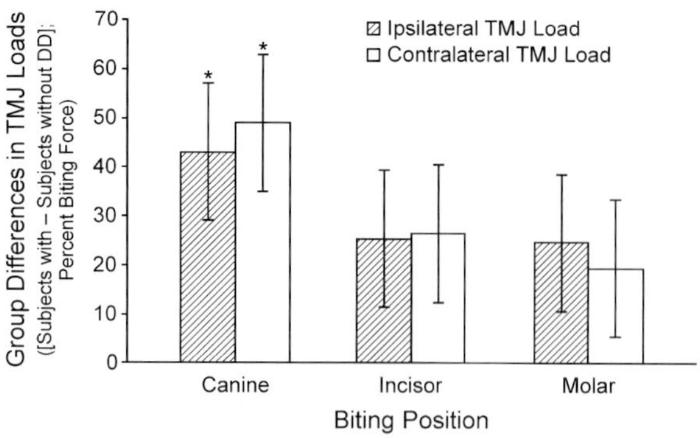

Figure 12.14 Between group differences in mean ipsilateral and contralateral TMJ loads for three biting positions. Mean differences between disc displacement (DD, $n = 17$) and normal disc position ($n = 17$) groups in ipsilateral and contralateral TMJ loads are plotted on the vertical axis. Differences in TMJ loads were expressed as a percentage of the applied bite force. Subjects with TMJ disc displacement had statistically higher joint loads of 40–50% (* indicates $P < 0.05$) during canine biting. During incisor and molar biting, joint loads in +DD subjects were >20% higher but were not statistically significant. (Reprinted with permission from Iwasaki *et al.*, 2009a.)

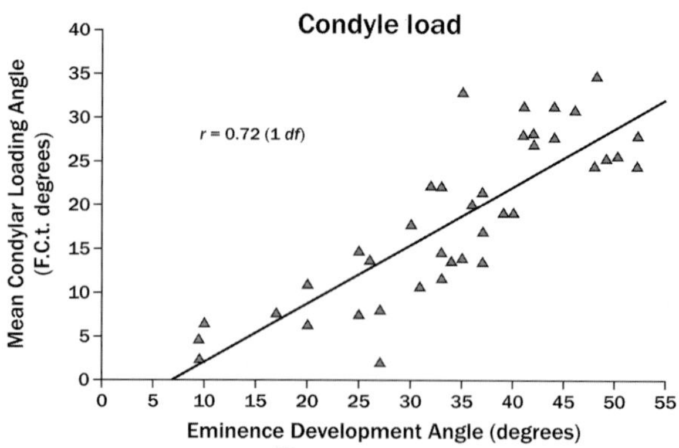

Figure 12.15 Mean condylar loading angle versus eminence development angle. The combination of CNS control of direction of joint load, together with changes in direction of joint load reflecting feeding behaviors, results in a linear relationship between the mean condylar loading angle and the eminence development angle. The data suggest that the development of the eminence is consistent with a CNS objective of minimization of joint loads. (Modified from Iwasaki *et al.*, 1997.)

involving genes such as ones that control inflammatory responses and sensitivity to pain.

3D space and time effects on TMJ growth, development, and degenerative joint disease

Development of the TMJ eminence begins before birth (Nickel *et al.*, 1988) and appears to develop in a manner that is consistent with minimization of joint loads (Iwasaki *et al.*, 2010). This objective and the previously described computer-assisted numerical models thus can be employed to predict individual-specific effective TMJ eminence shape based on the individual's 3D geometry. For a given geometry and this CNS objective, the model predicts joint load magnitude and direction for a specified jaw-loading situation, such as during suckling or biting. Modeling geometries and jaw-loading situations that reflected appropriate feeding behaviors (e.g., suckling, incisor biting, and unilateral molar biting) for a set of human craniomandibular specimens representing a range of developmental stages from pre- to post-natal showed a predictable linear relationship between the mean condylar loading angle and the eminence development angle (Figure 12.15). The maintenance of eminence morphology appears to depend on the 3D geometry of the muscles of mastication. Furthermore, asymmetries of muscle 3D geometry have been related to asymmetries in eminence morphology (de Zee *et al.*, 2009), phenomena that should be tested by validated numerical modeling in the future.

The mean age of onset of degenerative joint disease (DJD) in the TMJ is about 15–20 years earlier than the onset of DJD in other synovial joints such as the hip and knee (Lawrence *et al.*, 1989). The precocious breakdown of TMJ cartilages may reflect the energy densities imposed on these tissues compared with the tissues in other joints. Energy density is the mechanical work done to a tissue volume (mJ/mm^3) and has potential to effect the biomechanical and biochemical integrity of TMJ disc cartilage. The disc is a liability for degenerative joint changes because it is the primary mechanism for stress distribution and lubrication in the TMJ (Nickel *et al.*, 2001) with known sensitivities to loading rate and direction (Beatty *et al.*,

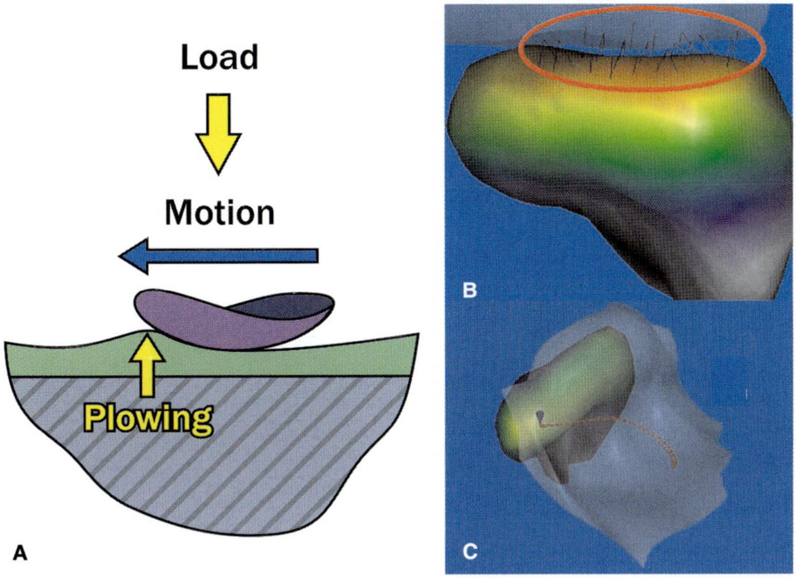

Figure 12.16 *A*: Plowing tractional forces associated with stress-field translation are a result of pressurization of the fluid within the cartilage matrix. Fluid pressurization results in application of mechanical strain on the collagen component of the cartilage. Rate of fatigue of the collagen fibers depends on the frequency and magnitude of strains applied. *B*: Frontal view of a subject's left TMJ, where the stress field was defined in the TMJ by finding the area of minimum condyle-fossa distance. For each sampling time of mandibular motion, the 30 smallest adjacent condyle-fossa distances, measured between polygon vertices, were identified. The centroid of this area was calculated and determined to be the mediolateral position of the stress field. *C*: Superior view of the path of the stress field during symmetrical opening and closing of a subject's left TMJ. The coordinates of the mediolateral position were smoothed over 30 ms, and the velocity of the stress-field translation (*V*, mm/s) was calculated. (Reproduced with permission from Nickel, J.C., Iwasaki, L.R., Gallo, L.M., *et al.* (2009) *Temporomandibular Disorders and Orofacial Pain: Separating Controversy from Consensus*. Monograph #46, The University of Michigan Craniofacial Growth Series, pp. 427–449.)

2001). The utility of 3D imaging when combined with real-time kinematics in a technique called dynamic stereometry (Palla *et al.*, 2003) has enabled the characterization of stress-field translation in synovial joints such as the TMJ (Figure 12.16; Gallo *et al.*, 2000, 2006) and the knee (Anderst & Tashman, 2010). Recent work has measured the variables involving TMJ stress-field translation and the consequent surface tractional forces that may contribute to disc wear and fatigue. Tractional forces on the surface of TMJ tissues are composed of plowing and frictional forces due to stress-field translation (Mow *et al.*, 1993). Laboratory studies have shown that frictional forces measured on the surface of the TMJ disc are low and tractional forces associated with plowing on the surface of the TMJ disc are 10 times greater than these frictional forces (Nickel *et al.*, 2006). Of particular note, the *in situ* translation of the TMJ stress field is mediolateral (Figure 12.16) in the direction where the TMJ disc has the lowest yield strength (Beatty *et al.*, 2001). This may be one of the reasons for the susceptibility of the TMJ disc to early failure.

Data recorded from human subjects suggest that average cumulative mechanical work done per open-close cycle of the mandible is higher significantly in TMJs of subjects with disc displacement by 18–23 times (Figure 12.17) compared with healthy subjects (Nickel *et al.*, 2009). Sex differences in average instantaneous work in TMJs with disc displacement were more than 350% higher in women compared with men. Average

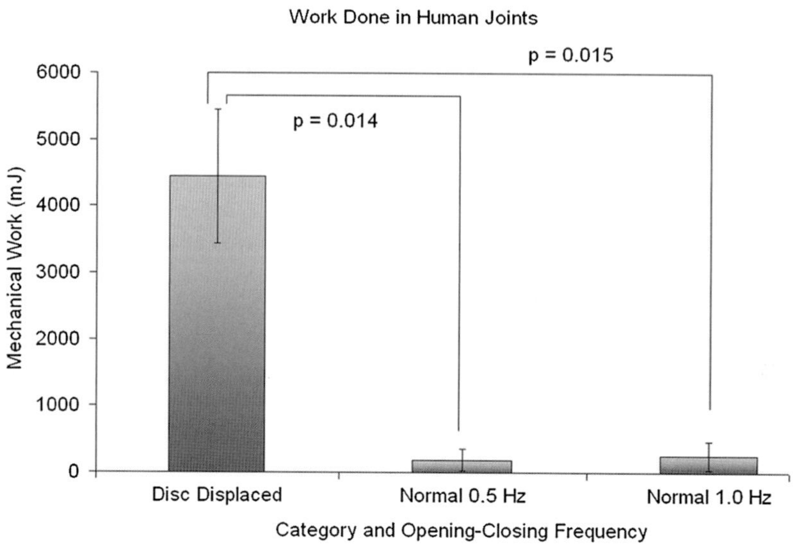

Figure 12.17 Average cumulative work done per cycle in healthy TMJs and TMJs with disc displacement. Data were calculated over 10 symmetrical opening/closing movements of the mandible at 0.5 and 1.0 Hz in healthy subjects and 1.0 Hz frequency in subjects with disc displacement. Subjects with disc displacement produced significantly more work during movement compared with healthy subjects. (Reproduced with permission from Nickel, J.C., Iwasaki, L.R., Gallo, L.M., *et al.* (2009) *Temporomandibular Disorders and Orofacial Pain: Separating Controversy from Consensus*. Monograph #46, The University of Michigan Craniofacial Growth Series, pp. 427–449.)

instantaneous energy densities per cycle (Figure 12.18) were relatively higher for females and the group with TMJ disc displacement, and were greater significantly by 3.4-fold in females with disc displacement compared with healthy males ($p < 0.04$). Within the TMJ disc displacement group, analysis of covariance showed that mean energy densities per cycle, adjusted for magnitude of joint loads, were greater significantly ($p < 0.05$) by 3.6-fold in females (4.3 mJ/mm^3) compared with males (1.2 mJ/mm^3). The differences in mechanical energy densities may be important to disc displacement and sex differences in the TMJ. These data provide further evidence of the sex bias in TMJD-related symptoms.

CONCLUSIONS

The capabilities of computer modeling, when combined with multidimensional imaging by means of CT, CBCT, and MRI technologies, will continue to produce new insights on the physiologic and pathologic changes of the TMJ structures as well as to CNS control of the masticatory muscles. Given the precocious development of TMJ arthritis, continuing investigations will focus on the interactions of biomolecular mechanisms, myofunctional dynamics and genetic factors in TMJ remodeling during growth, in tissue response to adaptive and orthopedic load, as well as risk assessments for degenerative reactions.

ACKNOWLEDGMENTS

The authors wish to thank the subjects who participated in the various protocols described. We thank Beatriz Paniagua and Martin Styner for their help in Shape Analysis and Mike Crosby, Luigi Gallo, Yoly Gonzalez, Jeff Kohlmeier, Dave Marx, Scott McCall, Gena McGivern, Matthew Moss, Tien Nguyen, Richard Ohrbach, Paul Robinson, and Laura Rothe for help in producing the data

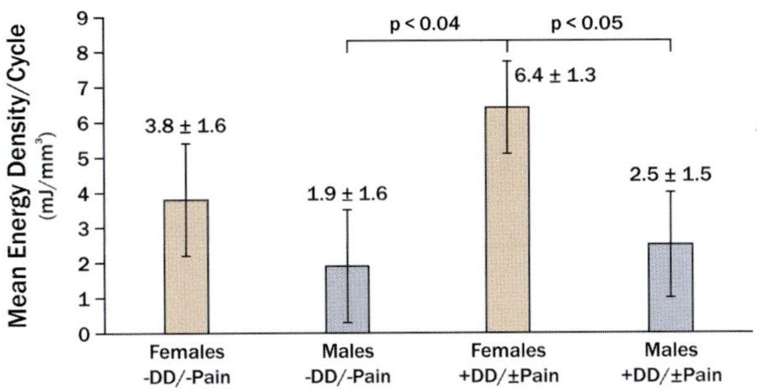

Figure 12.18 Sex differences in energy densities (ED) in healthy TMJs and subjects with TMJ disc displacement. This pilot study measured and compared energy densities in TMJs of 18 subjects (10 females, 8 males) with TMJ disc displacement (+DD) and 14 subjects (7 females, 7 males) without TMJ disc displacement (−DD). Imaging and kinematic data characterized each subject's intracapsular contact mechanics during symmetrical jaw closing. Numerical modeling was used to determine TMJ compressive loads (F_{normal}). Dynamic stereometry was used to measure the intracapsular variables required to estimate ED. ANOVA (group, sex) and ANCOVA (sex, single variable effects) were performed. Mean energy densities were higher relatively for females and the +DD group and were greater significantly in +DD females compared with −DD males ($p < 0.04$). Within the +DD group, ANCOVA showed that mean energy densities, adjusted for F_{normal}, were greater significantly ($p < 0.05$) in +DD females compared with +DD males.

presented on modeling geometries and jaw loading. Krista Evans, Aaron Jacobsen, Hongzeng Liu, Bobby Semitich, and Adam Shaver produced programs for data analysis. Theresa Speers and Elizabeth Piccolo helped in the recruitment and management of subjects. Kim Theesen, graphic artist, produced some of the figures. The data presented were made possible through funding from NIH/NIDCR (RO1DE016417 to J.N., RO3DE018962 to L.C., and RO1DE018455 to S.K.).

References

Abe, E., Ishimi, Y., Takahashi, N., *et al.* (1988) A differentiation-inducing factor produced by the osteoblastic cell line MC3T3-E1 stimulates bone resorption by promoting osteoclast formation. *Journal of Bone and Mineral Research*, 3 (6), 635–645.

Adams, R. & Bischof, L. (1994) Seeded region growing. *IEEE Transactions on Pattern Analysis and Machine Intelligence*, 16 (6), 641–647.

Ahmad, M., Hollender, L., Anderson, Q., *et al.* (2009) Research diagnostic criteria for temporomandibular disorders (RDC/TMD): development of image analysis criteria and examiner reliability for image analysis. *Oral Surgery, Oral Medicine, Oral Pathology, Oral Radiology, and Endodontics*, 107 (6), 844–860.

Aho, K., Heliövaara, M., Maatela, J., *et al.* (1991) Rheumatoid factors antedating clinical rheumatoid arthritis. *Journal of Rheumatology*, 18 (9), 1282–1284.

Aho, K., von Essen, R., Kurki, P., *et al.* (1993) Antikeratin antibody and antiperinuclear factor as markers for subclinical rheumatoid disease process. *Journal of Rheumatology*, 20 (8), 1278–1281.

Alexiou, K., Stamatakis, H., & Tsiklakis, K. (2009) Evaluation of the severity of temporomandibular joint osteoarthritic changes related to age using cone beam computed tomography. *Dentomaxillofacial Radiology*, 38 (3), 141–147.

Alkhader, M., Ohbayashi, N., Tetsumura, A., *et al.* (2010) Diagnostic performance of magnetic resonance imaging for detecting osseous abnormalities of the temporomandibular joint and its correlation with cone beam computed tomography. *Dentomaxillofacial Radiology*, 39 (5), 270–276.

Allaart, C.F., Goekoop-Ruiterman, Y.P., de Vries-Bouwstra, J.K., *et al.* (2006) Aiming at low disease activity in rheumatoid arthritis with initial combination therapy or initial monotherapy strategies: the BeSt study. *Clinical and Experimental Rheumatology*, 24 (6 Suppl 43), S77–S82.

Anderson, G.C., Gonzalez, Y.M., Ohrbach, R., *et al.* (2010) The research diagnostic criteria for temporomandibular disorders. VI: future directions. *Journal of Orofacial Pain*, 24 (1), 79–88.

Anderst, W.J. & Tashman, S. (2010) Using relative velocity vectors to reveal axial rotation about the medial and lateral compartment of the knee. *Journal of Biomechanics*, 43 (5), 994–997.

Andresen, R., Bookstein, F.L., Conradsen, K., *et al.* (2000) Surface-bounded growth modeling applied to human mandibles. *IEEE Transactions on Medical Imaging*, 19 (11), 1053–1063.

Beatty, M.W., Bruno, M.J., & Iwasaki, L.R. (2001) Strain rate dependent orthotropic properties of pristine and impulsively loaded porcine temporomandibular joint disk. *Journal of Biomedical Materials Research*, 57 (1), 25–34.

Bookstein, F.L. (1991) *Morphometric Tools for Landmark Data*. Cambridge University Press, Cambridge, UK.

Cairns, B.E. (2010) Pathophysiology of TMD pain: basic mechanisms and their implications for pharmacotherapy. *Journal of Oral Rehabilitation*, 37 (6), 391–410.

Carvalho Fde, A., Cevidanes, L.H., da Motta, A.T., *et al.* (2010) Three-dimensional assessment of mandibular advancement 1 year after surgery. *American Journal of Orthodontics and Dentofacial Orthopedics*, 137 (Suppl 4), S53.e1–S53e12.

Celiker, R., Gökce-Kutsal, Y., & Eryilmaz, M. (1995) Temporomandibular joint involvement in rheumatoid arthritis: relationship with disease activity. *Scandinavian Journal of Rheumatology*, 24 (1), 22–25.

Cevidanes, L.H., Bailey, L.J., Tucker, G.R., Jr., *et al.* (2005) Superimposition of 3D cone-beam CT models of orthognathic surgery patients. *Dentomaxillofacial Radiology*, 34 (6), 369–375.

Cevidanes, L.H.S., Hajati, A.-K., Paniagua, B., *et al.* (2010) Quantification of condylar resorption in temporomandibular joint osteoarthritis. *Oral Surgery, Oral Medicine, Oral Pathology, Oral Radiology, and Endodontics*, 110 (1), 110–117.

Conaghan, P.G., O'Connor, P., McGonagle, D., *et al.* (2003) Elucidation of the relationship between synovitis and bone damage: a randomized magnetic resonance imaging study of individual joints in patients with early rheumatoid arthritis. *Arthritis and Rheumatism*, 48 (1), 64–71.

Crow, H.C., Parks, E., Campbell, J.H., *et al.* (2005) The utility of panoramic radiography in temporomandibular joint assessment. *Dentomaxillofacial Radiology*, 34 (2), 91–95.

Dean, D., Hans, M.G., Bookstein, F.L., *et al.* (2000) Three-dimensional Bolton-Brush Growth Study landmark data: ontogeny and sexual dimorphism of the Bolton standards cohort. *Cleft Palate-Craniofacial Journal*, 37 (2), 145–155.

de Vos, W., Casselman, J., & Swennen, G.R. (2009) Cone-beam computerized tomography (CBCT) imaging of the oral and maxillofacial region: a systematic review of the literature: review. *International Journal of Oral and Maxillofacial Surgery*, 38 (6), 609–625.

De Zee, M., Cattaneo, P.M., Svensson, P., *et al.* (2009) Prediction of the articular eminence shape in a patient with unilateral hypoplasia of the right mandibular ramus before and after distraction osteogenesis: a simulation study. *Journal of Biomechanics*, 42 (8), 1049–1053.

Dworkin, S.F. & LeResche, L. (1992) Research diagnostic criteria for temporomandibular disorders: review, criteria, examinations and specifications, critique. *Journal of Craniomandibular Disorders*, 6 (4), 301–355.

Finzel, S., Rech, J., Schmidt, S., *et al.* (2011) Repair of bone erosions in rheumatoid arthritis treated with tumour necrosis factor inhibitors is based on bone apposition at the base of the erosion. *Annals of the Rheumatic Diseases*, 70 (9), 1587–1593.

Forslind, K., Ahlmen, M., Eberhardt, K., *et al.* (2004) Prediction of radiological outcome in early RA in clinical practice: role of antibodies to citrullinated peptides (anti-CCP). *Annals of the Rheumatic Diseases*, 63 (9), 1090–1095.

Forslind, K., Boonen, A., Albertsson, K., *et al.* (2009) Hand bone loss measured by digital X-ray radiogrammetry is a predictor of joint damage in early rheumatoid arthritis. *Scandinavian Journal of Rheumatology*, 38 (6), 431–438.

Galal, N., El Beialy, W., Deyama, Y., *et al.* (2008) Effect of estrogen on bone resorption and inflammation in the temporomandibular joint cellular elements. *International Journal of Molecular Medicine*, 21 (6), 785–790.

Gallo, L.M., Nickel, J.C., Iwasaki, L.R., *et al.* (2000) Stress-field translation in the healthy human temporomandibular joint. *Journal of Dental Research*, 79 (10), 1740–1746.

Gallo, L.M., Chiaravalloti, G., Iwasaki, L.R., *et al.* (2006) Mechanical work during stress-field translation in the human TMJ. *Journal of Dental Research*, 85 (11), 1006–1010.

Gerig, G., Jomier, M., & Chakos, M. (2001) Valmet: a new validation tool for assessing and improving 3D object segmentation. In Niessen, W. & Viergever, M. (eds.), *MICCAI 2001: Proceedings of the International Society and Conference Series on Medical Image Computing and Computer-Assisted Intervention 2001 October 14–17. Utrecht, Netherlands*. Springer, Berlin, pp. 516–528.

Gerig, G., Prastawa, M., Lin, W., *et al.* (2003) Assessing early brain development in neonates by segmentation of high-resolution 3T MRI. Short paper, Lecture Notes in Computer Science LNCS #2879, pp. 979–980.

Gonzalez, Y., Iwasaki, L.R., McCall, W.D., *et al.* (2011a) Reliability of electromyographic activity *vs.* bite-force from human masticatory muscles. *European Journal of Oral Sciences*, 119 (3), 219–224.

Gonzalez, Y.M., Schiffman, E., Gordon, S.M., *et al.* (2011b) Development of a brief and effective temporomandibular disorder pain screening questionnaire: reliability and validity. *Journal of the American Dental Association*, 142 (10), 1183–1191.

Greene, C.S. (2010) Management of patients with TMDs: a new "standard of care." *International Journal of Prosthodontics*, 23 (3), 190–191.

Gunz, P., Mitteroecker, P., & Bookstein, F.L. (2004) Semi-landmarks in three dimensions. In Slice, D.L. (ed.), *Modern Morphometrics in Physical Anthropology*. Kluwer Academic, New York.

Gynther, G.W., Tronje, G., & Holmlund, A.B. (1996) Radiographic changes in the temporomandibular joint in patients with generalized osteoarthritis and rheumatoid arthritis. *Oral Surgery, Oral Medicine, Oral Pathology, Oral Radiology, and Endodontics*, 81 (5), 613–618.

Hajati, A.K., Alstergren, P., Näsström, K., *et al.* (2009) Endogenous glutamate in association with inflammatory and hormonal factors modulates bone tissue resorption of the temporomandibular joint in patients with early rheumatoid arthritis. *Journal of Oral and Maxillofacial Surgery*, 67 (9), 1895–1903.

Hajati, A.K., Näsström, K., Alstergren, P., *et al.* (2010) Temporomandibular joint bone tissue resorption in patients with early rheumatoid arthritis can be predicted by joint crepitus and plasma glutamate level. *Mediators of Inflammation*, 2010, 627803.

Helenius, L.M., Hallikainen, D., Helenius, I., *et al.* (2005) Clinical and radiographic findings of the temporomandibular joint in patients with various rheumatic diseases: a case control study. *Oral Surgery, Oral Medicine, Oral Pathology, Oral Radiology, and Endodontics*, 99 (4), 455–463.

Honda, K., Larheim, T.A., Maruhashi, K., *et al.* (2006) Osseous abnormalities of the mandibular condyle: diagnostic reliability of cone beam computed tomography compared with helical computed tomography based on an autopsy material. *Dentomaxillofacial Radiology*, 35 (3), 152–157.

Honey, O.B., Scarfe, W.C., Hilgers, M.J., *et al.* (2007) Accuracy of cone-beam computed tomography imaging of the temporomandibular joint: comparisons with panoramic radiology and linear tomography. *American Journal of Orthodontics and Dentofacial Orthopedics*, 132 (4), 429–438.

Iwasaki, L.R., Nickel, J.C., & McLachlan, K.R. (1997) Relationship between growth, function, and stress in the temporomandibular joint. In McNeill, C. (ed.), *Science and Practice of Occlusion*. Quintessence, Chicago, IL.

Iwasaki, L.R., Baird, B.W., McCall, W.D., *et al.* (2003a) Muscle and temporomandibular joint forces associated with chincup loading predicted by numerical modeling. *American Journal of Orthodontics and Dentofacial Orthopedics*, 124 (5), 530–540.

Iwasaki, L.R., Petsche, P.E., McCall, W.D., *et al.* (2003b) Neuromuscular objectives of the human masticatory apparatus during static biting. *Archives of Oral Biology*, 48 (11), 767–777.

Iwasaki, L.R., Crosby, M.J., Gonzalez, Y., *et al.* (2009a) Temporomandibular joint loads in subjects with and without disc displacement. *Orthopedic Reviews (Pavia)*, 1 (2), 90–93.

Iwasaki, L.R., Uchida, S., Marx, D.B., *et al.* (2009b) Ipsilateral and contralateral human TMJ loads compared via validated numerical models. In Kapila, S.D. & McNamara, J.A., Jr. (eds.), *Temporomandibular Disorders and Orofacial Pain: Separating Controversy from Consensus*. Needham Press, Ann Arbor, MI, pp. 405–426.

Iwasaki, L.R., Crosby, M.J., Marx, D.B., *et al.* (2010) Human temporomandibular joint eminence shape and load minimization. *Journal of Dental Research*, 89 (7), 722–727.

Katzberg, R.W. (1990) Temporomandibular joint imaging. *Anesthesia Progress*, 37 (2–3), 121–126.

Koyama, J., Nishiyama, H., & Hayashi, T. (2007) Follow-up study of condylar bony changes using helical computed tomography in patients with temporomandibular disorder. *Dentomaxillofacial Radiology*, 36 (8), 472–477.

Lacey, D.L., Timms, E., Tan, H.L., *et al.* (1998) Osteoprotegerin ligand is a cytokine that regulates osteoclast differentiation and activation. *Cell*, 93 (2), 165–176.

Larheim, T.A. (2005) Role of magnetic resonance imaging in the clinical diagnosis of the temporomandibular joint. *Cells, Tissues, Organs*, 180 (1), 6–21.

Larheim, T.A., Westesson, P.L., Hicks, D.G., *et al.* (1999) Osteonecrosis of the temporomandibular joint: correlation of magnetic resonance imaging and histology. *Journal of Oral and Maxillofacial Surgery*, 57 (8), 888–898.

Larheim, T.A., Katzberg, R.W., Westesson, P.L., *et al.* (2001) MR evidence of temporomandibular joint fluid and condyle marrow alterations: occurrence in asymptomatic volunteers and symptomatic patients. *International Journal of Oral and Maxillofacial Surgery*, 30 (2), 113–117.

Lawrence, R.C., Hochberg, M.C., Kelsey, J.L., *et al.* (1989) Estimates of the prevalence of selected arthritic and musculoskeletal diseases in the United States. *Journal of Rheumatology*, 16 (4), 427–441.

Leeuw, R.D. (2008) *American Academy of Orofacial Pain. Orofacial Pain: Guidelines for Assessment, Diagnosis and Management*. 4th ed. Quintessence, Chicago, IL.

Lerner, U.H. (2006a) Bone remodeling in post-menopausal osteoporosis. *Journal of Dental Research*, 85 (7), 584–595.

Lerner, U.H. (2006b) Inflammation-induced bone remodeling in periodontal disease and the influence of postmenopausal osteoporosis. *Journal of Dental Research*, 85 (7), 596–607.

Lie, W.N. (1995) Automatic target segmentation by locally adaptive image thresholding. *IEEE Transactions on Image Processing*, 4 (7), 1036–1041.

Lieberman, J.M., Gardner, C.L., Motta, A.O., *et al.* (1996) Prevalence of bone marrow signal abnormalities observed in the temporomandibular joint using magnetic resonance imaging. *Journal of Oral and Maxillofacial Surgery*, 54 (4), 434–439.

List, T. & Axelsson, S. (2010) Management of TMD: evidence from systematic reviews and meta-analyses. *Journal of Oral Rehabilitation*, 37 (6), 430–451.

Look, J.O., John, M.T., Tai, F., *et al.* (2010a) The research diagnostic criteria for temporomandibular disorders. II: reliability of Axis I diagnoses and selected clinical measures. *Journal of Orofacial Pain*, 24 (1), 25–34.

Look, J.O., Schiffman, E.L., Truelove, E.L., *et al.* (2010b) Reliability and validity of Axis I of the research diagnostic criteria for temporomandibular disorders (RDC/TMD) with proposed revisions. *Journal of Oral Rehabilitation*, 37 (10), 744–759.

Ma, W.Y. & Manjunath, B.S. (2000) EdgeFlow: a technique for boundary detection and image segmentation. *IEEE Transactions on Image Processing*, 9 (8), 1375–1388.

Maixner, W., Diatchenko, L., Dubner, R., *et al.* (2011) Orofacial pain prospective evaluation and risk assessment study: the OPPERA study. *Journal of Pain*, 12 (Suppl 11), T4.e1-2–T11.e1-2.

McQueen, F.M., Benton, N., Perry, D., *et al.* (2003) Bone edema scored on magnetic resonance imaging scans of the dominant carpus at presentation predicts radiographic joint damage of the hands and feet six years later in patients with rheumatoid arthritis. *Arthritis and Rheumatism*, 48 (7), 1814–1827.

Michael, H., Härkönen, P.L., Väänänen, H.K., *et al.* (2005) Estrogen and testosterone use different cellular pathways to inhibit osteoclastogenesis and bone resorption. *Journal of Bone and Mineral Research*, 20 (12), 2224–2232.

Michelotti, A. & Iodice, G. (2010) The role of orthodontics in temporomandibular disorders. *Journal of Oral Rehabilitation*, 37 (6), 411–429.

Moon, N., Bullitt, E., Leemput, K., *et al.* (2002) Model-based brain and tumor segmentation. In *Proceedings of the 16th International Conference on Pattern Recognition 2002*, 1, pp. 528–531.

Motta, A.T., Cevidanes, L.H.S., Carvalho, F.A.R., *et al.* (2011) Three-dimensional regional displacements after mandibular advancement surgery: a 1-year follow-up. *Journal of Oral and Maxillofacial Surgery*, 69 (5), 1447–1457.

Mow, V.C., Ateshian, G.A., & Spilker, R.L. (1993) Biomechanics of diarthrodial joints: a review of twenty years of progress. *Journal of Biomechanical Engineering*, 115 (4B), 460–467.

National Institutes of Health Technology Assessment Conference on Management of Temporomandibular Disorders Bethesda, Maryland. April 29–May 1, 1996: proceedings. *Oral Surgery, Oral Medicine, Oral Pathology, Oral Radiology, and Endodontics*, 83 (1), 49–183.

Nickel, J.C., McLachlan, K.R., & Smith, D.M. (1988) Eminence development of the postnatal human temporomandibular joint. *Journal of Dental Research*, 67 (6), 896–902.

Nickel, J.C., Iwasaki, L.R., Feely, D.E., *et al.* (2001) The effect of disc thickness and trauma on disc surface friction in the porcine temporomandibular joint. *Archives of Oral Biology*, 46 (2), 155–162.

Nickel, J.C., Yao, P., Spalding, P.M., *et al.* (2002) Validated numerical modeling of the effects of combined orthodontic and orthognathic surgical treatment on TMJ loads and muscle forces. *American Journal of Orthodontics and Dentofacial Orthopedics*, 121 (1), 73–83.

Nickel, J.C., Iwasaki, L.R., Walker, R.D., *et al.* (2003) Human masticatory muscle forces during static biting. *Journal of Dental Research*, 82 (3), 212–217.

Nickel, J.C., Iwasaki, L.R., Beatty, M.W., *et al.* (2006) Static and dynamic loading effects on temporomandibular joint disc tractional forces. *Journal of Dental Research*, 85 (9), 809–813.

Nickel, J.C., Iwasaki, L.R., Gallo, L.M., *et al.* (2009) Tractional forces, work and energy densities in the human TMJ. In Kapila, S.D. & McNamara, J.A., Jr. (eds.), *Temporomandibular Disorders and Orofacial Pain: Separating Controversy from Consensus*. Needham Press, Ann Arbor, MI, pp. 427–450.

Nickel, J.C., Gonzalez, Y.M., McCall, W.D., *et al.* (2012) Muscle organization in individuals with and without pain and joint dysfunction. *Journal of Dental Research*, 91 (6), 568–573.

Ohrbach, R. (2010) Disability assessment in temporomandibular disorders and masticatory system rehabilitation. *Journal of Oral Rehabilitation*, 37 (6), 452–480.

Ohrbach, R., Turner, J.A., Sherman, J.J., *et al.* (2010) The research diagnostic criteria for temporomandibular disorders. IV: evaluation of psychometric properties of the Axis II measures. *Journal of Orofacial Pain*, 24 (1), 48–62.

Okeson, J.P. (1996) *Orofacial Pain: Guidelines for Assessment, Diagnosis and Management*. Quintessence, Chicago, IL.

Palla, S., Gallo, L.M., & Gossi, D. (2003) Dynamic stereometry of the temporomandibular joint. *Orthodontics & Craniofacial Research*, 6 (Suppl. 1), 37–47.

Paniagua, B., Cevidanes, L., Zhu, H., *et al.* (2010) Outcome quantification using SPHARM-PDM toolbox in orthognathic surgery. *International Journal of Computer Assisted Radiology and Surgery*, 6 (5), 617–626.

Paniagua, B., Cevidanes, L., Walker, D., *et al.* (2011) Clinical application of SPHARM-PDM to quantify temporomandibular joint osteoarthritis. *Computerized Medical Imaging and Graphics*, 35 (5), 345–352.

Peck, C.C., Murray, G.M., Gerzina, T.M., *et al.* (2008) How does pain affect jaw muscle activity? The Integrated Pain Adaptation Model. *Australian Dental Journal*, 53 (3), 201–207.

Peterfy, C.G., Schneider, E., & Nevitt, M. (2008) The osteoarthritis initiative: report on the design rationale for the magnetic resonance imaging protocol for the knee. *Osteoarthritis and Cartilage*, 16 (12), 1433–1441.

Petersson, A. (2010) What you can and cannot see in TMJ imaging: an overview related to the RDC/TMD diagnostic system. *Journal of Oral Rehabilitation*, 37 (10), 771–778.

Pfeilschifter, J., Köditz, R., Pfohl, M., *et al.* (2002) Changes in proinflammatory cytokine activity after menopause. *Endocrine Reviews*, 23 (1), 90–119.

Rantapää-Dahlqvist, S., de Jong, B.A., Berglin, E., *et al.* (2003) Antibodies against cyclic citrullinated peptide and IgA rheumatoid factor predict the development of rheumatoid arthritis. *Arthritis and Rheumatism*, 48 (10), 2741–2749.

Rohr, K. (2001) *Landmark-Based Image Analysis: Using Geometric and Intensity Models*. Volume 21 of Computational Imaging and Vision Series. Kluwer Academic, Dordrecht.

Ruf, S. & Pancherz, H. (1998) Temporomandibular joint growth adaptation in Herbst treatment: a prospective magnetic resonance imaging and cephalometric roentgenographic study. *European Journal of Orthodontics*, 20 (4), 375–388.

Ruf, S. & Pancherz, H. (1999) Temporomandibular joint remodeling in adolescents and young adults during Herbst treatment: a prospective longitudinal magnetic resonance imaging and cephalometric radiographic investigation. *American Journal of Orthodontics and Dentofacial Orthopedics*, 115 (6), 607–618.

Saccucci, M., Polimeni, A., Festa, F., *et al.* (2012) Do skeletal cephalometric characteristics correlate with condylar volume, surface and shape? A 3D analysis. *Head and Face Medicine*, 8 (1), 15.

Sanmartí, R., Gómez-Centeno, A., Ercilla, G., *et al.* (2007) Prognostic factors of radiographic progression in early rheumatoid arthritis: a two-year prospective study after a structured therapeutic strategy using DMARDs and very low doses of glucocorticoids. *Clinical Rheumatology*, 26 (7), 1111–1118.

Schiffman, E.L., Ohrbach, R., Truelove, E.L., *et al.* (2010a) The research diagnostic criteria for temporomandibular disorders. V: methods used to establish and validate revised Axis I diagnostic algorithms. *Journal of Orofacial Pain*, 24, 63–78.

Schiffman, E.L., Truelove, E.L., Ohrbach, R., *et al.* (2010b) The research diagnostic criteria for temporomandibular disorders. I: overview and methodology for assessment of validity. *Journal of Orofacial Pain*, 24 (1), 7–24.

Shevde, N.K., Bendixen, A.C., Dienger, K.M., *et al.* (2000) Estrogens suppress RANK ligand-induced osteoclast differentiation via a stromal cell independent mechanism involving c-Jun repression. *Proceedings of the National Academy of Sciences of the United States of America*, 97 (14), 7829–7834.

Shintaku, W.H., Venturin, J.S., Azevedo, B., *et al.* (2009) Applications of cone-beam computed tomography in fractures of the maxillofacial complex. *Dental Traumatology*, 25 (4), 358–366.

Smartt, J.M., Jr., Low, D.W., & Bartlett, S.P. (2005) The pediatric mandible. I: a primer on growth and development. *Plastic and Reconstructive Surgery*, 116 (1), 14e–23e.

Stoustrup, P., Küseler, A., Kristensen, K.D., *et al.* (2011) Orthopaedic splint treatment can reduce mandibular asymmetry caused by unilateral temporomandibular involvement in juvenile idiopathic arthritis. *European Journal of Orthodontics*, first published online October 3, 2011. doi:10.1093/ejo/cjr116.

Styner, M., Oguz, I., Xu, S., *et al.* (2006) Framework for the statistical shape analysis of brain structures using Spharm-PDM: special edition open science workshop at MICCAI. *Insight Journal*, 2006 (1071), 242–250.

Subsol, G., Thirion, J.P., & Ayache, N. (1998) A scheme for automatically building three-dimensional morphometric anatomical atlases: application to a skull atlas. *Medical Image Analysis*, 2 (1), 37–60.

Syversen, S.W., Gaarder, P.I., Goll, G.L., *et al.* (2008) High anticyclic citrullinated peptide levels and an algorithm of four variables predict radiographic progression in patients with rheumatoid arthritis: results from a 10-year longitudinal study. *Annals of the Rheumatic Diseases*, 67 (2), 212–217.

Tasaki, M.M., Westesson, P.L., Isberg, A.M., *et al.* (1996) Classification and prevalence of temporomandibular joint disk displacement in patients and symptom-free volunteers. *American Journal of Orthodontics and Dentofacial Orthopedics*, 109 (3), 249–262.

Trainor, P.G., McLachlan, K.R., McCall, W.D., *et al.* (1995) Modelling of forces in the human masticatory system with optimization of the angulations of the joint loads. *Journal of Biomechanics*, 28 (7), 829–843.

Truelove, E., Pan, W., Look, J.O., *et al.* (2010) The research diagnostic criteria for temporomandibular disorders. III: validity of Axis I diagnoses. *Journal of Orofacial Pain*, 24 (1), 35–47.

Uchida, S., Whittle, T., Wanigaratne, K., *et al.* (2002) Activity in the inferior head of the human lateral pterygoid muscle with different directions of isometric force. *Archives of Oral Biology*, 47 (11), 771–778.

Uchida, S., Iwasaki, L.R., Marx, D.B., *et al.* (2008) Variations in activities of human jaw muscles depend on tooth-tipping moments. *Archives of Oral Biology*, 53 (2), 199–205.

van der Heijde, D.M. (1995) Joint erosions and patients with early rheumatoid arthritis. *British Journal of Rheumatology*, 34 (Suppl 2), 74–78.

van der Heijde, D.M., van Leeuwen, M.A., van Riel, P.L., *et al.* (1992) Biannual radiographic assessments of hands and feet in a three-year prospective followup of patients with early rheumatoid arthritis. *Arthritis and Rheumatism*, 35 (1), 26–34.

van Dijke, C.F., Kirk, B.A., Peterfy, C.G., *et al.* (1997) Arthritic temporomandibular joint: correlation of macromolecular contrast-enhanced MR imaging parameters and histopathologic findings. *Radiology*, 204 (3), 825–832.

van Venrooij, W.J., van de Putte, L.B., & van den Hoogen, F.H. (2003) Anti-cyclic citrullinated peptide antibody in early rheumatoid arthritis: comment on the editorial by Scott. *Arthritis and Rheumatism*, 48 (3), 857.

Vittecoq, O., Incaurgarat, B., Jouen-Beades, F., *et al.* (2004) Autoantibodies recognizing citrullinated rat filaggrin in an ELISA using citrullinated and non-citrullinated recombinant proteins as antigens are highly diagnostic for rheumatoid arthritis. *Clinical and Experimental Immunology*, 135 (1), 173–180.

Wiese, M., Svensson, P., Bakke, M., *et al.* (2008a) Associations between temporomandibular joint symptoms, signs, and clinical diagnosis using the RDC/TMD and radiographic findings in temporomandibular joint tomograms. *Journal of Orofacial Pain*, 22 (3), 239–251.

Wiese, M., Wenzel, A., Hintze, H., *et al.* (2008b) Osseous changes and condyle position in TMJ tomograms: impact of RDC/TMD clinical diagnoses on agreement between expected and actual findings. *Oral Surgery, Oral Medicine, Oral Pathology, Oral Radiology, and Endodontics*, 106 (2), e52–e63.

Wiese, M., Wenzel, A., Hintze, H., *et al.* (2011) Influence of cross-sectional temporomandibular joint tomography on diagnosis and management decisions of patients with temporomandibular joint disorders. *Journal of Orofacial Pain*, 25 (3), 223–231.

Yura, S., Ooi, K., Kadowaki, S., *et al.* (2010) Magnetic resonance imaging of the temporomandibular joint in patients with skeletal open bite and subjects with no dentofacial abnormalities. *British Journal of Oral and Maxillofacial Surgery*, 48 (6), 459–461.

Zhao, N.N., Evans, R.W., Byth, K., *et al.* (2011) Development and validation of a screening checklist for temporomandibular disorders. *Journal of Orofacial Pain*, 25 (3), 210–222.

13 Characterization of the Upper Airway Morphology and Its Changes in the Apneic Patient Using Cone Beam Computed Tomography

R. Scott Conley, DMD, Paolo M. Cattaneo, MSc, PhD, and Bruce S. Haskell, DMD, MA, PhD

INTRODUCTION

The term "airway" refers to the air's path from the nose or mouth to the alveoli of the lungs, the conduit for which includes the nose, mouth, trachea, pharynx, bronchi, bronchioles, and lungs. The "upper" airway, which is the most frequently analyzed portion in orthodontics and oral maxillofacial surgery, is divided anatomically into three sections: the area from the nasal turbinate to the hard palate, called the nasopharyix; the retropalatal and retroglottal regions, known as the oropharynx; and the hypopharynx, which is contained between the tongue's base and the larynx (Schwab, 1998).

Since their discovery in the 1890s, X-rays have been utilized in many medical and dental disciplines for a wide variety of reasons. Since then, technological advances have resulted in an evolution of radiographic and nonradiographic methods for the diagnosis of airway diseases and malfunctions. Diagnostic imaging in orthodontics began in the late 1920s and early 1930s with the invention and widespread use of cephalometry (Broadbent, 1931). The "new technology of cephalometrics" adopted many of the direct anthropometric caliper-based measures performed on cadaveric skulls to radiographic projections of living patients that were obtained under standardized conditions of the lateral and frontal views. Since the end of World War II, cephalometrics has been applied widely and consistently to orthodontic diagnosis and has remained the gold standard for orthodontic imaging (Keim, 2009). Multiple angular and linear measurements are recorded and evaluated routinely for orthodontic diagnosis, treatment planning, assessment of treatment progress, and research purposes (Al-Balkhi, 2003). Although cephalometric images can be obtained in the posterior-anterior (PA) view, the lateral cephalometric view is the more common imaging method used for analyzing craniofacial and airway structures (White & Pae, 2009).

Cone Beam Computed Tomography in Orthodontics: Indications, Insights, and Innovations, First Edition. Sunil D. Kapila.

Cephalometric analysis has many limitations: perfect superimposition of bilateral structures is impossible to achieve, which, in turn, reduces the accuracy and validity of these films; magnification, distortion, and patient positioning errors limit traditional analysis (Quintero *et al.*, 1999); and airway analysis can be performed only in the anteroposterior but not in the lateral dimension (Ciscar *et al.*, 2001; Kim *et al.*, 2008). Due to the latter limitation, most cephalometric airway studies examine the hard and soft tissues surrounding the airway, rather than the airway space directly. The reproducibility of airway dimensions and tongue and hyoid positions on lateral cephalometric radiographs has proven to be unreliable (Malkoc *et al.*, 2005). These limitations have spurred the desire to create new imaging tools that represent the patient's airway anatomy more accurately and in a true three-dimensional (3D) manner.

The purpose of this chapter is to summarize several of the historical methods used to describe the airway, to discuss the limitations of these earlier methods, and to examine how new noninvasive low radiation dose and true 3D images enable the practitioner to better understand airway size, shape, and volume. Several initial investigations that have used this new technology to study the potential effects of clinical interventions on airway dimensional changes also are described.

TECHNOLOGICAL EVOLUTIONS IN AIRWAY ASSESSMENTS AND ANALYSES

In an attempt to overcome the deficiencies of assessing the airway on cephalograms, other nonradiographic methods of measuring upper airway including rhinometry, acoustic reflection, and magnetic resonance imaging (MRI) have been utilized. A rhinomanometer uses pressure transducers and miniaturized technology to provide data on both the nasal airflow and nasal pressures. Using this technology, researchers who have sought to identify whether there is any relationship between malocclusion and upper airway inadequacy have failed to demonstrate any such association (Solow *et al.*, 1984). With the failure of rhinometry to identify an association between compromised airway and malocclusion, investigators again turned to utilizing cephalometrics for studying the airway. A classic primate study performed to examine the effects of obligate mouth breathing induced by creating a nasal obstruction in primates showed inconsistent responses with the experimental animals, demonstrating variable adaptations and no direct correlation between oral or nasal respiration and type of malocclusion (Harvold *et al.*, 1981). This finding has held true for orthodontic patient populations as well. Thus, while practitioners may suspect oral breathing in some facial types such as long faces, vertical maxillary excess, and adenoid faces, the mode of respiration has not been correlated consistently and definitively to facial morphology (Kluemper *et al.*, 1995).

Acoustic reflection, which combines a rhinomanometer for nasal airway and a pharyngometer for upper airway patency determinations, is another nonradiographic method for assessing airway. The two are connected to a monitor that shows both the cross-sectional areas and volumetric data at different sites throughout the airway (El & Palomo, 2011). This method was popular due to the lack of radiation exposure and relative ease of use and is the only method used in multiple studies that have examined the airway of normal, healthy individuals (Brown *et al.*, 1986; Brooks & Strohl, 1992; Martin *et al.*, 2006). Martin and colleagues' study (1997) examined the effect of age, sex, obesity, and posture on upper airway size in both the upright and supine positions. It concluded that the upper airway decreases in size with increasing age in both men and women and that men have greater airway collapsibility in the supine position than women. While men may have a larger airway (Brooks & Strohl, 1992), this increased susceptibility to airway collapse may explain some of the differences in incidence of obstructive sleep apnea (OSA) between the two sexes. Additional studies show a negative correlation of pharyngeal airway cross-section with age in males and no differences between men and women when accounting for body size (Brown *et al.*, 1986).

Prior to the advent of cone beam computed tomography (CBCT), MRI and computed tomography (CT) were the only 3D imaging tools available. CT, which first emerged in the 1970s, transformed diagnostic radiology but subjected the patients to high radiation exposure levels (Brenner & Hall,

2007). Unfortunately, conventional CT scanners also are large and expensive and have limited resolution in the vertical plane of space (Maki *et al.*, 2003). Since CTs typically are available primarily in hospitals or imaging centers, they are not suitable for routine orthodontic records or airway surveys.

MRI creates both static and dynamic 3D images by using a magnetic field to manipulate hydrogen ions that are present in large quantities in the human body (Patel *et al.*, 2006). Some benefits of MRI include its capacity to convey high tissue contrast and accurate pictures, 3D flexibility, noninvasiveness, and the high sensitivity and specificity of the generated images, especially for soft tissues. An updated approach called volumetric MRI is capable not only of generating 3D images, but also of obtaining the volume of organs or systems. This approach has been demonstrated to be beneficial for the quantitative determination of certain airway risk factors (Schwab *et al.*, 2003). MRI also has some weaknesses, including the scatter produced by metal orthodontic appliances and isolated reports of significant complications such as injury from dislodgement of ferromagnetic materials as well as induced electrical currents and excessive heating (Patel *et al.*, 2006); however, methods for safe imaging have been described (Klocke *et al.*, 2005, 2006).

CBCT scanners enable a single rotation of the unit to generate a scan of the entire head and have significantly lower radiation levels relative to multi-slice CTs (MSCT) that make CBCT a practical choice for dentistry (Maki *et al.*, 2003; see also Chapter 2). By producing sagittal, axial, and coronal images, CBCT provides true 3D anatomically accurate views that are not attainable in traditional two-dimensional (2D) planar radiologic imaging. Using both proprietary and open-source software, the images can be viewed in any possible orientation. As discussed in several chapters of this book, images generated from these views already have proven to be useful in diagnosis and treatment planning of impacted teeth, surgical orthodontic care and temporomandibular joint (TMJ) pathology (Kapila *et al.*, 2011), planning of dental implants, pathological lesion identification, supernumerary teeth location, mixed dentition planning, and airway analysis (Kau *et al.*, 2005).

The limitations of cephalometry in the analyses of airway include the inherent errors in representing a 3D structure in 2D and lack of ability to provide information on cross-sectional area and volume. This has been validated further in the study by Lenza and associates (2010), who concluded that the morphology of the upper airway cannot be depicted accurately using sagittal or transversal linear measurements because these variables have a poor correlation with airway cross-sectional area and volume in CBCTs, findings that are verified further by ours, described below. Moreover, calculating upper airway volume alone does not give accurate information with respect to the most constricted cross-sectional area. Therefore, a complete analysis with linear measurements, area, and volume likely is necessary to assess the complex 3D structure of the upper airway correctly.

Prior to adapting a new technology such as CBCT to examine the airway, its measurement accuracy and reliability must be validated. Both linear and angular measurements from CBCTs have been shown to be highly accurate with a measurement accuracy of up to 0.1 mm, which is insignificant clinically (Lagravère *et al.*, 2008). Furthermore, analysis of the airway using an airway phantom has demonstrated excellent accuracy and reliability of CBCTs in airway area and volume measurements (Aboudara *et al.*, 2009; Schendel & Hatcher, 2010).

A second requirement for application of CBCT imaging to assess airways is establishing normative data on airway dimensions that would be highly valuable to serve as guidelines for diagnostics or therapeutics for airway disorders. Due to the relative inaccessibility of 3D images of the normal adult airway, there currently are no published norms for its dimensions and volume (Osorio *et al.*, 2008). However, because CBCT scans increasingly are being used to evaluate otherwise healthy individuals for various dental treatments, the availability of these scans will enable the determination of population normative values for the airway volume and cross-sectional areas. Thus, the application of CBCT in dental practices and the pooling of these resources likely will provide a good source of data to further our knowledge and to establish and refine normative values for the airways.

RELEVANCE OF THE AIRWAY TO ORTHODONTICS

Relationship of airway to skeletal morphology

The upper airway is surrounded, shaped, and supported by soft tissue and skeletal structures. The soft tissue structures that encompass the upper airway are the nasopharynx superiorly, the maxilla-mandibular complex and the posterior part of the soft palate anteriorly, the spinal column posteriorly, and the epiglottis inferiorly. The skeletal structures that delimit the upper airway include the cranial base superiorly, the vertebral column posteriorly, the nasal septum antero-superiorly, and the posterior aspect of the maxilla and mandible as well as the hyoid bone that partially embraces the oropharynx anteriorly. Therefore, it seems logical that the skeletal patterns should have a role in determining the morphology of the upper airway and vice versa (Solow & Kreiborg, 1977; Harvold *et al.*, 1981; Vig, 1998).

In an attempt to solve part of the controversy on any relationship between 2D and 3D airway dimensions as well as between upper airway morphology and craniofacial parameters, 30 CBCT scans of 14- to 35-year-old non-apneic subjects equally divided between Class I, II, and III were analyzed. An analysis was developed utilizing 41 cephalometric landmarks to describe maxillo-mandibular relationships and airway dimensions. The upper airway morphology was assessed by linear, surface, and volume measurements using a previously described procedure (Lenza *et al.*, 2010). Six sagittal linear measurements as described previously (Linder-Aronson, 1970; Holmberg & Linder-Aronson, 1979) and paired transverse (coronal) dimensions of the upper airway were determined (Figure 13.1A). To calculate the cross-sectional areas, total airway volume, and partial airway volumes, the upper airway was segmented from the CBCT using a semi-manual segmentation, as it has been shown to be more accurate and minimizes the systematic errors in "automated" volume segmentation (El & Palomo, 2010). The airway boundary and partial segmentations were divided into five partial volumes (Figure 13.1B) delineated by the six sagittal cross-sections described above (Figure 13.1A).

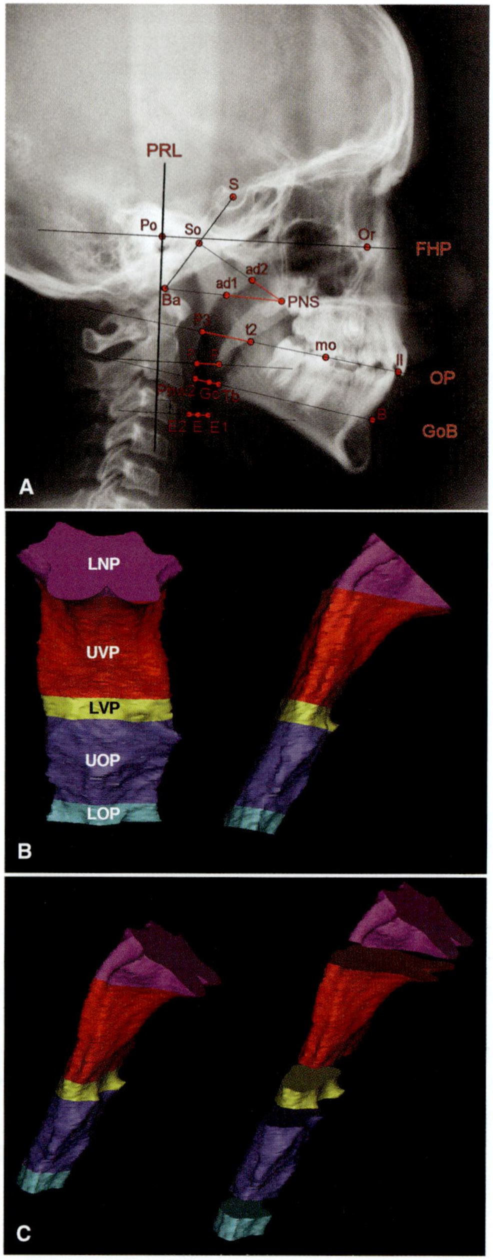

Figure 13.1 *A*: Six sagittal linear airway measurements from PNS to ad2, PNS to ad1, t2 to P3, P to P′, GoTb to PhW2, and E1 to E2. *B* and *C*: Using these landmarks, the airway volume can be divided into the lower nasopharynx (LNP), upper velopharynx (UVP), lower velopharynx (LVP), upper oropharynx (UOP), and lower oropharynx (LOP) and analyzed as one entire volume or subdivided into its component portions (left image in *C*).

Overall, the 2D sagittal and transverse dimensions were not correlated consistently with the cross-sectional areas of the airway at the six sites measured. The 2D sagittal measurements correlated with the 3D cross-section area only for the two most superior portions of the airway in the area of the nasopharynx. Although the linear transverse measurements at the level of upper velopharynx (UVP), lower velopharynx (LVP), upper oropharynx (UOP), and lower oropharynx (LOP) are fairly reliable, good correlation between sagittal and transverse measurements and the corresponding partial volumes exist only for the lower nasopharynx (LNP). Only a weak correlation between the minimum sagittal linear airway distance and the minimum cross-sectional area of the upper airway was found. This suggests that use of the antero-posterior (AP) linear dimensions alone is insufficient to predict the minimum cross-sectional area accurately. Neither the minimum cross-section nor the total volume of the upper airway correlated with Class I, II, or III skeletal pattern, a finding that may be attributable to the large variation in morphology of the airway (Figure 13.2). For this reason, a series of indices that describe the craniofacial proportions was made to

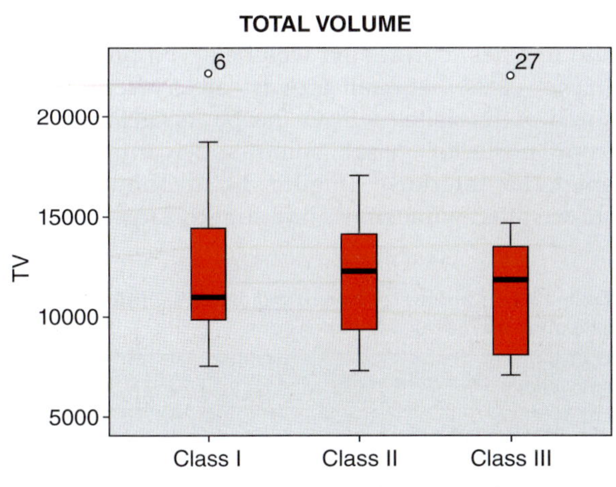

Figure 13.2 Box plot of the total volume (TV) of airway in Class I, II, and III subjects. The median value (black line) is not different significantly between the groups. Note the large variability in patient airway volumes among all three skeletal classifications and that the airway volume for Class III patients demonstrates less variability than that of Class I and Class II patients.

scale the measured airway volume of each subject to the craniofacial proportions and dimensions of the average subject. This adjustment resulted in slight improvement in the correlation between cross-sectional area, airway volume, and skeletal patterns, but still failed to reach statistical significance. The results strongly suggest that the craniofacial pattern on its own is insufficient to describe the morphology of the upper airway and that more sophisticated indices, possibly including other variables such as body mass index (BMI), height, and posture, may be necessary for better understanding the determinants of airway dimensions.

Effects of rapid palatal expansion (RPE) on airway

Because rapid palatal expansion (RPE) increases palatal width and has been advocated by some clinicians for alleviating OSA, the next logical question to address is whether this treatment modality has any effect on nasal cavity size, airway dimensions, and airway resistance. A study of 38 subjects (Oliviera De Felippe *et al.*, 2008) using 3D imaging and acoustic rhinometry demonstrated a mean short-term reduction in nasal airway resistance concomitant with a mean increase in palatal area, volume, and intermolar distance. In the long term, the mean palatal area and intermolar distances regressed toward pre-treatment values, but the nasal cavity volume and minimal cross-sectional airway increased. It is unclear why the nasal cavity dimensions continued to increase even though the palatal and molar dimensions reverted to pre-treatment levels. However, it is plausible that since the studies were performed in growing patients, the airway increases reflect growth of the nasal cavity, while the decreases in palatal and intermolar dimensions reflect post-expansion relapse. It also is possible that environmental factors such as allergens, allergic rhinitis, or seasonal viruses may have been more prevalent at pre-treatment, leading to an artificially reduced nasal volume. Clearly, additional work remains to be performed to address further the relationship, if any, between RPE and changes in nasal airway dimensions and into its possible therapeutic efficacy in OSA.

AIRWAY PARAMETERS IN HEALTHY AND APNEIC SUBJECTS

Obstructive sleep apnea (OSA)

OSA is one of the most widely studied airway diseases. Individuals with OSA experience recurrent collapse of the airway most often during sleep (Ogawa *et al.*, 2007). An apnea is defined as a breathing cessation of greater than 10 seconds; a hypopnea is a 50% breathing reduction or a significant drop in O_2 saturation (Ingman *et al.*, 2004). The clinical signs of OSA include morning headaches, sleepiness during daytime, impotence, lowered libido, mood swings, impaired memory and concentration, intensive snoring, and depression. Patients afflicted with OSA have a high risk of developing coronary artery stenosis, hypertension, and ischemic stroke due to frequent breathing cessation (Ingman *et al.*, 2004).

OSA is much more common in males than in females (Bixler *et al.*, 2001). One theory for this sex difference is that males and females have structurally and functionally different upper airways (Mohsenin, 2001). Another theory is that hormonal differences between men and women could influence the airway. This theory is supported by multiple studies that have demonstrated that post-menopausal women on hormone replacement therapy (HRT) have decreased risk of OSA compared with post-menopausal women not on HRT (Bixler *et al.*, 2001; Kapsimalis & Kryger, 2002). Since obesity is a significant risk factor for OSA (Guilleminault *et al.*, 1988) and animal studies show that ovariectomized rats in the absence of estrogen replacement gain weight (Zoth *et al.*, 2012), the higher risk of OSA in women not on HRT may result due to their greater potential for developing obesity than women undergoing HRT. While studies have been unable to pinpoint the factors contributing to these sex differences for OSA, they nevertheless indicate that these likely arise from variables other than age, BMI, or neck circumference (Dancey *et al.*, 2003).

Although medical and dental practitioners have attempted to describe changes in the airway associated with OSA for decades (Guilleminault *et al.*, 1976; Lowe *et al.*, 1995), research data and opinions continue to vary widely. Furthermore, there currently are inadequate data available to help distinguish normal from abnormal anatomical airway characteristics. One common etiology of this condition is obstruction or occlusion of the upper airway (Ogawa *et al.*, 2007). The fact that this compromised airway patency, as one etiologic factor of OSA, can be treated through orthodontics/orthognathic surgery, together with its high morbidity and mortality, have contributed to substantial interest in this disease among orthodontists and oral and maxillofacial surgeons in OSA (Ingman *et al.*, 2004).

Normal adult airway

To begin to address whether the airway dimension may be altered locally, regionally, or in its entirety, it is important to establish normative data, preferably that are age- and sex-specific. Toward this goal, a recent cross-sectional retrospective investigation determined airway dimensions of 539 females and 233 males aged between 18 and 69 years that provided an adequate sample size when divided by sex and by decade of life (Table 13.1; Smith *et al.*, 2009). These adult patients had undergone CBCT for either pre-prosthetic purposes, orthodontics, or occasionally to rule out TMJ pathology. Also, routine cephalometric projections of this sample demonstrated that both the males and females represented well-balanced profiles.

The cross-sectional airway areas were measured at five sites within the pharyngeal airway from posterior nasal spine superiorly to the epiglottis inferiorly (Figure 13.3). The findings showed that while males had slightly larger airway

Table 13.1 Sample size by sex and age of subjects used to determine normal airway dimensions.

	Age in years				
	18–29	30–39	40–49	50–59	60+
Number of male patients	41	40	51	45	56
Number of female patients	105	86	131	118	99

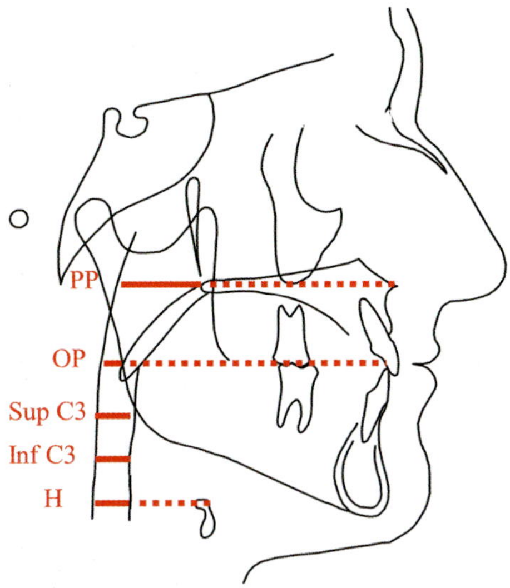

Figure 13.3 Sites at which airway cross-sectional areas were derived to determine normative airway values of adult male and female subjects. Airway cross-sectional dimensions were determined at five levels of the airway on a plane parallel to the palatal plane (PP) at PP, occlusal plane (OP), tangent to the superior aspect of C3 (Sup C3), tangent to the inferior of C3 (Inf C3), and tangent to the hyoid (H).

cross-sections than females in the lower pharynx, these differences were minor and not significant statistically (Figure 13.4). The male airway was longer and of a larger volume than the female airway. Few to no age-related changes were observed in airway cross-section at the palatal plane, inferior aspect of C3, and at the hyoid in both males and females. However, there were strong and consistent trends toward decreased airway cross-sections with age at the occlusal plane and superior aspect of C3, in both male and female subjects that, at the occlusal plane, was more marked for females than males. One interesting finding was the location of the minimum airway cross-section that moved more inferiorly in males than in females with age. The possible ramifications of this finding will be discussed in context of the abnormal airway, particularly in the OSA patient, later in this chapter.

This investigation provides valuable new data for age-related norms for the airway. Much like orthodontic cephalometric norms, these 2D and 3D airway normative values potentially can be used as an aid when examining patients with pathologic airway, such as those with OSA. While these normal airway values are important, studies correlating airway data with that from overnight polysomnography (PSG) are required to validate the sensitivity and specificity of CBCT airway imaging in the diagnosis of OSA and support relevance of these norms for diagnostic purposes. Until such a determination is made, these will remain a clinically useful guide only. If validated through functional studies, some potential future clinical applications of these airway norms include their use in assessing orthognathic surgery patients. For example, adult orthodontic/orthognathic surgery patients with decreased airway dimensions may require additional inquiries into clinical history, objective testing, and medical attention prior to definitive treatment plans being developed, which in the presence of OSA can be directed toward addressing various structural anatomical deficiencies in the airway. Thus, in an individual with mandibular prognathism and OSA, a preferred treatment option may be maxillary advancement rather than mandibular setback, which could aggravate the apnea further.

2D imaging and OSA

Most cephalometric studies examining the airway typically have compared OSA patients as verified by overnight PSG to matched controls. The findings on the differences between controls and OSA patients from these studies have been varied. Some of this variation can be explained by differences in control groups that were utilized, which included either age and/or sex-matched controls (Tangugsorn *et al.*, 2000; Finkelstein *et al.*, 2001), age- and size-matched controls (Mayer *et al.*, 1996), or an incompletely described control group, leaving the reader to infer the demographics and reliability of the comparisons. Overall, due to the limited sample sizes and varied types of controls utilized, the anatomic characteristics described in these control groups may not be applicable generally to the entire population.

Many differences have been reported in the anatomy of the structures neighboring or related to the airways between OSA and control groups. These include an increased distance between the

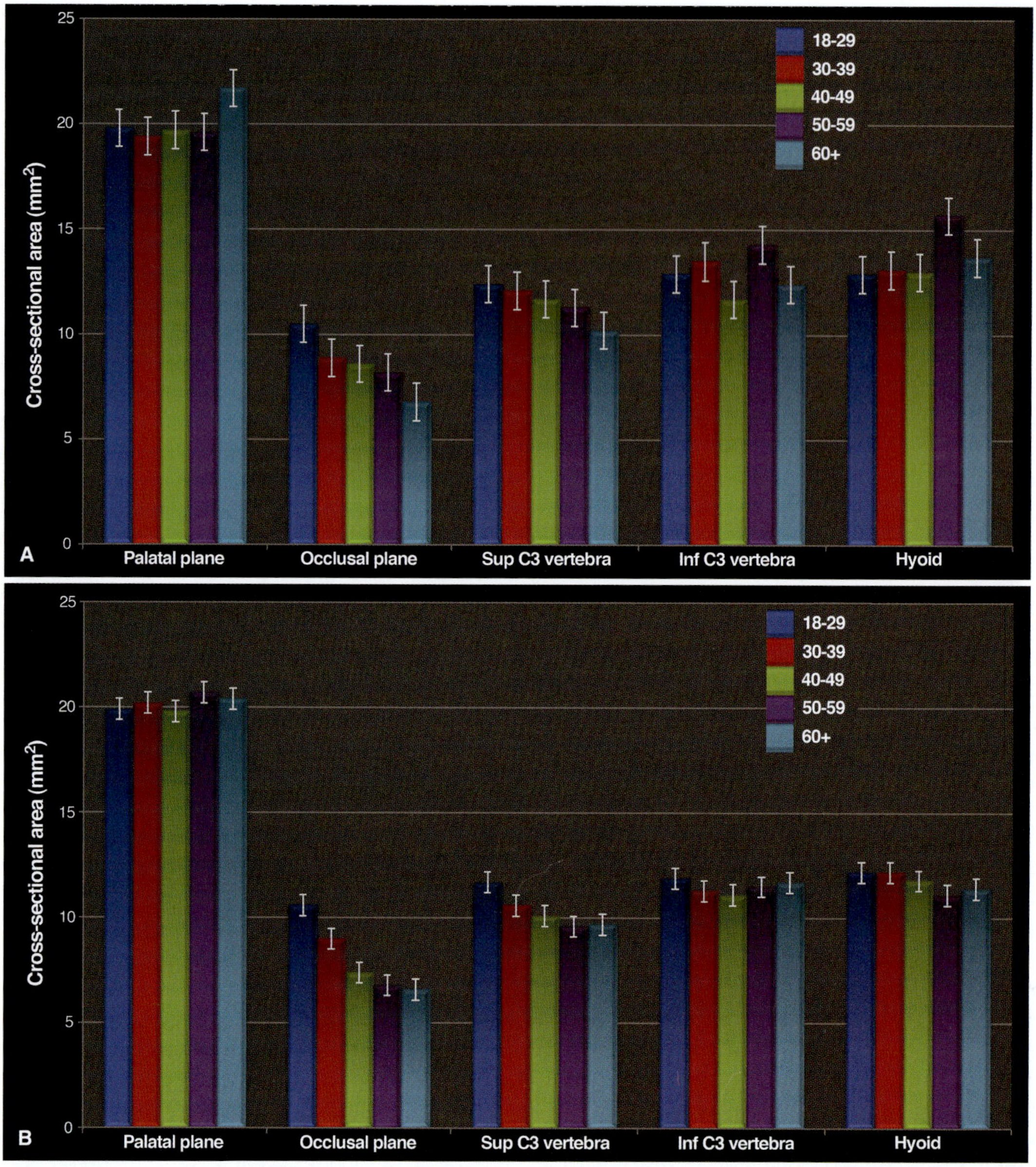

Figure 13.4 Mean (±SD) cross-sectional airway areas in (*A*) male and (*B*) female patients at five locations along the airway. While airway cross-sections at the palatal plane (PP), inferior aspect of the third cervical vertebra (Inf C3), and the hyoid remained relatively consistent over time, those at the occlusal plane (OP) and superior aspect of the third cervical vertebra (Sup C3) demonstrated a consistent decrease with age over each decade of life.

hyoid bone to the mandibular plane distance (Guilleminault *et al.*, 1984; deBerry-Borowiecki *et al.*, 1988; Partinen *et al.*, 1988; Strelzow *et al.*, 1988; Tangugsorn *et al.*, 1995a; Finkelstein *et al.*, 2001; Baik *et al.*, 2002; Cuccia *et al.*, 2007; Johal *et al.*, 2007; Tsai *et al.*, 2007), a general increase in thickness or length of the soft palate (deBerry-Borowiecki *et al.*, 1988; Strelzow *et al.*, 1988; Bacon *et al.*, 1990; Tangugsorn *et al.*, 1995b; Finkelstein *et al.*, 2001; Baik *et al.*, 2002; Yucel *et al.*, 2005; Johal *et al.*, 2007; Tsai *et al.*, 2007), small or retro-positioned mandibles and maxillas and shortened cranial bases (Rivlin *et al.*, 1984; Lowe *et al.*, 1986; Strelzow *et al.*, 1988; Andersson & Brattstrom, 1991; Tangugsorn *et al.*, 1995a; Baik *et al.*, 2002; Cuccia *et al.*, 2007; Johal *et al.*, 2007; Tsai *et al.*, 2007; Muto *et al.*, 2008), increased neck circumference (Yucel *et al.*, 2005), steeper mandibular planes (Lowe *et al.*, 1986; Tangugsorn *et al.*, 1995a), and larger tongues (Lowe *et al.*, 1986; deBerry-Borowiecki *et al.*, 1988; Tangugsorn *et al.*, 1995a; Tsuiki *et al.*, 2008) in OSA patients compared with controls.

In contrast to the above differences in airway-related structures and possibly due to the limitations of the lateral cephalogram, only a few studies have found statistically significant differences in the airway space between OSA and control subjects using this imaging methodology. A decreased posterior airway space measured from the base of the tongue to the posterior pharyngeal wall has been found in some populations of OSA patients (Guilleminault *et al.*, 1984; Partinen *et al.*, 1988; Andersson & Brattstrom, 1991). Others have noted that the length of the pharyngeal airway may be more important than a measure of the most constricted area in the airway in the diagnosis and treatment planning of OSA (Pae *et al.*, 1997).

Longitudinal changes in the normal airway using lateral cephalograms also have been studied. In one such study, the airways of 16 adults (11 male and five females) taken 32 years apart were analyzed to reveal an increase in maxillary prominence and upper and lower face heights, decreased AP depth of the oropharynx, and a longer and thicker soft palate with increasing age (Johnston & Richardson, 1999). Thus, it was postulated that these observations might explain the increased prevalence of OSA later in life. A similar longitudinal study examining airways in normal adults at 10-year intervals from 22 to 42 years of age found increased length, thickness, and sagittal area of the soft palate, a more upright and caudally extended tongue, and a decrease in the sagittal dimension of the oropharynx with age (Kollias & Krogstad, 1999b). Additionally, age-related increase in anterior and posterior face height, reduction in mandibular prognathism and increased mandibular plane angle in females, and a hyoid bone positioned more inferiorly has been noted (Kollias & Krogstad, 1999a). However, as stated previously, 2D studies do not capture the entirety of the anatomical features of the airway in health and disease, which require detailed 3D visualization of these structures.

3D airway image analyses in OSA

The initial 3D airway studies relied on medical MSCT, whose usefulness in airway analysis has been noted by several authors due to its capability to generate dimensionally accurate axial slices of the pharynx at multiple levels. Calculations of the pharynx's diameter, cross-sectional areas, and assessment of the nearby tissues and structures can be performed with the aid of CT imaging technology (Caballero *et al.*, 1998). Furthermore, 3D CT airway analysis has been shown to be precise and accurate for both linear and volumetric measurements (Cavalcanti *et al.*, 2004).

In a number of smaller sample size CT studies comparing OSA patients with controls, the OSA patients were found to have a smaller cross-sectional area in the location of the nasopharynx and/or oropharynx and/or hypopharynx (Haponik *et al.*, 1983; Galvin *et al.*, 1989; Schwab *et al.*, 1993; Avrahami & Englender, 1995; Avrahami *et al.*, 1996; Yucel *et al.*, 2005). A thicker soft palate (Yucel *et al.*, 2005) and increased retropharyngeal tissue have been found in OSA patients compared with controls (Caballero *et al.*, 1998). Not surprisingly, a difference in the general shape of the airway has been noted in OSA patients using CT that includes an airway that is wider in the AP dimensions in the OSA group versus an airway that is wider in the transverse dimension in the control group. The relationship of airway dimensions determined using CT with OSA remains equivocal since studies also have shown no statistically significant differences in these measurements between these two groups of subjects (Bhattacharyya *et al.*, 2000).

Due to the prevalence of obesity in OSA patients, it generally is assumed that obesity is a major risk factor in the development and progression of OSA. Therefore, researchers have examined the correlation of airway shape and BMI in the development of OSA. Studies by Mayer and colleagues (1996) have concluded that the shape changes of the pharynx are caused by the increase in BMI, which leads to the development of OSA, but OSA alone does not create an altered pharyngeal shape.

More recently, an increasing number of studies utilizing CBCT to evaluate the airway have been published. A study with a small sample size found that OSA patients had a lower total volume of the airway, smaller AP dimension of the airway at the minimum cross-sectional area, and a smaller minimum cross-sectional area than controls (Ogawa *et al.*, 2007). Also, while the OSA patients had concave or elliptically shaped airways, the non-OSA subjects had concave, round, or square-shaped airways. Another study evaluating the nasopharyngeal airway in adolescents and young adults found that a traditional 2D cephalogram could not identify the space taken up by large inferior turbinates and, therefore, led to an underestimation of the potential airway space (Aboudara *et al.*, 2009). The CBCT scans taken on these patients proved to be a simple and effective method for accurately analyzing the airway. Finally, a recent cross-sectional study of 239 "non-apneic" Taiwanese subjects aged 7–27 years found that pharyngeal airway depth increases from the mixed dentition to the permanent dentition, that there is sexual dimorphism in the lower pharyngeal airway depth, and that the vertical position of the hyoid bone changed with age (Sheng *et al.*, 2009). This study provides insights into the changes in the airway and supporting structures from childhood to early adulthood and could serve as a guide to studying whether OSA subjects in this age range have any developmental differences in the airways.

A sample of 50 adult dentate subjects with no previous history of surgery was studied in an investigation (Haskell, 2010) to determine the effects that the position and anatomy of the hyoid bone and vertical facial phenotype has on airway shape. For standardization, the images were rotated post-exposure so the patient's occlusal plane was established as the horizontal (or axial) reference plane, and measurements of the hyoid, the craniofacial complex, and the oropharyngeal airway were performed (Figure 13.5A; Table 13.2). The findings demonstrate that the more receded or closer the hyoid body is to the vertebrae, the more elliptical and laterally wide the airway, and the closer the hyoid is to the chin, the more elliptical the airway. This implies that in a mandibular deficient, vertically developed individual, the hyoid will be close to both the chin and the vertebrae resulting in a laterally wide and a highly elliptical airway. Also, the wider the greater and lesser cornu of the hyoid, the more elliptical and laterally wide is the airway. Finally, the steeper the pitch of the hyoid relative to the Frankfort Horizontal Plane, the more elliptical is the airway. Linear regression analysis demonstrated that the most significant craniofacial predictor for airway width were modified facial axis C1 (Figure 13.5A) and modified mandibular plane angle C2 (Figure 13.6). Other significant predictors for lateral airway width were greater and lesser cornu width (HI and H2), the distance of the hyoid to the nearest vertebra (H7), the angle of the hyoid plane to the occlusal plane (H3), and the angle of the hyoid plane to FH (H5; Table 13.3).

If long face individuals have elliptical airways that theoretically have greater volume and less airflow resistance and turbulence than round airways, why do long face patients have higher OSA rates? One explanation for this apparent discrepancy is that airway collapsibility is a function not only of lumen shape, but also of lumen size. Recent cross-sectional investigations have shown a narrowing of the airway with increasing numbers of "choke points" in aging non-OSA subjects. Long-face OSA patients with retrusive mandibles have been reported to have a smaller AP and transverse lumen size (Grauer *et al.*, 2009). As a result, the elliptical airway reported in these patients likely is "protective," reducing their likelihood of developing OSA compared with individuals who have round airways.

Sage and coworkers (2010) demonstrated several significant differences in airway dimensions between 32 OSA patients with age-, sex-, and size-matched controls. The airway was significantly

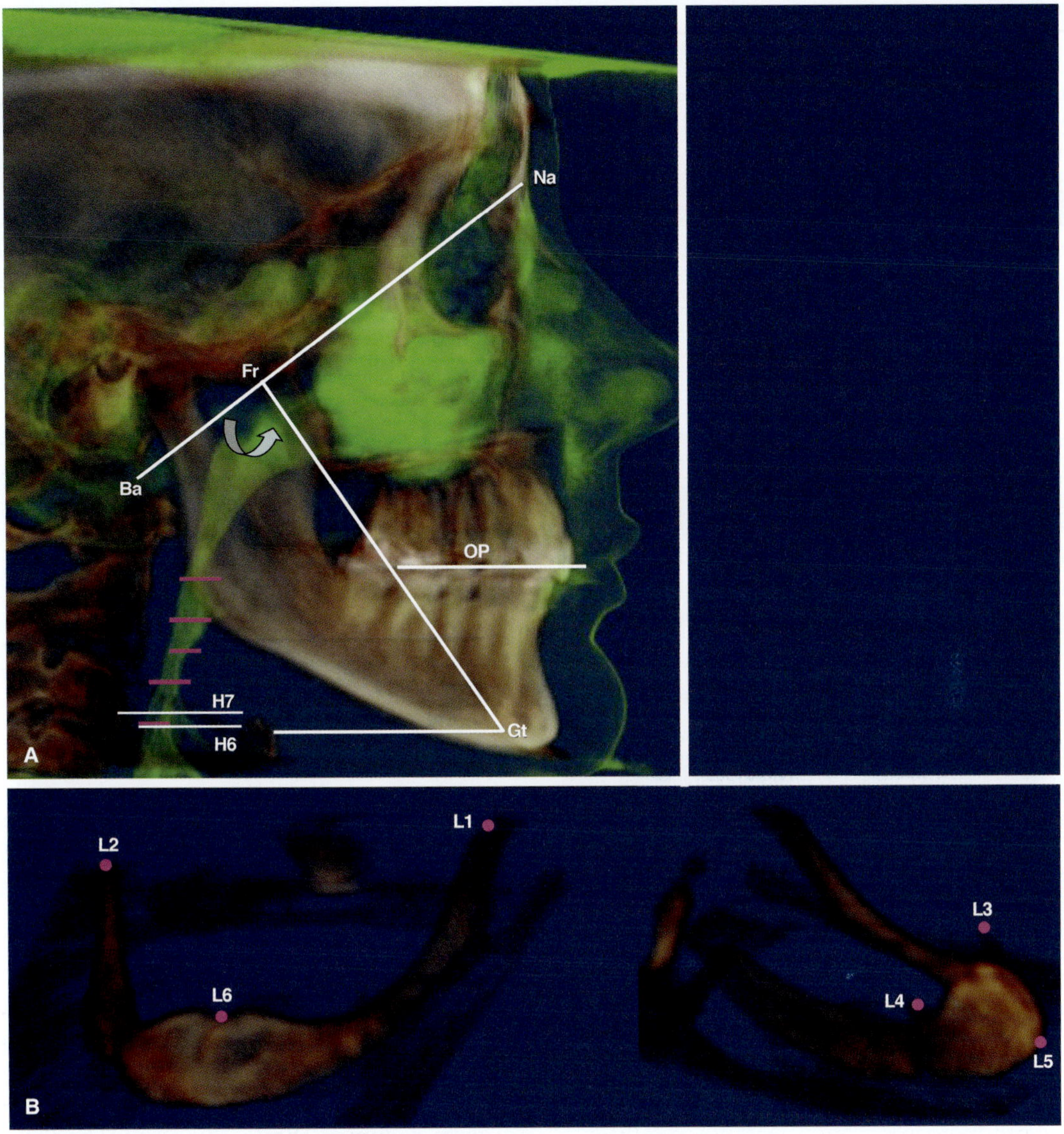

Figure 13.5 *A*: Depiction of the standard orientation performed on each of the 50 adult dentate patients using the occlusal plane (OP). The pink lines indicate the five sites where the cross-section of the airway was determined. The modified facial axis is defined as the angle created by the intersection of a plane extending from foramen rotundum (Fr) to the genial tubercles (Gt) to a line connecting nasion (Na) and basion (Ba). The modified facial axis (curved arrow), geniohyoid length (line parallel to the occlusal plane extending from the genial tubercle to the anterior aspect of the hyoid), hyoid distance to posterior of the pharynx (H6), and hyoid to anterior border of the vertebral column (H7) are illustrated. *B*: The hyoid bone consists of a main central body with a greater and lesser cornu. Points L1 and L2 represent the paired greater cornu, L3 and L4 represent the paired lesser cornu, L5 represents the most anterior-superior aspect of the hyoid body, and point L6 was used to define the most posterior-superior aspect of hyoid body.

Table 13.2 Definitions for hyoid bone landmarks and measurements made (see also Figure 13.5B for hyoid bone landmarks).

Label	Definition
L1	Greater cornu tip hyoid left
L2	Greater cornu tip hyoid right
L3	Lesser cornu tip hyoid left
L4	Lesser cornu tip hyoid right
L5	Most anterior-superior portion of hyoid body
L6	Most posterior-superior aspect of hyoid body
Measure	Definition
H1	Width between greater cornua: distance (mm) from L1-L2
H2	Width between lesser cornua: distance (mm) from L3-L4
H3	Pitch of hyoid to OP: angle of hyoid plane (L1, L2, L5) to occlusal plane
H4	Pitch of hyoid to MP: angle of hyoid plane (defined above) to mandibular plane
H5	Pitch of hyoid to FH: angle of hyoid plane (defined above) to Frankfort Horizontal Plane
H6	Anterior-posterior positioning of the hyoid from the posterior of the body of hyoid to the posterior of the pharynx: distance (mm)
H7	Anterior-posterior positioning of the hyoid from the posterior of the body of hyoid to the anterior of the vertebral column: distance (mm)

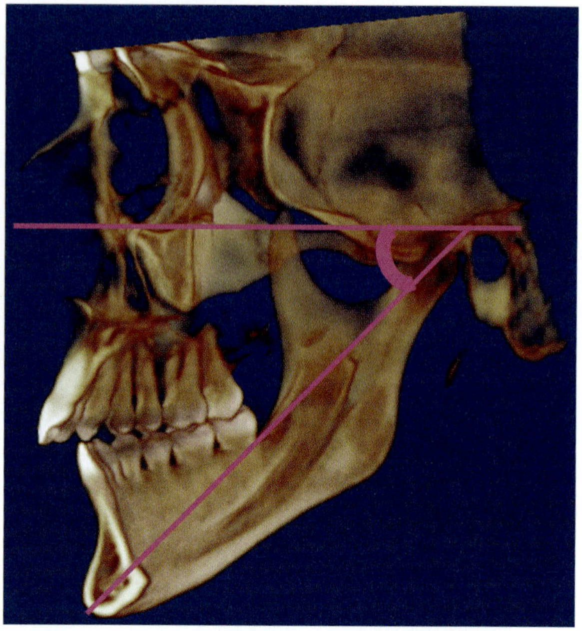

Figure 13.6 Modified mandibular plane angle (magenta) constructed as the interior angle formed by Frankfort horizontal plane and a line joining condylion and the genial tubercles. This angle more closely represents the orientation of the entire mandible rather than using the cephalometric mandibular planes, which represent the inferior border of the mandible.

longer in both male and female OSA patients determined by apnea hypopnea index (AHI) than in non-OSA subjects (Figure 13.7A). In male patients, increasing severity of OSA was associated with significantly smaller cross-sectional airway at the hyoid (Figure 13.7B). In the female study group with a smaller sample size, there was a statistically significant difference in cross-sectional airway at the hyoid between the least severe and most severe OSA. Finally, the airway minimum cross-sectional area correlated negatively with BMI (Figure 13.7C), which suggests that the minimum airway cross-sectional area decreases significantly with increasing weight. This finding seems to be logical since deposits of fat all over the body also would include the parapharyngeal areas with a concomitant increase in the pressure and greater chance of airway collapse. While this study had a small sample and future investigations are needed to validate these findings, it demonstrates the potential for CBCT to be a surrogate diagnostic test for OSA in patients requiring orthodontic or orthognathic surgery care.

Despite substantial progress on CBCT image-based analyses of the airway, several caveats and limitations of the currently published studies minimize the ability to make definitive connections between OSA and airway morphology. These include small sample sizes, inappropriate or small control samples, CBCTs performed in upright rather than supine position, and a lack of correlation of CBCT imaging with functional analyses of

Table 13.3 Predictors for lateral airway width including *p* value.

Outcome variable: Lateral width	Predictor variables	Regression coefficient	*p* value
At superior C2	Lesser cornu width	0.65	0.03
	Sagittal distance of the hyoid from nearest vertebra (along hyoid plane)	−2.65	0.01
At mid C2	Modified mandibular plane angle	0.27	0.03
	Lesser cornu width	0.82	0.006
	Sagittal distance of the hyoid from nearest vertebra (along hyoid plane)	−2.16	0.02
At inferior C2	Modified facial axis	−0.52	0.01
At superior C3	Modified facial axis	−19.66	0.04
	Hyoid plane to occlusal plane angle	−15.82	0.009
At mid C3	Greater cornu width	0.39	0.01
	Hyoid plane to occlusal plane angle	−0.29	0.003

Note: Regression coefficients were obtained from a multivariable linear regression in an effort to determine the relative importance of each variable. For example, the coefficient of −2.65 for the sagittal distance of the hyoid from nearest vertebra means that if all the other variables are kept constant, one unit of increase in the sagittal distance will lead a 2.65 unit decrease in lateral airway width.

apneic incidents through PSG. As in OSA studies that utilize different imaging modalities, conclusions of CBCT and CT airway studies are influenced by the selected control groups and the data available on normal adult airways. For example, Avrahami & Englender (1995) concluded that OSA patients had a smaller minimal axial pharyngeal cross-sectional area than controls. However, the control group used was both small in size and not matched for age or size with the OSA sample, making it difficult to draw any conclusions about the characteristics of the normal adult airway from this study. Similarly, studies by Bhattacharyya and associates (2000) using 3D CT found no differences in airway dimensions between OSA patients and controls (four females and six males) that again could have resulted from the small sample size of the control group. Finally, as is evident from this chapter, the use of different reference planes, landmarks, and sites for determining linear and volumetric dimensions remains a significant impediment to cross-study comparisons. Thus, it would serve the field well if experts in the field could define optimal and logical reference planes and landmarks for airway analyses for use in future research and clinical applications.

The physics of airway resistance and flow

Although studies performed to date have focused on key differences in shape and size of the upper airways, little consideration has been given to the physics of airway resistance and flow. In this context, the effect of cross-sectional shape on the type of flow within the airway needs specific consideration. When assuming laminar flow and an incompressible fluid, Poiseuille's law states that the flow $[V]$ in a tube is directly proportional to the driving pressure $[\Delta P]$ and inversely proportional with the resistance $[R]$ as in the following equation:

$$V = \Delta P / R.$$

And further that

$$R = 8nl/\pi r^4$$

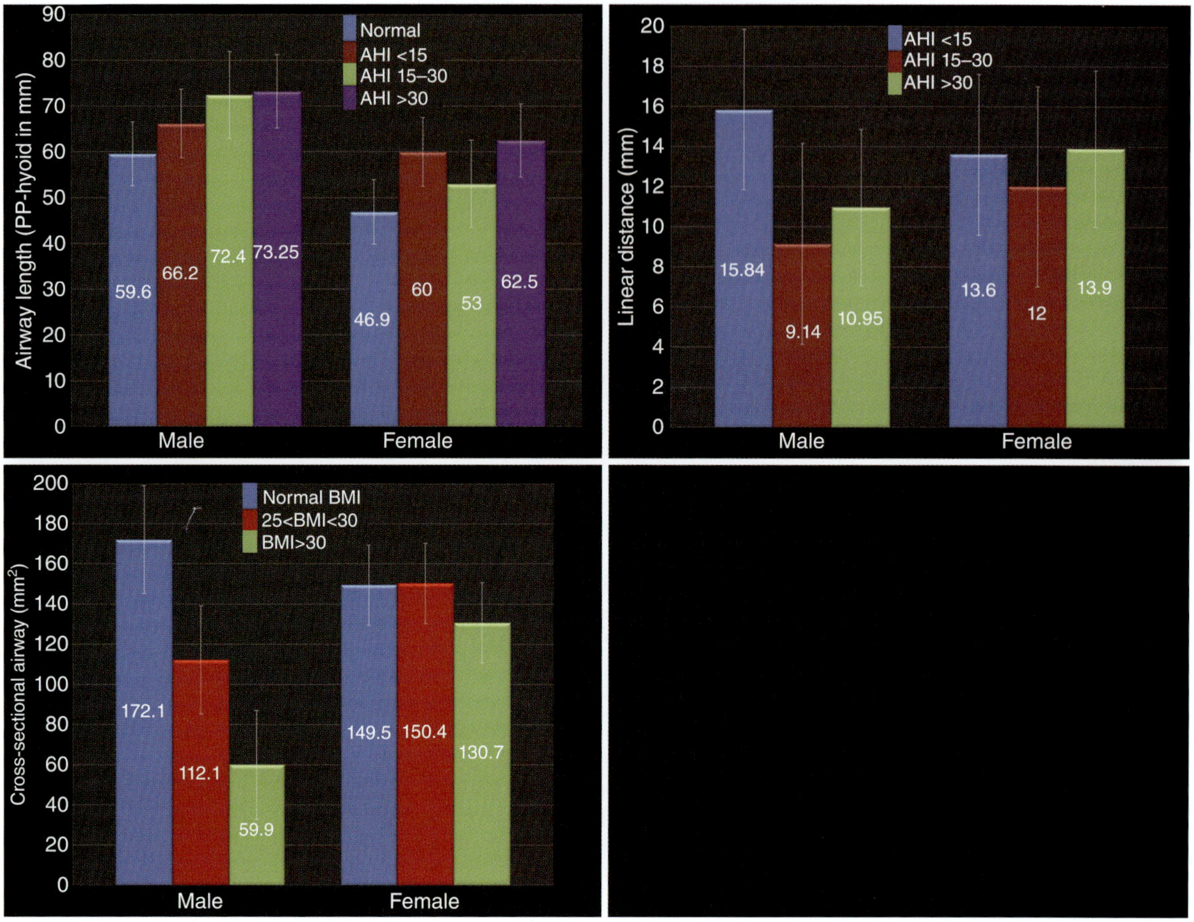

Figure 13.7 Means (±SD) for males and females depicting differences in (*A*) airway length and (*B*) airway cross-section tangent to hyoid in non-apneic individuals and apneic patients grouped by severity of OSA. *C*: Means (±SD) of minimum cross-sectional airway area in normal indviduals and those with BMI of between 25 and 30 or greater than 30.

where n is the viscosity of the fluid/gas; l is length of the tube, and r is radius of the tube.

Under these circumstances, it is obvious that the resistance is dependent not only on the radius (r) of the tube (R is proportional to l/r^4), but also the length (l) of the tube. This equation is supported by findings in OSA patients who have increased airway length and, at least in some studies, diminished minimum cross-sectional areas compared with controls (Tso, 2009; Abramson *et al.*, 2010; Schendel & Hatcher, 2010; Susarla *et al.*, 2010).

Because air is a compressible gas rather than an incompressible fluid and because fluid flow in most cases is turbulent rather than lamellar, Poiseuille's law must be modified to the following to be apply for airways:

$$V = (\Delta P/R)^n \text{ where } 1.7 < n < 2.0.$$

This implies that because gaseous flow (V) is proportional to the square root of the pressure (P), to double the flow, the pressure (P) now must nearly quadruple.

Besides the length and radius of the airway, the shape of the cross-section is another important variable that can affect airflow; indeed, the

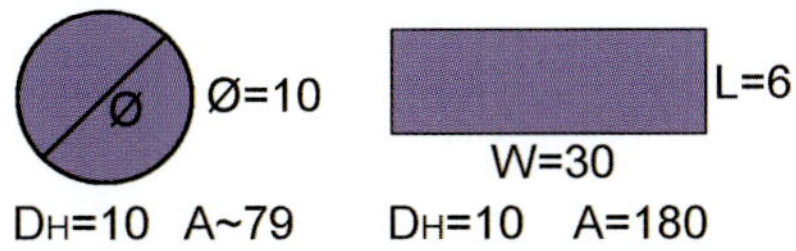

Figure 13.8 The shape of an object or "tube" can have a substantial effect on hydraulic diameter. The circle and the rectangle share the same hydraulic diameter yet have different cross-sectional dimensions. This effect likely plays a critical role in the airflow rate and airflow resistance in OSA patients.

measurement of the volume alone is inadequate to calculate the type of flow and the pressure loss, which is dependent on the hydraulic diameter of the airway. Hydraulic diameter is a measure of flow in noncircular tubes or channels. An example of the effect of airway shape on hydraulic diameter is depicted in Figure 13.8, which shows that although the two cross-sections have different areas—the one for the rectangle is more than twice that of the circle—both cross-sections are characterized by the same hydraulic diameter. Moreover, the equivalent diameter, defined as the diameter of a circular duct or pipe that gives the same pressure loss as an equivalent rectangular duct, is an important variable in airflow. Thus, for example, the equivalent diameter of the rectangular duct with a cross-section of 180 mm^2 will be a circular duct with a diameter of 13.6 mm, which is characterized by a cross-section area of about 145 mm^2, as depicted in Figure 13.8. Therefore, when comparing a round versus a rectangular tube of equivalent length and cross-sectional areas, the pressure drop will be smaller for the former than for the latter (Patil *et al.*, 2007; Susarla *et al.*, 2010), supporting the postulate that elliptical airways are less prone to OSA. This working hypothesis is based primarily on mathematical principles and requires further studies to validate or disprove.

CONCLUSIONS

Unlike in the past when 2D imaging was used predominantly, 3D techniques increasingly are becoming important for various orthodontic applications and in related fields, such as its potential uses in airway diagnostics. 3D imaging of the airway increasingly has become sophisticated using low dose radiation techniques as well as some noninvasive techniques. Most of the cross-sectional areas and volumes generated by these methods can be analyzed using refined computer software programs, and the presentation of images is user-friendly for the orthodontic practitioner. While much work has been performed on airway morphology, volume, and size, much remains to be investigated. Not surprisingly, initial forays into using CBCT imaging to address questions pertaining to airway patency, function, and disorders have answered some rudimentary questions while also creating new ones. To begin to understand the role that imaging may have in understanding the airway form and function, sensitivity and specificity tests will need to be performed in conjunction with overnight PSG on known OSA patients. With increasing multicenter collaborations, data can be pooled and more meaningful results likely are to be developed for a valid use of CBCT imaging in airway diagnostics.

References

Aboudara, C., Nielsen, I., Huang, J.C., *et al.* (2009) Comparison of airway space with conventional lateral headfilms and 3-dimensional reconstruction from cone-beam computed tomography. *American Journal of Orthodontics and Dentofacial Orthopedics*, 135 (4), 468–479.

Abramson, Z., Susarla, S., August, M., *et al.* (2010) Three-dimensional computed tomographic analysis of airway anatomy in patients with obstructive sleep apnea. *Journal of Oral and Maxillofacial Surgery*, 68 (2), 354–362.

Al-Balkhi, K.M. (2003) Orthodontic treatment planning: do orthodontists treat to cephalometric norms? *Journal of Contemporary Dental Practice*, 4 (4), 12–27.

Andersson, L. & Brattstrom, V. (1991) Cephalometric analysis of permanently snoring patients with and without obstructive sleep apnea syndrome. *International Journal of Oral and Maxillofacial Surgery*, 20 (3), 159–162.

Avrahami, E. & Englender, M. (1995) Relation between CT axial cross-sectional area of the oropharynx and obstructive sleep apnea syndrome in adults. *American Journal of Neuroradiology*, 16 (1), 135–140.

Avrahami, E., Solomonovich, A., & Englender, M. (1996) Axial CT measurements of the cross-sectional area of the oropharynx in adults with obstructive sleep apnea syndrome. *American Journal of Neuroradiology*, 17 (6), 1107–1111.

Bacon, W.H., Turlot, J.C., Krieger, J., *et al.* (1990) Cephalometric evaluation of pharyngeal obstructive factors in patients with sleep apneas syndrome. *The Angle Orthodontist*, 60, 115–122.

Baik, U.B., Suzuki, M., Ikeda, K., *et al.* (2002) Relationship between cephalometric characteristics and obstructive sites in obstructive sleep apnea syndrome. *The Angle Orthodontist*, 72 (2), 124–134.

Bhattacharyya, N., Blake, S.P., & Fried, M.P. (2000) Assessment of the airway in obstructive sleep apnea syndrome with 3-dimensional airway computed tomography. *Otolaryngology and Head and Neck Surgery*, 123 (4), 444–449.

Bixler, E.O., Vgontzas, A.N., Lin, H.M., *et al.* (2001) Prevalence of sleep-disordered breathing in women: effects of gender. *American Journal of Respiratory and Critical Care Medicine*, 163 (3 Pt 1), 608–613.

Brenner, D.J. & Hall, E.J. (2007) Computed tomography: an increasing source of radiation exposure. *New England Journal of Medicine*, 357 (22), 2277–2284.

Broadbent, H. (1931) A new X-ray technique and its application to orthodontia. *The Angle Orthodontist*, 1, 45–66.

Brooks, L.J. & Strohl, K.P. (1992) Size and mechanical properties of the pharynx in healthy men and women. *American Review of Respiratory Disease*, 146 (6), 1394–1397.

Brown, I.G., Zamel, N., & Hoffstein, V. (1986) Pharyngeal cross-sectional area in normal men and women. *Journal of Applied Physiology*, 61 (3), 890–895.

Caballero, P., Alvarez-Sala, R., Garcia-Rio, F., *et al.* (1998) CT in the evaluation of the upper airway in healthy subjects and in patients with obstructive sleep apnea syndrome. *Chest*, 113 (1), 111–116.

Cavalcanti, M.G., Rocha, S.S., & Vannier, M.W. (2004) Craniofacial measurements based on 3D-CT volume rendering: implications for clinical applications. *Dentomaxillofacial Radiology*, 33 (3), 170–176.

Ciscar, M.A., Juan, G., Martinez, V., *et al.* (2001) Magnetic resonance imaging of the pharynx in OSA patients and healthy subjects. *European Respiratory Journal*, 17 (1), 79–86.

Cuccia, A.M., Campisi, G., Cannavale, R. *et al.* (2007) Obesity and craniofacial variables in subjects with obstructive sleep apnea syndrome: comparisons of cephalometric values. *Head & Face Medicine*, 3, 41.

Dancey, D.R., Hanly, P.J., Soong, C., *et al.* (2003) Gender differences in sleep apnea: the role of neck circumference. *Chest*, 123 (5), 1544–1550.

Deberry-Borowiecki, B., Kukwa, A., & Blanks, R.H. (1988) Cephalometric analysis for diagnosis and treatment of obstructive sleep apnea. *The Laryngoscope*, 98 (2), 226–234.

El, H. & Palomo, J.M. (2010) Measuring the airway in 3 dimensions: a reliability and accuracy study. *American Journal of Orthodontics and Dentofacial Orthopedics*, 137 (Suppl 4), S50.e1–S50.e9.

El, H. & Palomo, J.M. (2011) Airway volume for different dentofacial skeletal patterns. *American Journal of Orthodontics and Dentofacial Orthopedics*, 139 (6), e511–e521.

Finkelstein, Y., Wexler, D., Horowitz, E., *et al.* (2001) Frontal and lateral cephalometry in patients with sleep-disordered breathing. *The Laryngoscope*, 111 (4 Pt 1), 634–641.

Galvin, J.R., Rooholamini, S.A., & Stanford, W. (1989) Obstructive sleep apnea: diagnosis with ultrafast CT. *Radiology*, 171 (3), 775–778.

Grauer, D., Cevidanes, L.S., Styner, M.A., *et al.* (2009) Pharyngeal airway volume and shape from cone-beam computed tomography: relationship to facial morphology. *American Journal of Orthodontics and Dentofacial Orthopedics*, 136, 805–814.

Guilleminault, C., Tilkian, A., & Dement, W.C. (1976) The sleep apnea syndromes. *Annual Review of Medicine*, 27, 465–484.

Guilleminault, C., Riley, R., & Powell, N. (1984) Obstructive sleep apnea and abnormal cephalometric measurements: implications for treatment. *Chest*, 86 (5), 793–794.

Guilleminault, C., Quera-Salva, M.A., Partinen, M., *et al.* (1988) Women and the obstructive sleep apnea syndrome. *Chest*, 93 (1), 104–109.

Haponik, E.F., Smith, P.L., Bohlman, M.E., *et al.* (1983) Computerized tomography in obstructive sleep apnea: correlation of airway size with physiology during sleep and wakefulness. *American Review of Respiratory Disease*, 127 (2), 221–226.

Harvold, E.P., Tomer, B.S., Vargervik, K., *et al.* (1981) Primate experiments on oral respiration. *American Journal of Orthodontics*, 79 (4), 359–372.

Haskell, J.A. (2010) Correlates of craniofacial form and the oropharyngeal airway with regard to hyoid position: a cone beam CT cephalometric study. Senior Resident thesis, Eastman Institute for Oral Health, University of Rochester.

Holmberg, H. & Linder-Aronson, S. (1979) Cephalometric radiographs as a means of evaluating the capacity of the nasal and nasopharyngeal airway. *American Journal of Orthodontics*, 76 (5), 479–490.

Ingman, T., Nieminen, T., & Hurmerinta, K. (2004) Cephalometric comparison of pharyngeal changes in subjects with upper airway resistance syndrome or obstructive sleep apnoea in upright and supine positions. *European Journal of Orthodontics*, 26 (3), 321–326.

Johal, A., Patel, S.I., & Battagel, J.M. (2007) The relationship between craniofacial anatomy and obstructive sleep apnoea: a case-controlled study. *Journal of Sleep Research*, 16 (3), 319–326.

Johnston, C.D. & Richardson, A. (1999) Cephalometric changes in adult pharyngeal morphology. *European Journal of Orthodontics*, 21 (4), 357–362.

Kapila, S., Conley, R.S., & Harrell, W.E., Jr. (2011) The current status of cone beam computed tomography imaging in orthodontics. *Dentomaxillofacial Radiology*, 40 (1), 24–34.

Kapsimalis, F. & Kryger, M.H. (2002) Gender and obstructive sleep apnea syndrome. Part 2: mechanisms. *Sleep*, 25 (5), 499–506.

Kau, C.H., Richmond, S., Palomo, J.M., *et al.* (2005) Three-dimensional cone beam computerized tomography in orthodontics. *Journal of Orthodontics*, 32 (4), 282–293.

Keim, R.G. (2009) A new dimension in diagnosis. *Journal of Clinical Orthodontics*, 43 (4), 213–214.

Kim, H.Y., Bok, K.H., Dhong, H.J., *et al.* (2008) The correlation between pharyngeal narrowing and the severity of sleep-disordered breathing. *Otolaryngology and Head and Neck Surgery*, 138 (3), 289–293.

Klocke, A., Kemper, J., Schulze, D., *et al.* (2005) Magnetic field interactions of orthodontic wires during magnetic resonance imaging (MRI) at 1.5 Tesla. *Journal of Orofacial Orthopedics*, 66 (4), 279–287.

Klocke, A., Kahl-Nieke, B., Adam, G., *et al.* (2006) Magnetic forces on orthodontic wires in high field magnetic resonance imaging (MRI) at 3 Tesla. *Journal of Orofacial Orthopedics*, 67 (6), 424–429.

Kluemper, G.T., Vig, P.S., & Vig, K.S. (1995) Nasorespiratory characteristics and craniofacial morphology. *European Journal of Orthodontics*, 17 (6), 491–495.

Kollias, I. & Krogstad, O. (1999a) Adult craniocervical and pharyngeal changes: a longitudinal cephalometric study between 22 and 42 years of age. Part I: morphological craniocervical and hyoid bone changes. *European Journal of Orthodontics*, 21 (4), 333–344.

Kollias, I. & Krogstad, O. (1999b) Adult craniocervical and pharyngeal changes: a longitudinal cephalometric study between 22 and 42 years of age. Part II: morphological uvulo-glossopharyngeal changes. *European Journal of Orthodontics*, 21 (4), 345–355.

Lagravère, M.O., Carey, J., Toogood, R.W., *et al.* (2008) Three-dimensional accuracy of measurements made with software on cone-beam computed tomography images. *American Journal of Orthodontics and Dentofacial Orthopedics*, 134 (1), 112–116.

Lenza, M.G., Lenza, M.M., Dalstra, M., *et al.* (2010) An analysis of different approaches to the assessment of upper airway morphology: a CBCT study. *Orthodontics & Craniofacial Research*, 13 (2), 96–105.

Linder-Aronson, S. (1970) Adenoids: their effect on mode of breathing and nasal airflow and their relationship to characteristics of the facial skeleton and the dentition: a biometric, rhino-manometric and cephalometro-radiographic study on children with and without adenoids. *Acta Otolaryngologica Supplementum*, 265, 1–132.

Lowe, A.A., Santamaria, J.D., Fleetham, J.A., *et al.* (1986) Facial morphology and obstructive sleep apnea. *American Journal of Orthodontics and Dentofacial Orthopedics*, 90 (6), 484–491.

Lowe, A.A., Fleetham, J.A., Adachi, S., *et al.* (1995) Cephalometric and computed tomographic predictors of obstructive sleep apnea severity. *American Journal of Orthodontics and Dentofacial Orthopedics*, 107 (6), 589–595.

Maki, K., Inou, N., Takanishi, A., *et al.* (2003) Computer-assisted simulations in orthodontic diagnosis and the application of a new cone beam X-ray computed tomography. *Orthodontics & Craniofacial Resesarch*, 6 (Suppl 1), 95–101.

Malkoc, S., Usumez, S., Nur, M., *et al.* (2005) Reproducibility of airway dimensions and tongue and hyoid positions on lateral cephalograms. *American Journal of Orthodontics and Dentofacial Orthopedics*, 128 (4), 513–516.

Martin, O., Muelas, L., & Vinas, M.J. (2006) Nasopharyngeal cephalometric study of ideal occlusions. *American Journal of Orthodontics and Dentofacial Orthopedics*, 130 (4), 436.e1–436.e9.

Martin, S.E., Mathur, R., Marshall, I., *et al.* (1997) The effect of age, sex, obesity and posture on upper airway size. *European Respiratory Journal*, 10 (9), 2087–2090.

Mayer, P., Pepin, J.L., Bettega, G., *et al.* (1996) Relationship between body mass index, age and upper airway measurements in snorers and sleep apnoea patients. *European Respiratory Journal*, 9 (9), 1801–1809.

Mohsenin, V. (2001) Gender differences in the expression of sleep-disordered breathing: role of upper airway dimensions. *Chest*, 120 (5), 1442–1447.

Muto, T., Yamazaki, A., & Takeda, S. (2008) A cephalometric evaluation of the pharyngeal airway space in patients with mandibular retrognathia and prognathia, and normal subjects. *International Journal of Oral and Maxillofacial Surgery*, 37 (3), 228–231.

Ogawa, T., Enciso, R., Shintaku, W.H., *et al.* (2007) Evaluation of cross-section airway configuration of obstructive sleep apnea. *Oral Surgery, Oral Medicine, Oral*

Pathology, Oral Radiology, and Endodontics, 103 (1), 102–108.

Oliviera De Felippe, N.L., Da Silveira, A.C., Viana, G., *et al.* (2008) Relationship between rapid maxillary expansion and nasal cavity size and airway resistance: short- and long-term effects. *American Journal of Orthodontics and Dentofacial Orthopedics*, 134 (3), 370–382.

Osorio, F., Perilla, M., Doyle, D.J., *et al.* (2008) Cone beam computed tomography: an innovative tool for airway assessment. *Anesthesia and Analgesia*, 106 (6), 1803–1807.

Pae, E.K., Lowe, A.A., & Fleetham, J.A. (1997) A role of pharyngeal length in obstructive sleep apnea patients. *American Journal of Orthodontics and Dentofacial Orthopedics*, 111 (1), 12–17.

Partinen, M., Guilleminault, C., Quera-Salva, M.A., *et al.* (1988) Obstructive sleep apnea and cephalometric roentgenograms: the role of anatomic upper airway abnormalities in the definition of abnormal breathing during sleep. *Chest*, 93 (6), 1199–1205.

Patel, A., Bhava, S., & O'Neill, J.R. (2006) MRI scanning and orthodontics. *Journal of Orthodontics*, 33 (4), 246–249.

Patil, S.P., Schneider, H., Schwartz, A.R., *et al.* (2007) Adult obstructive sleep apnea: pathophysiology and diagnosis. *Chest*, 132 (1), 325–337.

Quintero, J.C., Trosien, A., Hatcher, D., *et al.* (1999) Craniofacial imaging in orthodontics: historical perspective, current status, and future developments. *The Angle Orthodontist*, 69 (6), 491–506.

Rivlin, J., Hoffstein, V., Kalbfleisch, J., *et al.* (1984) Upper airway morphology in patients with idiopathic obstructive sleep apnea. *American Review of Respiratory Disease*, 129 (3), 355–360.

Sage, J.W., Conley, R.S., Edwards, S.P., *et al.* (2010) The evaluation of the adult pre-surgical obstructive sleep apnea airway using cone beam computed tomography: a retrospective analysis. MS thesis, University of Michigan.

Schendel, S.A. & Hatcher, D. (2010) Automated 3-dimensional airway analysis from cone-beam computed tomography data. *Journal of Oral and Maxillofacial Surgery*, 68 (3), 696–701.

Schwab, R.J. (1998) Upper airway imaging. *Clinics in Chest Medicine*, 19 (1), 33–54.

Schwab, R.J., Gefter, W.B., Hoffman, E.A., *et al.* (1993) Dynamic upper airway imaging during awake respiration in normal subjects and patients with sleep disordered breathing. *American Review of Respiratory Disease*, 148 (5), 1385–1400.

Schwab, R.J., Pasirstein, M., Pierson, R., *et al.* (2003) Identification of upper airway anatomic risk factors for obstructive sleep apnea with volumetric magnetic resonance imaging. *American Journal of Respiratory and Critical Care Medicine*, 168 (5), 522–530.

Sheng, C.M., Lin, L.H., Su, Y., *et al.* (2009) Developmental changes in pharyngeal airway depth and hyoid bone position from childhood to young adulthood. *The Angle Orthodontist*, 79 (3), 484–490.

Smith, J.M., Conley, R.S., Brooks, S.L., *et al.* (2009) The normal adult airway in 3-dimensions: a cone-beam computed tomography evaluation establishing normative values. MS thesis, University of Michigan.

Solow, B. & Kreiborg, S. (1977) Soft-tissue stretching: a possible control factor in craniofacial morphogenesis. *Scandinavian Journal of Dental Research*, 85 (6), 505–507.

Solow, B., Siersbaek-Nielsen, S., & Greve, E. (1984) Airway adequacy, head posture, and craniofacial morphology. *American Journal of Orthodontics*, 86 (3), 214–223.

Strelzow, V.V., Blanks, R.H., Basile, A., *et al.* (1988) Cephalometric airway analysis in obstructive sleep apnea syndrome. *The Laryngoscope*, 98 (11), 1149–1158.

Susarla, S.M., Thomas, R.J., Abramson, Z.R., *et al.* (2010) Biomechanics of the upper airway: changing concepts in the pathogenesis of obstructive sleep apnea. *International Journal of Oral and Maxillofacial Surgery*, 39 (12), 1149–1159.

Tangugsorn, V., Skatvedt, O., Krogstad, O., *et al.* (1995a) Obstructive sleep apnoea: a cephalometric study. Part I: cervico-craniofacial skeletal morphology. *European Journal of Orthodontics*, 17 (1), 45–56.

Tangugsorn, V., Skatvedt, O., Krogstad, O., *et al.* (1995b) Obstructive sleep apnoea: a cephalometric study. Part II: uvulo-glossopharyngeal morphology. *European Journal of Orthodontics*, 17 (1), 57–67.

Tangugsorn, V., Krogstad, O., Espeland, L., *et al.* (2000) Obstructive sleep apnea (OSA): A cephalometric analysis of severe and non-severe OSA patients. Part I: multiple comparison of cephalometric variables. *International Journal of Adult Orthodontics and Orthognathic Surgery*, 15 (2), 139–152.

Tsai, H.H., Ho, C.Y., Lee, P.L., *et al.* (2007) Cephalometric analysis of nonobese snorers either with or without obstructive sleep apnea syndrome. *The Angle Orthodontist*, 77 (6), 1054–1061.

Tso, H.H., Lee, J.S., Huang, J.C., *et al.* (2009) Evaluation of the human airway using cone-beam computerized tomography. *Oral Surgery Oral Medicine Oral Pathology Oral Radiology, and Endodontics*, 108 (5), 768–776.

Tsuiki, S., Isono, S., Ishikawa, T., *et al.* (2008) Anatomical balance of the upper airway and obstructive sleep apnea. *Anesthesiology*, 108 (6), 1009–1015.

Vig, K.W. (1998) Nasal obstruction and facial growth: the strength of evidence for clinical assumptions.

American Journal of Orthodontics and Dentofacial Orthopedics, 113, 603–611.

White, S. & Pae, E.K. (2009) Patient image selection criteria for cone beam computed tomography imaging. *Seminars in Orthodontics*, 15 (1), 19–28.

Yucel, A., Unlu, M., Haktanir, A., *et al.* (2005) Evaluation of the upper airway cross-sectional area changes in different degrees of severity of obstructive sleep apnea syndrome: Cephalometric and dynamic CT study. *American Journal of Neuroradiology*, 26 (10), 2624–2629.

Zoth, N., Weigt, C., Zengin, S., *et al.* (2012) Metabolic effects of estrogen substitution in combination with targeted exercise training on the therapy of obesity in ovariectomized Wistar rats. *Journal of Steroid Biochemistry and Molecular Biology*, 130 (1–2), 64–72.

14 Alveolar Boundary Conditions in Orthodontic Diagnosis and Treatment Planning

Sunil D. Kapila, BDS, MS, PhD, and Jeanne M. Nervina, DMD, PhD

INTRODUCTION

In orthodontics, alveolar boundary conditions are the depth, height, and morphology of alveolar bone relative to tooth root dimensions, angulation, and spatial position (Kapila *et al.*, 2011). Boundary conditions are defined not only by dentoalveolar anatomy prior to treatment, but also by their adaptability during tooth movement and their morphology following the final positioning of teeth. As such, the pre-treatment status of boundary conditions and their potential adaptation may dictate the limits of planned tooth movement, as well as the final desired spatial position and angulation of the tooth. Alveolar boundary conditions are not static; in fact, their remarkable dynamism can be both good and bad. Without remodeling of alveolar boundary conditions, orthodontic tooth movement would not be possible. Conversely, applying inappropriate orthodontic forces to a tooth can affect alveolar boundary conditions adversely, resulting in dehiscences and fenestrations. Maximizing alveolar boundary condition remodeling and minimizing unwanted sequelae for each patient is a desired orthodontic goal. Although not established yet, it is possible that cone beam computed tomography (CBCT) may offer a useful tool to meet this objective.

Alveolar boundary conditions impact diagnosis and treatment of various malocclusions, such as mild to moderately crowded nonextraction cases, dentoalveolar compensations due to transverse (Figure 14.1A,B) or sagittal skeletal discrepancies, situations with severely compromised bone (Figure 14.1C,D), bimaxillary protrusion (Figure 14.2), and inadequate or missing bone such as in cleft lip and palate (CL/P). Moreover, bone boundary conditions can affect treatment decisions and diminish the ability to provide ideal treatment in situations where neighboring structures, such as sinuses or transposed teeth, are likely to interfere with the planned tooth movement (Figure 14.3).

Prior to the introduction of CBCT, little was known about how alveolar boundary conditions

Cone Beam Computed Tomography in Orthodontics: Indications, Insights, and Innovations, First Edition. Sunil D. Kapila.

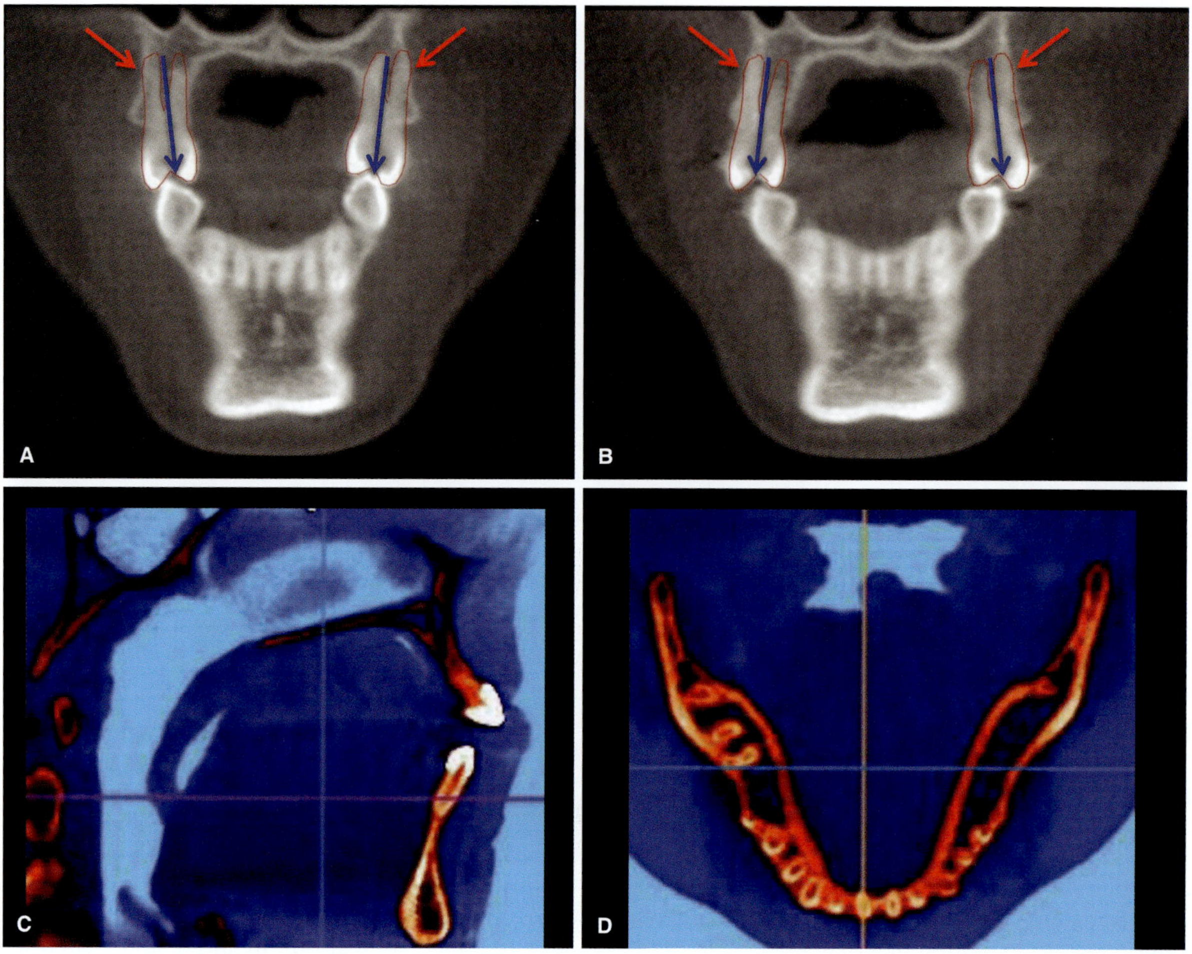

Figure 14.1 CBCT provides novel information on boundary conditions that are not discernible from routine radiographs or during clinical examination, which may impact treatment options. *A*: Pre-treatment coronal view showing the lingual inclination (blue arrows) of maxillary premolars and proximity of their buccal roots to the cortical bone margin (red arrows). *B*: Post-treatment coronal view demonstrating that the limitations established by the bone–root boundary conditions have been addressed through lingual torquing of the roots such that the torque of these teeth more closely matches the inclination of the cortical and alveolar process of the maxilla. Sagittal (*C*) and axial (*D*) sections from CBCT scans of an individual with severe limitations in boundary conditions where the cortical bone margins are incapable of sustaining orthodontic movements in any plane of space. Orthodontic treatment is contraindicated in this case. (Modified and reprinted with permission from Kapila *et al.*, 2011.)

restricted or responded to orthodontic treatment beyond the appearance of gingival recession or bony dehiscences. Because conventional two-dimensional (2D) radiographs do not image the dentoalveolar complex in all three planes of space, researchers often have drawn conflicting interpretations of morphological changes in the teeth and their supporting structures following orthodontic treatment. This chapter reviews the small and sometimes conflicting literature on alveolar boundary conditions with the goal of providing information on its implications to orthodontic diagnosis,

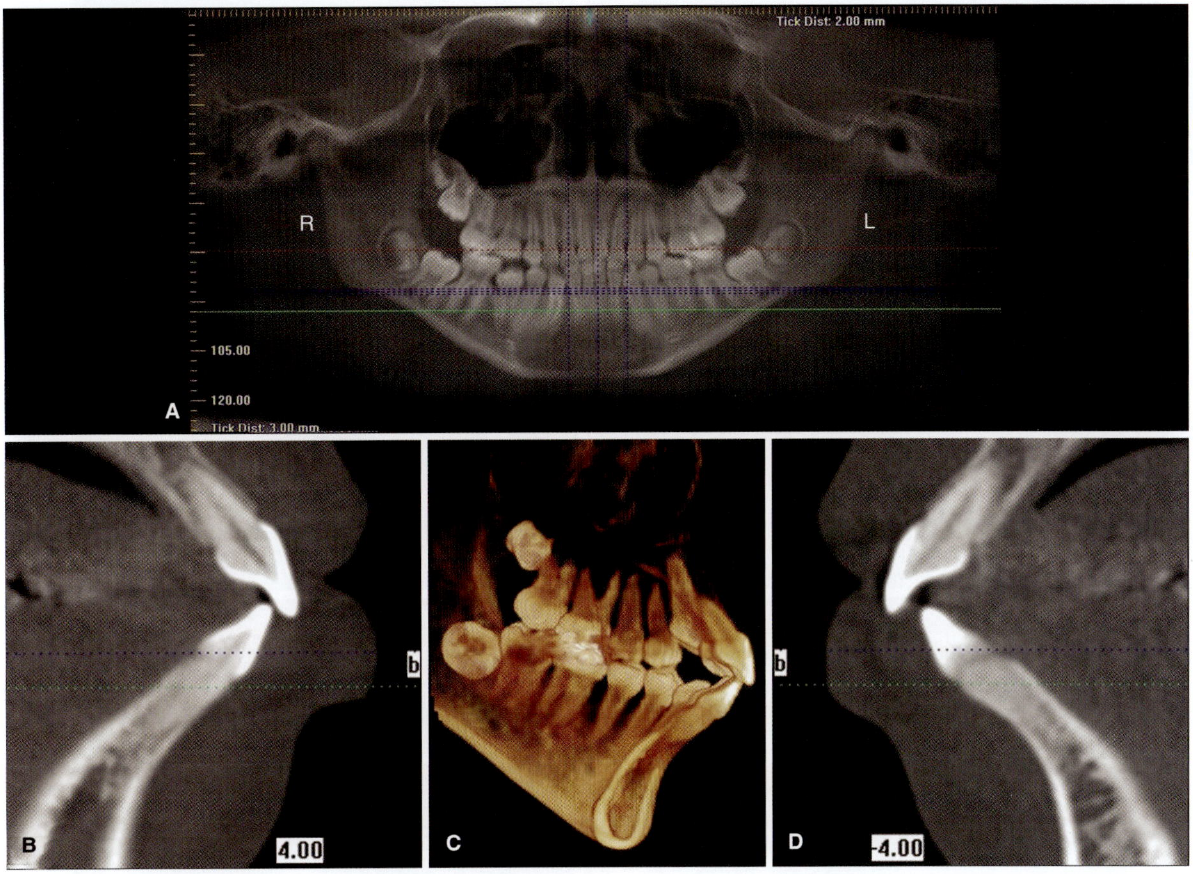

Figure 14.2 The utility of CBCT in diagnosis of boundary conditions and root morphology in bimaxillary protrusive patients. *A*: Panoramic view of a patient with bimaxillary protrusion which, due to the 2D perspective, does not provide information on any potential buccolingual boundary limitations and suggests a near normal length of the roots of the maxillary anterior teeth (crown-to-root ratio of about 1:2). In contrast, the sagittal cross-sections along the long axis of the central incisors (*B* and *D*) as well as the 3D reconstruction (*C*) show that the roots of the incisors are short (crown-to-root ratio of 1:1). The boundary conditions also likely would limit the clinician's ability to retract teeth, particularly in the mandible where the labio-lingual width of the roots of the anterior teeth approximate the width of the cortical bone. Despite orthodontic indications for extraction of four first premolars and high anchorage to retract maximally the incisors, the limits imposed by the short roots and bone boundary conditions resulted in a different treatment approach involving non-extraction treatment and a possible genioplasty at a later date. (Reprinted with permission from Kapila *et al.*, 2011.)

treatment planning, and treatment outcomes. More specifically, we have delineated the use of CBCT to classify patients by their alveolar boundary condition biotype and to identify patient- and treatment-specific risk factors that may compromise alveolar boundary conditions. Also discussed are advances in our understanding of extreme variations in morphologic boundary conditions most commonly associated with developmental anomalies as revealed through CBCT imaging. In addition, we describe an approach to analyzing and biotyping alveolar boundary conditions using CBCT images.

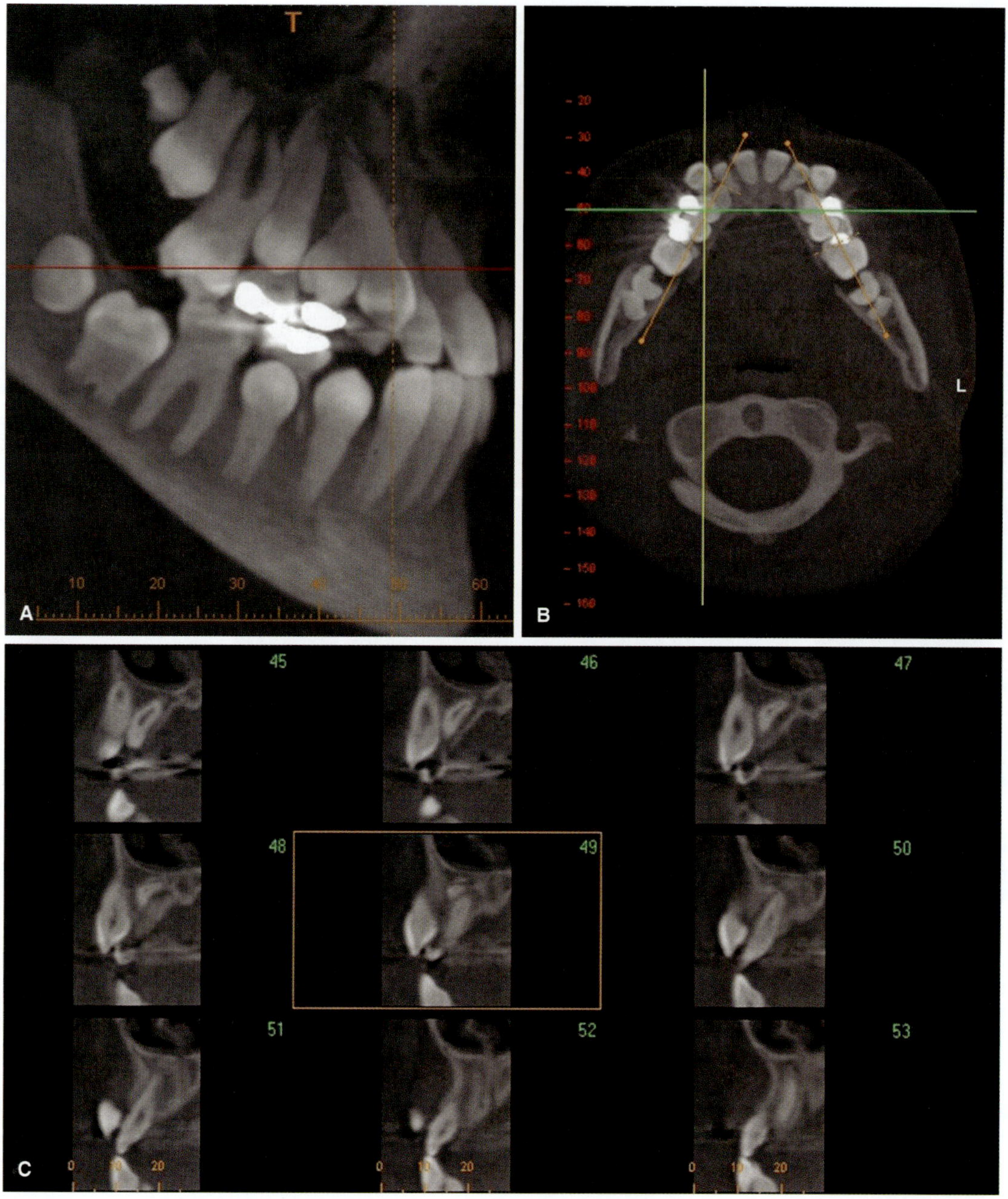

Figure 14.3 Utility of CBCT in diagnosis and treatment planning of transposed teeth help to define restrictions placed by boundary conditions for specific treatment options. This case demonstrates transposed roots of the maxillary canines and first premolars in which CBCT image reveals that the canine root is buccal and distal to the premolar root. Evaluation of these CBCT-derived 3D (*A*) and 2D cross-sectional images (*B* and *C*) may help the clinician to optimize treatment planning that includes proactively moving tooth roots out of the path to be used to relocate the transposed tooth or root, determining if the boundary conditions will permit such movement, and planning the biomechanics (including the force systems, types and direction of movements), which together define the prognosis of moving transposed teeth or roots past each other. (Reprinted with permission from Kapila *et al*., 2011.)

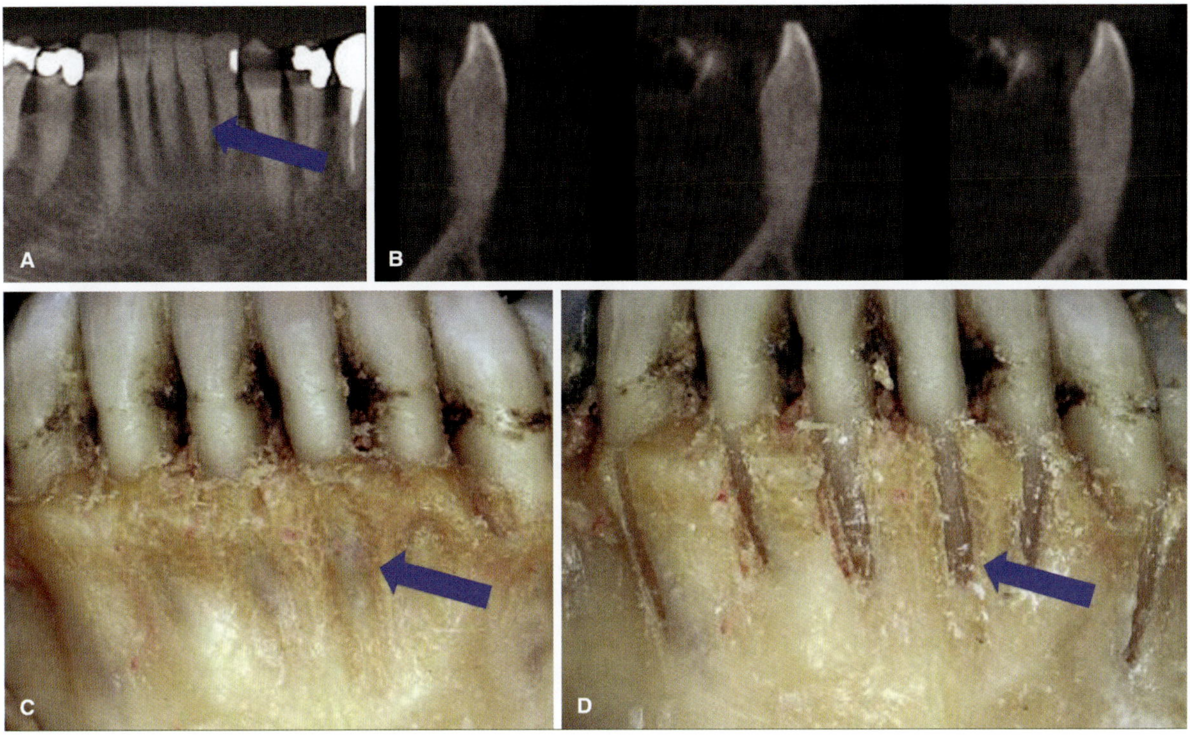

Figure 14.4 Dehiscences on mandibular incisors cannot be detected on panoramic radiographs (*A*), but are seen readily on serial sagittal CBCT radiographs (*B*). Human cadaver mandible after removal of gingiva (*C*) and after removal of the thin overlying alveolar bone (*D*) show compromised bone support on tooth roots. (Reprinted with permission from Patcas *et al.*, 2012.)

ALVEOLAR BOUNDARY CONDITION BIOTYPE: A POTENTIAL NEW DIAGNOSTIC CRITERIA

Orthodontic forces move teeth within the alveolar bone of the maxilla and mandible. Failure to stay within the alveolar bone has significant and often irreversible negative sequelae, such as dehiscences and fenestrations (Wennstrom, 1996). Assessing a patient's periodontal status before, during, and after orthodontic treatment generally is considered standard of care (Machen, 1989). While bleeding on probing and pocket depths are reliable indicators of active periodontal inflammation, they do not indicate if the alveolar bone is normal. There now is abundant evidence that bony dehiscences and fenestrations may be present in individuals who otherwise have unremarkable gingiva and who never had orthodontic treatment (Nauert & Berg, 1999; Mostafa *et al.*, 2009; Evangelista *et al.*, 2010; Lund, 2011; Ehnos *et al.*, 2012; Nahm *et al.*, 2012; Patcas *et al.*, 2012; Yagci *et al.*, 2012; Figure 14.4). Failure to diagnose compromised alveolar bone prior to treatment and to factor this into the treatment plan likely will lead to worsening of the problem if the involved teeth are moved orthodontically. Even if tooth movement does not necessarily position the teeth into more compromised bone sites, some bone loss can be expected during routine orthodontic treatment (Johnson, 2011; Welmerink, 2012). Thus, the more data we obtain on pre-treatment alveolar boundary conditions and on the magnitude of expected change in bone support during orthodontic tooth movement, the better our orthodontic diagnosis and treatment planning for our patients will be.

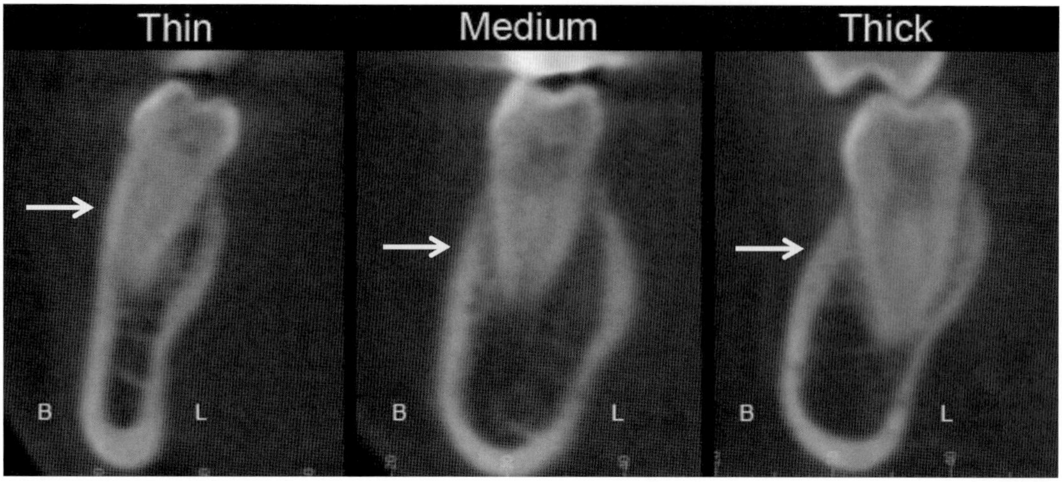

Figure 14.5 Demonstration of buccal and lingual alveolar bone biotypes. Coronal CBCT slices through the first molars of three patients demonstrate thin, medium, and thick buccal bone biotypes based on the distance between the buccal bone surface to the buccal root surface. A treatment plan to increase intermolar width in the thin biotype patient must take into account that pure crown torque is likely to cause dehiscence. B, buccal; L, lingual.

Studies demonstrating pre-existing dehiscences or fenestrations also demonstrate a considerable range of cortical bone thickness overlying tooth roots and total alveolar bone width in subjects with intact alveolar bone. This suggests that patients could be categorized into thin, medium, or thick alveolar bone biotypes based on CBCT images taken as part of the pre-treatment database, as discussed later (Figure 14.5). These data could improve orthodontic diagnosis and treatment planning greatly, especially in borderline non-extraction or camouflage patients where the treatment plan may require moving teeth close to the alveolar boundary or, in some cases, beyond the existing alveolar boundary with the hope or expectation that it will remodel to keep up with the repositioned teeth.

Patients with moderate crowding may be candidates for non-extraction treatment if sufficient arch length can be achieved by expansion, incisor proclination/protrusion, or molar distalization, provided that the boundary conditions will undergo the desired change concurrently. Estimates of how much arch length can be gained in non-extraction treatment vary. For every 1 mm of incisor proclination/protrusion, 2 mm of arch length can be gained. Canine expansion results in a 1:1 increase in arch length. The expected increase in arch length from the increases in both the incisor position and canine expansion is considered to be an overestimation of the actual change (Noroozi *et al.*, 2002 and references therein). Estimates also vary regarding rapid palatal expansion with reported increases in arch length of 0.5–0.7 times the amount of posterior expansion (Adkins *et al.*, 1990; Akkaya *et al.*, 1998; Claro *et al.*, 2006). While dental alignment certainly is achievable in crowded cases, as has been demonstrated over the past more than a century of orthodontics, the ability and limits of bone adaptability to follow suit has not been documented well. Furthermore, although conventional 2D radiograph studies are able to provide some insights into the ability of the alveolar bone to adapt or not adapt around incisors in the sagittal plane when using lateral cephalograms (Figure 14.6), they are unable to depict changes in periodontal status in most other dimensions and cases; this is important particularly for the borderline non-extraction or camouflage cases (Demir *et al.*, 2005; Isik *et al.*, 2005; Xu *et al.*, 2006; Kinzinger *et al.*, 2009; Troy *et al.*, 2009; Burns *et al.*, 2010; Germec-Cakan *et al.*, 2010; Turkoz & Iscan, 2011). Given the lack of consensus on the arch length changes in borderline non-extraction cases, it should not be a surprise that these cases generate

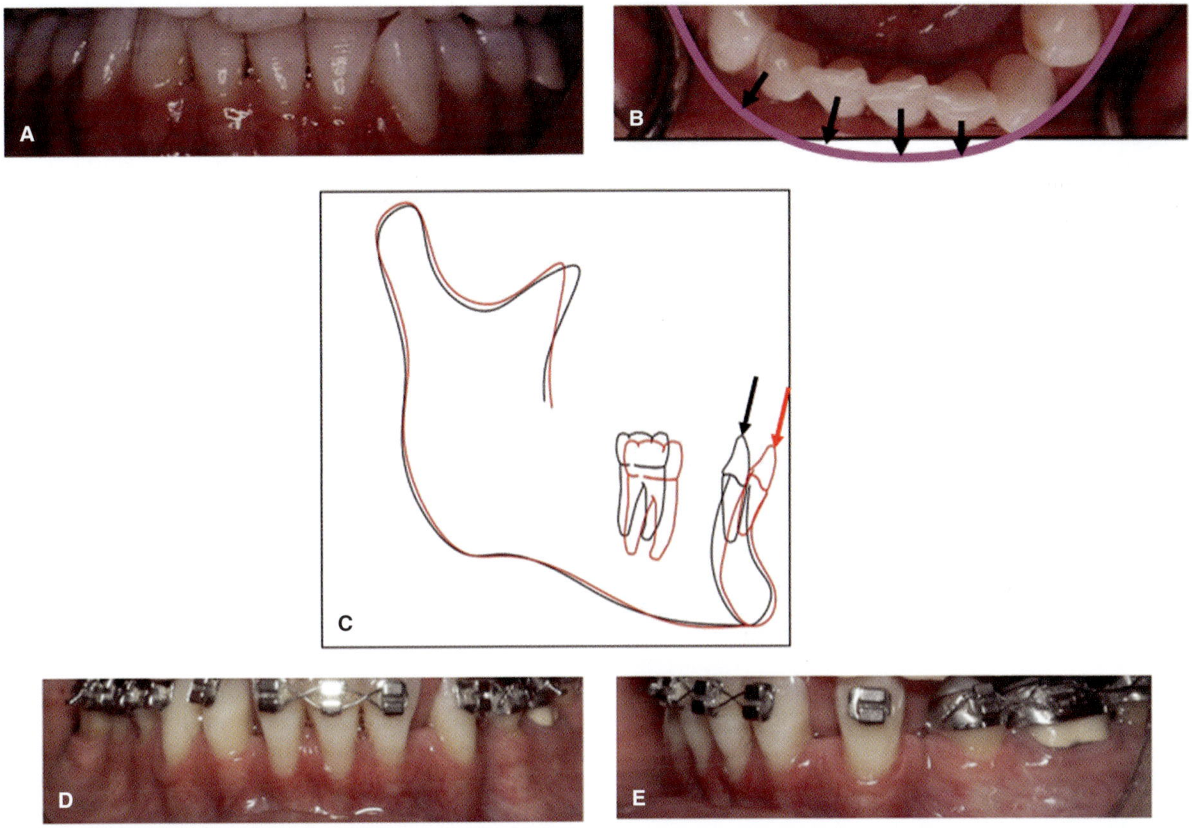

Figure 14.6 *A* and *B*: Pre-treatment intraoral frontal and lower occlusal photographs demonstrating crowding and thin attached gingiva on lower incisors. Placing a continuous archwire (simulated in *B*) would result in labial forces on the incisors and their resultant proclination. *C*: Regional superimpositions of pre-treatment and progress cephalograms showing proclination of incisors and inadequate adaptation of alveolar boundary conditions. *D* and *E*: In such a patient with thin pre-treatment alveolar boundary conditions and minimal attached gingiva, proclination of incisors may be accompanied by bone loss and gingival recession. (Modified and reprinted with permission from Kapila & Conley, 2009.)

significantly different treatment approaches among orthodontists (Baelum *et al.*, 2012). CBCT may offer additional relevant data for evidence-based treatment planning and better predict treatment outcomes for these patients.

Although, in general, a thin gingival biotype is likely to be an indicator of a similarly thin underlying bone biotype (Fu *et al.*, 2010; Cook *et al.*, 2011), the reverse, namely, that a thick gingival biotype is associated with a thick bone phenotype, may not always hold true. While little research has been performed to determine whether the latter is indeed the case, individuals with a thick and dense soft tissue sometimes can present with fenestrations in the underlying bone. This is demonstrated in a patient presenting with a bimaxillary anterior openbite associated with a long-standing thumb-sucking habit (Figure 14.7). The treatment involved extractions with corticotomies to facilitate tooth movement and bite closure. On reflecting the flap for the corticotomy, substantially compromised periodontal boundary conditions with fenestrations on the lateral incisors and canines were noted. Due to the thick gingival biotype, it was not

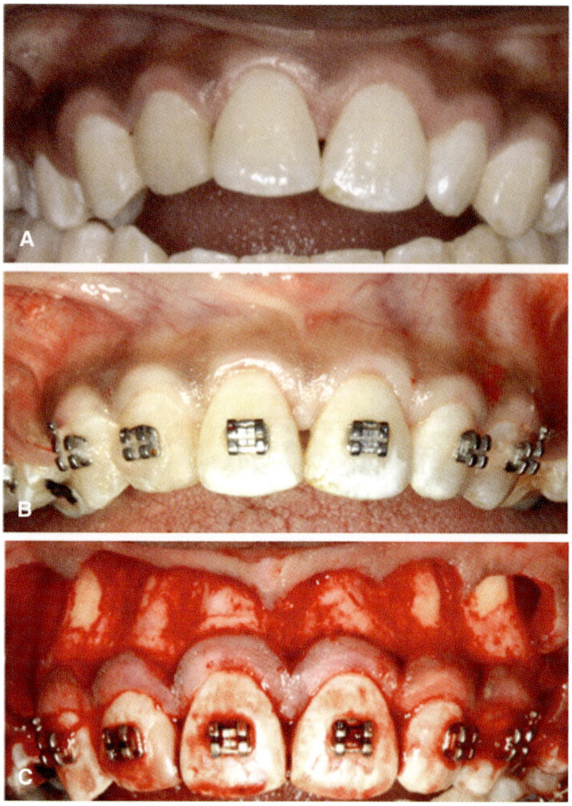

Figure 14.7 *A*: Pre-treatment photograph of patient presenting with a bimaxillary anterior openbite malocclusion associated with a long-standing thumb-sucking habit and a thick gingival biotype. *B*: Shortly after initiation of orthodontic treatment, the patient was referred for corticotomy to expedite treatment. *C*: Flap reflection during surgical preparation for corticotomy revealed fenestrations on maxillary canines and lateral incisors (arrows) that were not detectable clinically due to the thick gingival biotype.

possible to detect any root prominences clinically. It is plausible that the poor bone support around the roots of several teeth in this patient may have resulted from the high forces generated from the thumb-sucking habit. Thus, long-standing finger habits may be another indicator for CBCT imaging to determine the status of bone boundary conditions and for appropriate planning the treatment in these patients.

TECHNICAL CONSIDERATIONS FOR USING CBCT TO ASSESS ALVEOLAR BOUNDARY CONDITIONS

It is important to point out that there are several technical variables that alter the sensitivity and specificity of CBCT for diagnosing alveolar boundary condition biotypes (Leung *et al.*, 2010; Ising *et al.*, 2012; Patcas *et al.*, 2012). While details of these variables are beyond the scope of this chapter and are discussed elsewhere (see Chapter 2), it is sufficient to say that these affect all CBCT images and include machine-specific settings such as milliampere (mA), peak kilovoltage (kVp), exposure time, and sensor size, and patient-specific variables including age, bone density, and periodontal biotype (Molen, 2010). Of these variables, sensor size is the most logical candidate for manipulation if the objective of imaging is to obtain accurate measurements of alveolar boundary conditions. Sensor size influences the image resolution; thus, smaller sensors are indicated for alveolar bone imaging, yet clinicians should be aware that the highest available resolution images currently overestimate dehiscences and fenestrations (Patcas *et al.*, 2012). As sensor and software technologies improve, limited field of view (FOV) CBCTs possibly could provide adequate diagnostic information for this purpose and may be indicated for patients who are considered at risk for developing alveolar defects during orthodontic treatment.

RISK FACTORS FOR COMPROMISING ALVEOLAR BOUNDARY CONDITIONS

In general, risk factors for negative sequelae in orthodontics are categorized as patient- or treatment-specific. Potential risk factors that may compromise alveolar boundary conditions are no exception to this rule. Despite the limited research in this area, especially for CBCT-based studies, initial studies are providing significant insights into patient- and treatment-specific changes in alveolar boundary conditions following orthodontic treatment.

Patient-specific risk factors for compromised alveolar boundary conditions

Facial pattern and skeletal malocclusion have been the focus of early CBCT studies as potential risk factors for compromised alveolar boundary conditions. Several studies show that retraction or proclination of incisors in patients presenting with specific malocclusions or pre-existing alveolar boundary conditions are associated with adverse bone support at the end of treatment. Thus, a spiral CT-based study supports the conclusion that bimaxillary protrusive patients undergoing extraction treatment are at risk for significant alveolar bone loss by demonstrating that significant crestal and mid-root alveolar lingual bone loss occurs routinely around maxillary and mandibular incisors of these patients following incisor retraction (Sarikaya *et al.*, 2002). The maxillary lateral incisors lost 87% and 50% of their crestal and mid-root lingual alveolar bone, respectively. Also, maxillary central incisors lost 61% and 42% of their crestal and midroot alveolar lingual bone, respectively. Likewise, the mandibular lateral incisors lost 70% and 37%, and mandibular central incisors lost 94% and 44% of their crestal and midroot lingual alveolar bone, respectively. Moreover, of the 19 subjects in this study, eight had at least one palatal dehiscence in the maxilla and 11 had at least one lingual dehiscence in the mandible after treatment. Patients with bialveolar protrusion also were shown to start treatment with less than 1 mm of buccal bone covering over as much as 80% of the root length (Nahm *et al.*, 2012; Figure 14.7). Taken together, these studies strongly suggest that bimaxillary protrusive patients may be at risk for dehiscences following incisor retraction. Thus, if the treatment plan entails decreasing the bimaxillary protrusion through incisor retraction, pre-treatment CBCT images may be warranted to determine if sufficient palatal or lingual alveolar bone width is available to retract the incisors fully without compromising the alveolar boundary conditions (Figure 14.2).

Just as with bialveolar protrusive cases where bone boundary conditions may fail to adapt to the substantial orthodontic retraction of incisors, increases in incisal proclination are known to be a risk factor for development of dehiscence (Fuhrmann, 1996). Recession caused by proclination of the incisors has been hypothesized to be worse in patients with thin pre-treatment symphysis width (Wehrbein *et al.*, 1996; Artun & Grobety, 2001; Figure 14.8). These findings suggest that there may be limits to adaptability of bone on incisors undergoing proclination, particularly in patients with specific pre-treatment bone biotypes, and that it may be best to maintain incisal angulation during treatment, especially when thin bone is present.

Other possible patient-specific variables that might be related to presence of dehiscences and fenestrations are angle and skeletal classifications of the malocclusion. Two CBCT studies provide conflicting data regarding the effect of skeletal classification on the presence of fenestrations, but not dehiscences in patients without bidentoalveolar protrusion (Evangelista *et al.*, 2010; Yagci *et al.*, 2012). Both studies confirm that pre-treatment dehiscences are present across the spectrum of Class I, II, and III patients. Only the study by Evangelista and colleagues (2010) found that Class I patients have significantly more dehiscences compared with Class II division 1 patients. In this study, 51.1% of all teeth ($n = 4319$) had dehiscences, most of which are on the mandibular teeth (57.4%). Interestingly, dehiscences are equally likely on the buccal and lingual aspects of the mandibular incisors in Class I and Class II patients, but buccal dehiscences alone are present in 69.4% of the remaining teeth. In contrast, Yagci and colleagues (2012) found that dehiscences are common across all angle classifications, although they are more prevalent in Class II patients. In each Angle Class, dehiscences are found most often on the mandibular incisors (27.0%), and, unlike the findings by Evangelista and coworkers, buccal dehiscences are significantly more common than lingual dehiscences for all maxillary (86% buccal vs. 14% lingual) and mandibular (98.5% buccal vs. 1.54% lingual) teeth ($n = 3{,}976$).

Evangelista and associates (2010) and Yagci and coworkers (2012) also assessed fenestrations and noted that pre-treatment fenestrations are found in each angle class, but there were differences between the two studies in the locations of the fenestrations.

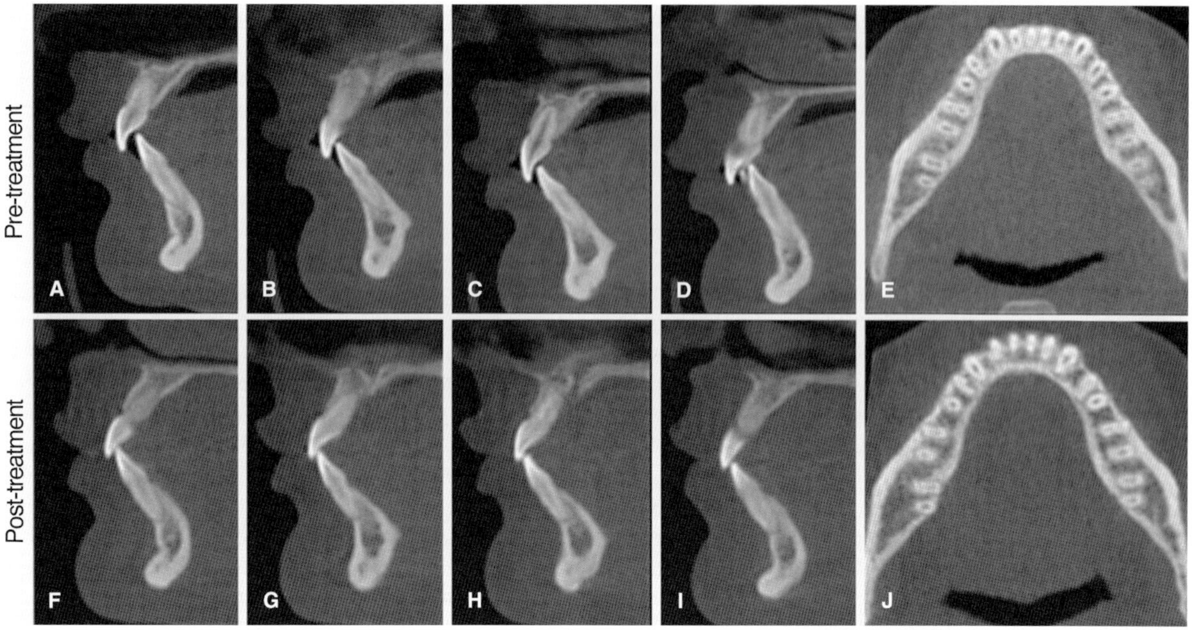

Figure 14.8 CBCT images of incisors with thin alveolar boundary condition biotype before (*A–E*) and after (*F–J*) nonextraction orthodontic treatment involving anterior expansion and flaring of the incisors. Sagittal sections along the long axis of the mandibular left lateral (*A* and *F*), left central (*B* and *G*), right central (*C* and *H*), and right lateral (*D* and *I*) incisors show considerable loss of alveolar buccal bone following treatment. Pre- and post-treatment axial slices (*E* and *J*) demonstrate protrusion of mandibular incisors at the end of orthodontic treatment. In order to make valid comparisons, the sections in post-treatment images were taken as close as possible to those in pre-treatment images.

Yagci's group found more fenestrations on mandibular teeth in Class II (18.3%) compared with Class I (1.73%) or Class III (2.38%) malocclusions. In contrast, Evangelista's group found no difference in fenestrations between Class I and Class II patients. Moreover, they found a greater prevalence of maxillary fenestrations (68.4%) compared with mandibular fenestrations (31.6%). There are no obvious reasons for the variations in the data collected in these studies, which points to the need for continued research on the presence of dehiscences and fenestrations in untreated Class I, II, and III patients.

Vertical facial patterning also may contribute to the occurrence of dehiscences, but not fenestrations. Hyper-, normo-, and hypo-divergent patients all have dehiscences, especially on the mandibular incisors. However, hypo-divergent patients have significantly fewer dehiscences than hyper- or normo-divergent patients (Ehnos *et al.*, 2012). This study also found that fenestrations are rare, but, when present, they are most common on maxillary first premolars, which confirms the findings of Yagci and colleagues (2012).

While there currently are only a small number of CBCT-based studies regarding patient-specific factors that may contribute to compromised alveolar boundary conditions, it appears that orthodontists would benefit from collecting pre-treatment CBCT data on specific types of patients where information on boundary conditions would be helpful for treatment planning. Treatment planning decisions—especially for borderline nonextraction or camouflage cases or cases where teeth are being decompensated (e.g., prior to surgery), which may require moving teeth close to the alveolar boundaries—clearly would be easier to make if the orthodontist knew precisely where the alveolar boundaries are for each patient. Although lateral cephalograms may provide some insights on alveolar boundary conditions in the incisor region (Figure 14.6), this can be complicated somewhat by any superimposition of structures. Thus, CBCT currently is the only means of obtaining information on boundary conditions relatively accurately in all areas of the mouth.

Treatment-specific effects on alveolar boundary conditions

CBCT imaging currently is being used to assess treatment outcomes following the use of different orthodontic appliances. Of particular importance to our discussion are appliances that affect alveolar boundary conditions by expanding the transverse dimension. Because palatal and mandibular expanders most often are tooth-borne and produce both orthopedic and dental expansion, it is logical to expect that the alveolar boundary conditions will change during expansion. This assumption has been confirmed through CBCT studies (see Chapter 17).

The effect of rapid palatal expansion with a four-banded hyrax expander on alveolar boundary conditions studied by CBCT confirms that alveolar tipping or bending toward the buccal occurs in the posterior region (Garrett *et al.*, 2008; Kartalian *et al.*, 2010). Garrett's group found that a net increase of 4.75° of alveolar buccal bending accounted for 6%, 9%, and 13% of the total expansion at the first premolar, second premolar, and first molar, respectively. Kartalian and associates measured expansion at the first molars only and found alveolar buccal bending of 5.6°. Interestingly, the two studies differed in their findings regarding dental expansion. While Garrett and coworkers reported that dental expansion at the first premolar, second premolar, and first molar accounted for 39%, 46%, and 49%, respectively, of the total expansion, Kartalian's group found no significant differences in dental expansion between these teeth.

The most likely explanation for why these studies differ in their conclusions regarding the contribution of dental tipping to total expansion is the way the angles were measured. While both studies measured alveolar bone angulation, only the investigation by Kartalian and colleagues directly measured dental angulation. Garrett's group calculated dental tipping by subtracting alveolar tipping (6%, 9%, and 13% at the first and second premolars and first molar, respectively) and sutural expansion (55%, 45%, and 38% at the first and second premolars and first molar, respectively) from the total expansion. Along the same line as these studies, the study by Ghoneima and associates (2010) used spiral CT images to measure dental angulation directly, but not alveolar bone angulation. The study derived conclusions on alveolar bone tipping indirectly by comparing changes in the transarch alveolar crest distance with those in the maxillary base width. The authors found that the increase in tip on first molars was 6.75°, the first premolars was 6°, and the canines was 4.3°, and the transarch alveolar bone distance increased more (4.5 mm) than the maxillary base width (1.7 mm). Thus, they concluded that palatal expansion produces both dental and alveolar tipping, which is in agreement with the findings of Garrett and associates.

While the studies on rapid palatal expansion focused on dental, alveolar, and skeletal changes following treatment, the only study on slow palatal expansion with a quadhelix specifically assessed the alveolar boundary conditions at the molars (Corbridge *et al.*, 2011). Essentially every measure of alveolar boundary conditions changed significantly following quad-helix treatment. More specifically, buccal and lingual bone thickness—measured as the distance from the root to the outermost point of the respective cortical plates—decreased and increased, respectively, following quad-helix treatment. Total alveolar width, measured from the outermost buccal to outermost lingual cortical plate, increased slightly, but significantly. Interestingly, buccal cortical plate thickness decreased at the end of expansion, and no measurable bone was present on at least one molar in one-third of the patients at the beginning of Phase II treatment. The latter finding points to potential adverse effects of dental expansion by the quad-helix on alveolar buccal bone boundary and integrity.

The effects of maxillary and mandibular expansion with a Schwarz appliance on alveolar boundary conditions also has been studied (Tai *et al.*, 2010a, 2010b). The Schwarz appliances are removable and, in these studies, were worn by the patients only at night for 12 months. Expansion was achieved in both arches through alveolar buccal tipping, although the effect was greater in the maxilla than in the mandible. Because Schwarz appliances and the quadhelix often are used in younger patients during Phase I treatment, these results require follow-up to determine if the remodeled alveolar boundary conditions relapse prior to Phase II treatment.

Some full-fixed appliances are claimed to provide optimized forces for biologically compatible expansion. The only CBCT-based study to evaluate such a claim was one comparing the difference between active (In-Ovation R) and passive (Damon 3 MX) self-ligating brackets on alveolar boundary conditions (Cattaneo *et al.*, 2011). The findings demonstrated that while first and second premolars had significant buccal tipping with both bracket systems, the amount of tipping was not different significantly between the systems. Likewise, buccal cortical bone thickness at the second premolars decreased significantly for both bracket systems and there was no difference in bucco-lingual tipping movements between the two appliances. Thus, these findings call into question the claims that specific appliances generate forces that produce biologically compatible expansion whereby the bone support is not compromised during treatment.

The few CBCT-based studies of patient- and treatment-specific effects on alveolar boundary conditions demonstrate several differences in their findings. One possible explanation for the inconsistencies in the 3D, as well as in previous 2D radiograph-based studies of alveolar boundary conditions is the use of small sample sizes. Significant variability in alveolar boundary conditions in individuals who have not had orthodontic treatment implies that large sample sizes may be required to ensure that the study population truly represents the population at large and that significant differences, if present, can be detected (Johnson, 2011; Welmerink, 2012). These findings and those on the presence of dehiscences and fenestrations in untreated patients also suggest that we need a much more detailed understanding of alveolar boundary conditions in the untreated population to decipher any adverse effects that orthodontic treatment may have on the bone supporting the teeth.

From a clinical perspective, the studies on treatment-specific effects on alveolar boundary conditions suggest that while standard use of common orthodontic appliances is unlikely to produce adverse effects on bone support, these effects should not be considered in isolation. Instead, they must take into account existing bone boundary conditions as well as the magnitude of dental movements expected during treatment and the potential adaptability of the bone to remodel adequately with these movements (Figure 14.8 and Figure 14.9). Thus, CBCT imaging may be warranted for orthodontists who are concerned that an appliance they are considering may compromise existing boundary conditions or where the expected or planned orthodontic movements are substantial enough such that the bone anatomy is not likely to adapt to these movements (Figure 14.1C,D, Figure 14.2, Figure 14.6, Figure 14.8, and Figure 14.9). As CBCT technology continues to improve and research provides more details on treatment outcomes in a broad spectrum of patients, it will be possible to design biomechanic plans or to utilize specific appliances that take the individualized limitations of specific boundary conditions as well as their adaptability into consideration.

BONE BOUNDARY CONDITIONS ADAPTABILITY IN RESPONSE TO NON-EXTRACTION ORTHODONTIC TREATMENT

Based on recent CBCT studies, it appears that patients with thin gingival biotype are the most likely to have thin underlying alveolar bone, especially in the anterior region (Fu *et al.*, 2010; Cook *et al.*, 2011). From an orthodontics perspective, this is critical information if incisor proclination or protrusion is part of the treatment plan. Thin alveolar biotype is not a phenomenon of just the anterior maxilla or mandible, however. Recent studies using CBCT images demonstrate the variability in the presenting alveolar boundary conditions in the posterior mandible and why this information is critical for accurate orthodontic diagnosis and treatment planning.

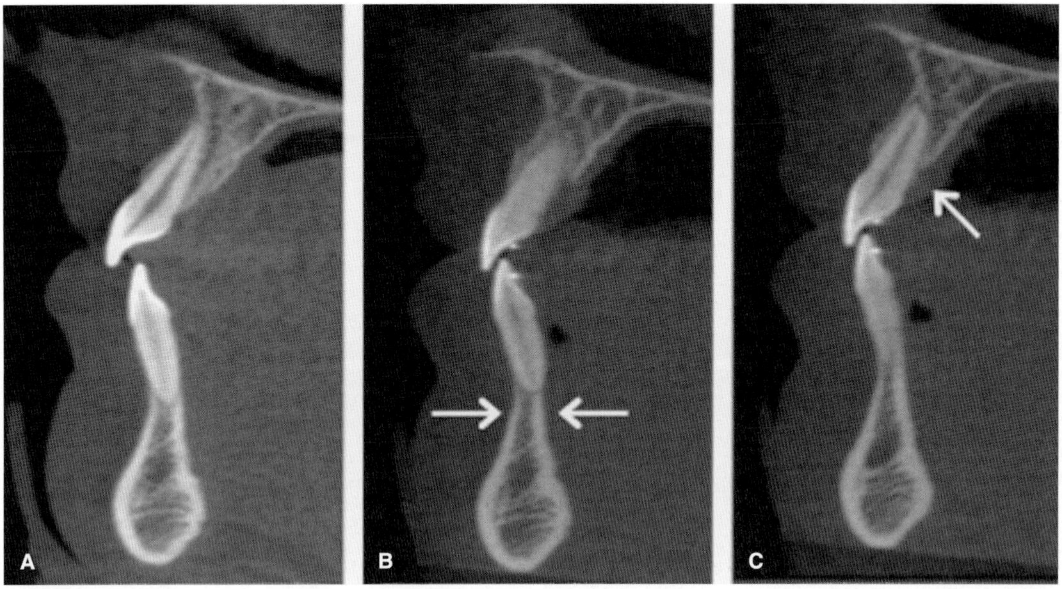

Figure 14.9 Effect of 20-month full-fixed appliance treatment on maxillary and mandibular central incisors with thin pre-treatment boundary condition biotype. *A*: CBCT images of alveolar bone supporting the maxillary and mandibular left central incisors prior to the start of treatment. Note the thin buccal alveolar bone on the apical third of the maxillary central incisor and the undetectable alveolar bone on both the buccal and lingual of the mandibular left central incisor. *B*: Sagittal section from post-treatment CBCT made along the long axis of the mandibular central incisor showing narrowing of alveolar bone at the apex and slight blunting of the left mandibular central incisor root (arrows). *C*: Sagittal section from post-treatment CBCT made along the long axis of the maxillary central incisor showing loss of palatal alveolar bone height (arrow) and moderate external apical root resorption of the left maxillary central incisor.

Methodology for measuring alveolar boundary conditions

Whether your interest is in patient- or treatment-specific factors that affect alveolar boundary conditions, the approach to collecting the data from CBCT images requires careful attention to image orientation and landmark placement. The measurements being made in CBCT-based studies often are in the millimeter or submillimeter range. Any inconsistency in image orientation or landmark placement can skew the data significantly. In general, the commercially available software and free shareware packages that are suitable to view the DICOM files generated by CBCT machines are user friendly and, with some practice, permit clinicians and researchers to measure treatment outcomes accurately. Dolphin 3D (Dolphin Imaging and Management Solutions, Los Angeles, CA) is used commonly by orthodontists and radiologists and will be used here to demonstrate the use of CBCT images for assessing changes in mandibular alveolar boundary conditions following orthodontic treatment.

Image orientation is key to ensuring accurate and consistent measurements from pre- and post-treatment CBCT images. All scans should be oriented in three planes of space using the triplane view (Figure 14.10). Landmarks of interest now can be identified and measurements can be made in all three planes of space at the region of interest (e.g., the molar or canine) after appropriate secondary orientation (Figure 14.11). To determine dental changes resulting from orthodontic treatment and their association with changes in bone boundary conditions, it is necessary to measure changes in tooth angulations and movements through inter-tooth measurements (Figure 14.12). Additionally, the width of the buccal and lingual bone at specific distances from the cemento-enamel junction (CEJ)

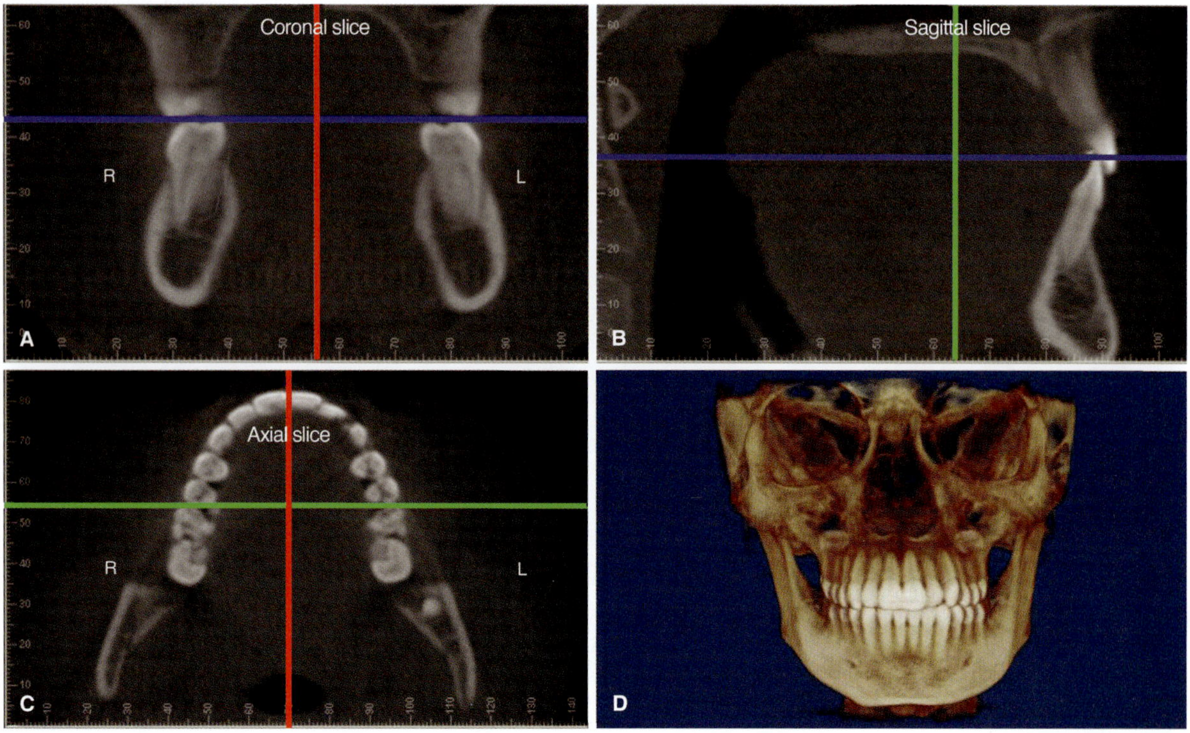

Figure 14.10 CBCT scan in triplane view of Dolphin Imaging Software demonstrating the coronal (*A*), sagittal (*B*), and axial (*C*) planes and the 3D volumetric rendering (*D*). Repeatable image orientation in all three planes of space must be performed for accurate pre- and post-treatment CBCT comparisons. As demonstrated here, the image first is oriented to align the intermolar occlusal plane to the blue line in the coronal slice (*A*). Generating the image for panel *B* is a two-step process. First, the right posterior occlusal plane is aligned with the blue line in panel *B*. Then, the sagittal plane (red line in panel *C*) is moved to the tooth of interest. Panel *C* is used to align the molars to the coronal plane (green line) and to the sagittal midplane (red line; Welmerink, 2012).

and the area of bone can be measured for various teeth after correct orientation and selection of reproducible locations at which these thicknesses are measured (Figure 14.13). With images oriented as described, posterior alveolar boundary conditions can be measured before and after orthodontic treatment (Welmerink, 2012).

Clinical consideration of alveolar boundary conditions and biotype

Using these methods on a sample of 35 adolescents with a mean age of 13.5 years (SD = 1.3) and mild crowding (mean = 2 mm; SD = 2.88) treated without extractions with full fixed appliances, it was noted that significant expansion occurred at the molars ($p < 0.001$) and canines ($p = 0.004$), and the incisors were proclined ($p = 0.004$) and moved anteriorly ($p < 0.001$) during orthodontic treatment. Consistent with reports that untreated patients can present with dehiscences and fenestrations (Nauert & Berg, 1999; Mostafa *et al.*, 2009; Evangelista *et al.*, 2010; Lund, 2011; Ehnos *et al.*, 2012; Nahm *et al.*, 2012; Yagci *et al.*, 2012), our observations also revealed that posterior alveolar boundary conditions have a broad range from thin to thick (Figure 14.5). The change in incisor and molar positions were correlated highly with resolution of arch length deficiency ($r > 0.55$; $p < 0.001$). Significant buccal alveolar bone loss occurred on the molars, canines, and incisors ($p < 0.01$; Figure

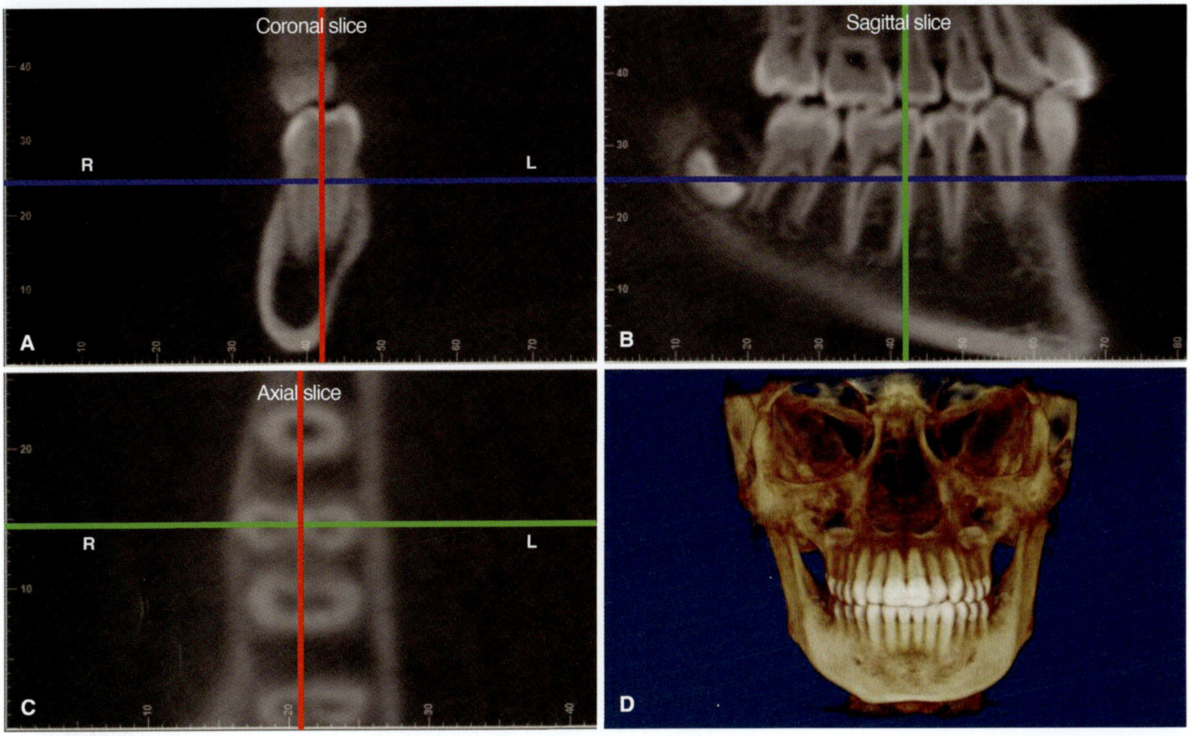

Figure 14.11 Secondary orientation of the mandibular right first molar in the coronal (*A*), sagittal (*B*), and axial (*C*) slices and 3D volumetric rendering (*D*) prior to alveolar bone measurements. First, the axial slice (*C*) is rotated until the green line representing the coronal plane bisects the mesial root of the molar at the mesiodistal center. Next, the image is rotated so the sagittal plane (red line) bisects the mesial root. The coronal slice (*A*) then is rotated to bisect the long axis of the tooth with the sagittal plane (red line). Finally, the blue axial line in panel *B* is moved to the level of the first molar CEJ. With this orientation, the molar then can be magnified to make measurements of the alveolar bone in the coronal and axial slices (Welmerink, 2012).

14.14). With the exception of an increase in lingual bone width at 9 mm from the CEJ, the lingual boundary conditions decreased on the molar and canine and remained largely unchanged on the incisor. The findings of bone loss, particularly on the buccal surfaces of all teeth in a sample with mild crowding, suggest possible compromised periodontal tissues even in cases with small amounts of crowding. Additional studies on cases with greater crowding treated with or without extractions will provide further insights on the effects of orthodontic treatment on the adaptability of bone boundary conditions to orthodontic tooth movement.

Given the range of buccal bone thicknesses defined by the quantity of alveolar bone present on the buccal surface of the first molars, canines, and central incisors, patients were classified into thick, medium, or thin bone biotypes (Figure 14.13B,C), and the responses of each bone phenotype to orthodontic treatment was determined. Significant differences between the amount but not the percentage of buccal bone changes between patients with different bony biotypes were noted. Specifically, individuals with a thick biotype underwent the greatest magnitude of buccal bone loss. These findings suggest that while any bone loss is undesirable, thick bone biotype patients still retain bone support following resolution of mild crowding; individuals with thin biotypes appear to compensate better in trying to retain bone in this type of sample. Caution should be exercised, however, in extrapolating

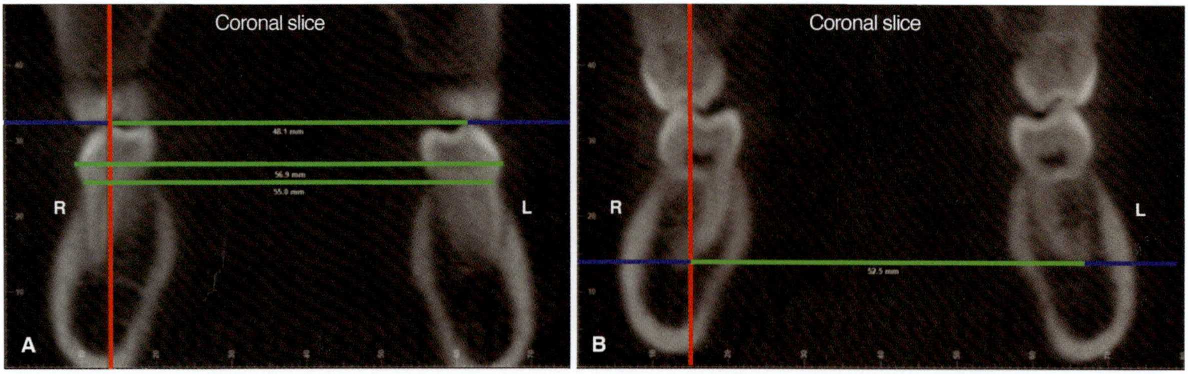

Figure 14.12 Measures of intermolar width at the mesiobuccal cusp tip, most buccal crown concavity (MBCC), CEJ (*A*), and root apex (*B*; Welmerink, 2012).

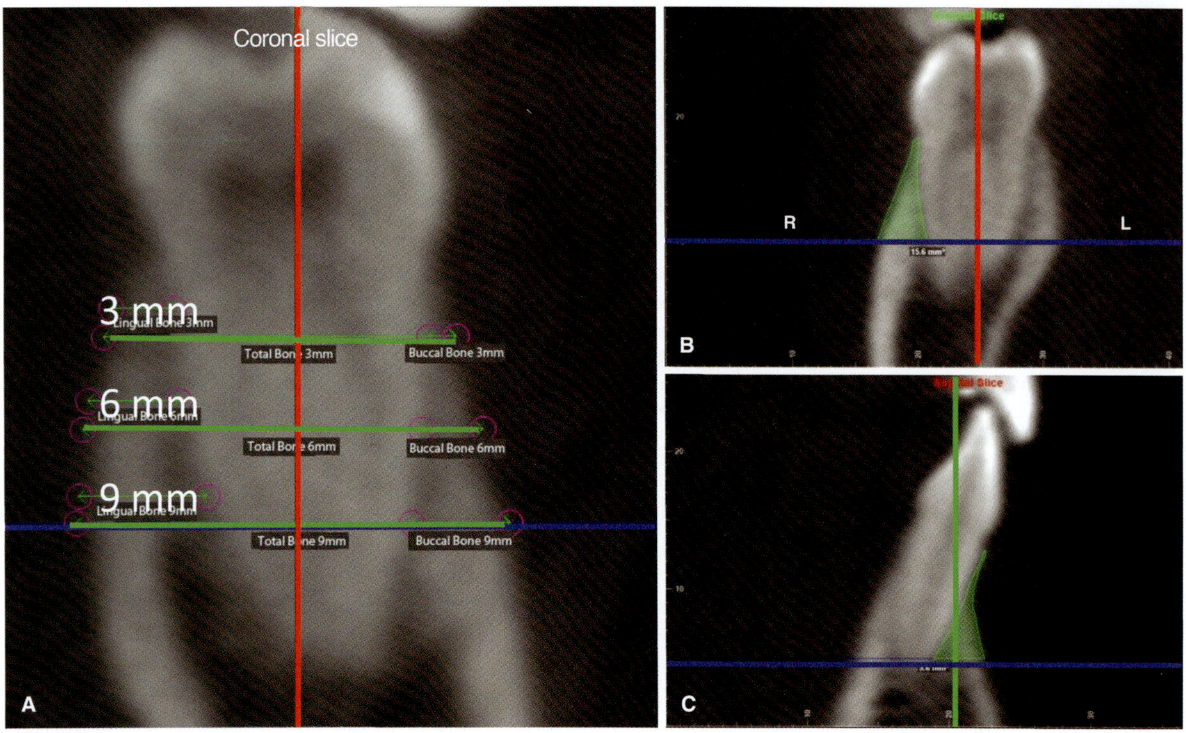

Figure 14.13 Measures of buccal, lingual, and total alveolar bone width at 3, 6, and 9 mm from the respective CEJ. *A*: A line parallel to the axial plane is constructed 3 mm apical to the CEJ and a linear measurement is made from the root surface to the most buccal or lingual point on the alveolar bone. The process is repeated for the 6 and 9 mm levels. Similarly, the total alveolar bone thickness is measured at the 3, 6, and 9 mm levels from the most buccal point of alveolar bone to the most lingual point. The bone biotype is determined by calculating the area of bone represented by the green triangle for the first molar (*B*) and the central incisor (*C*), determined as the surface area of bone between the alveolar crest and 9 mm from the CEJ (Welmerink, 2012).

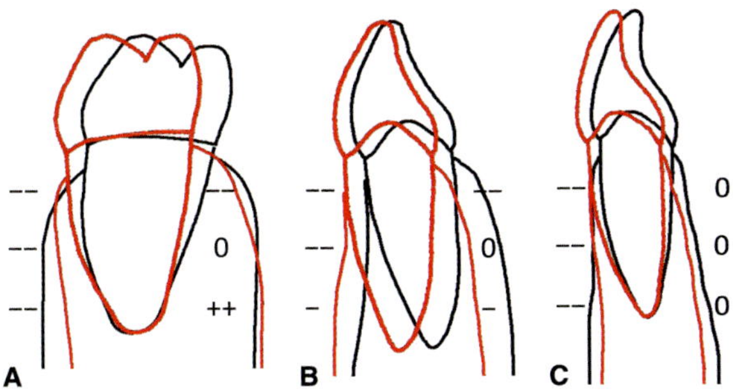

Figure 14.14 Composites of mean changes in tooth positions and boundary conditions in mildly crowded non-extraction treated cases at the mandibular molar (*A*), canine (*B*), and central incisor (*C*) measured at 3, 6, and 9 mm from the CEJ. Buccal movement of the teeth is accompanied by significant decreases in bone width, particularly close to the alveolar ridge area on all three teeth. Black lines: pretreatment tooth position; red lines: post-treatment tooth position; −: bone loss; 0: no bone loss; +: increase in bone thickness (Welmerink, 2012).

these findings to a different sample. For example, it is likely that there is a limit to the bone compensation such that the similar adaptability of bone may not occur in more severely crowded cases, resulting in adverse post-treatment periodontal status. Also, it is likely that the adaptability of boundary conditions to orthodontic tooth movement is subject to significant individual variation and variation by type of treatment mechanics utilized.

Finally, the study identified the pre-treatment variables that are most predictive of bone loss. This analysis demonstrated that initial bone width at 3 mm from the CEJ was the strongest predictor of change in bone width at 3 mm from the CEJ for the molars, canines, and incisors. Inter-molar width and arch length deficiency also were predictors of change in bone width at the incisors. Predictive equations were correlated highly with measured values for the molars ($r = 0.53$) and incisors ($r = 0.76$). The prediction equation derived from this sample can be used by a clinician to predict the amount of bone loss that might occur on the buccal surface of the molars and incisors when treating mildly crowded cases with a non-extraction treatment protocol. Further studies along these lines are likely to provide a basis for identifying specific orthodontic cases where the use of CBCT may be beneficial in deciding between an extraction or non-extraction protocol.

Given the uncertainty of achieving sufficient arch length using non-extraction or camouflage treatment, it is not surprising that these cases produce the greatest range of potential treatment plans or possible treatment options among orthodontists (Baelum *et al.*, 2012). The question then arises whether a clinician can determine confidently that non-extraction is the best treatment approach without knowing the patient's alveolar bone biotype or the ability of bone to adapt to an expanded dentition for it to retain its support around the entire root. Available evidence suggests that patients with thin gingival biotype are likely to present with thin alveolar bone (Fu *et al.*, 2010; Cook *et al.*, 2011) and be at risk for developing bony dehiscences (Melsen & Allais, 2005; Yared *et al.*, 2006). If proven to be efficacious for this purpose, CBCT could become a useful tool for assessing alveolar bone biotype and may be indicated in patients who are suspected of having a low alveolar bone biotype.

COMPLEX CASES WITH SUBSTANTIAL CHALLENGES POSED BY BOUNDARY CONDITIONS

As with all pathologies, malocclusions present as mild, moderate, or severe, depending on the complexity of the case. Severe malocclusions take many forms, but arise most commonly from abnormal dentoalveolar and craniofacial development. CBCT is a powerful tool for orthodontists and craniofacial teams to better diagnose and plan treatment of patients where the boundary conditions fall outside the normal limits.

Transposed and ectopic teeth

Alveolar boundary conditions may provide important insights into tooth development and ectopic eruption. In the majority of cases, tooth development follows a genetically driven program that results in the well-known bud-cap-bell stages of crown formation followed by root formation and eruption (Jussila & Thesleff, 2012). The alveolar bone and periodontal ligament complex develops along with the tooth. If this is successful, the full complement of primary and secondary teeth will appear in the proper sequence and location; however, there are times when teeth fail to develop, fail to erupt, or erupt ectopically. The molecular mechanisms responsible for these developmental anomalies are being investigated, and the data highlight the remarkable complexity of spatial and temporal choreography needed for normal dento-alveolar development.

While specific genes are important regulators of individual tooth development, it has been proposed that abnormal tooth development, especially transposed, ectopic, and impacted teeth, may result from abnormal maxillary or mandibular boundary conditions (Plunkett *et al.*, 1998, and references therein). Restricted space in the developing maxilla or mandible may force tooth buds to develop in abnormal locations, resulting in anomalous eruption patterns. Because the scientific literature on transposed, ectopic, and impacted teeth and their potential etiologies is extensive, these topics have been given their own chapter in this book (Chapter 16). It should be of little surprise that the need for a chapter dedicated to these developmental anomalies is, in large part, the result of CBCT-based studies that investigate tooth development and the alveolar boundary conditions in which this happens. The relationship of abnormally positioned transposed or impacted teeth to the bone boundary may dictate how the case is treated (Figure 14.3; see also Chapter 16). For example, in a case of canine–first premolar transposition, the teeth either can be extracted if space needs dictate, moved to their rightful positions, or maintained transposed close to their pre-treatment locations, depending on the complexity of the treatment and the limitations imposed by existing boundary conditions on each treatment option. In cases treated with the non-extraction option, the decision on where the teeth finally are placed ultimately is determined by the relationship of the teeth to the bone boundary both at the beginning of the treatment and during the entire phase of moving the teeth.

Camouflage treatment of compensated dentoalveolar structures

Compensated dentoalveolar structures are common in skeletal malocclusions. For example, in skeletal Class III patients with a prognathic mandible, the mandibular incisors are retroclined, while the maxillary incisors either are positioned ideally or proclined (Figure 14.15). In some of these cases where nonsurgical treatment offers a viable option, the treatment planning challenge is to determine if camouflage treatment is feasible whereby compensated dentoalveolar structures and bone boundaries can be maintained throughout and at the end of treatment. Extracting lower premolars followed by coordinating the arches and removing the compensations even transiently using continuous archwire mechanics presents one of the greatest threats to alveolar boundary condition integrity. This is true particularly for patients with thin alveolar bone biotype who would be at risk for dehiscences or fenestrations if compensations were eliminated beyond the limits of the ability of the bone to adapt. As demonstrated in the case presented in Figure 14.15, the pre-treatment lateral cephalograph shows the patient has a thin anterior boundary biotype (Figure 14.16A) that was not compromised during treatment (Figure 14.16B), primarily through careful proactive planning to maintain lower incisor compensations throughout treatment (Figure 14.17). Looking ahead, cases such as these could benefit from CBCT imaging-driven refinements in treatment and biomechanics plans.

Dilacerated teeth

As discussed at greater length in Chapter 15, dilacerated teeth offer challenges that may be diagnosed best and treated optimally after all relevant and required information first is derived through CBCT imaging.

Boundary conditions in cleft lip and palate

Cleft lip and palate (CL/P) represents one of the most severe forms of compromised alveolar boundary conditions. Given the need for extensive alveolar reconstruction to ensure optimal tooth eruption or intraosseous implant placement (Hynes & Earley, 2003), it is clear that the demand for accurate CBCT imaging is great for CL/P patients.

Several researchers have confirmed that CBCT's 3D volumetric analysis greatly increases our ability

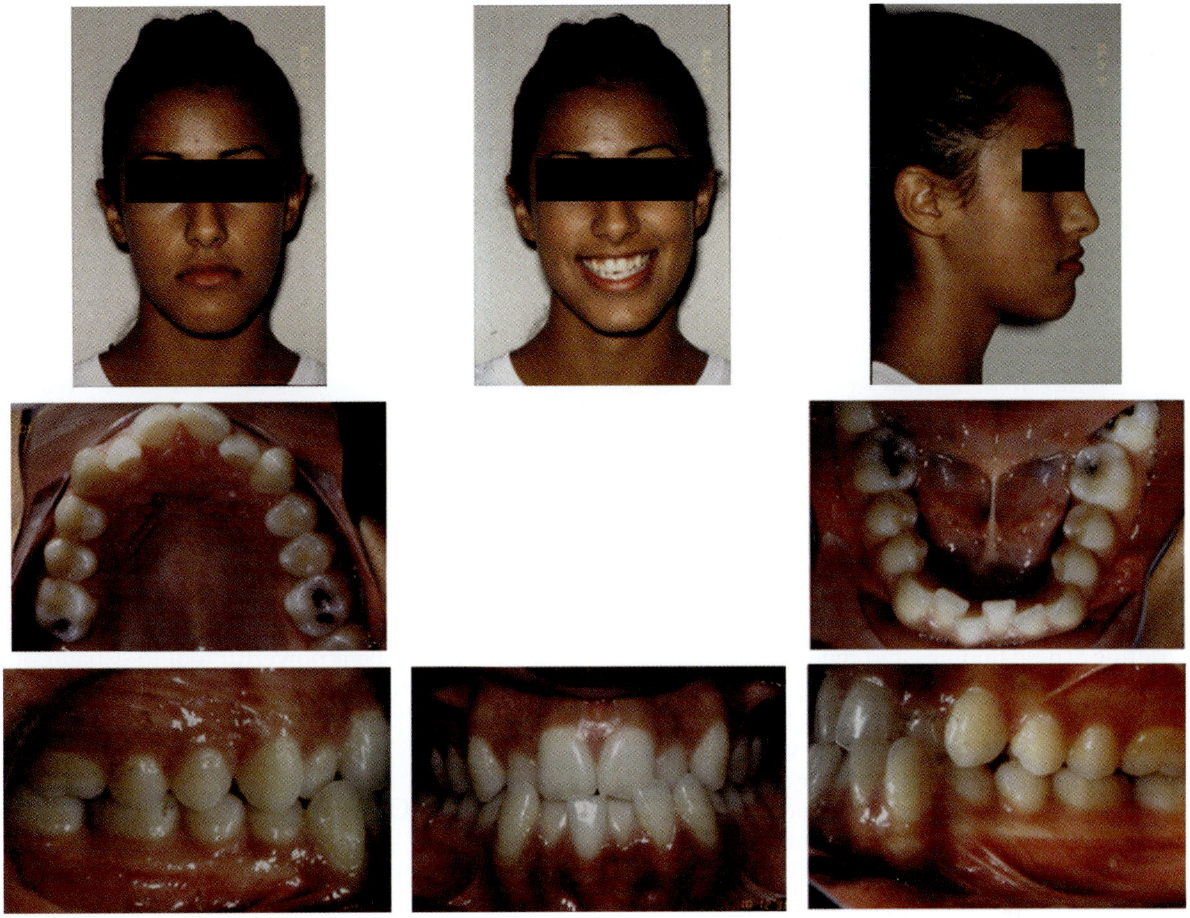

Figure 14.15 Maintaining dentoalveloar compensations within existing boundary conditions in skeletal malocclusions. Pre-treatment photographs of a patient with skeletal and dental Class III malocclusion. A nonsurgical treatment was undertaken. To aid in maintaining the incisor compensations and keep these teeth within the narrow alveolar boundaries, non-continuous archwire mechanics were utilized in the lower arch from start to finish of treatment. (Reprinted with permission from Kapila & Conley, 2009.)

to assess treatment planning and treatment outcomes in CL/P patients (Hamada *et al.*, 2002; Oberoi *et al.*, 2009, 2010; Quereshy *et al.*, 2011; Garib *et al.*, 2012; Zhang *et al.*, 2012). Of special interest to clinicians is the volume of graft material needed to fill the cleft and adequately facilitate canine eruption through the graft site. Two studies have reported a broad range for graft volume at cleft sites from a low of 6.1 mm^3 (Oberoi *et al.*, 2009) to a high of 489 mm^3 (Quereshy *et al.*, 2011) for unilateral CL/P patients. Bilateral CL/P patients have a combined total graft volume of 8.2 mm^3 (Oberoi *et al.*, 2009). The most likely reason for the large discrepancy between the volumes calculated for the unilateral CL/P patients is the approach used to measure the cleft site. Oberoi's group used axial and sagittal slices through the CBCT volume, while Quereshy's group made cleft measurements on the 3D volume. More research is needed to determine which of the two approaches is more accurate in analyzing the amount of regenerative bone in CL/P. Nevertheless, these findings point to the pre-treatment diagnostic value of CBCT imaging for planning of graft site reconstruction and bone

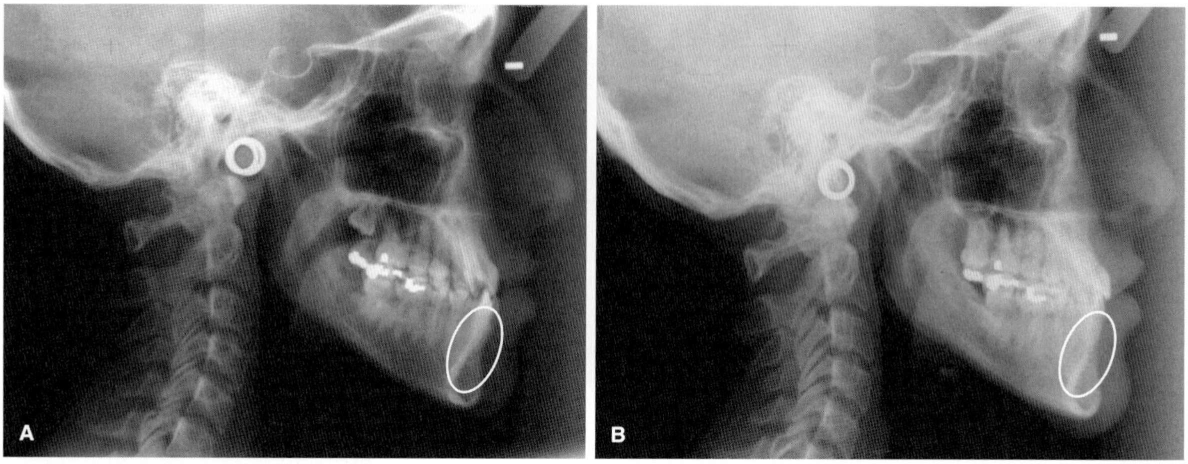

Figure 14.16 Maintaining dentoalveloar compensations within existing boundary conditions in skeletal malocclusions. *A*: Pre-treatment cephalograph of the patient presented in Figure 14.12 showing that retroclined lower incisors have limited boundary conditions. *B*: Post-treatment cephalograph showing the maintenance of dentoalveolar compensations and sound boundary conditions around incisor roots.

grafting. These findings and their implications are presented in greater detail in Chapter 23.

The canine eruption path also is important to evaluate in CL/P patients; again, CBCT is invaluable in providing this insight. If the secondary graft does not restore the alveolar boundary conditions adequately, then canine eruption may not occur or may be ectopic (Bergland *et al.*, 1986). In what currently is the only CBCT-based study of canine eruption in CL/P patients, Oberoi and coworkers (2010) quantified the 3D movements of erupting canines in unilateral and bilateral CL/P patients. They found no significant differences in the absolute incisal, facial, and mesial distances traveled when comparing the cleft-side canine following grafting and the non-cleft-side canine. However, there are differences in the number of cleft-side canines that mimicked the movements of the non-cleft-side canines. They found that 20 cleft-side canines moved facially, while only 10 non-cleft-side canines moved facially. Twenty-two cleft-side canines moved mesially, while only 10 non-cleft-side canines moved mesially. Moreover, the cleft-side canines are more likely to be impacted compared with the non-cleft-side canines. How, or if the alveolar boundary conditions and bone quality at the graft site contribute to these differences has yet to be determined, but clearly CBCT imaging would be a powerful tool to expand our ability to construct ideal alveolar boundary conditions in CL/P patients.

CONCLUSIONS

Alveolar boundary conditions represent morphologic limits on orthodontic tooth movement. CBCT provides a powerful tool for orthodontists to map alveolar boundary conditions accurately prior to treatment. This information is important especially to identify patients with pre-existing compromised boundary conditions and to plan treatment for borderline non-extraction cases where the possibility of dehiscences may arise if restrictive boundary conditions prevent ideal dental alignment. Ongoing and future studies also are likely to provide insights on the limits of adaptability of bone boundary conditions in response to orthodontic tooth movement and whether differences in pre-treatment bone biotypes may contradict specific treatment approaches. CBCT imaging in patients with complex dentoalveolar situations such as transposed, ectopic, and impacted teeth may be helpful in refining treatment plans and mechanics for successful treatments (see Chapter 16). Finally, craniofacial anomalies including CL/P represent

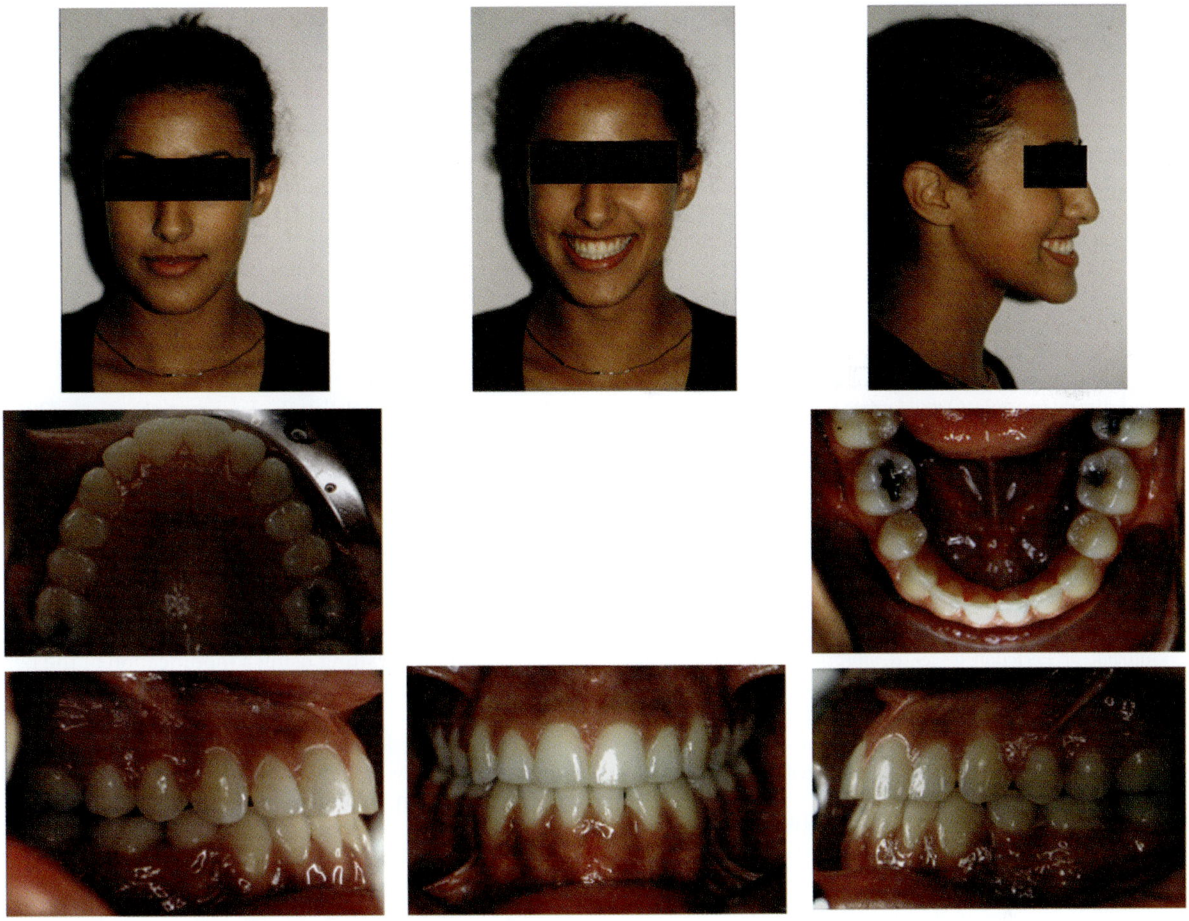

Figure 14.17 Maintaining dentoalveloar compensations within existing boundary conditions in skeletal malocclusions. Post-treatment photographs of the patient presented in Figure 14.12 demonstrate excellent maxillary and mandibular alignment and preservation of the mandibular incisor compensations. (Reprinted with permission from Kapila & Conley, 2009.)

the extremes of pre-existing compromised boundary conditions for which 3D image rendering capabilities of CBCTs have improved interdisciplinary treatment planning greatly.

References

Adkins, M.D., Nanca, R.S., & Currier, G.F. (1990) Arch perimeter changes on rapid palatal expansion. *American Journal of Orthodontics and Dentofacial Orthopedics*, 97 (3), 194–199.

Akkaya, S., Lorenzon, S., & Ucem, T.T. (1998) Comparison of dental arch and arch perimeter changes between bonded rapid and slow maxillary expansion procedures. *European Journal of Orthodontics*, 20 (3), 255–261.

Artun, J. & Grobety, D. (2001) Periodontal status of mandibular incisors after pronounced orthodontic advancement during adolescence: a follow-up evaluation. *American Journal of Orthodontics and Dentofacial Orthopedics*, 119, 2–10.

Baelum, V., Borchorst, E., Buch, H., *et al.* (2012) Inter-examiner variability in orthodontic treatment decisions for Danish children with "borderline" treatment need. *European Journal of Orthodontics*, 34 (2), 250–256.

Bergland, O., Semb, G., & Abyholm, F.E. (1986) Elimination of the residual alveolar cleft by secondary bone grafting and subsequent orthodontic treatment. *Cleft Palate Journal*, 23 (3), 175–205.

Burns, N.R., Musich, D.R., Martin, C., *et al.* (2010) Class III camouflage treatment: what are the limits? *American Journal of Orthodontics and Dentofacial Orthopedics*, 137 (1), 9.e1–9e13.

Cattaneo, P.M., Treccani, M., Carlsson, K., *et al.* (2011) Transversal maxillary dento-alveolar changes in patients treated with active and passive self-ligating brackets: a randomized clinical trial using CBCT-scans and digital models. *Orthodontics & Craniofacial Research*, 14 (4), 222–233.

Claro, C.A., Abrao, J., Reis, S.A., *et al.* (2006) Correlation between transverse expansion and increase in the upper arch perimeter after rapid maxillary expansion. *Brazilian Oral Research*, 20 (1), 76–81.

Cook, D.R., Mealey, B.L., Verrett, R.G., *et al.* (2011) Relationship between clinical periodontal biotype and labial plate thickness: an *in vivo* study. *International Journal of Periodontics & Restorative Dentistry*, 31 (4), 345–354.

Corbridge, J.K., Campbell, P.M., Taylor, R., *et al.* (2011) Transverse dentoalveolar changes after slow maxillary expansion. *American Journal of Orthodontics and Dentofacial Orthopedics*, 140 (3), 317–325.

Demir, A., Uysal, T., Sari, Z., *et al.* (2005) Effects of camouflage treatment on dentofacial structures in Class II division 1 mandibular retrognathic patients. *European Journal of Orthodontics*, 27 (5), 524–531.

Ehnos, S., Uysal, T., Yaggi, A., *et al.* (2012) Dehiscence and fenestration in patients with different vertical growth patterns assessed with cone-beam computed tomography. *Angle Orthodontist*, 82 (5), 868–874.

Evangelista, K., Vasconcelos Kde, F., Bumann, A., *et al.* (2010) Dehiscence and fenestration in patients with Class I and Class II Division 1 malocclusion assessed with cone-beam computed tomography. *American Journal of Orthodontics and Dentofacial Orthopedics*, 138 (2), 133.e1–133.e7.

Fu, J.H., Yeh, C.Y., Chan, H.L., *et al.* (2010) Tissue biotype and its relation to the underlying bone morphology. *Journal of Periodontology*, 81 (4), 569–574.

Fuhrmann, R. (1996) Three-dimensional interpretation of periodontal lesions and remodeling during orthodontic treatment: part III. *Journal of Orofacial Orthopedics*, 57 (4), 224–237.

Garib, D.G., Yatabe, M.S., Ozawa, T.O., *et al.* (2012) Alveolar bone morphology in patients with bilateral complete cleft lip and palate in the mixed dentition: cone beam computed tomography evaluation. *Cleft Palate-Craniofacial Journal*, 49 (2), 208–214.

Garrett, B.J., Caruso, J.M., Rungcharassaeng, K., *et al.* (2008) Skeletal effects to the maxilla after rapid maxillary expansion assessed with cone-beam computed tomography. *American Journal of Orthodontics and Dentofacial Orthopedics*, 134 (1), 8–9.

Germec-Cakan, D., Taner, T.U., & Akan, S. (2010) Arch-width and perimeter changes in patients with borderline Class I malocclusion treated with extractions or without extractions with air-rotor stripping. *American Journal of Orthodontics and Dentofacial Orthopedics*, 137 (6), 734.e1–734.e7.

Ghoneima, A., Abdel-Fattah, E., Eraso, F., *et al.* (2010) Skeletal and dental changes after rapid maxillary expansion: a computed tomography study. *Australian Orthodontic Journal*, 26 (2), 141–148.

Hamada, H., Kitamura, K., Chosa, E., *et al.* (2002) Adrenomedullin stimulates the growth of cultured normal human osteoblasts as an autocrine/paracrine regulator. *Peptides*, 23 (12), 2163–2168.

Hynes, P.J. & Earley, M.J. (2003) Assessment of secondary alveolar bone grafting using a modification of the Bergland grading system. *British Journal of Plastic Surgery*, 56 (7), 630–636.

Isik, F., Sayinsu, K., Nalbantgil, D., *et al.* (2005) A comparative study of dental arch widths: extraction and non-extraction treatment. *European Journal of Orthodontics*, 27 (6), 585–589.

Ising, N., Kim, K.B., Araujo, E., *et al.* (2012) Evaluation of dehiscences using cone beam computed tomography. *Angle Orthodontist*, 82 (1), 122–130.

Johnson, D.P. (2011) Effects of curve of Wilson correction and pre-treatment boundary conditions on quantitative changes in alveolar bone morphology. Master of Science thesis, University of Michigan.

Jussila, M. & Thesleff, I. (2012) Signaling networks regulating tooth organogenesis and regeneration, and the specification of dental mesenchymal and epithelial cell lineages. *Cold Spring Harbor Perspectives in Biology*, 4 (4), a008425.

Kapila, S. & Conley, R.S. (2009) Optimizing biomechanics in complex and compromised cases. In Nanda, R. & Kapila, S. (eds.), *Current Therapy in Orthodontics*. Mosby, Philadelphia.

Kapila, S., Conley, R.S., & Harrell, W.E., Jr. (2011) The current status of cone beam computed tomography imaging in orthodontics. *Dentomaxillofacial Radiology*, 40 (1), 24–34.

Kartalian, A., Gohl, E., Adamian, M., *et al.* (2010) Cone-beam computerized tomography evaluation of the maxillary dentoskeletal complex after rapid palatal expansion. *American Journal of Orthodontics and Dentofacial Orthopedics*, 138 (4), 486–492.

Kinzinger, G., Frye, L., & Diedrich, P. (2009) Class II treatment in adults: comparing camouflage orthodontics, dentofacial orthopedics and orthognathic surgery: a cephalometric study to evaluate various therapeutic effects. *Journal of Orofacial Orthopedics*, 70 (1), 63–91.

Leung, C.C., Palomo, L., Griffith, R., *et al.* (2010) Accuracy and reliability of cone-beam computed tomography for measuring alveolar bone height and detecting bony dehiscences and fenestrations. *American Journal of Orthodontics and Dentofacial Orthopedics*, 137 (Suppl. 4), S109–S119.

Lund, H. (2011) Cone beam computed tomography in evaluations of some side effects of orthodontic treatment. *Swedish Dental Journal. Supplement*, 219, 4–78.

Machen, D.E. (1989) Legal aspects of orthodontic practice: risk management concepts: periodontal disease in orthodontic practice. *American Journal of Orthodontics and Dentofacial Orthopedics*, 95 (5), 445–447.

Melsen, B. & Allais, D. (2005) Factors of importance for the development of dehiscences during labial movement of mandibular incisors: a retrospective study of adult orthodontic patients. *American Journal of Orthodontics and Dentofacial Orthopedics*, 127 (5), 552–561.

Molen, A.D. (2010) Considerations in the use of cone-beam computed tomography for buccal bone measurements. *American Journal of Orthodontics and Dentofacial Orthopedics*, 137 (Suppl 4), S130–S135.

Mostafa, Y.A., El Sharaby, F.A., & El Beialy, A.R. (2009) Do alveolar bone defects merit orthodontists respect? *World Journal of Orthodontics*, 10 (1), 16–20.

Nahm, K.Y., Kang, J.H., Moon, S.C., *et al.* (2012) Alveolar bone loss around incisors in Class I bidentoalveolar protrusion patients: a retrospective three-dimensional cone beam CT study. *Dentomaxillofacial Radiolology*, 41 (6), 481–488.

Nauert, K. & Berg, R. (1999) Evaluation of labio-lingual bony support of lower incisors in orthodontically untreated adults with the help of computed tomography. *Journal of Orofacial Orthopedics*, 60 (5), 321–334.

Noroozi, H., Djavid, G.E., Moeinzad, H., *et al.* (2002) Prediction of arch perimeter changes due to orthodontic treatment. *American Journal of Orthodontics and Dentofacial Orthopedics*, 122 (6), 601–607.

Oberoi, S., Chigurupati, R., Gill, P., *et al.* (2009) Volumetric assessment of secondary alveolar bone grafting using cone beam computed tomography. *Cleft Palate-Craniofacial Journal*, 46 (5), 503–511.

Oberoi, S., Gill, P., Chigurupati, R., *et al.* (2010) Three-dimensional assessment of the eruption path of the canine in individuals with bone-grafted alveolar clefts using cone beam computed tomography. *Cleft Palate-Craniofacial Journal*, 47 (5), 507–512.

Patcas, R., Muller, L., Ullrich, O., *et al.* (2012) Accuracy of cone-beam computed tomography at different resolutions assessed on the bony covering of the mandibular anterior teeth. *American Journal of Orthodontics and Dentofacial Orthopedics*, 141 (1), 41–50.

Plunkett, D.J., Dysart, P.S., Kardos, T.B., *et al.* (1998) A study of transposed canines in a sample of orthodontic patients. *British Journal of Orthodontics*, 25 (3), 203–208.

Quereshy, F.A., Barnum, G., Demko, C., *et al.* (2011) Use of cone beam computed tomography to volumetrically assess alveolar cleft defects: preliminary results. *Journal of Oral and Maxillofacial Surgery*, 70 (1), 188–191.

Sarikaya, S., Haydar, B., Ciger, S., *et al.* (2002) Changes in alveolar bone thickness due to retraction of anterior teeth. *American Journal of Orthodontics and Dentofacial Orthopedics*, 122 (1), 15–26.

Tai, K., Hotokezaka, H., Park, J.H., *et al.* (2010a) Preliminary cone-beam computed tomography study evaluating dental and skeletal changes after treatment with a mandibular Schwarz appliance. *American Journal of Orthodontics and Dentofacial Orthopedics*, 138 (3), 262.e1–262e11.

Tai, K., Park, J.H., Mishima, K., *et al.* (2010b) Using superimposition of 3-dimensional cone-beam computed tomography images with surface-based registration in growing patients. *Journal of Clinical Pediatric Dentistry*, 34 (4), 361–367.

Troy, B.A., Shanker, S., Fields, H.W., *et al.* (2009) Comparison of incisor inclination in patients with Class III malocclusion treated with orthognathic surgery or orthodontic camouflage. *American Journal of Orthodontics and Dentofacial Orthopedics*, 135 (2), 146.e1–146.e9.

Turkoz, C. & Iscan, H.N. (2011) Evaluation of extraction and non-extraction treatment effects by two different superimposition methods. *European Journal of Orthodontics*, 33 (6), 691–699.

Wehrbein, H., Bauer, W., & Diedrich, P. (1996) Mandibular incisors, alveolar bone, and symphysis after orthodontic treatment: a retrospective study. *American Journal of Orthodontics and Dentofacial Orthopedics*, 110 (3), 239–246.

Welmerink, A.D. (2012) Effects of non-extraction orthodontic therapy and boundary conditions on quantitative changes in alveolar bone morphology. Master of Science thesis, The University of Michigan.

Wennstrom, J.L. (1996) Mucogingival considerations in orthodontic treatment. *Seminars in Orthodontics*, 2 (1), 46–54.

Xu, T.M., Liu, Y., Yang, M.Z., *et al.* (2006) Comparison of extraction *versus* nonextraction orthodontic treatment outcomes for borderline Chinese patients. *American Journal of Orthodontics and Dentofacial Orthopedics*, 129 (5), 672–677.

Yagci, A., Veli, I., Uysal, T., *et al.* (2012) Dehiscence and fenestration in skeletal Class I, II, and III malocclusions assessed with cone-beam computed tomography. *Angle Orthodontist*, 82 (1), 67–74.

Yared, K.F., Zenobio, E.G., & Pacheco, W. (2006) Periodontal status of mandibular central incisors after orthodontic proclination in adults. *American Journal of Orthodontics and Dentofacial Orthopedics*, 130 (1), 6.e1–6.e8.

Zhang, W., Shen, G., Wang, X., *et al.* (2012) Evaluation of alveolar bone grafting using limited cone beam computed tomography. *Oral Surgery, Oral Medicine, Oral Pathology and Oral Radiology*, 113 (4), 542–548.

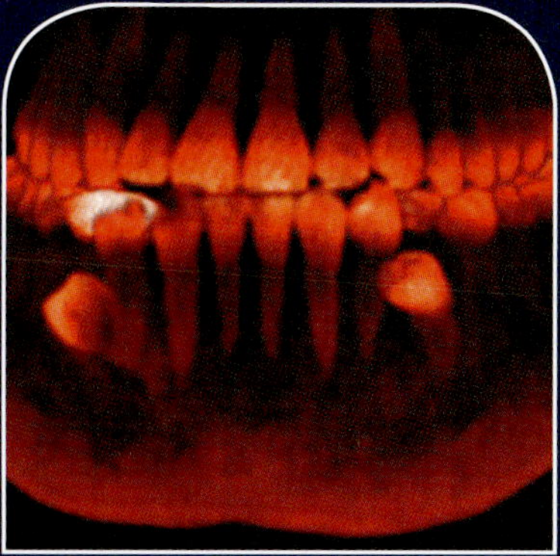

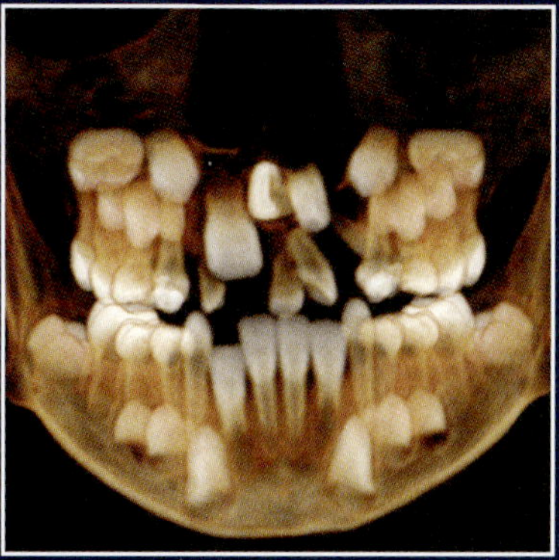

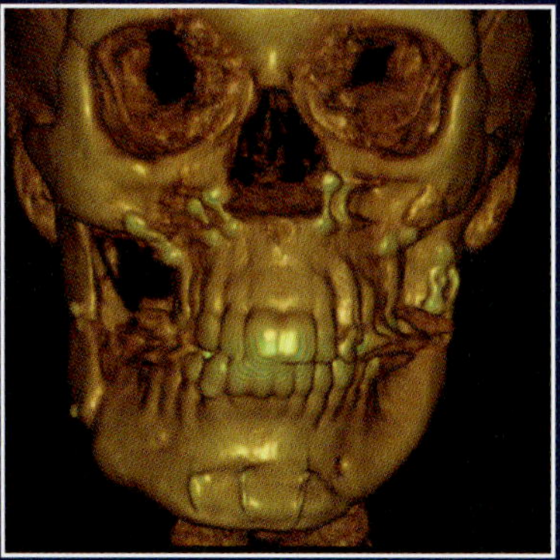

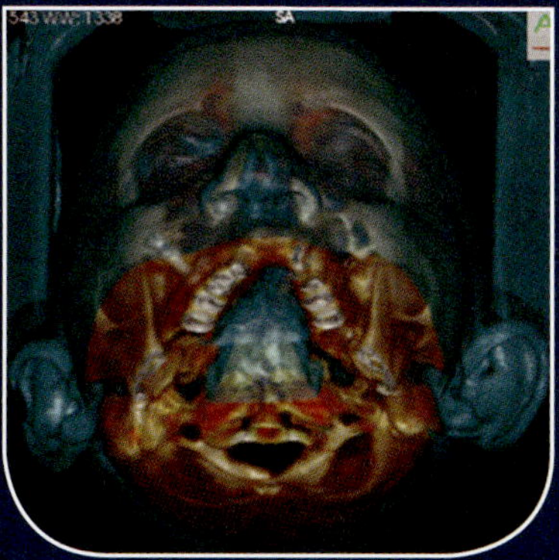

PART 4

Clinical Applications and Treatment Outcomes

15 Assessment of Root Position and Morphology by Cone Beam Computed Tomography

Jeanne M. Nervina, DMD, PhD, and Sunil D. Kapila, BDS, MS, PhD

INTRODUCTION

Following the groundbreaking invention of X-ray technology by W.C. Roentgen, C.E. Kells wasted no time in adapting it to dentistry. Roentgen introduced radiology to the world in November 1895, and Kells began using dental radiographs in the spring of 1896 (Hubar, 2000). Not long afterward, dental radiography was commercialized for use in every dental specialty. R. Ottolengui was one of radiography's early adopters and he published a manuscript entitled *The Physiological and Pathological Resorption of Tooth Roots* (1914), complete with startling images of severely resorbed roots in an orthodontics patient (Figure 15.1). F.C. Kemple, who opened the discussion of Ottolengui's paper, set the trajectory on inquiry in this field for future clinicians and researchers:

> The radiographs shown by Dr. Ottolengui seem to open up a new field of difficulty and complication and study, not only for the orthodontist, but also for the physiologist and the pathologist.... [T]he absorption of the roots of permanent teeth, which are to all appearances perfectly healthy, is a phase of the subject that has not been studied, or at least it has not been discussed in the dental literature. It is this phase of the subject that so vitally interests the orthodontists, and I hope that Dr. Ottolengui and others will continue to study and discuss this question from year to year until a satisfactory solution of the question has been reached.

Kemple would no doubt be surprised to learn that 100 years of study and discussion have not yielded the satisfactory solution he eagerly sought to the problem of root resorption.

This historical snippet serves two purposes. First, it emphasizes the indispensable role radiology plays in diagnosing pathology, thereby justifying continued research to improve radiographic technology to ensure safe high quality imaging of our patients. Second, it serves as a cautionary

Cone Beam Computed Tomography in Orthodontics: Indications, Insights, and Innovations, First Edition. Sunil D. Kapila.

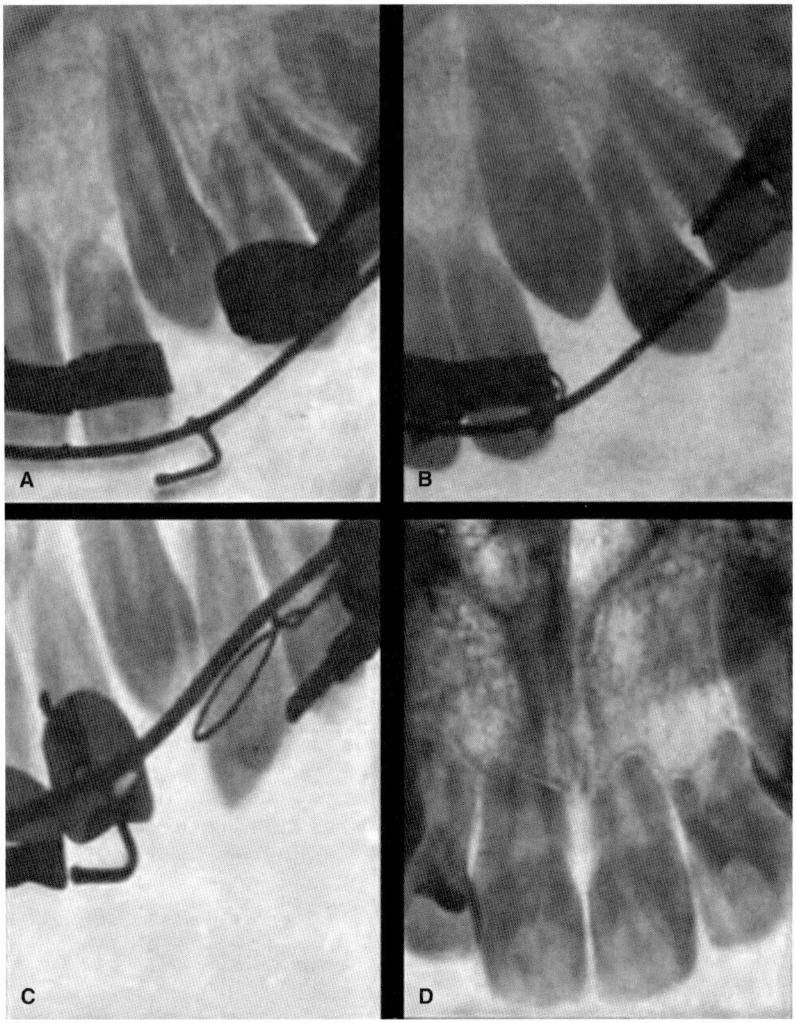

Figure 15.1 Intraoral radiographs taken on an orthodontics patient in the early 20th century. Radiographs taken on (*A*) October 26, 1909, (*B*) January 11, 1910, (*C*) March 18, 1910, and (*D*) February 6, 1911. (Reprinted with permission from Ottolengui, 1914.)

tale for researchers, clinicians, and patients who misjudge the promise of powerful new technologies. Cone beam computed tomography (CBCT), like two-dimensional (2D) radiography in Ottolengui's day, offers unprecedented images of teeth before and after orthodontic treatment. But, as clearly demonstrated by the past 100 years of imaging, radiography alone is powerless to solve the problem of understanding and preventing root resorption. Radiographs, regardless of their dimensionality, map the resulting topography of ectopic eruption or orthodontic forces but offer no insight into the complex biological processes and genetics that account for the pathology. In this chapter, we will continue what Ottolengui and Kemple began in 1914 by discussing how the latest radiographic technology—CBCT—contributes to our understanding of physiological and pathological root resorption, with a special focus on orthodontics patients. This discussion traces CBCT's emergence as an accurate and reliable methodology for assessing root angulation and morphology, which are among the most well-studied risk factors for root resorption. In addition, we will discuss the contribution of CBCT to our understanding of other clinically relevant aspects of root morphology, such as dentoalveolar compensations and dilacerations, as well as the emerging use of CBCT root imaging to gain insights into the biological connections between root morphology and complex craniofacial anomalies.

ACCURACY OF ROOT ANGULATION AND LENGTH MEASUREMENTS ON 2D AND 3D RADIOGRAPHS

Any emerging technology must be put through its paces before it can be incorporated into the clinician's armamentarium rightfully. CBCT has been available commercially for more than 10 years, and its value to dentists for diagnosis and treatment planning is now accepted widely (Scarfe *et al.*, 2012). Orthodontists have embraced CBCT imaging because its three-dimensional (3D) rendering capability is suited ideally for imaging skeletal and dental malocclusions, which are 3D problems. Moreover, combining 3D radiographs with clinically observable dental crowding, spacing, or anomalies gives a much more complete picture of how the teeth develop, erupt, and take their final positions as the primary and permanent occlusions emerge. This information is vital for orthodontic diagnosis and treatment planning because correcting malocclusion is not a simple matter of aligning the crowns. Root position and morphology are critical considerations for ideal orthodontic treatment for two reasons: (1) root position and parallelism are considered critical for an ideal stable occlusion (Bert, 1981; Mayoral, 1982; Casko *et al.*, 1998); and (2) external apical root resorption (EARR) is one of the few common adverse side effects of orthodontic treatment. As will be discussed, one risk factor for EARR is the magnitude of apical root movement, which can be determined only from radiographs. CBCT radiographs are valuable especially because they allow precise measurements of root angulation and length before and after orthodontic treatment. Given the importance of angular and linear root measurements for orthodontic diagnosis, treatment planning, and outcomes assessment, we will compare measurement accuracies of 2D and 3D radiographs.

Methodological approaches to measuring root angulations

Before proceeding to a discussion of radiographic studies of root angulation, it is important to understand how root angles are measured on radiographs, typodonts, and living human subjects. Root angulation measurements on radiographs methodologically are the simplest. Most often, root angulation is assessed on either conventional 2D or CBCT-extracted panoramic radiographs and is defined as the angle formed by the tooth's long axis and the occlusal plane (Figure 15.2). Ideally, this angle is 90° on a conventional 2D panoramic radiograph. When periapical radiographs are used, the tooth's long axis again is used to form an angle with some other researcher-defined reference line or plane. These approaches are used both for typodont- and human subject–based studies.

In typodont-based studies, root angles measured directly on the typodont are compared with the corresponding angles on the radiograph. The question that arises with this approach is this: How does one measure root angles on a typodont? A common method employs a coordinate measuring machine (CMM), which uses a probe to digitize researcher-determined landmarks on the typodont teeth (McKee *et al.*, 2002; Garcia-Figueroa *et al.*, 2008; Owens & Johal, 2008; Tong *et al.*, 2012a, 2012b). This establishes a tooth's x, y, and z coordinates, which are input into a computer program that then calculates the tooth's angle relative to a reference archwire that was placed on the teeth prior to digitizing.

Root angulation measurements in living human subjects cannot be obtained directly without surgical intervention. This highlights a caveat that must be acknowledged when designing or evaluating root angulation studies. Regardless of the medium from which root angles are measured—whether 2D radiographs, 3D radiographs, or dental casts—all of the measurements are indirect, and there currently is no way to verify the accuracy of these measurements. The best a clinician or researcher

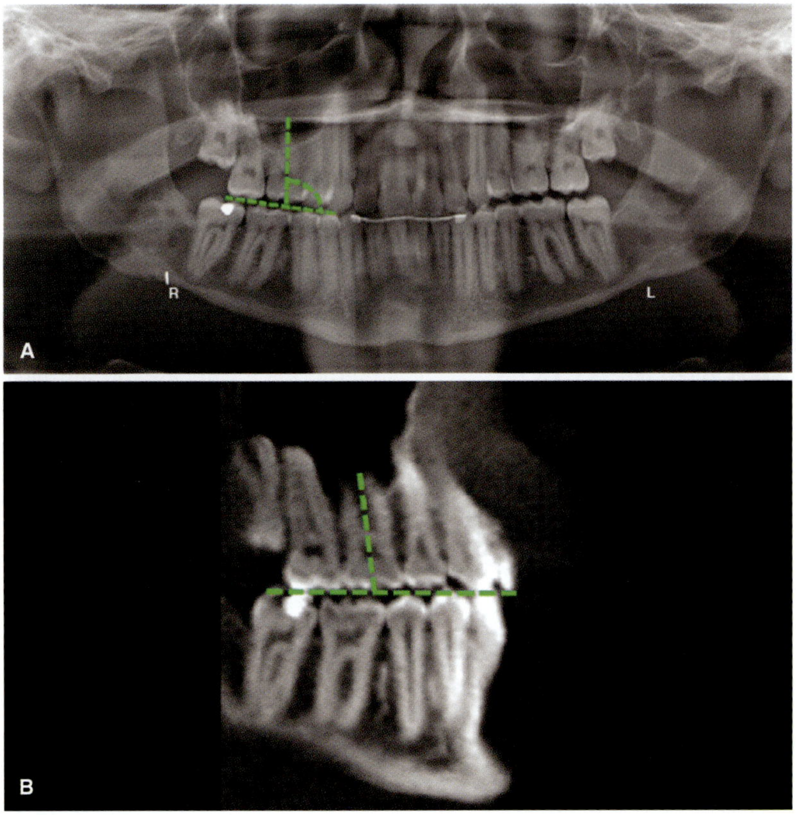

Figure 15.2 Maxillary first molar angulation measured from (*A*) a conventional 2D panoramic radiograph viewed in VixWin software and (*B*) a CBCT-extracted sagittal section viewed with InvivoDental software. Ideal tooth angulation generally is defined as the long axis of the tooth being perpendicular to the occlusal plane, as demonstrated here. (Reprinted with permission from Bouwens *et al.*, 2011.)

can hope for in human subject–based studies is to determine how the measurements obtained from different media compare with each other (e.g., 2D vs. 3D radiographs) or to determine how the measurements taken from a single medium change over time or after a specific treatment regimen. However, dried skull phantoms can serve as proxies for living human subjects to assess radiographic accuracy, but obviously not to assess treatment outcomes.

Accuracy of root angulation measurements on 2D and 3D radiographs

Andrews (1972) proposed six keys to normal occlusion based on his analysis of 120 dental casts from individuals with an ideal occlusion; among these keys is crown angulation and crown tip. Since crown-to-root angulations can range from normal to severely dilacerated (Carlsson & Rönnerman, 1973; Knösel *et al.*, 2009; Xuan *et al.*, 2010), the need for radiographic data on root angulation to diagnose accurately and plan treatment for orthodontics cases now is recognized widely (Tong *et al.*, 2012a). Root angulations are assessed to ensure that the teeth are positioned stably in the alveolus. Proclined or retroclined incisors and lingually/palatally or buccally inclined posterior teeth are considered unstable and potentially harmful as dehiscences or fenestrations may result (see also Chapter 14). In this section, we will discuss the importance of radiographic accuracy when assessing root angulations.

Root parallelism typically is assessed on conventional 2D panoramic radiographs. Unfortunately, parallelism on these radiographs is an optical illusion due to multiple confounding problems (McKee *et al.*, 2001; Hardy *et al.*, 2009; Dholakia & Bhat, 2011; Pfeiffer *et al.*, 2012). The preset arc of the panoramic X-ray machine, highly variable craniofacial geometries, and inconsistent head positioning prior to imaging all distort and magnify anatomic structures on 2D panoramic radiographs. While CBCT machines also have a preset arc, the collection of multiple images throughout that arc allows a volumetric or 3D image to be generated, rather than the single flattened image on conventional films. Using specialized software, the 3D volumes can be rotated to visualize structures directly, place landmarks, and take measurements that are free of the distortion and magnification artifacts that plague conventional 2D radiographs.

The magnitude of angular distortion that affects our perception of root parallelism on 2D panoramic radiographs is assessed readily on radiographs of typodonts or dried skull phantoms. This approach not only allows for precise manipulation of tooth angulation within the arch, but also (1) allows for manipulating how specific root features (dilacerations, resorbed areas, multiple roots) are oriented relative to the X-ray beam, (2) enables the measurement of root length and width, and (3) permits the rotation of the phantoms within the X-ray unit to assess the effect of head tilt on geometric distortion. Using this approach, approximately 73% of the root angulations measured from conventional 2D panoramic radiographs of typodonts are inaccurate (Owens & Johal, 2008). Whether the inaccuracy skews larger or smaller than the actual angulation depends on which teeth are being evaluated and greatly affects the perceived parallelism. The roots of all mandibular teeth appear tipped more mesially on the radiograph than they actually are (McKee *et al.*, 2002; Garcia-Figueroa *et al.*, 2008; Owens & Johal, 2008). In the maxillary arch, roots of the anterior teeth also project as tipped more mesially, but roots of the posterior teeth appear distally tipped relative to their true angulations. As a result, maxillary canines and first premolars that are parallel to each other appear excessively divergent on conventional 2D panoramic films. Orthodontic correction of this apparent divergence would result in roots that are approximated too closely. In fact, because the canine angulation is distorted in particular, the American Board of Orthodontics explicitly states that canine root angulations are not to be scored when assessing root parallelism on panoramic radiographs. Thus, clinicians must be aware that root positions are distorted significantly on conventional 2D panoramic radiographs (Lucchesi *et al.*, 1988).

Given CBCT's 3D rendering capacity, it should surprise no one that root angulation measurements taken from CBCT images are significantly more accurate than measurements taken from conventional 2D radiographs. While statistically significant angulation error was measured for 16 of 28 typodont teeth on a CBCT image relative to the true angulations, the errors are less than comparable angulation errors measured on 2D radiographs (Van Elslande *et al.*, 2010). Part of the measurement error in this and all radiographic studies is the result of human error in identifying and connecting landmarks to make linear or angular measurements. To help overcome this, typodonts also have been used to develop a computer algorithm that improves the accuracy of angular measurements on CBCT images (Tong *et al.*, 2012a). When compared with the gold standard of CMM-generated angular measurements, the algorithm accurately measured root angulation on 23 of 28 teeth on CBCT images (Figure 15.3). While this methodology currently is not available to clinicians, this study establishes the groundwork for computerized analysis of root angulation that should eliminate or at least greatly reduce measurement inaccuracies.

An important point must be made concerning the measurement error in these typodont-based CBCT studies. While angular measurements taken from CBCT radiographs of typodont teeth are more accurate than angular measurements taken from 2D radiographs, the CBCT-generated measurements are not always accurate. In fact, the angles measured from the CBCT images were different statistically from the actual angles measured on the CMM in the studies by Tong and associates (2012a) and Van Elslande and colleagues (2010). However, most of the differences were not considered to be significant clinically because they were

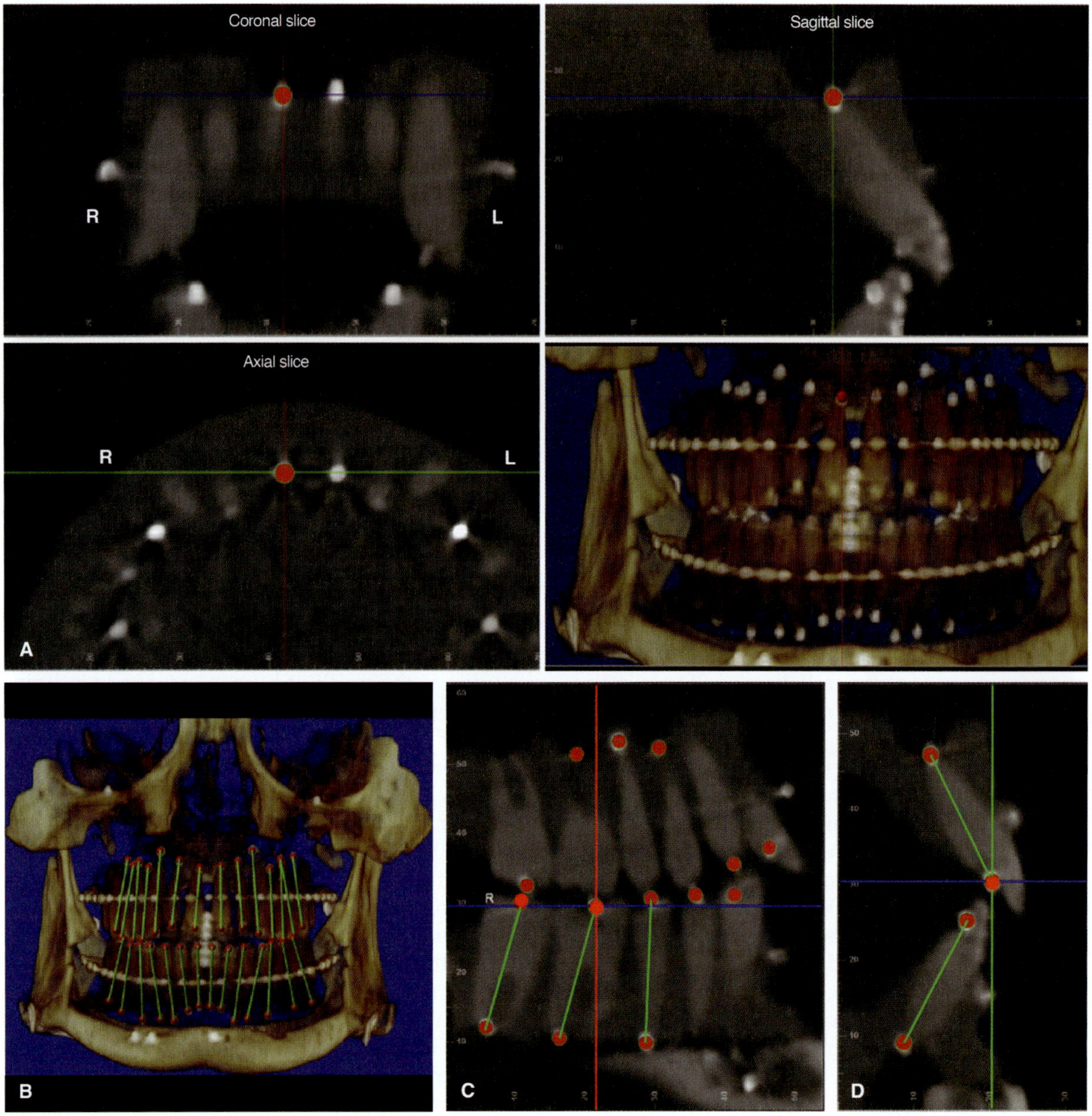

Figure 15.3 Tooth angulations determined from CBCT images of typodont teeth. A typodont studded with stainless steel balls centered at the mesiodistal and faciolingual occlusal surfaces and root apices (single rooted teeth) or midfurcation (multirooted teeth) is used to delineate the long axis of each tooth. In addition, each arch had an archwire for use as a horizontal reference plane. *A*: Triplanar view and volumetric rendering of typodont and angulation markers. *B*: Volumetric radiograph of root angulations with a typodont fixed in a dried skull phantom. *C*: Root apices and occlusal markers (red dots) are connected to generate long axis lines (green). The tooth axis line intersects a vertical line (red) that is perpendicular to a line (blue) that parallels the occlusal plane to generate an angle that describes the mesiodistal tooth angulation. *D*: The faciolingual angle of the incisors is determined in the same manner. (Modified and reprinted with permission from Tong *et al.*, 2012a.)

within ±2.5° of the true angulation; indeed, only measurements of the maxillary lateral incisor angles appear to be the most consistently erroneous in these studies. Why these teeth in particular differ from the actual measurement is not clear, although it is possible that differences in the buccolingual angulation or torque may contribute to these variances (Garcia-Figueroa *et al.*, 2008; Van Elslande *et al.*, 2010).

Accurate angular measurements are important clinically because root torque rarely is a treatment plan when a tooth's mesiodistal angulation is within ±2.5° of its standard reference plane as measured on conventional 2D radiograph (Sämfors & Welander, 1974; Tronje *et al.*, 1981; McKee *et al.*, 2001; Stramotas *et al.*, 2002; Hardy *et al.*, 2009). However, if the mesiodistal angulation exceeds ±2.5° from normal in 2D radiography, then torquing of the roots often is factored into the treatment plan toward correcting this discrepancy. Thus, in a direct comparison of 2D panoramic and CBCT radiographs, root torque would be planned unnecessarily as treatment for 34% of the maxillary teeth and 38% of the mandibular teeth for which the tooth angulation exceeds ±2.5° of normal on the 2D panoramic, but within ±2.5° of normal on the CBCT radiographs (Bouwens *et al.*, 2011). In fact, consistent with the studies of Tong and colleagues (2012a) and Van Elslande and coworkers (2010), Bouwens and associates (2011) suggested that because the lateral incisor angulations on 2D and 3D radiographs differ so significantly from the actual angle, the American Board of Orthodontics should consider eliminating the radiographic scoring of lateral incisor angulations from finished cases, as is done for canine angulations.

Similar to findings on typodonts, angles measured from CBCT images of patients differ significantly from those measured on 2D panoramic radiographs. Emphasizing the need to assess root parallelism accurately at the end of orthodontics treatment, contact between adjacent roots was assessed on CBCT and 2D panoramic radiographs (Leuzinger *et al.*, 2010). Of the 235 sites examined, root contact was detected in 47 sites on 2D panoramic radiographs. When those same 235 sites were examined by CBCT, only five sites had actual root-to-root contact, giving an 89% false-positive rate on 2D images. This raises the possibility that a clinician who diagnoses root contacts on a 2D panoramic radiograph taken near the end of treatment may continue treatment unnecessarily in trying to address a perceived root proximity or contact.

Using an intriguing study design, Peck and coworkers (2007) assessed angular measurements on five subjects who wore splints studded with radiopaque markers at the occlusal plane and root surfaces. Conventional 2D panoramic and CBCT radiographs were taken of each subject wearing his or her splint. Linear and angular measurements were made on each radiograph and compared with dental casts for each subject. CBCT-derived root angulation measurements consistently were more accurate than those taken from 2D panoramic radiographs. Similar to findings of Bouwens and associates (2011), there are significant differences (75% of the time) between tooth angulation measurements taken from CBCTs and 2D radiographs. While it remains to be determined conclusively if head position adversely affects the accuracy of angular measurements on CBCT images (El-Beialy *et al.*, 2011; Frongia *et al.*, 2012), it is clear that 2D radiographs cannot be considered a reliable medium for assessing root angulation in patients.

Another clinical application of CBCT not only demonstrates the accuracy of 3D imaging for measuring root angulation, but also highlights the ability of 3D imaging to capture angulations that 2D imaging simply cannot. Mandibular canine and first molar root buccolingual angulations were assessed on CBCT radiographs taken on Class I and II subjects prior to orthodontics treatment (Shewinvanakitkul *et al.*, 2011). Mandibular canine angulation had a mean of 98° relative to a line connecting the inferior border of the right and left mandible in the coronal plane and did not differ between the Angle groups. However, the buccolingual angulation of the first molar was higher in Class I patients (76°) compared with Class II patients (74°). Whether a 2° difference in first molar buccolingual angulation between Class I and Class II is relevant clinically depends on whether buccolingual crown torque is considered in the treatment plan. This decision, in turn, may depend on the boundary conditions around the roots of these teeth for which CBCT assessment may improve diagnosis and treatment planning decisions further (see Chapter 14).

While analysis of buccolingual angulation currently is not a standard part of the orthodontics evaluation, either before or after treatment, there are cases where this knowledge would prove invaluable. Decision making in borderline cases where orthodontics treatment alone is a potential treatment option without extractions, camouflage, or surgery certainly would be improved by knowing the amount of buccal or lingual tipping of the teeth that the alveolar bone may tolerate or to which it may adapt. Since the only way to obtain this information is by analyzing relative buccolingual dimensions of teeth and bone on CBCT radiographs, clinicians could justify taking the radiographs in these cases if it helps them decide whether or not extractions or surgery are necessary. This topic is covered in more detail in Chapter 14.

In an elegant example of translational research, Tong and associates applied their CBCT-based approach to tooth angulation measurements on a typodont (2012a) to human subjects (2012b). Using root apex and mid-occlusal markers to define the tooth's long axis, the whole tooth angulation relative to the occlusal plane in the CBCT images could be determined (Figure 15.4). Equally important, this approach allows interdental angulations to be determined from both the mesiodistal and faciolingual perspectives. These data offer an exciting opportunity to introduce individualized treatment planning objectives for our orthodontics patients. If we are to believe that Andrews's six keys to ideal occlusion (1972) are correct, then it should follow that tooth angulations are most stable in the context of strong supporting alveolar boundary conditions (see Chapter 14). By collecting and combining angulation data with alveolar boundary condition data from long-term follow-up studies of occlusal stability in orthodontics patients, we could define individualized ideal tooth positions for every patient, based on his or her pre-treatment dentoalveolar relationships.

In closing this section on the accuracy of angular measurements taken from 2D and 3D radiographs, one last caveat is offered. As CBCT studies proliferate, readers wanting to compare data from CBCT studies with each other and with data from conventional 2D radiographic studies face a potential danger in doing so if they fail to recognize the importance of the reference lines used to make the angular measurements. In general, lines through the long axis of the tooth and a clearly defined reproducible vertical or horizontal plane form the angle of interest. Unfortunately, the vertical or horizontal reference planes rarely are the same across studies. This has important implications if cross-study comparisons or meta-analyses are to be conducted. For example, the maxillary right lateral incisor in mixed dentition subjects (mean age 8.6–8.9 years old) is tipped distally at 88.4° relative to the right posterior occlusal plane on the conventional 2D panoramic image, but tipped mesially at 16.8° relative to the sagittal plane when viewed in the coronal CBCT image (Jesuino *et al.*, 2010; Baratieri *et al.*, 2011). There is no way for the reader to determine if these two measurements are equivalent because the reference lines used in each study generate unrelated angles. Moreover, there is no way for the reader to calculate or measure the corresponding angle directly in each study. This is a significant issue because it prevents us from developing a cohesive picture of root positioning. In all likelihood, this problem will be resolved at least partially when standardized 3D CBCT analyses are developed and researchers begin publishing data in which measurements are made relative to accepted, well-defined, and reproducible reference planes.

EXTERNAL APICAL ROOT RESORPTION IN ORTHODONTICS PATIENTS

External apical root resorption (EARR) is a type of pathologic root resorption unique to orthodontically moved teeth. As Kemple stated and as every orthodontist knows, there is another reason for turning our focus to EARR:

> When an orthodontist discovers a beautifully developed permanent tooth, strong and of good structure, becoming very loose—apparently almost ready to drop out of its socket—he is suddenly seized with something very akin to heart-failure. (Ottolengui, 1914)

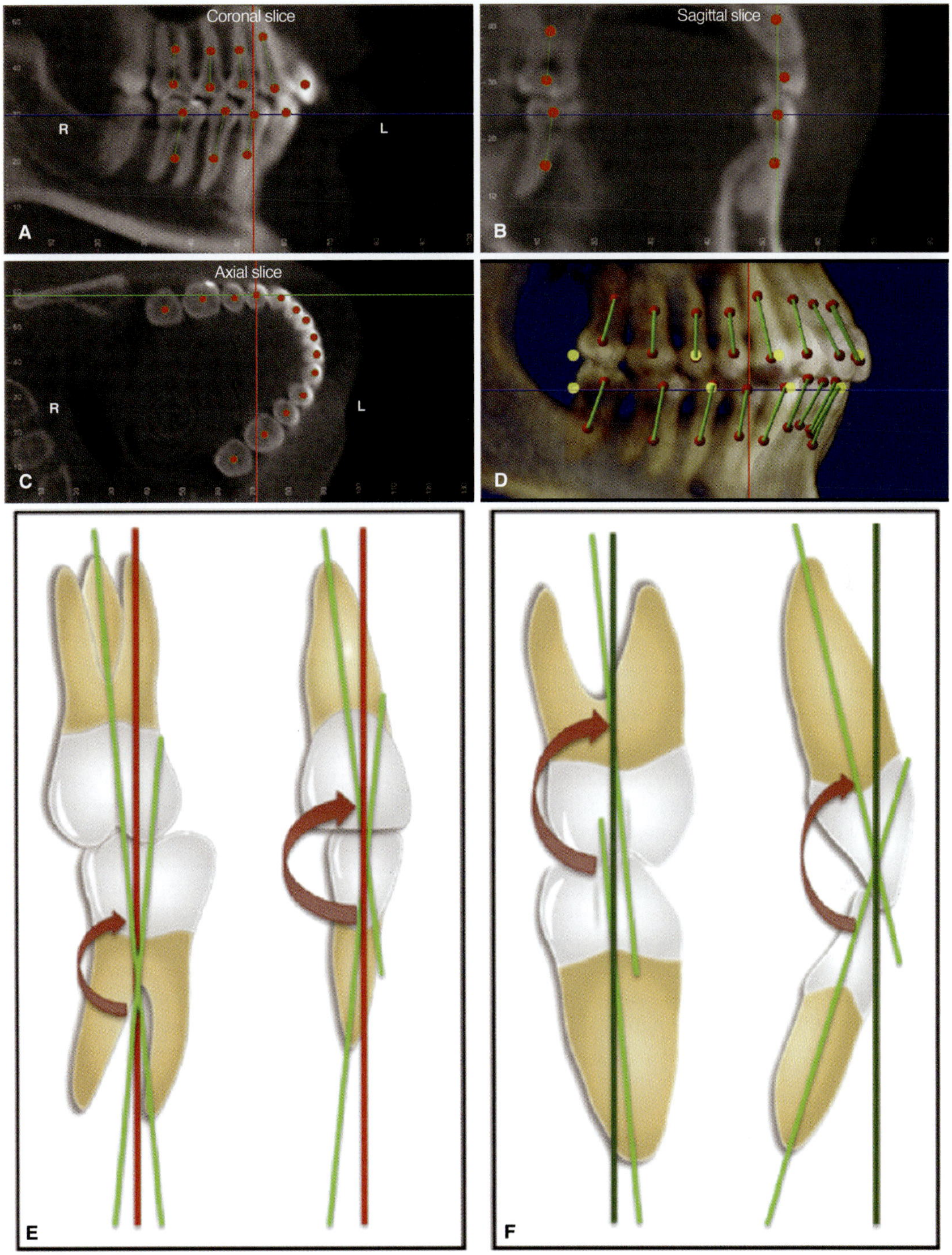

Figure 15.4 Tooth angulations determined from CBCT images of human subjects. *A–C*: In the translational application of their angulation studies on typodonts, the investigators used root and mid-occlusal points to define the long axis of each tooth in live subjects. *D*: Each tooth's long axis intersects a line perpendicular to the occlusal plane (red line) to generate a mesiodistal or faciolingual angle. Mesiodistal and faciolingual (*E*) and interdental (*F*) angulations also can be determined from these data. (Reprinted with permission from Tong *et al.*, 2012a, 2012b.)

EARR is the most common sequelae of orthodontic treatment (Harris, 2000). Irreversible and unpredictable, EARR occurs in 60–95% of orthodontics patients; in 2–5% of EARR cases, it is severe enough to diminish the prognosis of effected teeth (Spurrier *et al.*, 1990; Baumrind *et al.*, 1996; Kurol *et al.*, 1996; Taithongchai *et al.*, 1996). Conventional 2D periapical or panoramic radiographs taken within the first year of orthodontic treatment usually are the first time the orthodontist becomes aware that a patient is at risk for severe resorption. It has been proposed that if moderate EARR is detected on progress radiographs taken within the first year of orthodontic treatment, then severe EARR is likely if treatment is continued (Artun *et al.*, 2005, 2009; Smale *et al.*, 2005). Temporarily stopping orthodontic treatment for 2–3 months followed by treatment using the lightest forces possible appears to be the best approach to managing these cases (Weltman *et al.*, 2010).

EARR can range from mild (less than 1 mm on any tooth regardless of initial root length) to severe (more than 20% of initial root length; Kokich, 2008). Given the inability of conventional 2D radiographs to capture 3D anatomy accurately, it should not be surprising that root resorption cannot be measured accurately from 2D radiographs. EARR is diagnosed correctly only 44% of the time from digitized 2D periapical radiographs (Dudic *et al.*, 2008), and 2D panoramic radiographs overestimate the magnitude of EARR by 20% or more (Sameshima & Asgarifar, 2001). CBCT captures root anatomy in all three planes of space, and researchers have invested considerable time and effort validating the accuracy of root resorption measurements on the 3D images.

Accuracy of root defects measurement in 2D and 3D radiographs

Simulated root resorption is the approach used most often in radiographic accuracy studies (Lund *et al.*, 2010; Alqerban *et al.*, 2011a, 2011b; Durack *et al.*, 2011; Kumar *et al.*, 2011; Bernardes *et al.*, 2012; de Azevedo Vaz *et al.*, 2012; Neves *et al.*, 2012a, 2012b; Ponder *et al.*, 2012; Ren *et al.*, 2013). Resorption defects of varying sizes, shapes, and locations are placed on typodont or cadaver tooth roots with a dental bur. Compared with 2D radiographs, CBCT radiographs consistently generate more accurate images of defects ranging in size from 0.15 to 3.6 mm (Alqerban *et al.*, 2009, 2011b; Durack *et al.*, 2011; Ren *et al.*, 2013). Interestingly, one group did not find any difference between 2D and 3D imaging for detecting root resorption *in vitro* due to regression toward the mean as examiners overestimated defect size on CBCT images and underestimated defect size on periapical images (Kumar *et al.*, 2011).

One *in vivo* study diagnosing post-orthodontic root resorption on conventional 2D panoramic radiographs compared with CBCT radiographs supports the conclusion that panoramic radiographs underestimate EARR (Dudic *et al.*, 2009). In this study, orthodontics patients were referred for CBCT imaging to assess root parallelism that was not visible clearly on the 2D panoramic radiographs. EARR was diagnosed on 43% of all teeth on the panoramic radiographs and 69% of all teeth on the CBCT radiographs. Similarly, EARR of the maxillary incisors, which are the teeth most likely to undergo EARR (Segal *et al.*, 2004, and references therein), was not diagnosed 20% of the time on the panoramic radiographs and 14% of the time on the CBCT radiographs. Moreover, three cases of severe EARR were diagnosed on the CBCT images, but not on the panoramic radiographs. Overall, it is clear that CBCT is better significantly than conventional 2D radiographs for diagnosing EARR.

Regardless of the radiographic modality being used, optimizing the X-ray machine settings is critical for generating diagnostically acceptable radiographs. CBCT machines have variable voxel sizes that usually range from 0.2 to 0.4 mm^3 in size. Clinicians considering using CBCT to assess EARR should select a small voxel size to improve EARR diagnostic sensitivity, specificity, and accuracy (Liedke *et al.*, 2009; Neves *et al.*, 2012b). In addition to small voxel size, limited volume exposure is an option for obtaining high-resolution radiographs at a relatively low radiation dose (Durack *et al.*, 2011). The easiest way to do this is to use the smallest sensor to image the region of suspected localized root resorption, rather than the larger sensors that image the whole craniofacial complex. Another limited volume exposure option being tested is to collect images from a 180° rather than a 360° sweep of the skull. Images collected from the shorter scan are equally as accurate as the longer scan for diagnosing periapical bone loss *in vitro* (Lennon *et al.*, 2011) and may guide the development of targeted imaging protocols for suspected EARR in orthodontics patients. Finally, software development to improve the resolution of post-capture CBCT data is an active area of research (de Azevedo Vaz *et al.*, 2012; see also Chapter 5) that could enhance the capabilities of CBCT further in diagnosis of EARR.

Potential risk factors for orthodontically-induced external apical root resorption based on 2D and 3D data

Despite decades of research, consensus on the predisposing risk factors of EARR has not been reached. While it is agreed that EARR results from the combined influences of biology (patient susceptibility) and mechanics or orthodontic treatment (Weltman *et al.*, 2010), and abundant data on potential risk factors for EARR are available, much of that data are contradictory (Table 15.1). This is not surprising, as most of the existing data were collected from conventional 2D radiographs. Ironically, the amount of contradictory data from studies based on 2D radiographs supports the conclusion that these radiographs are inappropriate for assessing risk factors for EARR. This is not a trivial problem. EARR is an irreversible process that decreases the long-term prognosis of a tooth if rigorous effort is not expended to maintain a healthy periodontal status for the tooth or if the tooth is subjected to trauma, whether extraoral (e.g., blunt force) or intraoral (e.g., fremitus; Kokich, 2008). Yet the need for radiographic evidence of EARR cannot be overstated, as early detection of minor EARR (within the first 6 months of orthodontic treatment) is correlated highly with severe EARR at the end of treatment (Levander *et al.*, 1998a; Artun *et al.*, 2005; Weltman *et al.*, 2010). The conflicting radiographic data on EARR risk factors also highlight the need for combining imaging data with genetic and molecular biological data to identify EARR risk factors definitively in orthodontics patients.

3D imaging certainly offers significant power to measure changes accurately in root length during orthodontic treatment. Because of its relative newness to the field, however, few CBCT-based studies on orthodontically induced EARR are available. Such studies serve several important functions. First, they help to verify the accuracy of CBCT imaging in making and analyzing the submillimeter measurements common in subject-based EARR studies. Second, they help establish protocols for orienting and superimposing CBCT images to ensure reproducibility of these studies. Finally, they provide insight into selected risk factors for orthodontically-induced EARR.

As shown in Table 15.1, relatively few CBCT-based studies have been performed to evaluate EARR risk factors in orthodontics patients. Of all the potential risk factors, CBCT-based studies support patient age, tooth type, excessive overjet, and molar classification as potential risk factors, although, intriguingly, the 2D studies do not support excessive overjet or molar classification as risk factors. Conversely, CBCT-based studies do not support appliance type, patient sex, initial root/tooth length, root shape, finger habits, or history of dental trauma as potential risk factors. The jury is still out on treatment time as a risk factor for EARR in studies utilizing CBCT. None of the other potential risk factors for EARR in Table 15.1 thus far has been assessed with CBCT.

Among the treatment-related risk factors for EARR, two CBCT studies do not support the inclusion of appliance type. One study examined EARR in patients treated with the SureSmile® and conventional edgewise techniques (Patel *et al.*, 2012). The SureSmile® technique utilizes robots to bend custom archwires based on 3D intraoral scans of the patient's dentition and generally has been found to shorten overall treatment time for most orthodontics cases treated with full-fixed appliances (Sachdeva *et al.*, 2005). Pre- and post-treatment CBCT images of the subjects in each treatment group ($n = 14$; mean age 12.7 years) were used to assess EARR. The mean EARR for the maxillary incisors was 0.79 mm with SureSmile® and 0.57 mm with conventional edgewise appliances. Similarly, for mandibular incisors SureSmile® and edgewise appliance therapy was associated with a mean EARR of 0.41 mm and 0.48 mm, respectively. These differences were not significant statistically and given that they are all less than 1 mm, also are

Table 15.1 Conventional 2D radiograph and CBCT studies investigating potential treatment- and patient-related risk factors associated with EARR in orthodontics patients.

Treatment-related risk factors				
Potential risk factor	Conventional 2D radiographs		CBCT radiographs	
	Supports	Does not support	Supports	Does not support
Appliance type	Goldson & Henrikson, 1975 Ten Hoeve & Mulie, 1976 Janson *et al.*, 2000 Mavragani *et al.*, 2000 McNab *et al.*, 2000 Nigul & Jagomagi, 2006 Deguchi *et al.*, 2008 Liou & Chang, 2010 Kinzinger *et al.*, 2011 Motokawa *et al.*, 2012	Malmgren *et al.*, 1982 Lew, 1990 Beck & Harris, 1994 Blake *et al.*, 1995 Mohandesan *et al.*, 2007 Pandis *et al.*, 2008 Scott *et al.*, 2008	No studies	Leite *et al.*, 2012 Patel *et al.*, 2012
Treatment time	DeShields, 1969 McFadden *et al.*, 1989 Linge & Linge, 1991 Baumrind *et al.*, 1996 Levander *et al.*, 1998b Mavragani *et al.*, 2000 Segal *et al.*, 2004 Nigul & Jagomagi, 2006 Apajalahti & Peltola, 2007 Mohandesan *et al.*, 2007 Jung & Cho, 2011 Sunku *et al.*, 2011 Motokawa *et al.*, 2012	Dermaut & De Munck, 1986 Levander & Malmgren, 1988 Beck & Harris, 1994 Hendrix *et al.*, 1994 Mirabella & Artun, 1995 Taner *et al.*, 1999 Fritz *et al.*, 2003 Makedonas *et al.*, 2009	Patel *et al.*, 2012	Lund *et al.*, 2012
Extraction treatment	Kennedy *et al.*, 1983 McNab *et al.*, 2000 Sameshima & Sinclair, 2001b De Freitas *et al.*, 2007 Mohandesan *et al.*, 2007 Artun *et al.*, 2009 Marques *et al.*, 2010 Jung & Cho, 2011 Sunku *et al.*, 2011 Motokawa *et al.*, 2012 Rakhshan *et al.*, 2012	Hendrix *et al.*, 1994 Nigul & Jagomagi, 2006 Nishioka *et al.*, 2006 Makedonas *et al.*, 2009 Ioannidou-Marathiotou *et al.*, 2010	No studies	No studies
Type or direction of tooth movement	Stenvik & Mjör, 1970 Kaley & Phillips, 1991 Beck & Harris, 1994 Mirabella & Artun, 1995 Parker & Harris, 1998	Fritz *et al.*, 2003 van Loenen *et al.*, 2007 Huang *et al.*, 2010	No studies	No studies
Distance of tooth movement	Segal *et al.*, 2004 Motokawa *et al.*, 2012	No studies	No studies	No studies
Force level used to move teeth	Rygh & Reitan, 1972	No studies	No studies	No studies
Intermittent vs. continuous force during treatment	King *et al.*, 1991 Acar *et al.*, 1999 Konoo *et al.*, 2001	No studies	No studies	No studies

Table 15.1 *(Continued)*

Patient-related risk factors				
Potential risk factor	Conventional 2D radiographs		CBCT radiographs	
	Supports	Does not support	Supports	Does not support
Patient age	Reitan, 1974 Linge & Linge, 1983 Mavragani *et al.*, 2000 Sameshima & Sinclair, 2001a	Levander & Malmgren, 1988 McFadden *et al.*, 1989 Harris & Baker, 1990 Linge & Linge, 1991 Harris *et al.*, 1993 Beck & Harris, 1994 Hendrix *et al.*, 1994 Baumrind *et al.*, 1996 McNab *et al.*, 1999 Sameshima & Sinclair, 2001a Fritz *et al.*, 2003 Nigul & Jagomagi, 2006 Makedonas *et al.*, 2009 Ioannidou-Marathiotou *et al.*, 2010 Jung & Cho, 2011 Sunku *et al.*, 2011	Lund *et al.*, 2012	No studies
Patient sex	Newman, 1975 Spurrier *et al.*, 1990 Baumrind *et al.*, 1996 Horiuchi *et al.*, 1998 Kjaer, 1995 Mohandesan *et al.*, 2007 Rakhshan *et al.*, 2012	Newman, 1975 Levander & Malmgren, 1988 McFadden *et al.*, 1989 Hendrix *et al.*, 1994 Harris *et al.*, 1997 Parker & Harris, 1998 Mavragani *et al.*, 2000 Sameshima & Sinclair, 2001a Fritz *et al.*, 2003 Nigul & Jagomagi, 2006 Makedonas *et al.*, 2009 Ioannidou-Marathiotou *et al.*, 2010 Sunku *et al.*, 2011	No studies	Lund *et al.*, 2012 Patel *et al.*, 2012
Initial root/ tooth length	Newman, 1975 McFadden *et al.*, 1989 Mirabella & Artun, 1995 Otis *et al.*, 2004 Artun *et al.*, 2009 Makedonas *et al.*, 2009 Marques *et al.*, 2010	Ngan *et al.*, 2004	No studies	Lund *et al.*, 2012
Tooth type	McNab *et al.*, 1999 Mavragani *et al.*, 2000 Sameshima & Sinclair, 2001a Fritz *et al.*, 2003 Apajalahti & Peltola, 2007 Jung & Cho, 2011 Rakhshan *et al.*, 2012	Artun *et al.*, 2009	Lund *et al.*, 2012	Makedonas *et al.*, 2012

(Continued)

Table 15.1 *(Continued)*

Patient-related risk factors				
Potential risk factor	Conventional 2D radiographs		CBCT radiographs	
	Supports	Does not support	Supports	Does not support
Excessive overjet	Sameshima & Sinclair, 2001a Rakhshan *et al.*, 2012	Mirabella & Artun, 1995 Mavragani *et al.*, 2000 Nigul & Jagomagi, 2006 Ioannidou-Marathiotou *et al.*, 2010 Jung & Cho, 2011	No studies	Patel *et al.*, 2012
Molar classification	Taner *et al.*, 1999	Fritz *et al.*, 2003 Ioannidou-Marathiotou *et al.*, 2010 Sunku *et al.*, 2011	No studies	Patel *et al.*, 2012
Root shape	Levander & Malmgren, 1988 Kjaer, 1995 Mirabella & Artun, 1995 Levander *et al.*, 1998b Sameshima & Sinclair, 2001a Nigul & Jagomagi, 2006 Nishioka *et al.*, 2006 Marques *et al.*, 2010	Lee *et al.*, 1999 Mavragani *et al.*, 2000 Van Parys *et al.*, 2011	No studies	Makedonas *et al.*, 2012
Finger habits	Odenrick & Brattström, 1983, 1985 Linge & Linge, 1991	Mavragani *et al.*, 2000 Nishioka *et al.*, 2006 Makedonas *et al.*, 2009	No studies	Makedonas *et al.*, 2012
History of dental trauma	Malmgren *et al.*, 1982 Brin *et al.*, 1991 Mavragani *et al.*, 2000	Nishioka *et al.*, 2006	No studies	Makedonas *et al.*, 2012
Excessive overbite	Chiqueto *et al.*, 2008 Martins *et al.*, 2012	Mirabella & Artun, 1995 Mavragani *et al.*, 2000 Sameshima & Sinclair, 2001a Nigul & Jagomagi, 2006 Makedonas *et al.*, 2009 Ioannidou-Marathiotou *et al.*, 2010 Jung & Cho, 2011	No studies	No studies
Patient ethnicity	Sameshima & Sinclair, 2001a	No studies	No studies	No studies
Patient genetics	Al-Qawasmi *et al.*, 2003a, 2003b Ngan *et al.*, 2004 Iglesias-Linares *et al.*, 2012a, 2012b	Harris *et al.*, 1997	No studies	No studies

Table 15.1 *(Continued)*

Patient-related risk factors				
Potential risk factor	Conventional 2D radiographs		CBCT radiographs	
	Supports	Does not support	Supports	Does not support
Endodontically treated tooth	No studies	Mirabella & Artun, 1995 Llamas-Carreras *et al.*, 2010, 2012	No studies	No studies
Anomalous tooth	Kjaer, 1995 Thongudomporn & Freer, 1998 Mavragani *et al.*, 2000	Lee *et al.*, 1999 Mavragani *et al.*, 2006 Makedonas *et al.*, 2009	No studies	No studies
Root-to-bone distance	Kaley & Phillips, 1991 Taithongchai *et al.*, 1996 Horiuchi *et al.*, 1998 Motokawa *et al.*, 2012	Mirabella & Artun, 1995 Otis *et al.*, 2004	No studies	No studies
High bone density	Rygh & Reitan, 1972 Midgett *et al.*, 1981	Goldie & King, 1984	No studies	No studies
Cortical bone thickness	No studies	Taithongchai *et al.*, 1996 Otis *et al.*, 2004	No studies	No studies
Allergies or asthma	McNab *et al.*, 1999 Nishioka *et al.*, 2006	Mavragani *et al.*, 2000	No studies	No studies
Alveolar width	Handelman, 1996	No studies	No studies	No studies

not relevant clinically. In fact, when data for all of the maxillary incisors in both treatment groups were pooled, sex, Angle classification, overjet, and use of Class II elastics had no effect on EARR. The only variable that increased the risk of EARR was treatment time and this only on root resorption on the maxillary lateral incisors. The average root loss was 0.46 mm for treatment shorter than 12 months, 0.91 mm for treatment between 13 to 24 months, and 1.38 mm for treatment longer than 25 months.

In a second study assessing appliance type and EARR using CBCT radiographs (Leite *et al.*, 2012), subjects were treated with self-ligating and conventional edgewise brackets. In this prospective study, 19 subjects (mean age 20.0 years) were assigned randomly to the self-ligating bracket (SLB) group ($n = 11$) or the conventional edgewise group ($n = 8$). CBCT scans were taken before treatment and 6 months after the start of treatment. EARR was detected on all of the incisors in both groups, but the magnitude of the root loss did not differ between the groups. The maxillary incisors lost an average of 0.39 mm in both SLB and conventional edgewise bracket groups, while the mandibular incisors lost 0.31 mm and 0.36 mm in the SLB and conventional edgewise bracket groups, respectively.

Along with appliance type, treatment time is another treatment-related factor whose effect on EARR also has been assessed with CBCT. As mentioned above, increased treatment time increases the risk for EARR on the maxillary lateral incisors (Patel *et al.*, 2012). However, Lund and colleagues (2012) did not find a correlation between EARR and treatment time in Class I orthodontics patients treated with four premolar extractions. Importantly, this study measured root length on CBCT images of all teeth at pre-treatment, 6 months after treatment began, and at the end of treatment. After 6 months of treatment, more than

1 mm of EARR was detectable on many teeth, with maxillary double-rooted premolars (29.5%), maxillary and mandibular lateral incisors (16%), and maxillary single-rooted premolars (16%) being affected the most frequently. At 6 months, no teeth had more than 4 mm of EARR. By the end of orthodontic treatment, EARR was detected most often on the maxillary lateral incisors (56.3%), mandibular lateral incisors (43.1%), and maxillary central incisors (41.4%). Importantly, 94% of all subjects had EARR of at least 1 mm and 6.6% had more than 4 mm of EARR by the end of treatment. The latter group had severe EARR on the maxillary incisors, canines, double-rooted premolars, and the distal root of the mandibular first molars. Thus, this study demonstrates that treatment time and tooth type both are risk factors for EARR.

Taking full advantage of CBCT's 3D rendering capacity, Lund and associates (2012) also demonstrated that root resorption does not occur evenly around the root. The palatal/lingual surface showed a slanted resorption in 15.1% of the maxillary central incisors, 11.5% of the maxillary lateral incisors, 4.9% of the mandibular central incisors, and 2.3% of the mandibular lateral incisors. Interestingly, the maxillary canine roots were slanted on the palatal/lingual surface 4.1% of the time, but this nearly was matched by slanting on the proximal surface, which occurred on 3.7% of the upper canines. Mandibular canines were slanted most often on the proximal surface (4.4%). The findings show that the surfaces most prone to this type of root resorption are consistent with the general direction of movement of the anterior teeth during space closure in premolar extraction cases.

Finally, methodological approaches to studying factors associated with EARR using sensitive technologies such as CBCT need to be refined for extracting reliable and useful results. This fact is demonstrated by the apparently inconsistent findings from two recent CBCT studies performed by the same group (Lund *et al.*, 2012; Makedonas *et al.*, 2012) regarding tooth type as an EARR risk factor (Table 15.1). While it appears that both studies presumably were performed on the same subjects, the findings contradict one another for several potential reasons, including the differences between the two studies in the methodology for determining root resorption and the time point selected for this analysis. Makedonas and colleagues studied patients treated up to 6 months, and the study by Lund and associates followed the subjects through to the end of their treatment. Furthermore, the Makedonas study assessed root length using the qualitative index proposed by Malmgren and coworkers (1982), which categorizes root loss as <2 mm, 2 mm to 1/3 of the initial root length and >1/3 of the initial root length, while in the Lund study, resorption was categorized into root loss in 1 mm increments. The latter approach splits the data into much finer groups than the former approach, which makes it much more likely that subtle differences between tooth type susceptibility to EARR will be detected. This is not a trivial distinction for a radiographic approach that is able to detect submillimeter changes in root length. As shown in Table 15.1, the Makedonas study concluded that CBCT analysis does not support several potential risk factors as contributing to EARR—a conclusion that may have resulted partially from the lack of sensitivity of the index used for assessing root resorption. Again, by using both the powerful CBCT imaging technique together with sensitive and reliable methods for measuring root loss, it may be possible that future CBCT-based studies will conclude that variables such as root shape or history of dental trauma are, in fact, risk factors for EARR.

CBCT-BASED DIAGNOSIS OF DILACERATED ROOTS

Of note, a clinical entity involving roots as a possible indicator for using CBCT is dysmorphic roots. CBCT imaging is valuable for identifying dysmorphic or dilacerated teeth prior to eruption (Figure 15.5). While conventional 2D images may show an abnormal crown or dilacerated root, the true structure often is not appreciated until the tooth is extracted or exposed surgically. This is important especially in children who are prone to dental trauma that may lead to crown and/or root malformation and eruption failure (Sahai *et al.*, 2011).

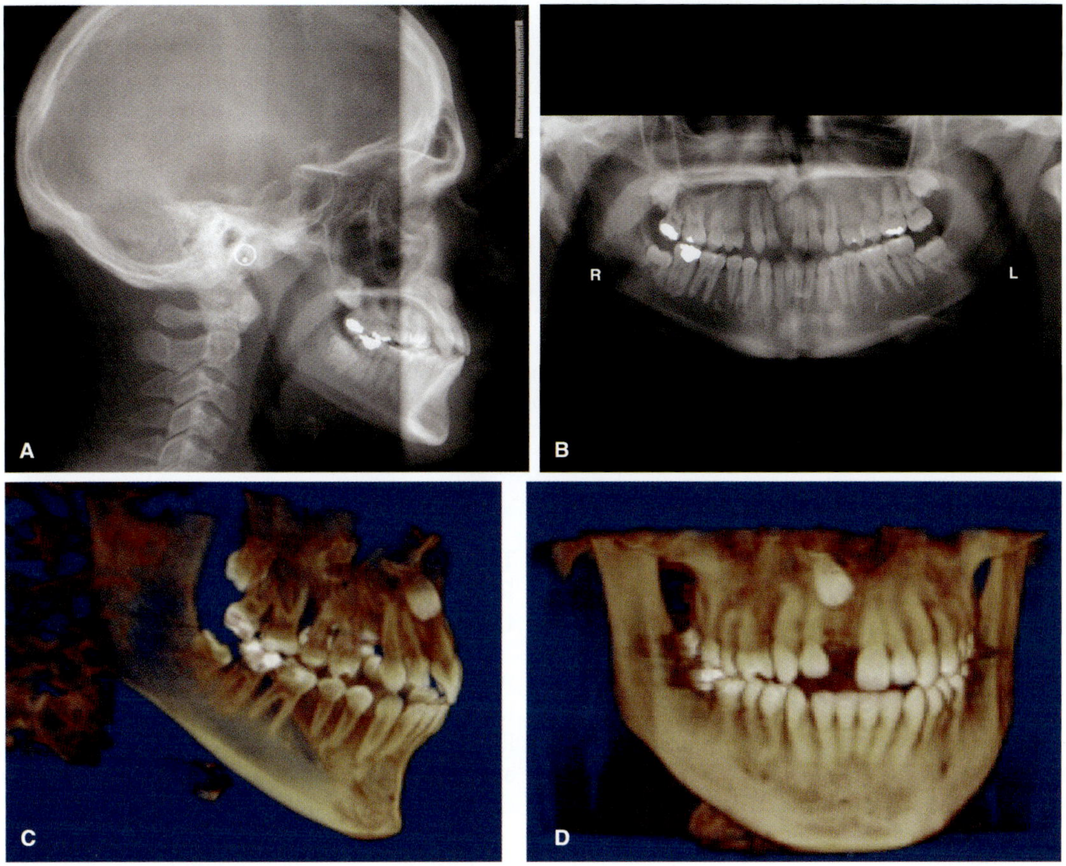

Figure 15.5 CBCT imaging of dilacerated teeth provides refined diagnostic information that can be valuable in treatment planning. Lateral cephalograph (*A*) and panoramic views (*B*) do not provide adequate information on the precise location and morphology of the impacted maxillary right central incisor. Sagittal (*C*) and coronal (*D*) volumetric CBCT renderings provide detailed insights into the severity of the dilacerations and what challenges await should surgical exposure and forced eruption be considered as a treatment option. Root proximity to the palatal cortex and to the adjacent lateral incisor root can be incorporated into a visual treatment and biomechanics plan to determine the feasibility of retrieving the impacted tooth with the dilacerated root.

Knowing that an unerupted tooth is developing abnormally will provide time for the dentist and family to consider treatment options, should the tooth need prosthetic treatment, surgical exposure, forced eruption, or extraction.

If crown exposure and forced eruption are considered as a treatment option for an impacted tooth with a dilacerated root, CBCT images not only provide a 3D view of how the tooth and dilacerated root are positioned, they also provide information on the quality and quantity of alveolar bone at the site where the tooth will be moved (see Chapter 14). Knowing if the alveolar boundary conditions are sufficient for housing a dilacerated tooth is critical in the treatment planning decision. While sufficient alveolar bone may be present to support the crown, the root may be angulated so severely that it will damage the palatal or buccal alveolar bone or adjacent teeth if the crown is brought into the arch. In these cases, there is a clear need for the information that only CBCT images can provide.

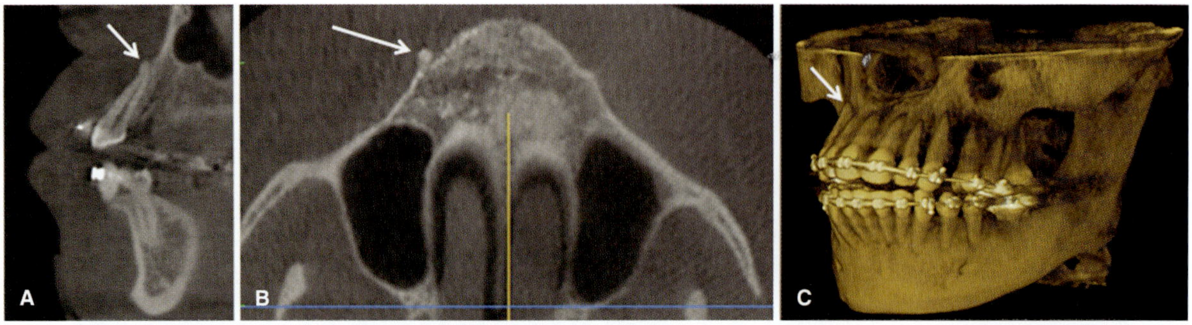

Figure 15.6 CBCT images of dilacerated maxillary right canine during orthodontic treatment for anterior openbite and dental protrusion. *A*: Sagittal view showing apical dilaceration of the maxillary right canine (arrow), possibly contributing to the perforation of the buccal alveolar bone and sensitivity of the tooth. *B*: Axial view showing maxillary right canine apex outside the alveolar housing (arrow). *C*: 3D volumetric image showing maxillary right canine apex (arrow) in relation to the alveolar bone and adjacent incisor roots.

The importance of assessing the boundary conditions that limit movement of dilacerated teeth now is being appreciated because of the unique images that CBCT generate. Dilacerations can go undiagnosed if the root curves directly toward or away from a conventional 2D radiographic film. CBCT images overcome this problem and permit detailed information on root location relative to the alveolar boundary conditions. This is valuable especially if a patient has thick gingiva that may prevent palpation of prominent roots at risk for dehiscences or fenestrations if excessive or improper torque is applied. An example of this is shown in Figure 15.6 where a bimaxillary protrusive patient with an anterior openbite had an undiagnosed buccal dilaceration of the apex of the maxillary right canine. The agreed-upon treatment plan was four premolar extractions followed by *en masse* retraction of the upper six anterior teeth. One month after *en masse* retraction began, the patient complained of discomfort around the maxillary right canine. Palpation of the affected area did not reveal any abnormal signs of root prominence. However, CBCT images revealed that due to the apical dilaceration on the canine, the apex of the tooth had penetrated through the alveolar cortical bone. This case demonstrates how the lack of detectable finding of root anomaly by conventional 2D radiographs can be overcome through CBCT imaging and can influence the next stage of treatment greatly.

THE FUTURE: CBCT RADIOGRAPHIC ROOT MAPPING AS AN INDICATOR OF DISEASE

As previously noted, CBCT radiography allows us to measure treatment-related changes in root length with high precision. While assessing root angulation and root length has obvious applications to orthodontic diagnosis and treatment planning, there is a growing realization that root positioning and morphology are indicators of disease. The importance of a patient's genetic background on tooth formation and eruption, susceptibility to oral diseases, and EARR is unquestioned. Indeed, short roots are not simply the sequelae of physiological exfoliation of primary teeth or pathological EARR. Short roots and other root anomalies are common phenotypic presentations of numerous genetic disorders (Table 15.2). It would be careless to think that all short or anomalous roots are the same. In fact, one CBCT-based study demonstrates the power of this radiographic technology to generate detailed images of highly anomalous roots in syndromic patients (Figure 15.7; Nawa *et al.*, 2008). Combining detailed mapping of root phenotypes with point-of-care genetic testing, such as salivary diagnostics (Giannobile, 2012; Wong, 2012), would establish the broad scientific foundation upon which solutions could be based for the problem of root resorption that Ottolengui and Kemple described a century ago. For this reason, it

Table 15.2 Root anomalies associated with medical syndromes.

Syndrome (OMIM #)	Inheritance and presentation	Root anomaly	Report type	Reference
Dentin dysplasia Type I (125400)	AD; abnormal dentin	1. Short roots 2. Short roots with taurodontism in one quadrant	1. Case report 2. Case report	1. Rocha *et al.*, 2011 2. Kosinski *et al.*, 1999
Ellis-van Creveld (225500)	AR; short limbs, post-axial polydactyly, ectodermal dysplasia, missing mandibular incisors, slight serrations of the alveolar ridge, multiple small alveolar notches	Single-rooted primary molars and taurodontism	Case report	Kalaskar & Kalaskar, 2012
Kenny-Caffey-Type 1 (244460)	AD; osteosclerotic bone dysplasia, hypocalcemia, short stature, ophthalmological features, hypo/oligodontia, microdontia	Short roots	Case report	Moussaid *et al.*, 2012
Axenfeld-Rieger Type 1 (180500) Type 2 (601499) Type 3 (602482)	AD; hypodontia, microdontia	1. Short roots 2. Short roots 3. Short, dilacerated roots	1. Case report 2. Case report 3. Case report	1. Berenstein-Aizman *et al.*, 2011 2. O'Dwyer & Jones, 2005 3. Jena & Kharbanda, 2005
Fraser (219000)	AR; cryptophthalmos, syndactyly, genital abnormalities, facial asymmetry, cleft lip and palate, high arched palate, dental crowding, fusion of primary teeth	Short roots	Case report	Keene & Day, 2011
Hallermann-Streiff (234100)	UI; bird-like face, hypotrichosis, ophthalmic disorders, hypo/oligodontia, natal teeth, enamel hypoplasia, supernumerary teeth, delayed eruption	Short roots	Case report	Robotta & Schafer, 2011
Oculo-facio-cardio-dental (300166)	X-linked dominant congenital cataracts, dysmorphic facial features, congenital heart disease	1. Canines with extremely large roots (radiculomegaly) 2. Maxillary central incisors, maxillary canines, mandibular canines with radiculomegaly 3. Radiculomegaly	1. Case report 2. Case report 3. Case report	1. Maden *et al.*, 2010 2. Altug-Atac, 2007 3. McGovern *et al.*, 2006
Robinow AR (26831) AD (18700)	AR, AD; short stature, mesomelic limb shortening, vertebral anomalies, dysmorphic facial features	1. Short roots on mandibular incisors 2. Short roots	1. Case report 2. Case report	1. Eronat *et al.*, 2009 2. Kantaputra *et al.*, 1999

(Continued)

Table 15.2 (*Continued*)

Syndrome (OMIM #)	Inheritance and presentation	Root anomaly	Report type	Reference
Van der Woude Type 1 (119300) Type 2 (606713)	AD; lip pits, cleft lip and/or palate	Taurodontism in mandibular 1st molars (35%), hypodontia (27%), mesodent (8%)	Retrospective, cross-sectional	Nawa *et al.*, 2008
Dyskeratosis congenital (305000)	AD/AR/x-linked; bone marrow failure, lacey reticular hyperpigmentation of the skin, dystrophic nails, mucous membrane leukoplakia, pancytopenia	Taurodontism, short roots	Cross-sectional	Atkinson *et al.*, 2008
Bardet-Biedl (209900)	AR; polydactyly, hypogonadism, retinopathy, renal failure, hypodontia, microdontia, high palatal vault	1. Short roots 2. Short roots	1. Case report 2. Cross-sectional	1. Drugowick *et al.*, 2007 2. Borgström *et al.*, 1996
Rothmund-Thomson (268400)	AR; poikilodermatous rash, juvenile cataracts, short stature, skeletal anomalies, predisposition to skin and bone cancers	Short roots	Case report	Roinioti & Stefanopoulos, 2007
Familial osteodysplasia-Anderson type (259250)	AR; osteogenesis disorder affecting primarily facial bones, impacted teeth, incomplete crown formation	Bulbous roots	Case report	Deger *et al.*, 2006
Ehlers-Danlos type I (130000)	AD; Skin hyperextensibility, articular hypermobility, tissue fragility, easily bruised	Bulbous roots	Case report	Pope *et al.*, 1992
Ehlers-Danlos type VIIC (225410)	AR; extreme skin fragility, easy bruising, large fontanels, blue sclera, puffy eyelids, micrognathia, umbilical hernia, short fingers, joint hypermobility, increased risk for internal organ rupture, generalized tooth dysmorphology	1. Dysplastic roots 2. Dysplastic roots	1. Case report 2. Case report	1. Malfait *et al.*, 2004 2. Ooshima *et al.*, 1990
Williams-Beuren (194050)	AD; supravalvular stenosis, mental retardation, "elfin facies," tooth agenesis	Taurodontism of mandibular permanent molars, short roots	Cross-sectional	Axelsson *et al.*, 2003
Marfan (154700)	AR; increased height, disproportionally long limbs and digits, anterior chest deformity, joint laxity, vertebral	Root deformity	Cross-sectional	De Coster *et al.*, 2002
Seckel (210600)	UI; extreme growth retardation, severe microcephaly, bird-like face, mental retardation, extremely delayed skeletal maturation, normal growth hormone and pituitary-thyroid axis function, tooth agenesis	Taurodontism in girls only	Case report of four siblings (two boys, two girls)	Kjaer *et al.*, 2001

Table 15.2 (*Continued*)

Syndrome (OMIM #)	Inheritance and presentation	Root anomaly	Report type	Reference
GAPO (growth retardation, alopecia, pseudoanodontia, optic atrophy; 230740)	AR; short stature, dysmorphic facial features, total alopecia, pseudoanodontia, absence of facial pneumatization, deficient cranial base	Unerupted permanent teeth with extensive ankylosis of extracted primary incisor	Case report	Bacon *et al.*, 1999
Stevens-Johnson (erythema multiforme; no OMIM entry)	No information available	1. Short roots 2. Short roots 3. Generalized abnormal root development 4. Delayed root development 5. Short roots	1. Case report 2. Case report 3. Case report 4. Case report 5. Case report	1. Brook, 1994 2. Thornton & Worley, 1991 3. Bimstein & Bystrom, 1984 4. Ranalli *et al.*, 1984 5. De Man, 1979
Parry-Romberg (hemifacial atrophy; 141300)	UI; delayed tooth eruption	Short roots	Case report	Fayad & Steffensen, 1994
Turner (no OMIM entry)	UI; microdontia, advanced dental age	Short roots	Cross-sectional	Ogiuchi *et al.*, 1985
X chromosome aneuploidy (no OMIM entry)	UI; bifid uvula, macroglossia, enamel defects	1. Taurodontism and abnormal roots 2. Taurodontism 3. Elongated mandibular, but not maxillary, roots	1. Cross-sectional 2. Cross-sectional 3. Case report	1. Farge *et al.*, 1985 2. Jaspers & Witkop, 1980 3. Lahdesmäki & Alvesalo, 2010
Cystinosis (219800)	AR: lysosomal storage disease, developmental and mineralization anomalies, mandibular deficiency, increased face height, reduced airway space, enamel defects	Taurodontism	Cross-sectional	Bassim *et al.*, 2010
Klinefelter (no OMIM entry)	UI; most common sex chromosome disorder in males, XXY genotype with inactivation of most genes on the extra X chromosome	Increased root length	Cross-sectional	Lahdesmäki & Alvesalo, 2007
Unclassified: severe short-limbed dwarfism (no OMIM entry)	No information available	Short conical roots with obliterated pulp chambers	Case report	Shaw, 1995

AD, autosomal dominant; AR, autosomal recessive; UI, unknown inheritance; OMIM #, Online Mendelian Inheritance in Man number. Note that not all syndromes are in the OMIM database. Numbers in the reference column correspond with those in the report type column.

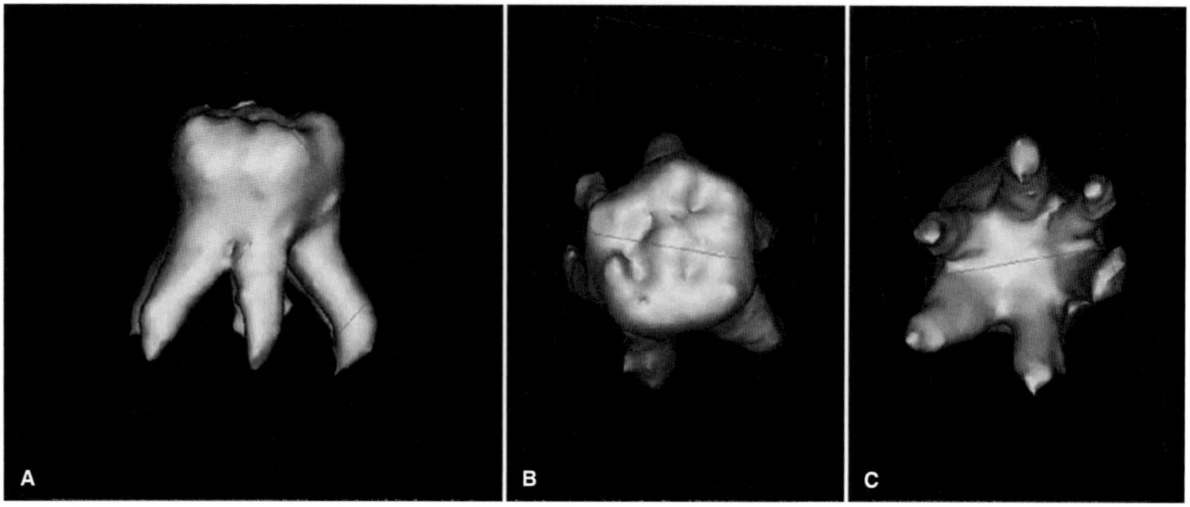

Figure 15.7 Sagittal (*A*), coronal (*B*), and apical (*C*) views of a six-rooted molar from patient with Van der Woude Syndrome imaged with CBCT. As our database of CBCT images expands, we are learning that abnormal root morphology may be an indicator of genetic or systemic disease. Detailed morphometric mapping of anomalous roots and how these maps correlate to molecular anomalies will broaden our understanding of tooth development as an integral part of overall embryogenesis. (Reprinted with permission from Nawa *et al.*, 2008.)

is perhaps most fitting that we let Ottolengui (1914) have the last word on the topic of root morphology:

> I trust that this rather hastily compiled record of radiographic data may result in inspiring some brighter and more scientific mind to take up these problems for us.

CONCLUSIONS

Radiographs of root angulation and morphology have held the attention of orthodontists for 100 years—and for good reason. Root parallelism is a primary objective in orthodontic treatment, as it is considered one of the keys to an ideal occlusion. Conventional 2D radiographs are fraught with technical problems that make accurate root angulation measurements nearly impossible. Rigorous tests of 2D and 3D imaging accuracy overwhelmingly demonstrate improved, albeit not perfect, angular measurements using CBCT images. New software advances and translational studies are advancing the application of 3D imaging to root positioning in orthodontics patients. Advances also are being made in CBCT analysis of root resorption in orthodontics patients. The finding that root loss is not symmetrical, but rather slanting, highlights the requirement for CBCT's 3D rendering capacity for accurate diagnosis of this type of root resorption. Finally, CBCT imaging will be critical for elucidating anomalous root morphology in genetic and systemic diseases. Overall, CBCT is a powerful radiographic technology that, when combined with the equally powerful genetic testing, will enable orthodontists to generate more accurate diagnoses and individualized treatment plans for their patients.

References

Acar, A., Canyurek, U., Kocaaga, M., *et al.* (1999) Continuous vs. discontinuous force application and root resorption. *Angle Orthodontist*, 69 (2), 159–163.

Al-Qawasmi, R.A., Hartsfield, J.K., Jr., Everett, E.T., *et al.* (2003a) Genetic predisposition to external apical root resorption. *American Journal of Orthodontics and Dentofacial Orthopedics*, 123 (3), 242–252.

Al-Qawasmi, R.A., Hartsfield, J.K., Jr., Everett, E.T., *et al.* (2003b) Genetic predisposition to external apical root resorption in orthodontic patients: linkage of chromosome-18 marker. *Journal of Dental Research*, 82 (5), 356–360.

Alqerban, A., Jacobs, R., Souza, P.C., *et al.* (2009) *In-vitro* comparison of two cone-beam computed tomography systems and panoramic imaging for detecting simulated canine impaction-induced external root resorption in maxillary lateral incisors. *American Journal of Orthodontics and Dentofacial Orthopedics*, 136 (6), 764. e1–764.11.

Alqerban, A., Jacobs, R., Fieuws, S., *et al.* (2011a) Comparison of six cone-beam computed tomography systems for image quality and detection of simulated canine impaction-induced external root resorption in maxillary lateral incisors. *American Journal of Orthodontics and Dentofacial Orthopedics*, 140 (3), e129–e139.

Alqerban, A., Jacobs, R., Fieuws, S., *et al.* (2011b) Comparison of two cone beam computed tomographic systems versus panoramic imaging for localization of impacted maxillary canines and detection of root resorption. *European Journal of Orthodontics*, 33 (1), 93–102.

Altug-Atac, A.T. (2007) Oculofaciocardiodental syndrome and orthodontics. *American Journal of Orthodontics and Dentofacial Orthopedics*, 131 (1), 83–88.

Andrews, L.F. (1972) The six keys to normal occlusion. *American Journal of Orthodontics*, 62 (3), 296–309.

Apajalahti, S. & Peltola, J.S. (2007) Apical root resorption after orthodontic treatment: a retrospective study. *European Journal of Orthodontics*, 29 (4), 408–412.

Artun, J., Smale, I., Behbehani, F., *et al.* (2005) Apical root resorption six and 12 months after initiation of fixed orthodontic appliance therapy. *Angle Orthodontist*, 75 (6), 919–926.

Artun, J., Van't Hullenaar, R., Doppel, D., *et al.* (2009) Identification of orthodontic patients at risk of severe apical root resorption. *American Journal of Orthodontics and Dentofacial Orthopedics*, 135 (4), 448–455.

Atkinson, J.C., Harvey, K.E., Domingo, D.L., *et al.* (2008) Oral and dental phenotype of dyskeratosis congenita. *Oral Diseases*, 14 (5), 419–427.

Axelsson, S., Bjørnland, T., Kjaer, I., *et al.* (2003) Dental characteristics in Williams syndrome: a clinical and radiographic evaluation. *Acta Odontologica Scandinavica*, 61 (3), 129–136.

Bacon, W., Hall, R.K., Roset, J.P., *et al.* (1999) GAPO syndrome: a new case of this rare syndrome and a review of the relative importance of different phenotypic features in diagnosis. *Journal of Craniofacial Genetics and Developmental Biology*, 19 (4), 189–200.

Baratieri, C., Canongia, A.C., & Bolognese, A.M. (2011) Relationship between maxillary canine intra-alveolar position and maxillary incisor angulation: a cone beam computed tomography study. *Brazilian Dental Journal*, 22 (2), 146–150.

Bassim, C.W., Gautam, P., Domingo, D.L., *et al.* (2010) Craniofacial and dental findings in cystinosis. *Oral Diseases*, 16 (5), 488–495.

Baumrind, S., Korn, E.L., & Boyd, R.L. (1996) Apical root resorption in orthodontically treated adults. *American Journal of Orthodontics and Dentofacial Orthopedics*, 110 (3), 311–320.

Beck, B.W. & Harris, E.F. (1994) Apical root resorption in orthodontically treated subjects: analysis of edgewise and light wire mechanics. *American Journal of Orthodontics and Dentofacial Orthopedics*, 105 (4), 350–361.

Berenstein-Aizman, G., Hazan-Molina, H., Drori, D., *et al.* (2011) Axenfeld-Rieger syndrome: dentofacial manifestation and oral rehabilitation considerations. *Pediatric Dentistry*, 33 (5), 440–444.

Bernardes, R.A., de Paulo, R.S., Pereira, L.O., *et al.* (2012) Comparative study of cone beam computed tomography and intraoral periapical radiographs in diagnosis of lingual-simulated external root resorptions. *Dental Traumatology*, 28 (4), 268–272.

Bert, J.D. (1981) Differential diagnosis and treatment of root angulation problems. *Dental Clinics of North America*, 25 (1), 85–93.

Bimstein, E. & Bystrom, E.B. (1984) Idiopathic, late, slow, and irregular dental development: report of case. *ASDC Journal of Dentristry for Children*, 51 (4), 302–304.

Blake, M., Woodside, D.G., & Pharoah, M.J. (1995) A radiographic comparison of apical root resorption after orthodontic treatment with the edgewise and Speed appliances. *American Journal of Orthodontics and Dentofacial Orthopedics*, 108 (1), 76–84.

Borgström, M.K., Riise, R., Tornqviste, K., *et al.* (1996) Anomalies in the permanent dentition and other oral findings in 29 individuals with Laurence-Moon-Bardet-Biedl syndrome. *Journal of Oral Pathology and Medicine*, 25 (2), 86–89.

Bouwens, D.G., Cevidanes, L., Ludlow, J.B., *et al.* (2011) Comparison of mesiodistal root angulation with posttreatment panoramic radiographs and cone-beam computed tomography. *American Journal of Orthodontics and Dentofacial Orthopedics*, 139 (1), 126–132.

Brin, I., Ben-Bassat, Y., Heling, I., *et al.* (1991) The influence of orthodontic treatment on previously traumatized permanent incisors. *European Journal of Orthodontics*, 13 (5), 372–377.

Brook, U. (1994) Stevens-Johnson syndrome and abnormal root development: a case report. *International Journal of Paediatric Dentistry*, 4 (2), 101–103.

Carlsson, R. & Rönnerman, A. (1973) Crown-root angles of upper central incisors. *American Journal of Orthodontics*, 64 (2), 147–154.

Casko, J.S., Vaden, J.L., Kokich, V.G., *et al.* (1998) Objective grading system for dental casts and panoramic radiographs: American Board of Orthodontics. *American Journal of Orthodontics and Dentofacial Orthopedics*, 114 (5), 589–599.

Chiqueto, K., Martins, D.R., & Janson, G. (2008) Effects of accentuated and reversed curve of Spee on apical root resorption. *American Journal of Orthodontics and Dentofacial Orthopedics*, 133 (2), 261–268.

De Azevedo Vaz, S.L., Vasoncelos, T.V., Neves, F.S., *et al.* (2012) Influence of cone-beam computed tomography enhancement filters on diagnosis of simulated external root resorption. *Journal of Endodontics*, 38 (3), 305–308.

De Coster, P.J., Martens, L.C., & De Paepe, A. (2002) Oral manifestations of patients with Marfan syndrome: a case-control study. *Oral Surgery, Oral Medicine, Oral Pathology, Oral Radiology and Endodontics*, 93 (5), 564–572.

de Freitas, M.R., Beltrão, R.T., Janson, G., *et al.* (2007) Evaluation of root resorption after open bite treatment with and without extractions. *American Journal of Orthodontics and Dentofacial Orthopedics*, 132 (2), 143.15–143e22.

De Man, K. (1979) Abnormal root development, probably due to erythema multiforme (Stevens-Johnson syndrome). *International Journal of Oral Surgery*, 8 (5), 381–385.

Deger, S., Tabar, G., Sermet, B., *et al.* (2006) Dental findings and rehabilitation in familial osteodysplasia (Anderson type): a case report. *Oral Diseases*, 12 (2), 208–212.

Deguchi, T., Murakami, T., Kuroda, S., *et al.* (2008) Comparison of the intrusion effects on the maxillary incisors between implant anchorage and J-hook headgear. *American Journal of Orthodontics and Dentofacial Orthopedics*, 133 (5), 654–660.

Dermaut, L.R. & De Munck, A. (1986) Apical root resorption of upper incisors caused by intrusive tooth movement: a radiographic study. *American Journal of Orthodontics and Dentofacial Orthopedics*, 90 (4), 321–326.

DeShields, R.W. (1969) A study of root resorption in treated Class II, Division I malocclusions. *Angle Orthodontist*, 39 (4), 231–245.

Dholakia, K.D. & Bhat, S.R. (2011) Assessment of the reliability of root angulations on panoramic radiographs. *Orthodontics: The Art and Practice of Dentofacial Enhancement*, 12 (2), 96–107.

Drugowick, R.M., Da Rós Goncalves, L., Barrôso, A.S., *et al.* (2007) Treatment of gingival overgrowth in a child with Bardet-Biedl syndrome. *Journal of Periodontology*, 78 (6), 1159–1163.

Dudic, A., Giannopoulou, C., Martinez, M., *et al.* (2008) Diagnostic accuracy of digitized periapical radiographs validated against micro-computed tomography scanning in evaluating othodontically induced apical root resorption. *European Journal of Oral Sciences*, 116 (5), 467–472.

Dudic, A., Giannopoulou, C., Leuzinger, M., *et al.* (2009) Detection of apical root resorption after orthodontic treatment by using panoramic radiography and cone-beam computed tomography of super-high resolution. *American Journal of Orthodontics and Dentofacial Orthopedics*, 135 (4), 434–437.

Durack, C., Patel, S., Davies, J., *et al.* (2011) Diagnostic accuracy of small volume cone beam computed tomography and intraoral periapical radiography for the detection of simulated external inflammatory root resorption. *International Endodontic Journal*, 44 (2), 136–147.

El-Beialy, A.R., Fayed, M.S., El-Bialy, A.M., *et al.* (2011) Accuracy and reliability of cone-beam computed tomography measurements: influence of head orientation. *American Journal of Orthodontics and Dentofacial Orthopedics*, 140 (2), 157–165.

Eronat, N., Cogulu, D., & Ozkinay, F. (2009) A case report on autosomal recessive Robinow syndrome. *European Journal of Paediatric Dentistry*, 10 (3), 147–150.

Farge, P., Dallaire, L., Albert, G., *et al.* (1985) Oral and dental development in X chromosome aneuploidy. *Clinical Genetics*, 27 (2), 122–126.

Fayad, S. & Steffensen, B. (1994) Root resorptions in a patient with hemifacial atrophy. *Journal of Endodontics*, 20 (6), 299–303.

Fritz, U., Diedrich, P., & Wiechmann, D. (2003) Apical root resorption after lingual orthodontic therapy. *Journal of Orofacial Orthopedics*, 64 (6), 434–442.

Frongia, G., Piancino, M.G., & Bracco, P. (2012) Cone-beam computed tomography: accuracy of three-dimensional cephalometry analysis and influence of patient scanning position. *Journal of Craniofacial Surgery*, 23 (4), 1038–1043.

Garcia-Figueroa, M.A., Raboud, D.W., Lam, E.W., *et al.* (2008) Effect of buccolingual root angulation on the mesiodistal angulation shown on panoramic radiographs. *American Journal of Orthodontics and Dentofacial Orthopedics*, 134 (1), 93–99.

Giannobile, W.V. (2012) Salivary diagnostics for periodontal diseases. *Journal of the American Dental Association*, 143 (10 Suppl), 6S–11S.

Goldie, R.S. & King, G.J. (1984) Root resorption and tooth movement in orthodontically treated, calcium-deficient, and lactating rats. *American Journal of Orthodontics*, 85 (5), 424–430.

Goldson, L. & Henrikson, C.O. (1975) Root resorption during Begg treatment: a longitudinal Roentgenologic study. *American Journal of Orthodontics*, 68 (1), 55–66.

Handelman, C.S. (1996) The anterior alveolus: its importance in limiting orthodontic treatment and its influence on the occurrence of iatrogenic sequelae. *Angle Orthodontist*, 66 (2), 95–109.

Hardy, T.C., Suri, L., & Stark, P. (2009) Influence of patient head positioning on measured axial tooth inclination in panoramic radiography. *Journal of Orthodontics*, 36 (2) 103–110.

Harris, E.F. (2000) Root resorption during orthodontic therapy. *Seminars in Orthodontics*, 6 (3) 183–194.

Harris, E.F. & Baker, W.C. (1990) Loss of root length and crestal bone height before and during treatment in adolescent and adult orthodontic patients. *American Journal of Orthodontics and Dentofacial Orthopedics*, 98 (5), 463–469.

Harris, E.F., Robinson, Q.C., & Woods, M.A. (1993) An analysis of causes of apical root resorption in patients not treated orthodontically. *Quintessence International*, 24 (6), 417–428.

Harris, E.F., Kineret, S.E., & Tolley, E.A. (1997) A heritable component for external apical root resorption in patients treated orthodontically. *American Journal of Orthodontics and Dentofacial Orthopedics*, 111 (3), 301–309.

Hendrix, I., Carels, C., Kuijpers-Jagtman, A.M., *et al.* (1994) A radiographic study of posterior apical root resorption in orthodontic patients. *American Journal of Orthodontics and Dentofacial Orthopedics*, 105 (4), 345–349.

Horiuchi, A., Hotokezaka, H., & Kobayashi, K. (1998) Correlation between cortical plate proximity and apical root resorption. *American Journal of Orthodontics and Dentofacial Orthopedics*, 114 (3), 311–318.

Huang, Y., Wang, X.X., Zhang, J., *et al.* (2010) Root shortening in patients treated with two-step and *en masse* space closure procedures with sliding mechanics. *Angle Orthodontist*, 80 (3), 492–497.

Hubar, J.S. (2000) C. Edmund Kells, Jr., pioneer in the field of dental X-rays. *Journal of the History of Dentistry*, 48 (1), 11–15.

Iglesias-Linares, A., Yañez-Vico, R., Ballesta-Mudarra, S., *et al.* (2012a) Postorthodontic external root resorption is associated with IL1 receptor antagonist gene variations. *Oral Diseases*, 18 (2), 198–205.

Iglesias-Linares, A., Yañez-Vico, R., Ortiz-Ariza, E., *et al.* (2012b) Postorthodontic external root resorption in root-filled teeth is influenced by interleukin-1beta polymorphism. *Journal of Endodontics*, 38 (3), 283–287.

Ioannidou-Marathiotou, I., Papadopoulos, M.A., Kondylidou-Sidira, A., *et al.* (2010) Digital subtraction radiography of panoramic radiographs to evaluate maxillary central incisor root resorption after orthodontic treatment. *World Journal of Orthodontics*, 11 (2), 142–152.

Janson, G.R., De Luca Canto, G., Martins, D.R., *et al.* (2000) A radiographic comparison of apical root resorption after orthodontic treatment with three different fixed appliance techniques. *American Journal of Orthodontics and Dentofacial Orthopedics*, 118 (3), 262–273.

Jaspers, M.T. & Witkop, C.J., Jr. (1980) Taurodontism: an isolated trait associated with syndromes and X-chromosomal aneuploidy. *American Journal of Human Genetics*, 32 (3), 396–413.

Jena, A.K. & Kharbanda, O.P. (2005) Axenfeld-Rieger syndrome: report on dental and craniofacial findings. *Journal of Clinical Pediatric Dentistry*, 30 (1), 83–88.

Jesuino, F.A., Costa, L.R., & Valladares-Neto, J. (2010) Mesiodistal root angulation of permanent teeth in children with mixed dentition and normal occlusion. *Journal of Applied Oral Science*, 18 (6), 625–629.

Jung, Y.H. & Cho, B.H. (2011) External root resorption after orthodontic treatment: a study of contributing factors. *Imaging Science in Dentistry*, 41 (1), 17–21.

Kalaskar, R. & Kalaskar, A.R. (2012) Oral manifestations of Ellis-van Creveld syndrome. *Contemporary Clinical Dentistry*, 3 (Suppl 1), S55–S59.

Kaley, J. & Phillips, C. (1991) Factors related to root resorption in edgewise practice. *Angle Orthodontist*, 61 (2), 125–132.

Kantaputra, P.N., Gorlin, R.J., Ukarapol, N., *et al.* (1999) Robinow (fetal face) syndrome: report of a boy with dominant type and an infant with recessive type. *American Journal of Medical Genetics*, 84 (1), 1–7.

Keene, E.J. & Day, P.F. (2011) Case report: hypodontia and short roots in a child with Fraser syndrome. *European Archives of Paediatric Dentistry*, 12 (4), 216–218.

Kennedy, D.B., Joondeph, D.R., Osterberg, S.K., *et al.* (1983) The effect of extraction and orthodontic treatment on dentoalveolar support. *American Journal of Orthodontics*, 84 (3), 183–190.

King, G.J., Keeling, S.D., McCoy, E.A., *et al.* (1991) Measuring dental drift and orthodontic tooth movement in response to various initial forces in adult rats. *American Journal of Orthodontics and Dentofacial Orthopedics*, 99 (5), 456–465.

Kinzinger, G.S., Savvaidis, S., Gross, U., *et al.* (2011) Effects of Class II treatment with a banded Herbst appliance on root lengths in the posterior dentition.

American Journal of Orthodontics and Dentofacial Orthopedics, 139 (4), 465–469.

Kjaer, I. (1995) Morphological characteristics of dentitions developing excessive root resorption during orthodontic treatment. *European Journal of Orthodontics*, 17 (1), 25–34.

Kjaer, I., Hansen, N., Becktor, K.B., *et al.* (2001) Craniofacial morphology, dentition, and skeletal maturity in four siblings with Seckel syndrome. *Cleft Palate-Craniofacial Journal*, 38 (6), 645–651.

Knösel, M., Jung, K., Attin, T., *et al.* (2009) On the interaction between incisor crown-root morphology and third-order angulation. *Angle Orthodontist*, 79 (3), 454–461.

Kokich, V.G. (2008) Orthodontic and nonorthodontic root resorption: their impact on clinical dental practice. *Journal of Dental Education*, 72 (8), 895–902.

Konoo, T., Kim, Y.J., Gu, G.M., *et al.* (2001) Intermittent force in orthodontic tooth movement. *Journal of Dental Research*, 80 (2), 457–460.

Kosinski, R.W., Chaiyawat, Y., & Rosenberg, L. (1999) Localized deficient root development associated with taurodontism: case report. *Pediatric Dentistry*, 21 (3), 213–215.

Kumar, V., Gossett, L., Blattner, A., *et al.* (2011) Comparison between cone-beam computed tomography and intraoral digital radiography for assessment of tooth root lesions. *American Journal of Orthodontics and Dentofacial Orthopedics*, 139 (6), e533–e541.

Kurol, J., Owman-Moll, P., & Lundgren, D. (1996) Time-related root resorption after application of a controlled continuous orthodontic force. *American Journal of Orthodontics and Dentofacial Orthopedics*, 110 (3), 303–310.

Lahdesmäki, R. & Alvesalo, L. (2007) Root lengths in the permanent teeth of Klinefelter (47,XXY) men. *Archives of Oral Biology*, 52 (9), 822–827.

Lahdesmäki, R.E. & Alvesalo, L.J. (2010) Root length in the permanent teeth of women with an additional X chromosome (47,XXX females). *Acta Odontologica Scandinavica*, 68 (4), 223–227.

Lee, R.Y., Artun, J., & Alonzo, T.A. (1999) Are dental anomalies risk factors for apical root resorption in orthodontic patients? *American Journal of Orthodontics and Dentofacial Orthopedics*, 116 (2), 187–195.

Leite, V., Conti, A.C., Navarro, R., *et al.* (2012) Comparison of root resorption between self-ligating and conventional preadjusted brackets using cone-beam computed tomography. *Angle Orthodontist*, 82 (6), 1078–1082.

Lennon, S., Patel, S., Foschi, F., *et al.* (2011) Diagnostic accuracy of limited-volume cone-beam computed tomography in the detection of periapical bone loss: 360° scans *versus* 180° scans. *International Endodontic Journal*, 44 (12), 1118–1127.

Leuzinger, M., Dudic, A., Giannopoulou, C., *et al.* (2010) Root-contact evaluation by panoramic radiography and cone-beam computed tomography of super-high resolution. *American Journal of Orthodontics and Dentofacial Orthopedics*, 137 (3), 389–392.

Levander, E. & Malmgren, O. (1988) Evaluation of the risk of root resorption during orthodontic treatment: a study of upper incisors. *European Journal of Orthodontics*, 10 (1), 30–38.

Levander, E., Bajka, R., & Malmgren, O. (1998a) Early radiographic diagnosis of apical root resorption during orthodontic treatment: a study of maxillary incisors. *European Journal of Orthodontics*, 20 (1), 57–63.

Levander, E., Malmgren, O., & Stenback, K. (1998b) Apical root resorption during orthodontic treatment of patients with multiple aplasia: a study of maxillary incisors. *European Journal of Orthodontics*, 20 (4), 427–434.

Lew, K. (1990) Intrusion and apical resorption of mandibular incisors in Begg treatment: anchorage bend or curve? *Australian Orthodontic Journal*, 11 (3), 164–168.

Liedke, G.S., Da Silveira, H.E., Da Silveira, H.L., *et al.* (2009) Influence of voxel size in the diagnostic ability of cone beam tomography to evaluate simulated external root resorption. *Journal of Endodontics*, 35 (2), 233–235.

Linge, B.O. & Linge, L. (1983) Apical root resorption in upper anterior teeth. *European Journal of Orthodontics*, 5 (3), 173–183.

Linge, L. & Linge, B.O. (1991) Patient characteristics and treatment variables associated with apical root resorption during orthodontic treatment. *American Journal of Orthodontics and Dentofacial Orthopedics*, 99 (1), 35–43.

Liou, E.J. & Chang, P.M. (2010) Apical root resorption in orthodontic patients with *en masse* maxillary anterior retraction and intrusion with miniscrews. *American Journal of Orthodontics and Dentofacial Orthopedics*, 137 (2), 207–212.

Llamas-Carreras, J.M., Amarilla, A., Espinar-Escalona, E., *et al.* (2012) External apical root resorption in maxillary root-filled incisors after orthodontic treatment: a split-mouth design study. *Medicina Oral Patologia Oral y Cirugía Bucal*, 17 (3), e523–e527.

Llamas-Carreras, J.M., Amarilla, A., Solano, E., *et al.* (2010) Study of external root resorption during orthodontic treatment in root filled teeth compared with their contralateral teeth with vital pulps. *International Endodontic Journal*, 43 (8), 654–662.

Lucchesi, M.V., Wood, R.E., & Nortjé, C.J. (1988) Suitability of the panoramic radiograph for assessment of mesiodistal angulation of teeth in the buccal segments of the mandible. *American Journal of Orthodontics and Dentofacial Orthopedics*, 94 (4), 303–310.

Lund, H., Gröndahl, K., & Gröndahl, H.G. (2010) Cone beam computed tomography for assessment of root length and marginal bone level during orthodontic treatment. *Angle Orthodontist*, 80 (3), 466–473.

Lund, H., Gröndahl, K., Hansen, K., *et al.* (2012) Apical root resorption during orthodontic treatment: a prospective study using cone beam CT. *Angle Orthodontist*, 82 (3), 480–487.

Maden, M., Savgat, A., & Görgül, G. (2010) Radiculomegaly of permanent canines: report of endodontic treatment in OFCD syndrome. *International Endodontic Journal*, 43 (12), 1152–1161.

Makedonas, D., Odman, A., & Hansen, K. (2009) Management of root resorption in a large orthodontic clinic. *Swedish Dental Journal*, 33 (4), 173–180.

Makedonas, D., Lund, H., Grondahl, K., *et al.* (2012) Root resorption diagnosed with cone beam computed tomography after six months of orthodontic treatment with fixed appliance and the relation to risk factors. *Angle Orthodontist*, 82 (2), 196–201.

Malfait, F., De Coster, P., Hausser, I., *et al.* (2004) The natural history, including orofacial features of three patients with Ehlers-Danlos syndrome, dermatosparaxis type (EDS type VIIC). *American Journal of Medical Genetics, Part A*, 131 (1), 18–28.

Malmgren, O., Goldson, L., Hill, C., *et al.* (1982) Root resorption after orthodontic treatment of traumatized teeth. *American Journal of Orthodontics*, 82 (6), 487–491.

Marques, L.S., Ramos-Jorge, M.L., Rey, A.C., *et al.* (2010) Severe root resorption in orthodontic patients treated with the edgewise method: prevalence and predictive factors. *American Journal of Orthodontics and Dentofacial Orthopedics*, 137 (3), 384–388.

Martins, D.R., Tibola, D., Janson, G., *et al.* (2012) Effects of intrusion combined with anterior retraction on apical root resorption. *European Journal of Orthodontics*, 34 (2), 170–175.

Mavragani, M., Vergari, A., Selliseth, N.J., *et al.* (2000) A radiographic comparison of apical root resorption after orthodontic treatment with a standard edgewise and a straight-wire edgewise technique. *European Journal of Orthodontics*, 22 (6), 665–674.

Mavragani, M., Apisariyakul, J., Brudvik, P., *et al.* (2006) Is mild dental invagination a risk factor for apical root resorption in orthodontic patients? *European Journal of Orthodontics*, 28 (4), 307–312.

Mayoral, G. (1982) Treatment results with light wires studied by panoramic radiography. *American Journal of Orthodontics*, 81 (6), 489–497.

McFadden, W.M., Engstrom, C., Engstrom, H., *et al.* (1989) A study of the relationship between incisor intrusion and root shortening. *American Journal of Orthodontics and Dentofacial Orthopedics*, 96 (5), 390–396.

McGovern, E., Al-Mudaffer, M., McMahon, C., *et al.* (2006) Oculo-facio-cardio-dental syndrome in a mother and daughter. *International Journal of Oral and Maxillofacial Surgery*, 35 (11), 1060–1062.

McKee, I.W., Glover, K.E., Williamson, P.C., *et al.* (2001) The effect of vertical and horizontal head positioning in panoramic radiography on mesiodistal tooth angulations. *Angle Orthodontist*, 71 (6), 442–451.

McKee, I.W., Williamson, P.C., Lam, E.W., *et al.* (2002) The accuracy of four panoramic units in the projection of mesiodistal tooth angulations. *American Journal of Orthodontics and Dentofacial Orthopedics*, 121 (2), 166–175.

McNab, S., Battistutta, D., Taverne, A., *et al.* (1999) External apical root resorption of posterior teeth in asthmatics after orthodontic treatment. *American Journal of Orthodontics and Dentofacial Orthopedics*, 116 (5), 545–551.

McNab, S., Battistutta, D., Taverne, A., *et al.* (2000) External apical root resorption following orthodontic treatment. *Angle Orthodontist*, 70 (3), 227–232.

Midgett, R.J., Shaye, R., & Fruge, J.F., Jr. (1981) The effect of altered bone metabolism on orthodontic tooth movement. *American Journal of Orthodontics*, 80 (3), 256–262.

Mirabella, A.D. & Artun, J. (1995) Risk factors for apical root resorption of maxillary anterior teeth in adult orthodontic patients. *American Journal of Orthodontics and Dentofacial Orthopedics*, 108 (1), 48–55.

Mohandesan, H., Ravanmehr, H., & Valaei, N. (2007) A radiographic analysis of external apical root resorption of maxillary incisors during active orthodontic treatment. *European Journal of Orthodontics*, 29 (2), 134–139.

Motokawa, M., Sasamoto, T., Kaku, M., *et al.* (2012) Association between root resorption incident to orthodontic treatment and treatment factors. *European Journal of Orthodontics*, 34 (3), 350–356.

Moussaid, Y., Griffiths, D., Richard, B., *et al.* (2012) Oral manifestations of patients with Kenny-Caffey Syndrome. *European Journal of Medical Genetics*, 55 (8–9), 441–445.

Nawa, H., Oberoi, S., & Vargervik, K. (2008) Taurodontism and Van der Woude syndrome: is there an association? *Angle Orthodontist*, 78 (5), 832–837.

Neves, F.S., Vasconcelos, T.V., Vaz, S.L., *et al.* (2012a) Evaluation of reconstructed images with different voxel sizes of acquisition in the diagnosis of simulated external root resorption using cone beam computed tomography. *International Endodontic Journal*, 45 (3), 234–239.

Neves, F.S., de Freitas, D.Q., Campos, P.S., *et al.* (2012b) *In vitro* comparison of cone beam computed tomography with different voxel sizes for detection of simulated external root resorption. *Journal of Oral Science*, 54 (3), 219–225.

Newman, W.G. (1975) Possible etiologic factors in external root resorption. *American Journal of Orthodontics*, 67 (5), 522–539.

Ngan, D.C., Kharbanda, O.P., Byloff, F.K., *et al.* (2004) The genetic contribution to orthodontic root resorption: a retrospective twin study. *Australian Orthodontic Journal*, 20 (1), 1–9.

Nigul, K. & Jagomagi, T. (2006) Factors related to apical root resorption of maxillary incisors in orthodontic patients. *Stomatologija*, 8 (3), 76–79.

Nishioka, M., Ioi, H., Nakata, S., *et al.* (2006) Root resorption and immune system factors in the Japanese. *Angle Orthodontist*, 76 (1), 103–108.

O'Dwyer, E.M. & Jones, D.C. (2005) Dental anomalies in Axenfeld-Rieger syndrome. *International Journal of Paediatric Dentistry*, 15 (6), 459–463.

Odenrick, L. & Brattström, V. (1983) The effect of nailbiting on root resorption during orthodontic treatment. *European Journal of Orthodontics*, 5 (3), 185–188.

Odenrick, L. & Brattström, V. (1985) Nailbiting: frequency and association with root resorption during orthodontic treatment. *British Journal of Orthodontics*, 12, 78–81.

Ogiuchi, H., Takano, K., Tanaka, M., *et al.* (1985) Oromaxillofacial development in patients with Turner's syndrome. *Endocrinologica Japonica*, 32 (6), 881–890.

Ooshima, T., Abe, K., Kohno, H., *et al.* (1990) Oral manifestations of Ehlers-Danlos syndrome type VII: histological examination of a primary tooth. *Pediatric Dentistry*, 12 (2), 102–106.

Otis, L.L., Hong, J.S., & Tuncay, O.C. (2004) Bone structure effect on root resorption. *Orthodontics & Craniofacial Research*, 7 (3), 165–177.

Ottolengui, R. (1914) The physiological and pathological resorption of tooth roots. *Dental Items of Interest*, 36, 332–362.

Owens, A.M. & Johal, A. (2008) Near-end of treatment panoramic radiograph in the assessment of mesiodistal root angulation. *Angle Orthodontist*, 78 (3), 475–481.

Pandis, N., Nasika, M., Polychronopoulou, A., *et al.* (2008) External apical root resorption in patients treated with conventional and self-ligating brackets. *American Journal of Orthodontics and Dentofacial Orthopedics*, 134 (5), 646–651.

Parker, R.J. & Harris, E.F. (1998) Directions of orthodontic tooth movements associated with external apical root resorption of the maxillary central incisor. *American Journal of Orthodontics and Dentofacial Orthopedics*, 114 (6), 677–683.

Patel, N., Currier, G.F., Kadioglu, O., *et al.* (2012) A CBCT comparison of anterior root resorption in SureSmile and conventional edgewise treatments. *Orthodontics: The Art and Practice of Dentofacial Enhancement*, 13 (1), 100–109.

Peck, J.L., Sameshima, G.T., Miller, A., *et al.* (2007) Mesiodistal root angulation using panoramic and cone beam CT. *Angle Orthodontist*, 77 (2), 206–213.

Pfeiffer, P., Bewersdorf, S., & Schmage, P. (2012) The effect of changes in head position on enlargement of structures during panoramic radiography. *International Journal of Oral & Maxillofacial Implants*, 27 (1), 55–63.

Ponder, S., Benavides, E., Kapila, S., *et al.* (2012) Quantification of external root resorption by low- vs. high-resolution cone beam computed tomography and periapical radiography: a volumetric and linear analysis. *American Journal of Orthodontics and Dentofacial Orthopedics*, 143 (1), 77–91.

Pope, F.M., Komorowska, A., Lee, K.W., *et al.* (1992) Ehlers Danlos syndrome type I with novel dental features. *Journal of Oral Pathology and Medicine*, 21 (9), 418–421.

Rakhshan, V., Nateghian, N., & Ordoubzazri, M. (2012) Risk factors associated with external apical root resorption of the maxillary incisors: a 15-year retrospective study. *Australian Orthodontic Journal*, 28 (1), 51–56.

Ranalli, D.N., Elliott, M.A., Whaley, T.M., *et al.* (1984) Stevens-Johnson syndrome: report of case with abnormal root development. *ASDC Journal of Dentristry for Children*, 51 (4), 298–301.

Reitan, K. (1974) Initial tissue behavior during apical root resorption. *Angle Orthodontist*, 44 (1), 68–82.

Ren, H., Chen, J., Deng, F., *et al.* (2013) Comparison of cone-beam computed tomography and periapical radiography for detecting simulated apical root resorption. *Angle Orthodontist*, 83 (2), 189–195.

Robotta, P. & Schafer, E. (2011) Hallermann-Streiff syndrome: case report and literature review. *Quintessence International*, 42 (4), 331–338.

Rocha, C.T., Nelson-Filho, P., Silva, L.A., *et al.* (2011) Variation of dentin dysplasia type I: report of atypical findings in the permanent dentition. *Brazilian Dental Journal*, 22 (1), 74–78.

Roinioti, T.D. & Stefanopoulos, P.K. (2007) Short root anomaly associated with Rothmund-Thomson syndrome. *Oral Surgery, Oral Medicine, Oral Pathology, Oral Radiology and Endodontics*, 103 (1), e19–e22.

Rygh, P. & Reitan, K. (1972) Ultrastructural changes in the periodontal ligament incident to orthodontic tooth movement. *Transactions: European Orthodontic Society*, 393–405.

Sachdeva, R., Frugé, J.F., Frugé, A.M., *et al.* (2005) Sure-Smile: a report of clinical findings. *Journal of Clinical Orthodontics*, 39 (5), 297–314.

Sahai, S., Kaveriappa, S., Arora, H., *et al.* (2011) 3-D imaging in post-traumatic malformation and eruptive disturbance in permanent incisors: a case report. *Dental Traumatology*, 27 (6), 473–477.

Sameshima, G.T. & Asgarifar, K.O. (2001) Assessment of root resorption and root shape: periapical vs. panoramic films. *Angle Orthodontist*, 71 (3), 185–189.

Sameshima, G.T. & Sinclair, P.M. (2001a) Predicting and preventing root resorption. Part I: diagnostic factors. *American Journal of Orthodontics and Dentofacial Orthopedics*, 119 (5), 505–510.

Sameshima, G.T. & Sinclair, P.M. (2001b) Predicting and preventing root resorption. Part II: treatment factors. *American Journal of Orthodontics and Dentofacial Orthopedics*, 119 (5), 511–515.

Sämfors, K.A. & Welander, U. (1974) Angle distortion in narrow beam rotation radiography. *Acta Radiologica: Diagnosis*, 15 (5), 570–576.

Scarfe, W.C., Li, Z., Aboelmaaty, W., *et al.* (2012) Maxillofacial cone beam computed tomography: essence, elements and steps to interpretation. *Australian Dental Journal*, 57 (Suppl 1), 46–60.

Scott, P., DiBiase, A.T., Sherriff, M., *et al.* (2008) Alignment efficiency of Damon3 self-ligating and conventional orthodontic bracket systems: a randomized clinical trial. *American Journal of Orthodontics and Dentofacial Orthopedics*, 134 (4), 470.e1–470.e8.

Segal, G.R., Schiffman, P.H., & Tuncay, O.C. (2004) Meta-analysis of the treatment-related factors of external apical root resorption. *Orthodontics & Craniofacial Research*, 7 (2), 71–78.

Shaw, L. (1995) Short root anomaly in a patient with severe short-limbed dwarfism. *International Journal of Paediatric Dentistry*, 5 (4), 249–252.

Shewinvanakitkul, W., Hans, M.G., Narendran, S., *et al.* (2011) Measuring buccolingual inclination of mandibular canines and first molars using CBCT. *Orthodontics & Craniofacial Research*, 14 (3), 168–174.

Smale, I., Artun, J., Behbehani, F., *et al.* (2005) Apical root resorption six months after initiation of fixed orthodontic appliance therapy. *American Journal of Orthodontics and Dentofacial Orthopedics*, 128 (1), 57–67.

Spurrier, S.W., Hall, S.H., Joondeph, D.R., *et al.* (1990) A comparison of apical root resorption during orthodontic treatment in endodontically treated and vital teeth. *American Journal of Orthodontics and Dentofacial Orthopedics*, 97 (2), 130–134.

Stenvik, A. & Mjör, I.A. (1970) Pulp and dentine reactions to experimental tooth intrusion: a histologic study of the initial changes. *American Journal of Orthodontics*, 57 (4), 370–385.

Stramotas, S., Geenty, J.P., Petocz, P., *et al.* (2002) Accuracy of linear and angular measurements on panoramic radiographs taken at various positions *in vitro*. *European Journal of Orthodontics*, 23 (1), 43–52.

Sunku, R., Roopesh, R., Kancherla, P., *et al.* (2011) Quantitative digital subtraction radiography in the assessment of external apical root resorption induced by orthodontic therapy: a retrospective study. *Journal of Contemporary Dental Practice*, 12 (6), 422–428.

Taithongchai, R., Sookkorn, K., & Killiany, D.M. (1996) Facial and dentoalveolar structure and the prediction of apical root shortening. *American Journal of Orthodontics and Dentofacial Orthopedics*, 110 (3), 296–302.

Taner, T., Ciğer, S., & Sençift, Y. (1999) Evaluation of apical root resorption following extraction therapy in subjects with Class I and Class II malocclusions. *European Journal of Orthodontics*, 21 (5), 491–496.

Ten Hoeve, A. & Mulie, R.M. (1976) The effect of antero-postero incisor repositioning on the palatal cortex as studied with laminagraphy. *Journal of Clinical Orthodontics*, 10 (11), 804–822.

Thongudomporn, U. & Freer, T.J. (1998) Anomalous dental morphology and root resorption during orthodontic treatment: a pilot study. *Australian Orthodontic Journal*, 15 (3), 162–167.

Thornton, J.B. & Worley, S.L. (1991) Short root anomaly in a patient with a history of Stevens-Johnson syndrome: report of case. *ASDC Journal of Dentistry for Children*, 58 (3), 256–259.

Tong, H., Enciso, R., Van Elslande, D., *et al.* (2012a) A new method to measure mesiodistal angulation and faciolingual inclination of each whole tooth with volumetric cone-beam computed tomography images. *American Journal of Orthodontics and Dentofacial Orthopedics*, 142 (1), 133–143.

Tong, H., Kwon, D., Shi, J., *et al.* (2012b) Mesiodistal angulation and faciolingual inclination of each whole tooth in 3-dimensional space in patients with near-normal occlusion. *American Journal of Orthodontics and Dentofacial Orthopedics*, 141 (5), 604–617.

Tronje, G., Welander, U., McDavid, W.D., *et al.* (1981) Image distortion in rotational panoramic radiography. III: inclined objects. *Acta Radiologica: Diagnosis*, 22 (5), 585–592.

Van Elslande, D., Heo, G., Flores-Mir, C., *et al.* (2010) Accuracy of mesiodistal root angulation projected by cone-beam computed tomographic panoramic-like images. *American Journal of Orthodontics and Dentofacial Orthopedics*, 137 (4 Suppl.), S94–S99.

van Loenen, M., Dermaut, L.R., Degrieck, J., *et al.* (2007) Apical root resorption of upper incisors during the torquing stage of the tip-edge technique. *European Journal of Orthodontics*, 29 (6), 583–588.

Van Parys, K., Aartman, I.H., Kuitert, R., *et al.* (2011) Assessment of dental anomalies on panoramic radiographs: inter- and intra-examiner agreement. *European Journal of Orthodontics*, 33 (3), 250–255.

Weltman, B., Vig, K.W., Fields, H.W., *et al.* (2010) Root resorption associated with orthodontic tooth movement: a systematic review. *American Journal of Orthodontics and Dentofacial Orthopedics*, 137 (4), 462–476.

Wong, D.T. (2012) Salivaomics. *Journal of the American Dental Association*, 143 (10 Suppl), 19S–24S.

Xuan, K., Zhang, Y.F., Liu, Y.L., *et al.* (2010) Comprehensive and sequential management of an impacted maxillary central incisor with severe crown-root dilacerations. *Dental Traumatology*, 26 (6), 516–520.

16 3D Image-Aided Diagnosis and Treatment of Impacted and Transposed Teeth

Sunil D. Kapila, BDS, MS, PhD, and Jeanne M. Nervina, DMD, PhD

INTRODUCTION

Because impacted and transposed teeth often are difficult to diagnose accurately or treat predictably, they remain some of the most challenging cases in orthodontics. Some hurdles or limitations in treating these cases include existing and/or treatment-related root resorption, extended treatment time, failure to retrieve the tooth, and ankylosis. Part of the complexity in treating these cases is related to the inability of the clinician to accurately visualize the location, angulation, spatial position, and relationships of the tooth in three dimensions using conventional two-dimensional (2D) radiographs. Furthermore, even with the availability of three-dimensional (3D) cone beam computed tomography (CBCT), there currently remains a gap in knowledge and abilities of clinicians on how best to extract and utilize all the information available in the 3D dataset for precision diagnosis and how to use this evidence to plan and execute treatment and biomechanics strategies optimally. To achieve these capabilities, it is important for clinicians to acquire the skill set needed to utilize imaging software and to manipulate and interpret 3D images. It is expected that with ongoing improvements in 3D imaging and software, and increasing hands-on experience of clinicians in using this new technology, this hurdle also will be overcome. This chapter provides important insights toward achieving this goal.

Since its introduction into dentistry in 1999, CBCT increasingly has become a valuable aid in diagnosis and treatment planning in orthodontics (Kapila *et al.*, 2011). However, despite substantial research discoveries with CBCT, many of which are highlighted in this book, the profession is still in the early phases of developing approaches and protocols that help us to utilize the information contained in 3D volumes optimally to enhance diagnosis or treatment planning of cases, optimize biomechanics, and ultimately improve the treatment outcomes for our patients. Of the many clinical situations presenting to the orthodontist, the

Cone Beam Computed Tomography in Orthodontics: Indications, Insights, and Innovations, First Edition. Sunil D. Kapila.

one with the strongest research evidence justifying the use of CBCT is impacted teeth. While there currently is considerable information available on the application of CBCT to impacted teeth, a cohesive and comprehensive approach to applying information derived from CBCT and optimal protocols for its utilization in these cases have not been established.

In this chapter, we provide insights into evidence-based use of CBCT for treating impacted and transposed teeth and how best to utilize the information thus derived for predictable and efficient treatment of these teeth. Specifically, we provide the foundational background on impacted and transposed teeth and extend this to contemporary insights gained by imaging these teeth with CBCT. We then discuss protocols for CBCT imaging, interpretation, and treatment planning for impacted and transposed teeth. Finally, we use cases to demonstrate the potential pitfalls of suboptimal diagnosis and treatments resulting partially from the limitations of 2D radiographs and to demonstrate approaches for individualized 3D image-based biomechanics for efficient and predictable treatment of impacted and transposed teeth while minimizing damage to neighboring roots or periodontium.

PREVALENCE AND ETIOLOGY OF IMPACTED AND TRANSPOSED TEETH

Maxillary canines are the second most commonly impacted teeth after third molar impactions (Bedoya & Park, 2009; Manne *et al.*, 2012, and references therein). Approximately 1–3% of the population has an impacted maxillary canine, which occurs twice as frequently in females than in males. The majority of maxillary impacted canines are unilateral (90–92%), and palatally (85%) rather than buccally (15%) displaced (Peck *et al.*, 1994; Quirynen *et al.*, 2000). Mandibular canine impactions are rare, with an incidence of 0.35% (Dachi & Howell, 1961).

Transposition is defined as the partial or complete positional exchange of adjacent teeth (Shapira & Kuftinec, 2001). Less commonly, a tooth can erupt in the position of a nonadjacent tooth (Peck *et al.*, 1993; Peck & Peck, 1995). Transpositions are more rare than maxillary canine impactions, occurring in less than 1% of the population (Peck *et al.*, 1993; Peck & Peck, 1995). When present, transpositions are most likely to occur in the maxilla and most often involve the canine (Plunkett *et al.*, 1998; Shapira & Kuftinec, 2001; Ely *et al.*, 2006). In the maxilla, the canine is transposed most commonly with the first premolar followed by the lateral incisor (Joshi & Bhatt, 1971; Shapira, 1980; Gholston & Williams, 1984; Peck & Peck, 1995; Wasserstein *et al.*, 1997). Interestingly, all reported cases of mandibular transpositions involve the canine and lateral incisor (Peck *et al.*, 1998). As with impactions, females are more likely to have transposed teeth, and the majority of these will be unilateral and left-sided (Shapira, 1980; Peck & Peck, 1995). Not surprisingly, transpositions also are more common in cleft lip and palate (CL/P) patients than in non-cleft patients (Oberoi *et al.*, 2010).

Because both impactions and transpositions represent ectopic eruption, it commonly is accepted that their etiologies are multifactorial, involving local, systemic, and genetic factors (Peck *et al.*, 1993, 1998, 2002; Frazier-Bowers *et al.*, 2010). Supporting this concept are the growing number of studies showing the concomitant presence of dental anomalies, especially peg lateral incisors and/or dental agenesis, especially second premolars, with canine impactions (Peck *et al.*, 1996a, 1996b; Peck & Peck, 1997; Peck, 1998; Shalish *et al.*, 2002; Leonardi *et al.*, 2003; Garib *et al.*, 2009). Genome-wide association studies have yet to be performed specifically on patients with impactions or transpositions, but it is likely that this approach will yield significant information on the genes responsible for normal or abnormal developmental positioning of teeth. This could help clinicians diagnose and treat impactions early, which is important for improving outcomes for these patients (Manne *et al.*, 2012).

While current research on tooth eruption relies heavily on understanding the molecular regulation of eruption, conventional 2D radiographs, especially periapical and panoramic radiographs, have allowed us to identify several local factors that may contribute to ectopic or impacted canines. These factors include enlarged crown, retained primary canines, ankylosis, cysts, neoplasms, root dilacerations, and missing or peg lateral incisor (Manne *et al.*, 2012). Identifying the presence of these local factors is important for accurate diagnosis and treatment planning for impactions and transpositions. As noted below, 3D radiography has broadened our understanding of normal and ectopic tooth development and eruption that likely will contribute to further refinements in diagnostics and treatment approaches. Furthermore, the knowledge gained through these studies will be critical for focusing future research efforts on the pathophysiological mediators of impactions and transpositions.

2D AND 3D RADIOGRAPHIC FINDINGS ON NORMAL CANINE DEVELOPMENT AND ERUPTION

Since the maxillary canine is the most commonly impacted tooth, it has received the majority of attention from researchers interested in the process of dental impactions. For this reason, the following section focuses on studies, particularly those using 2D and 3D radiographs, that have broadened our understanding of normal canine development and eruption.

While conventional 2D radiographs have given us important data on normal tooth development, their accuracy for assessing tooth position falls significantly below the accuracy of 3D radiographs (see also Chapter 15). Knowing this, a critical reader of the scientific literature on radiographic mapping of maxillary canine development and eruption rightly would be wary of existing literature because it is based overwhelmingly on conventional 2D radiographs. Moreover, as Broadbent (1941) advised early on, researchers and clinicians must recognize the technical limitations of 2D radiographs to describe a 3D process. He suggested that useful information on canine development and eruption can be gleaned only from both a lateral and posterior-anterior cephalograph of the subject, which then was the best available approach to "representing" a structure in 3D. Investigations using this approach to assess 3D canine position have shown that, on average, the maxillary canines move incisally 18.6 mm in children between ages 5 and 13, distally 11.5 mm from ages 7 to 13 years, and palatally until about 2 years prior to eruption, at which point the canines reverse direction, eventually moving 2.7 mm buccal to their starting position (Coulter & Richardson, 1997). The question regarding this study is how accurate the data are given that the measurements were taken from conventional 2D radiographs, which inherently are inaccurate. It is clear that CBCT offers a much clearer and far more accurate picture than 2D radiographs of how canines develop and erupt.

To date, the only published 3D study focused on canine eruption was conducted on CL/P patients (Oberoi *et al.*, 2010). Unlike the Coulter and Richardson study (1997), which tracked canine eruption annually between the ages of 5 and 15, the CBCT scans in this study were taken only twice, once at age 10 years 6 months and then again at age 11 years 9 months. Therefore, we do not have a complete 3D picture of maxillary canine development in these children. Nonetheless, this study traces canine movement prior to eruption on both the cleft and non-cleft sides. Both the cleft- and non-cleft-side canines move incisally, mesially, and buccally, albeit at different rates. The cleft-side canine moves incisally 0.8 mm more than the non-cleft-side canine (6.8 mm and 5.9 mm, respectively), mesially 1.6 mm more than the non-cleft-side canine (3.2 mm and 1.6 mm, respectively) and the same distance buccally as the non-cleft-side canine (2.5 mm). By comparison, strikingly smaller maxillary canine movements of 0.2 mm incisally, 0.6 mm buccally, and none in the mesio-distal axis were reported in children ages 10–11 and 11–12 using 2D lateral and posterior-anterior cephalographs (Coulter & Richardson, 1997). Thus, not only are the measurements made from 2D radiographs far smaller than those derived from CBCT, but they essentially show that the canines do not move in 10- to 12-year-old children, which, besides contradicting the 3D observations, is highly unlikely.

With the introduction of CBCT and its 3D rendering capacity, it now is becoming common practice for orthodontists to prescribe CBCT for patients with an impacted canine diagnosed clinically and/or on conventional 2D radiographs, providing a database of 2D and 3D radiographs taken on the same patient. This allows direct comparison of the diagnostic quality of each image and, more importantly, enables the assessment of how CBCT images effect a clinician's treatment planning decisions;

this will be discussed later. These 3D data also have enabled researchers to determine if impacted canines have a unique 3D positional signature relative to that of a normally erupting canine. Thus, analyses of CBCT scans from 29 consecutively treated orthodontics patients (mean age = 16.6 years) who presented with at least one impacted canine showed that the average distance of the unerupted canine cusp was 10.1 mm mesial, 1.8 mm palatal, and 10 mm vertical from the position it would occupy if positioned ideally in the arch (Oberoi & Knueppel, 2012). Whether this pattern is detectable earlier in development is not known yet, but if it is, it would be helpful for early diagnosis of impacted canines and implementation of case-specific interceptive strategies or treatment approaches.

Another distinction between 2D and 3D radiography is in their capacity to detect resorption of roots of teeth that are in close proximity to impacted teeth (Alqerban *et al.*, 2009a, 2011). Diagnosing root resorption with conventional 2D radiographs can be challenging due to superimposition of structures and the other pitfalls of 2D images (Figure 16.1). Thus, while periapical and panoramic radiographs enable the detection of root resorption in about 33–50% of the incisors associated with impacted canines, CBCT facilitates the detection of root resorption on an additional 65% of these roots than are detectable with 2D imaging (Alqerban *et al.*, 2011; see also Chapter 15). These findings and their clinical implications are discussed below in greater depth.

EFFICACY OF CBCT IN DIAGNOSIS AND TREATMENT PLANNING OF IMPACTED TEETH AND ASSOCIATED ROOT RESORPTION

As pointed out in Chapters 1 and 6, the use of CBCT imaging ideally should be determined by evidence showing its efficacy in enhancing diagnosis and treatment decisions, and ultimately in improving treatment efficiency and outcomes. In the absence of such research-based support for using CBCT, a secondary justification for imaging is when, on the basis of clinical or other diagnostic aids, the clinician determines that the benefits of CBCT outweigh its risks. In this context, there now is substantial research evidence to support the use of CBCT imaging for diagnosing and treatment planning impacted teeth. Indeed, it is one of the few clinical situations in orthodontics that has this level of research evidence to support the use of CBCT (Haney *et al.*, 2010; Katheria *et al.*, 2010; Botticelli *et al.*, 2011). The most supportive research evidence for the use of CBCT radiographs for diagnosing and treatment planning impacted canines arises from comparison studies that demonstrate differences between 2D and 3D imaging in the accuracy of localizing impacted canines, identification of canine-induced root resorption on adjacent teeth, and pinpointing the site for surgical access to the impacted canine. Importantly, some of these studies also demonstrate that CBCT images increase the clinician's confidence in treatment planning. In the following sections, we will review the lines of research that support the use of CBCT imaging on patients with impacted teeth.

2D versus 3D radiography for diagnosing impacted teeth

Prior to the introduction of CBCT imaging, localizing and diagnosis for impacted canines were performed primarily from 2D radiographs (Power & Short, 1993; Stivaros & Mandall, 2000; Warford *et al.*, 2003). Occlusal and periapical radiographs traditionally have been utilized to localize the position of the canine using the "same lingual, opposite buccal" (SLOB) rule, which generally focuses on localizing the impacted tooth crown's 2D buccolingual position rather than detailing the entire tooth's 3D spatial position and relationship to surrounding structures. With the growing body of research on CBCT imaging to localize impacted canines, the limitations of making treatment decisions using the SLOB rule and conventional 2D radiographs is becoming increasingly evident, as will be discussed later.

While using conventional 2D panoramic radiographs for localizing an impacted canine is not advised (Nagpal *et al.*, 2009), it has been proposed that panoramic radiographs can be used for early diagnosis of canine impaction in patients as young as 5–9 years old (Novak *et al.*, 2012; Sajnani & King,

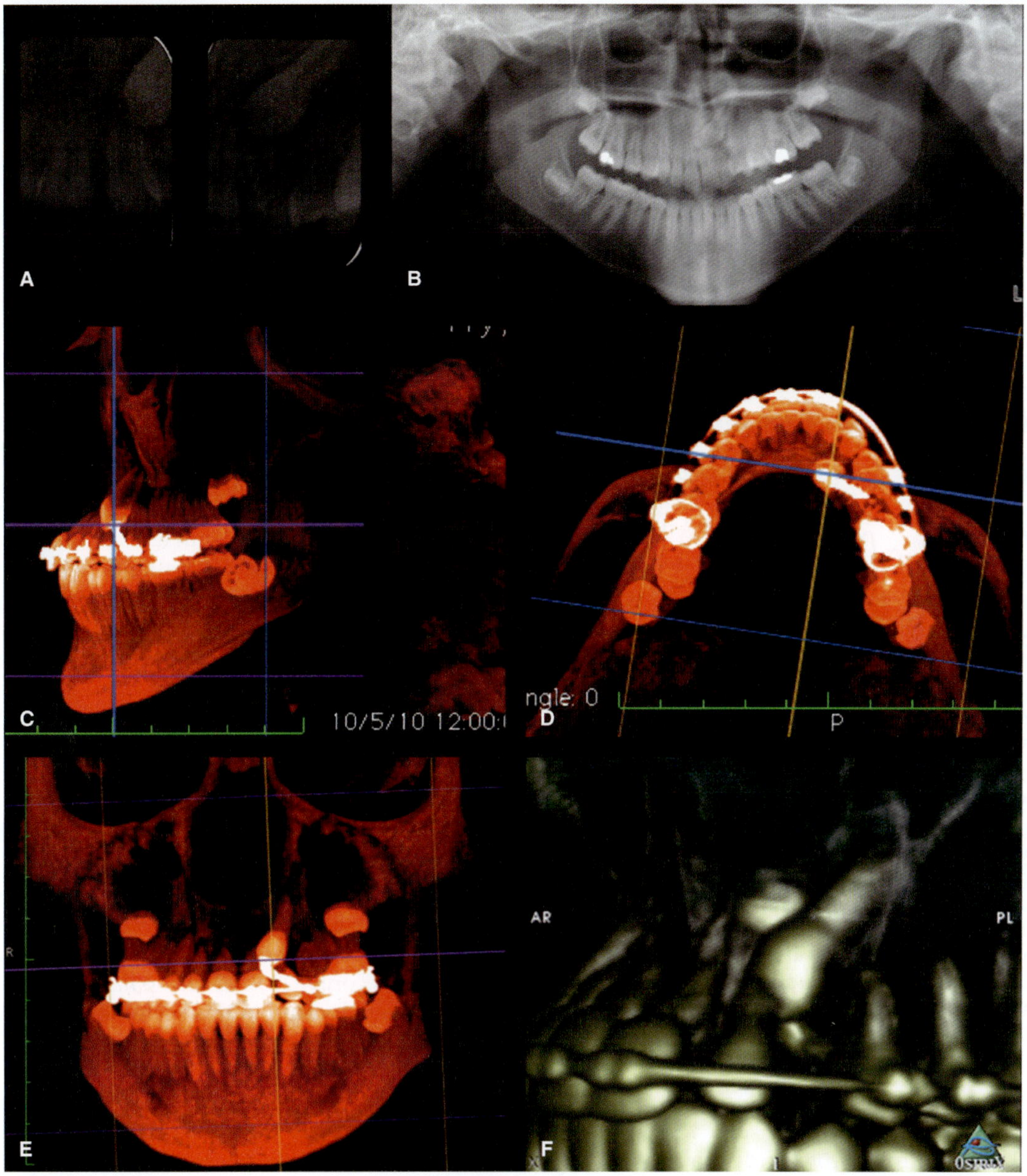

Figure 16.1 Diagnosis of root resorption associated with impacted teeth. *A* and *B*: Pre-treatment periapical and panoramic radiographs do not provide optimal information on the presence of existing root damage. *C–F*: Following treatment over several months in which the impacted tooth was not visible clinically, a CBCT was taken to determine the possible reason for the failure of guided eruption treatment. Sagittal (*C*), axial (*D*), coronal (*E*), and lateral (*F*) volumetric representations demonstrate the proximity of the impacted tooth to the lateral incisor and the substantial root resorption on the lateral incisor. Given the lack of pre-treatment CBCT, it is not possible to determine the extent of pre-treatment root resorption or the contributions of treatment to the current magnitude of root damage. However, because of the position of the bond on the tooth cingulum and despite desirable force vectors, it is likely that the cusp tip has continued to move along the root of the lateral incisor, contributing to root resorption and difficulty in canine retrieval.

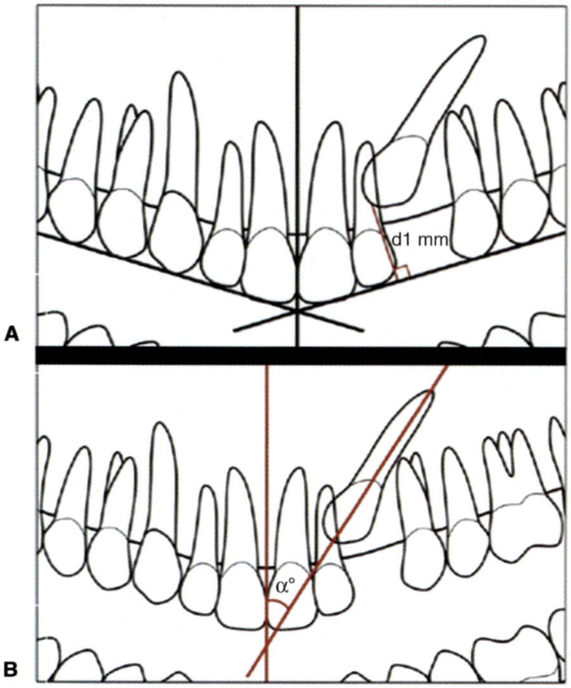

Figure 16.2 Approaches to assessing the risk of canine impaction using conventional 2D panoramic radiographs. *A*: Canine cusp distance is measured as the perpendicular distance to the occlusal plane. The longer this distance, the more likely the canine will be impacted. *B*: Canine angulation is measured as the angle formed by the intersection of the canine long axis and the midline vertical. The more obtuse this angle, the more likely the canine will be impacted horizontally. It also means that the canine eruption is toward the incisor roots, which puts the incisor roots at risk for resorption. (Modified and reprinted with permission from Sajnani & King, 2012.)

2012). Thus, a retrospective study (Sajnani & King, 2012) of 2D panoramic radiographs of 442 patients between 3 years of age to adulthood with at least one impacted maxillary canine demonstrated that the perpendicular distance of the canine cusp tip to the occlusal plane is significantly larger for the impacted than normally erupting canines from age 5 years and up (Figure 16.2A). Also, whereas the normal canine cusp tip did not appear to overlap any part of the lateral incisor, that of the impacted canine overlapped the distal of the lateral incisor root at age 9 years and, on average, eventually overlapped the mesial of the lateral incisor root. Finally, the canine angle relative to the midline was significantly larger for the impacted canine (28.4°) compared with the normal canine (11.3°) beginning at 9 years of age (Figure 16.2B). Moreover, this angulation of the impacted canine increases with age, while the non-impacted canine angle decreases with age. These findings indicate that the canine cusp location relative to the occlusal plane and the lateral incisor and its angulation relative to the midline may be used to predict whether the canine is at risk for impaction.

Early diagnosis of potential canine impaction from conventional 2D lateral cephalographs in combination with panoramic radiographs also has been reported in a prospective controlled study of 35 orthodontics patients with at least one palatally displaced canine and 50 patients with normal canine eruption in subjects with a mean age of slightly over 10 years (Novak *et al.*, 2012). The panoramic radiographs were utilized to assess the canine mesial angulation relative to the midline and canine cusp tip distance from the occlusal plane using the same approach as shown in Figure 16.2. In addition, the position of the canine cusp tip relative to the lateral and central incisors was assigned a sector value (Figure 16.3A). The mesial angle of the palatally displaced canine to the midline was significantly larger (27.5°) than the normal canine (7.6°). As opposed to nearly all (92%) of the normal canine cusps being positioned in sector 1, only 23% of the palatally displaced canines were located in this sector. These palatally displaced canines more often were distributed in sectors 2 (43%), 3 (23%), and 4 (11%). There was no significant difference in the distance from the occlusal plane between the palatally displaced and normal canines on the panoramic radiographs. The lateral cephalographs (Figure 16.3B,C) were used to evaluate the vertical angle of the canine to the Frankfort and palatal planes and to the central incisor. The canine cusp tip distance from the central incisor vertical axis parallel to Frankfort Horizontal, anterior alveolar ridge parallel to Frankfort Horizontal, and the functional occlusal plane also were measured from the lateral cephalographs. Each of the angular measurements was smaller, while the linear measurements all were larger for the palatally displaced canines compared with the normally developing canines. These

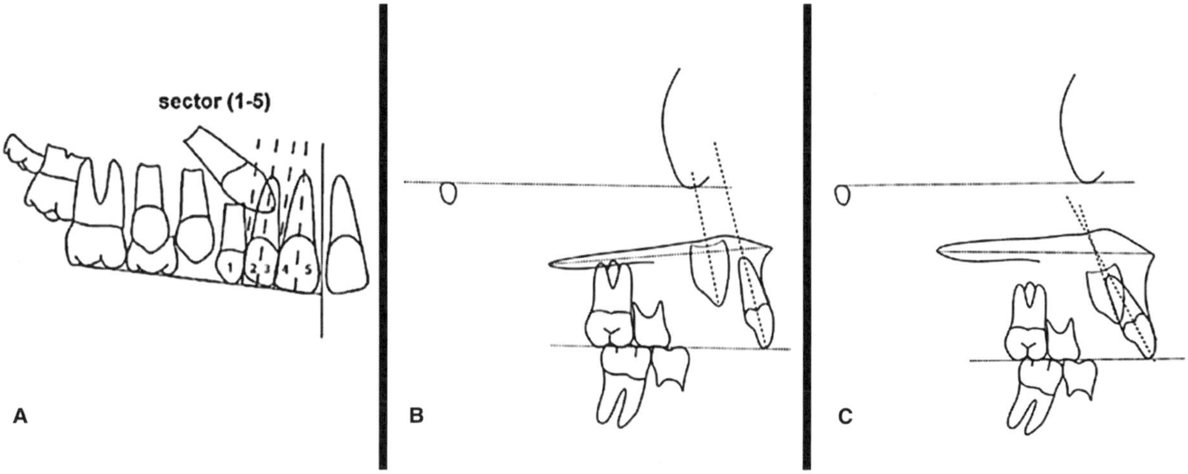

Figure 16.3 Assessing the risk of maxillary canine impaction from conventional 2D radiographs. *A*: Characterization of canine cusp sector position from a panoramic radiograph used to assess the likelihood of impaction. Sectors are labeled as shown, with sector 1 being the primary canine and sector 5 being the mesial half of the central incisor. The higher the sector in which the canine cusp is located, the higher the likelihood of impaction. *B* and *C*: Tracing of a canine on a lateral cephalograph that likely is to be displaced palatally (*B*) and in position for normal eruption (*C*). Using this approach, the canine angle relative to Frankfort Horizontal Plane, palatal plane and long axis of the central incisor are measured. The linear distance of the canine cusp from the central incisor along a line parallel to Frankfort Horizontal Plane, from the alveolar ridge parallel to Frankfort Horizontal, and from the functional occlusal plane also are measured. Impacted canines are likely to have smaller angular measurements, but larger linear measurements than normally erupting canines. (Reprinted with permission from Novak *et al.*, 2012.)

findings provide a guide to assessing the potential for canine impactions using panoramic and cephalometric radiographs.

Assessing impacted canine position on 2D radiographs has been the gold standard for decades largely because 3D radiographs were not available. Also, although previous studies indicate a 92% accuracy of localizing impacted canines from 2D radiographs (Ericson & Kurol, 1986a, 1986b, 1987), recent findings demonstrate a substantial discrepancy between 2D and 3D images in localizing canines and in the detection of root resorption (Alqerban *et al.*, 2009a, 2011; Haney *et al.*, 2010; Katheria *et al.*, 2010; Botticelli *et al.*, 2011). More important, a key question regarding CBCT imaging of impacted teeth is whether the information obtained from these images improves diagnosis, aids in refining treatment plan(s), and, in the long term, improves treatment outcomes. The answer to the first two questions is provided by several recent studies that have demonstrated significant differences in diagnosis and treatment planning and improved confidence in these decisions for impacted teeth when comparing 3D with 2D radiography (Haney *et al.*, 2010; Katheria *et al.*, 2010; Botticelli *et al.*, 2011; Alqerban *et al.*, 2013).

In a study by Haney and colleagues (2010), the investigators sought responses from a group of orthodontists and oral and maxillofacial surgeons on the location and site of surgical access for impacted canines in routine 2D radiographs (panoramic, occlusal, and two periapicals) versus printouts of 3D CBCT images. There was an approximate 20% lack of agreement among clinicians on the palatal versus labial location of the tooth tip between the two imaging modalities. The same lack of agreement was found when determining on which side to start the surgical access, implying that an accurate identification of tooth tip location has a direct effect on site of surgical access. When the treatment plan included forced recovery of the tooth, then the initial force vector selected was influenced significantly by the radiographic modality. Specifically, when these teeth were evaluated with 3D images, the vector was changed for 11 of 12 teeth judged to have an initial distal recovery vector on 2D images. Interestingly, clinicians generated the same orthodontic treatment plan using CBCT and 2D radiographs for only 36% of the impacted teeth, demonstrating large differences in treatment approaches when the two imaging methods were compared. Furthermore, CBCT contributed to significantly higher confidence in diagnosis and treatment planning relative to the combination of panoramic, periapical, and occlusal radiographs. Similar, and in some instances larger, differences in determination of canine or supernumerary positions and treatment decisions between CBCT and conventional imaging have been reported by others (Katheria *et al.*, 2010; Botticelli *et al.*, 2011). Observers in the Katheria study scored a significantly higher proportion of CBCT examinations as "very useful" in treatment planning than conventional radiographic examinations (Katheria *et al.*, 2010). The treatment decisions made differed between the two imaging modalities for 27–30% of the subjects (Haney *et al.*, 2010; Botticelli *et al.*, 2011). While these studies provide sound support for the efficacy of CBCT in diagnosing and treatment planning impacted teeth, it is plausible that the findings would have been strengthened further if virtual images on a computer monitor were used, rather than printouts of the 3D images.

2D and 3D findings on root resorption associated with impacted canines

An ectopic or impacted tooth presents a risk for resorbing roots of nearby teeth, which in the case of impacted canines typically affects the lateral incisor and less frequently the central incisor (Alqerban *et al.*, 2009b; Bjerklin & Guitirokh, 2011; Bertl *et al.*, 2013; Strbac *et al.*, 2013). Because of this, any improved efficacy in detecting root resorption using CBCT rather than 2D radiography that contributes to better and informed treatment decisions could prove to be valuable to the patient and clinician, providing further justification for the use of CBCT for treatment of impacted teeth. Indeed, research findings show not only a 22–36% lack of agreement in the perception of root resorption of teeth adjacent to impacted teeth between 2D versus 3D imaging (Haney *et al.*, 2010; Botticelli *et al.*, 2011), but that the incidence and magnitude of root resorption detected in association with impacted teeth is greater in 3D versus conventional radiographs. Specifically, CBCT is more sensitive than 2D radiographs in detecting root resorption associated with impacted canines (Alqerban *et al.*, 2009a). Furthermore, whereas 2D radiographs reveal root resorption in 30–50% of lateral incisors in individuals with impacted canines, the detection of lateral incisor root resorption increases by at least another 65% when using CBCT (Alqerban *et al.*, 2011). Thus, it is not surprising that 71% of clinicians consider CBCT to be "very useful" for diagnosing root resorption, while only 9% of clinicians say the same about conventional 2D radiographs (Katheria *et al.*, 2010).

In summary, the findings of several studies (Walker *et al.*, 2005; Haney *et al.*, 2010; Katheria *et al.*, 2010; Botticelli *et al.*, 2011) suggest that the use of 2D versus 3D images of impacted maxillary canines contributes to different diagnoses and treatment plans in a significant number of subjects. Specifically, these studies show that CBCT enhances the ability to localize impacted canines accurately, evaluate their proximity to other teeth, determine the follicle size and presence of pathology, estimate space needs, detect root resorption of adjacent teeth, contribute to modifications in treatment plan, and improve the confidence in diagnosis and treatment plans (Walker *et al.*, 2005; Haney *et al.*, 2010; Katheria *et al.*, 2010; Bjerklin & Guitirokh, 2011; Botticelli *et al.*, 2011).

Treatment outcomes as the gold standard evidence for utilizing CBCT

Despite the current evidence on the value of CBCT in enhancing diagnosis and treatment planning of impacted teeth, additional supporting evidence that CBCT translates into overall better treatment outcomes and efficiency than those resulting from conventional 2D radiographs still is lacking. For this purpose, it is important to specifically determine if information obtained from CBCT imaging improves the success rate in retrieving teeth, contributes to more efficient treatment with shorter treatment times, and decreases morbidity including root resorption and poor soft and hard tissue support better than treatments based on conventional 2D radiography. Derivation of such evidence requires longer-term follow-up studies. While we await treatment outcome–based justification for the use CBCT in treating impacted teeth, the findings that CBCT contributes to changes in treatment decisions in approximately 30% of these cases (Haney *et al.*, 2010; Botticelli *et al.*, 2011) may provide adequate rationale for utilizing CBCT in diagnosis and treatment planning of impacted teeth.

Although data on the efficacy of CBCT in enhancing treatment outcomes and efficiency for impacted teeth are pending, it is reasonable to assume that if the orthodontist or surgeon fails to utilize the information available from CBCT images optimally and instead implements the same or similar treatment approaches and mechanics as done with conventional 2D radiographs, no improvements in treatment outcomes should be expected. Indeed, for improved treatment outcomes and efficiencies, it is imperative that the data from CBCT be utilized fully to refine or modify treatment plans and to implement optimal retrieval mechanics. It is likely that if CBCT-derived information truly is used to comprehend the precise spatial location of the entire tooth and its relationship to neighboring structures and to define optimal surgical access, bond position, and mechanics, enhanced outcomes that include decreased treatment time, improved success rate, and decreased damage to neighboring teeth should result. The sections below outline the recommended imaging, diagnostic, treatment, and biomechanical protocols that can help in achieving the goals of improved treatment outcomes and efficiencies for impacted and transposed teeth.

PROTOCOLS FOR CBCT IMAGING OF IMPACTED AND TRANSPOSED TEETH

Determining imaging needs and field of view (FOV)

As discussed in Chapter 1, before obtaining a CBCT, it is important first to perform a thorough clinical examination to extract and synthesize all pertinent diagnostic information needed for determining whether to take a CBCT and, if needed, which region and FOV will facilitate treatment planning best. The appropriately selected optimal FOV in turn will determine if additional conventional 2D radiographs are needed (see Figure 1.5 in Chapter 1). In general, if the clinical exam reveals that the only reason to prescribe a CBCT image is an impacted tooth, then a small FOV CBCT, which captures the canine, adjacent teeth, and surrounding bony structures, would suffice. On the other hand, if the clinical examination reveals impacted teeth in different quadrants or other significant findings requiring further 3D radiographic information, then the prescribed FOV should be modified accordingly. For example, if the patient is a candidate for orthognathic surgery, then an extended FOV may be preferred. Since a panoramic radiograph can be reconstructed from medium and extended FOV CBCTs and a cephalogram can be derived from an extended FOV, the need for these two types of conventional 2D radiographs will be determined by the preferred CBCT FOV prescribed for the patient. When uncertain about the optimal FOV for a particular patient, consulting an oral and maxillofacial radiologist is recommended. Overall, as with other clinical scenarios, an individualized rather than a routine radiographic protocol should be followed for imaging impacted or transposed teeth (see also Chapters 1 and 6).

Protocols for CBCT image interpretation

Given the high percentage of missed lesions and false-positive errors in reading and interpreting CBCT images by orthodontists (Ahmed *et al.*, 2012), it is advisable that the services of an oral and maxillofacial radiologist be utilized to provide a report on the region of interest (ROI) and on any significant incidental findings (see Figure 1.14 in Chapter 1). If clinically significant incidental findings are noted, it is important to refer the patient to the appropriate healthcare provider(s) for follow-up and treatment.

A careful review by the orthodontist of the oral and maxillofacial radiologist's report and images may aid in making decisions on how to proceed with treating the impacted or transposed tooth.

Given that the radiologist may not be aware of the precise information required for surgical and biomechanical decisions and the high level of diagnostically valuable data contained in the CBCT, however, it is important that the orthodontist review and manipulate CBCT images directly on the computer to derive all the pertinent information. This process is performed best through a careful review of 3D volumetric rendering and multiplanar reconstructions (MPR) using one of various commercial software (Dolphin, QuickCeph) or freeware (e.g., Osirix, ViewBox, LightningCeph). This, in turn, entails that the orthodontist achieve a sound level of skill in software utilization and image interpretation to enable him or her to extract as much information as possible to compile a highly refined treatment plan and sophisticated biomechanical plan in three planes of space. Thus, the evaluation of the CBCT volume by the orthodontist ensures that all possible information relevant to providing optimal and efficient orthodontic treatment is available to and utilized by the orthodontist, while the radiologist's evaluation ensures that nothing of clinical significance including incidental findings present in the CBCT dataset is overlooked (see Figure 1.14 in Chapter 1). Together, this combined and collaborative interpretation of the CBCT provides the patient the "best of both worlds" with maximal utilization of the wealth of information available in the CBCT to the benefit of the patient.

CURRENT APPROACHES TO TREATING IMPACTED TEETH

Before discussing the clinical applications of CBCT to planning and implementing treatment for impacted teeth, we provide a synopsis of current approaches to treating impacted teeth. Several case-specific approaches are utilized for treating impacted teeth, all of which require radiographs that are critical for accurate diagnosis and treatment planning. When impacted teeth are identified at an early age or stage of development and are in a relatively favorable position, extraction of the primary canine and developing arch dimension if indicated can help the canine to erupt in a favorable position (Ngan *et al.*, 2005; Schmidt & Kokich, 2007). When sufficient arch length is available, this interceptive approach requires that the deciduous canines be extracted between the ages of 10 and 13. This is thought to encourage the permanent canines to spontaneously erupt into their normal position (Ericson & Kurol, 1988; Parkin *et al.*, 2009). In these patients, accurate early diagnosis of canine impaction is critical because unnecessary early extraction of primary teeth can adversely affect space availability as the permanent teeth erupt.

When the impacted tooth is identified at a later age and/or when it is in a relatively poor position and angulation, surgical exposure of the canine crown with or without guided eruption is indicated (Cooke & Wang, 2006; Bedoya & Park, 2009, and references therein). The surgical approach used depends primarily on where the impacted canine is located. Labially impacted canines can be exposed using gingivectomy, apically positioned flap, or conventional window. Gingivectomy rarely is followed by guided orthodontic eruption, as these teeth usually erupt spontaneously. Nevertheless, these canines often require orthodontic treatment to achieve proper alignment within the arch. Guided eruption on canines exposed with an apically positioned flap or conventional window can begin within 1–3 weeks following surgery.

Palatally impacted canines are treated most commonly with either open or closed exposures with or without guided orthodontic eruption. Open eruption is indicated when the canine cusp is close to the occlusal plane. Both open window eruptions and closed flaps are utilized for canines in close proximity to the incisors, or those that are horizontally impacted, or located high in the palate. It should be noted that there is no evidence of the superiority of open versus closed surgical exposure in the dental health, esthetic, economic, surgical, periodontal health, or patient-assessed outcomes to date (Parkin *et al.*, 2008, 2009, 2012, 2013), suggesting that the preferred method of exposing canines may be based largely on personal preferences of the surgeon and/or orthodontist (Parkin *et al.*, 2008). Finally, tunnel traction in which the permanent canine is guided into the arch through the "tunnel" created by the extraction of a primary canine is the surgical approach best used when the impacted canine is in close proximity to the retained primary canine.

Like the numerous surgical options available to uncover an impacted canine crown, there are numerous options for guided or forced eruption of impacted teeth (Caprioglio *et al.*, 2007; Parkin *et al.*, 2008; Manne *et al.*, 2012, and references therein). Well-planned guided eruption is necessary for teeth that are positioned adversely and/or are in close proximity to other teeth and require to be "disengaged" from adjacent structures. An improperly applied traction vector in closed guided eruption can contribute to root resorption, long treatment duration, and even a lack of success in retrieving the canine. Given the information now available from CBCT, combined with its optimal utilization to develop rational treatment and biomechanical approaches, most of these consequences may be minimized or avoided by virtual treatment planning and careful implementation of these plans. Here we highlight the maximal utilization of CBCT-based diagnostic information for improved treatment outcomes and efficiency in retrieving impacted teeth.

VIRTUAL DIAGNOSIS AND TREATMENT PLANNING OF IMPACTED TEETH

The virtual review of the CBCT images by the orthodontist should include viewing the images in 3D from all relevant angles to obtain a big picture, followed by viewing images in at least two planes from MPR. This evaluation provides comprehensive 3D information on the spatial position of the impacted tooth in its entirety and its relationships to neighboring structures. The objectives of this detailed review of the CBCT by the orthodontist are (1) to finalize diagnosis; (2) to determine existing or potential for damage to roots of neighboring teeth; (3) to refine or modify the treatment plan, including which teeth to extract in extraction cases, surgical access, and bond position; (4) to define existing and any potential limits during tooth movement of alveolar boundary conditions; and (5) to generate a detailed biomechanics plan in 3D. When these objectives are fulfilled, the process can be considered analogous to a virtual diagnosis and treatment planning of the impacted tooth that should contribute to improved treatment outcomes.

By extracting information from the CBCT images to arrive at a customized virtual treatment plan, the clinician can delineate proactively the shortest route of movement in three planes of space while avoiding damage to neighboring structures. Proactive virtual treatment planning also allows the clinician to determine a safe tractional path and, if needed, to plan for the movement of any interfering tooth and root out of the tractional path(s) so as to avoid damage. This information, in turn, is utilized to design spring(s) for delivering optimal direction(s) and magnitude of forces. The type of tooth movement desired and the proximity of the impacted tooth to neighboring roots also enables the clinician to determine the optimal location for bond placement on the impacted tooth, which, in turn, provides information on the ideal site for accessing the tooth. An accurate determination of tooth size with CBCT can aid in proactively developing the space needed to fit the tooth into the arch. Finally, planning of the 3D biomechanics to retrieve the impacted tooth also enables the orthodontist to preemptively plan strategies to minimize adverse movements of anchor teeth. If applied diligently, these approaches should contribute to improved success of retrieval, enhanced treatment efficiency, and minimization of damage to adjacent structures including roots and bone.

One of the key steps in virtual 3D biomechanic planning for guided eruption involves the predetermination of ideal force directions and preplanning of the needed sequential changes in force directions as the tooth erupts to guide it safely and efficiently into the arch. This virtual biomechanic plan in turn allows clinicians to design and fabricate one or more customized springs and levers specifically for each patient that can achieve moving the impacted tooth into the arch efficiently. The proactive planning of force directions also provides the clinician with a sense of the stage of treatment when force directions need to be changed. In general, the earlier stages of retrieval require that the tooth crown be guided away from nearby roots or bony structures that would be damaged if the impacted tooth is moved in a direct line from its initial to final position. Subsequent stages usually require movement of the tooth into the arch that is accomplished by changing the spring or its direction of activation. For patients in whom a retained primary canine is extracted, the force may be directed to correspond with the bone tunnel left following its extraction to expedite and guide eruption of the impacted permanent canine.

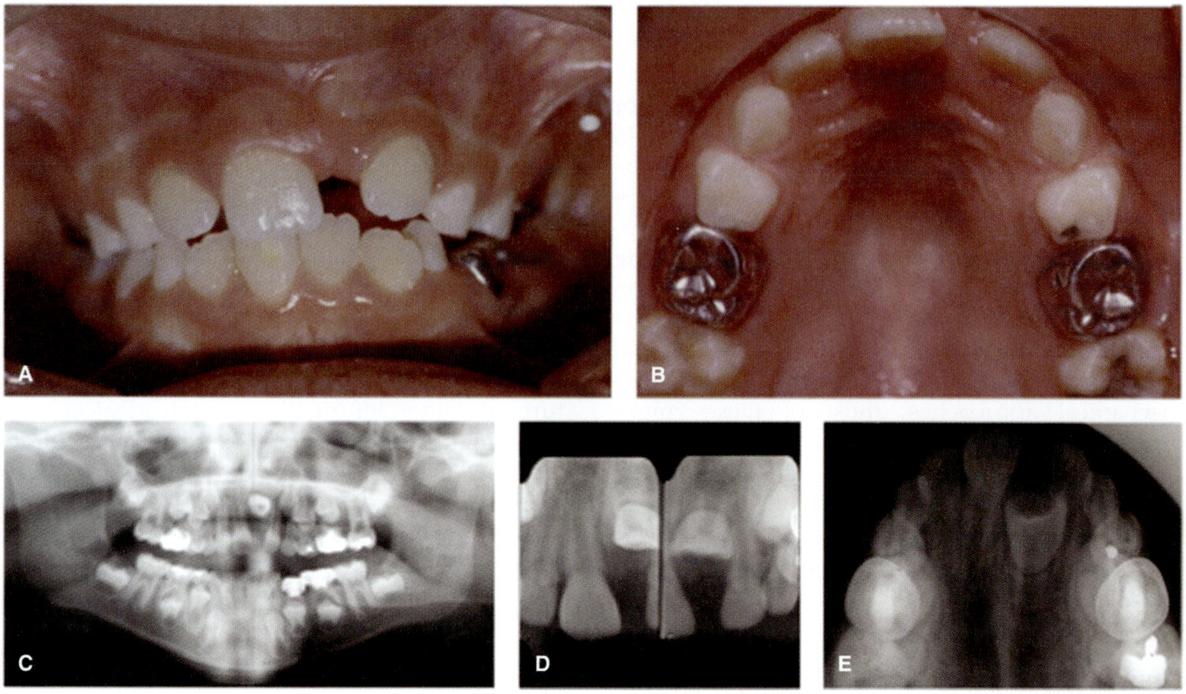

Figure 16.4 Pre-treatment photographs (*A* and *B*) and panoramic (*C*), periapical (*D*), and occlusal (*E*) radiographs of an 8-year-old patient presenting with a horizontally impacted maxillary left central incisor.

These protocols for determining the need for CBCT imaging, interpreting these images, and generating a virtual diagnosis and treatment plan offer general principles in managing impacted and transposed teach. However, since every patient presents with unique clinical problems, these general protocols and procedures must be customized for each patient. To demonstrate how this can be done, we provide cases showing ways to incorporate CBCT imaging for optimized and efficient treatment of impacted and transposed teeth.

IMPLEMENTING 3D IMAGE-AIDED TREATMENT OF IMPACTED TEETH

Diagnosis of spatial position and proximity to neighboring structures for optimal surgical access and bond placement

Prior to the introduction of the CBCT, clinical examination together with two or more 2D radiographs were used to localize and treat impacted teeth. The limitations of conventional 2D radiographs, including 2D representation of 3D anatomy and structural superimposition and the inability to visualize the entire tooth, necessitated that clinicians focus on using this information primarily to localize the 2D bucco-lingual position of the crown rather than the entire tooth. This is evident in the case shown in Figure 16.4, in which pre-treatment periapical, occlusal, and panoramic radiographs were used to localize the crown, bond it, and start applying forces. It is not possible to define clearly the entire impacted tooth due to superimposition of structures or to visualize its precise spatial position and relationships to neighboring teeth in 3D using conventional 2D radiographs. Following approximately 1 year of treatment in which the tooth did not appear in the oral cavity, but a noticeable swelling was observed in the palatal vault, CBCT was performed. This imaging revealed several causes of concern, including the proximity or contact of the impacted tooth with roots of neighboring teeth, possible root resorption, and breach of the palatal alveolar boundaries by the apical part of the root of the impacted tooth (Figure 16.5). The sagittal MPR images also revealed that the major reason for this undesirable treatment outcome was the position of the bond and, therefore, the point of force application at the cingulum of the impacted incisor. Since the center of resistance of a tooth that is embedded entirely in bone is close to the cemento-enamel junction that, in this case, is near the bond location, application of forces at this site would result in bodily movement of the entire tooth rather than the preferred uncontrolled tipping. In this case, the desirable palatal movement of the crown and labial movement of the root apex would be achieved better by placing the bond close to the incisal edge and then applying optimal mechanics. The CBCT information available at this stage of treatment also can be useful in midcourse corrections in treatment to include repositioning the bond and reconfiguring the mechanics for subsequent successful tooth retrieval.

The case in Figure 16.4 and Figure 16.5 also highlights another important difference and emerging terminology for the 3D location of impacted teeth using CBCT. Because of the enhanced information obtained from CBCT, the use of the term *localization* previously used with 2D images to describe the location of the cusp tip may no longer be considered an accurate descriptor of the diagnostic outcome derived from CBCT of impacted teeth. Indeed the detailed information provided by CBCT contributes to the determination of the *spatial position of the entire impacted tooth and its relationships to its neighboring structures in 3D*, which is the preferred descriptor to utilize for defining impacted teeth when using CBCT.

The previous case also highlights the importance of CBCT to position the bond accurately for optimizing treatment outcomes. Since not all clinicians who expose and place bonds on impacted teeth have access to CBCT imaging software, our preferred referral protocol includes a written prescription for exposure and bond placement together with a composite image identifying the desired position of bond placement (Figure 16.6). Typically, the preferred bond location is at the incisal edge or cusp tip, but there may be instances that require the bond to be placed at a slightly different location for biomechanical advantages. Placing the bond at the incisal edge or cusp tip provides a higher tolerance to errors in force vectors than if the bond is placed further away from this location (Figure 16.7). In contrast, placing the bond and, therefore, the force at some distance from the cusp tip decreases the *error tolerance range* of the force vector due to limited ability to control the movement of the tip and can have adverse consequences such as encroaching into tooth roots, root resorption, long treatment time, or failure to retrieve the tooth. Given the ability to control force directions with a reasonable level of accuracy using spring designs derived through virtual treatment planning, as described later, the caveat of applying poorly controlled force directions that are likely to result with traditional biomechanical approaches becomes less of a concern. The ability to control the direction of the forces more accurately using approaches discussed below also provides the latitude to position bonds at other suitable locations on the tooth crown for biomechanical advantages that facilitate achieving the desired tooth movements during guided eruption of the tooth (Figure 16.8).

Designing springs and implementing appropriate anchorage

While there is no single standardized spring design for forced eruption of impacted teeth into the oral cavity and aligning them into the arch, successful guided eruption must adhere to basic biomechanical principles. One of the most important of these principles is anchorage. Careful planning of anchorage during guided eruption is highly desirable because the force needed to erupt the impacted tooth can easily overwhelm inadequately anchored teeth. One example of this is a biomechanical approach using NiTi wires engaged to the impacted tooth without stabilizing the anchorage teeth that results in the forces and moments placed on anchor teeth contributing to their undesirable movements and worsening of the occlusion (Figure 16.9). The use of a stiff base wire in conjunction with an overlay wire minimizes such adverse movements of neighboring teeth but is likely to be inefficient because the overlay wire must overcome unraveling through the brackets it is engaged into

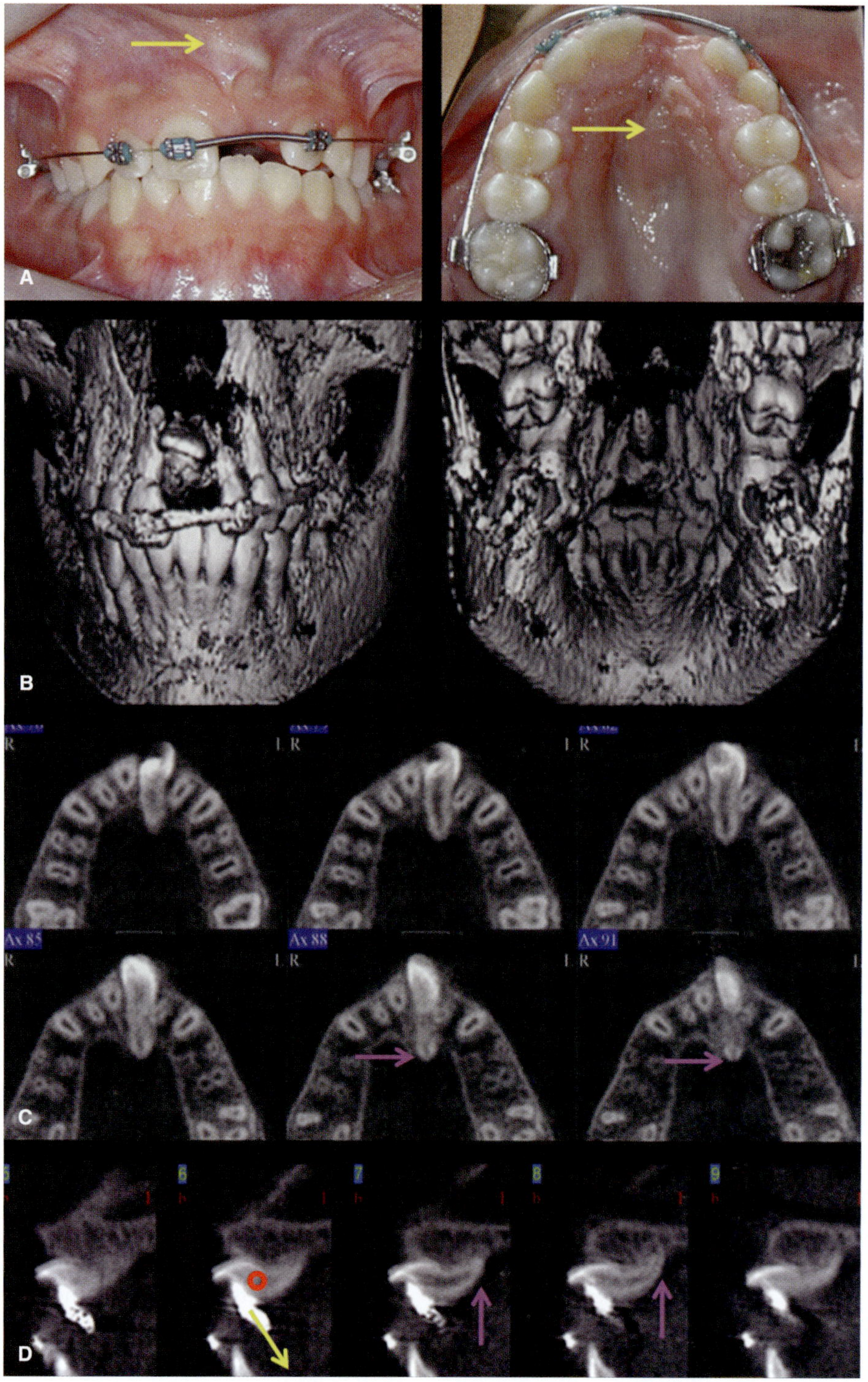
A
B
Ax 85
Ax 88
Ax 91
C
D

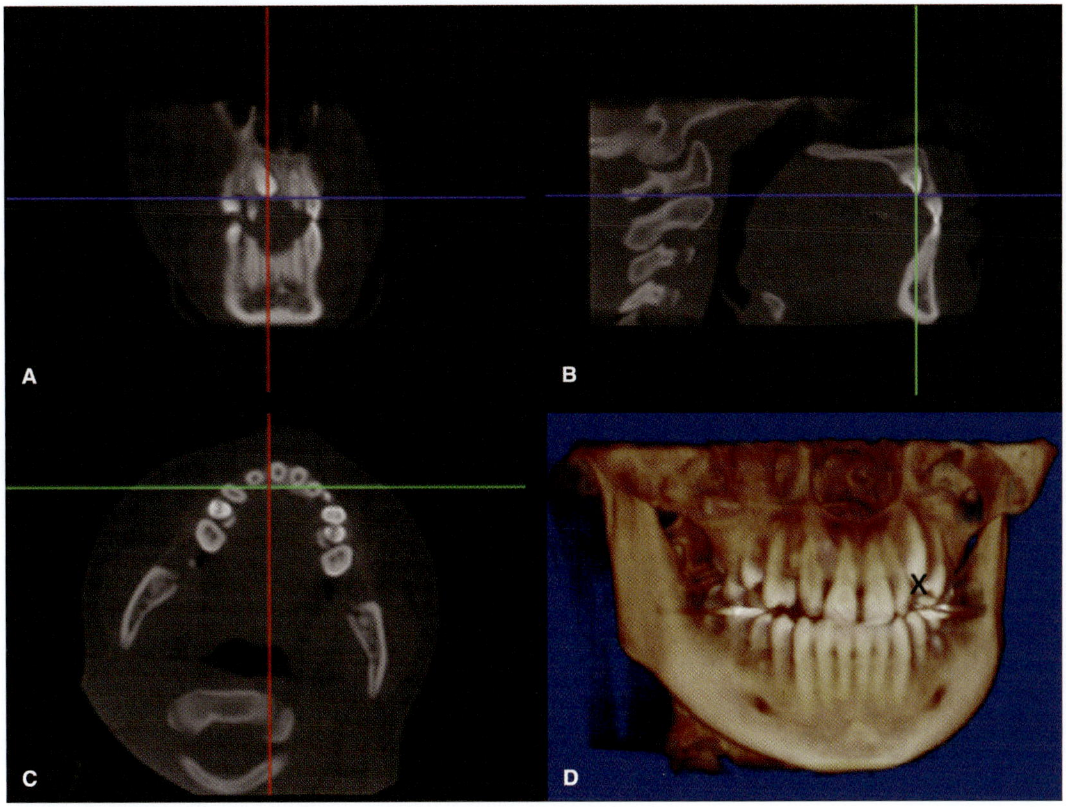

Figure 16.6 Example of a composite image printout that is included in the prescription sent to the clinician who will expose and bond the impacted teeth. It is important to depict the desired location of the bond placement in coronal (*A*), sagittal (*B*), and axial (*C*) sections, depicted where the horizontal and vertical axis intersect, and in 3D volumetric reconstruction (*D*), marked with an "X."

Figure 16.5 Photographs and CBCT radiographs taken during treatment of patient in Figure 16.4 to determine the spatial position and relationship to neighboring teeth of the impacted left central incisor. *A*: Photographs demonstrating incisal edge of the impacted incisor that is visible in the buccal vestibule and palatal swelling (yellow arrows). *B*: Volumetric renderings showing the horizontal position of the impacted left central incisor with proximity of its crown to the roots of the neighboring central and lateral incisors. *C*: Axial sections confirm the proximity of the impacted tooth crown and its root to neighboring tooth roots, as well as the possible fenestration of the root apex through the palatal bone (purple arrows). *D*: Sagittal sections confirm the lack of bone around the lingual surface of the root apex (purple arrows) and demonstrate the position of the bond on the cingulum. Since the center of resistance (red circle) is close to the cemento-enamel junction in cases where the tooth is encased completely in bone, placing the bond and forces (yellow arrow) on the cingulum close to this location would result in bodily extrusion of the impacted tooth.

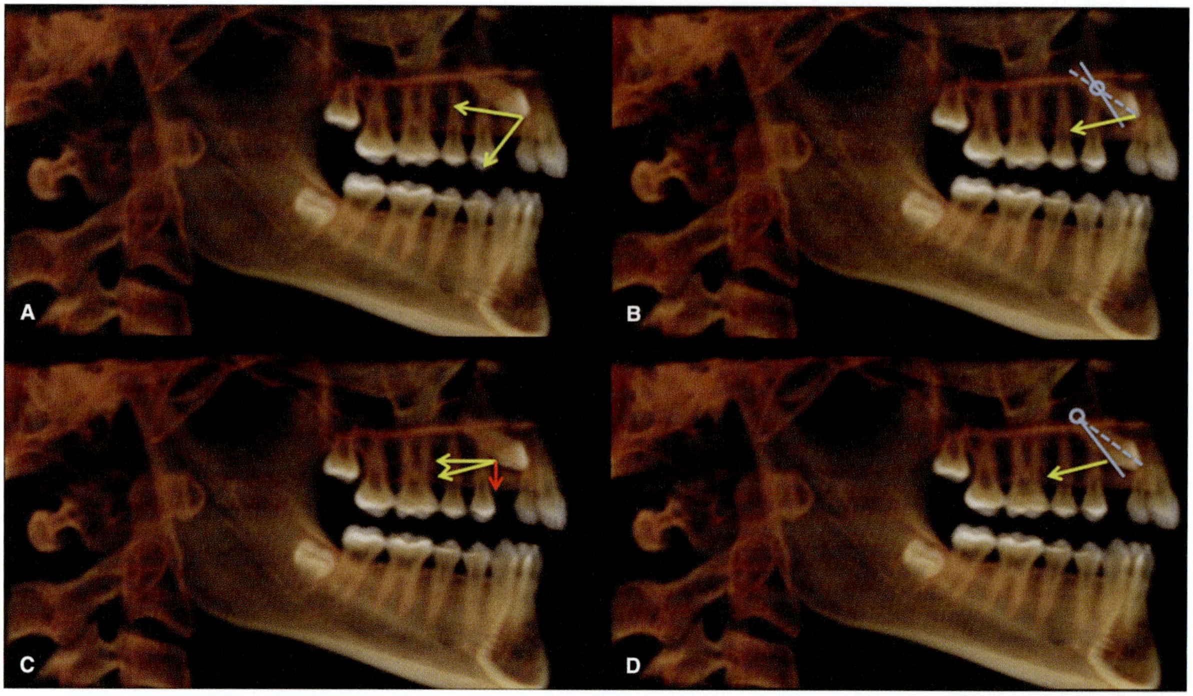

Figure 16.7 Effects of bond position on error tolerance range or angle and type of resultant tooth movement. *A*: Placing the bond at the cusp tip results in a high tolerance to any errors in force vectors placed on the tooth depicted here by the angle between the two lines such that less accuracy in force vector is necessary. *B*: Placing the bond close to the cusp tip results in a large distance between the point of force application from the center of resistance, which would contribute to greater tipping movements as depicted by dashed and solid lines than if the bond was placed closer to the center of resistance. *C*: When the bond is placed closer to the cemento-enamel junction by accident or by design, the error tolerance range is diminished, approximating that between the two yellow arrows, such that even a small error in the force vector can result in undesirable movement of the cusp tip toward the roots of neighboring teeth (red arrow). *D*: Bond placement closer to the cemento-enamel junction places the point of force application closer to the center of resistance, which would result in tooth movement approximating controlled tipping, as depicted by dashed and solid blue lines, or translation. The blue circle depicts the center of rotation; dashed blue lines represent pre-movement; and solid blue lines represent post-movement long axis of the impacted tooth.

and because of a lack of directional control of the eruption forces (Figure 16.10A,B). For these reasons, this approach may be applicable largely to canines that are mildly malpositioned buccally or palatally and are in relatively close proximity to their final positions.

Every patient with impacted teeth presents with unique clinical findings and biological variables including bone density and the spatial position and proximity of the impacted tooth to adjacent structures. Thus the orthodontist must implement customized biomechanics and spring design with the understanding that while this may suffice in most cases, each case must be followed closely for signs of optimal tooth movement and anchorage, and the biomechanics plan reconfigured if necessary. A number of approaches to achieve guided eruption are utilized commonly, but many of these are less than ideal in most situations. Besides use of overlay wires in conjunction with stiff base wires (Figure 16.10A,B), various types of springs in continuous archwires (e.g., continuous archwires with a loop facing occlusally that is activated palatally), springs soldered on the archwires, and power

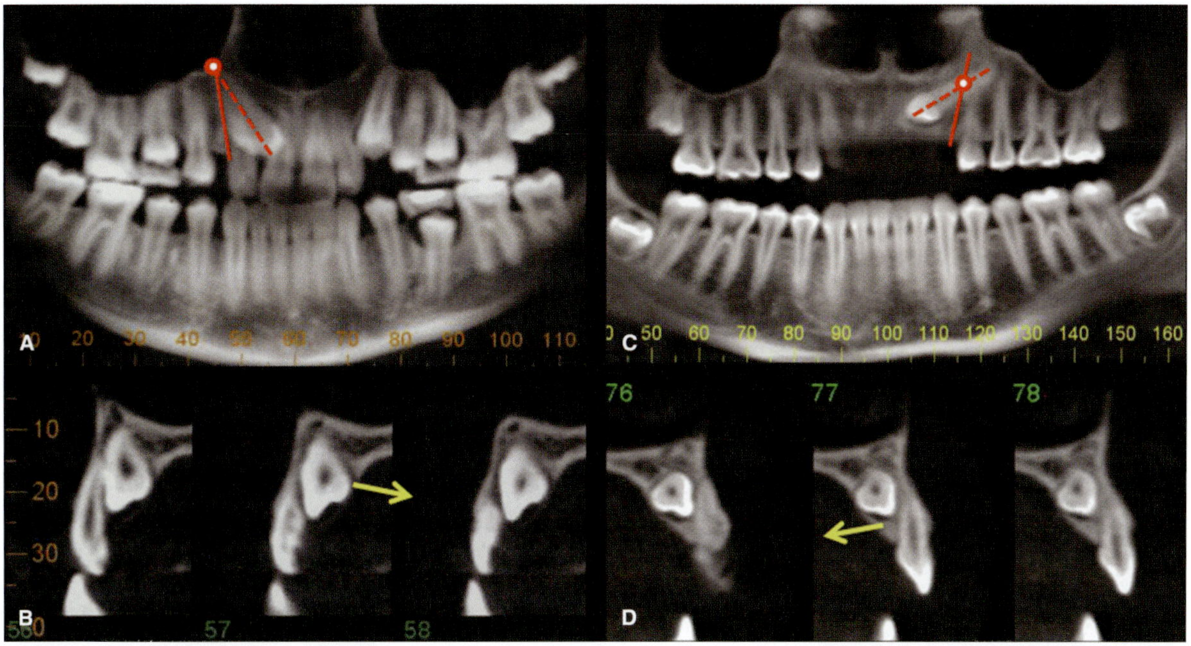

Figure 16.8 Optimizing bond position and point of force application to obtain desired movement of impacted teeth. Given that impacted teeth often are embedded almost completely in bone, their centers of resistance will be closer to the cemento-enamel junction than for an erupted tooth. Thus, placing a bond or point of force application close to this location will result in controlled tipping or translational movement, rather than tipping movement. Thus, in situations where the root apex is lying close to the desired final position of the tooth when controlled tipping is desired (*A*), the bond can be placed on the cingulum (*B*), provided that the force vectors can be controlled optimally to move the crown without damaging adjacent tooth roots. In situations requiring uncontrolled tipping where the root apex needs to be moved in the direction opposite to the movement of the crown (*C*), the bond should be placed as far from the center of resistance as possible, such as at the cusp tip (*D*). The red circle depicts the center of rotation; dashed red lines represent pre-movement; and solid red lines represent post-movement long axis of the impacted tooth; yellow arrows indicate direction of forces originating from the point of force application.

chains to a transpalatal arch or the archwire (Figure 16.10C–F) are used frequently for guided eruption of impacted canines. Most of these approaches have limitations, including the inability to provide multidimensional control on force directions and the lack of flexibility to change direction of forces when needed or to apply forces to the teeth that dissipate quickly after activation. Such relatively unrefined approaches to guided eruption may be considered adequate when there already is a given amount of guesswork in locating and accessing the canines from conventional 2D radiographs. However, given the ability to visualize precisely the spatial position and relationships to neighboring structures of the entire impacted tooth in 3D makes the use of these less-refined approaches *passé*. Indeed, the visualization of impacted teeth in 3D offers a new paradigm for defined and efficient treatment of these teeth involving a proactive determination of optimal path(s) of traction and efficient movement of the entire tooth in 3D. This new paradigm is analogous to developing a virtual treatment plan, which in turn can be used to design individualized springs for the patient's specific challenge.

Given the various caveats of routine biomechanical approaches to retrieve impacted teeth and using sound mechanical principles and information gained from the CBCT, it would be ideal to deliver the most desirable direction and magnitude of force to move the impacted tooth optimally in three planes of space. Optimal movements

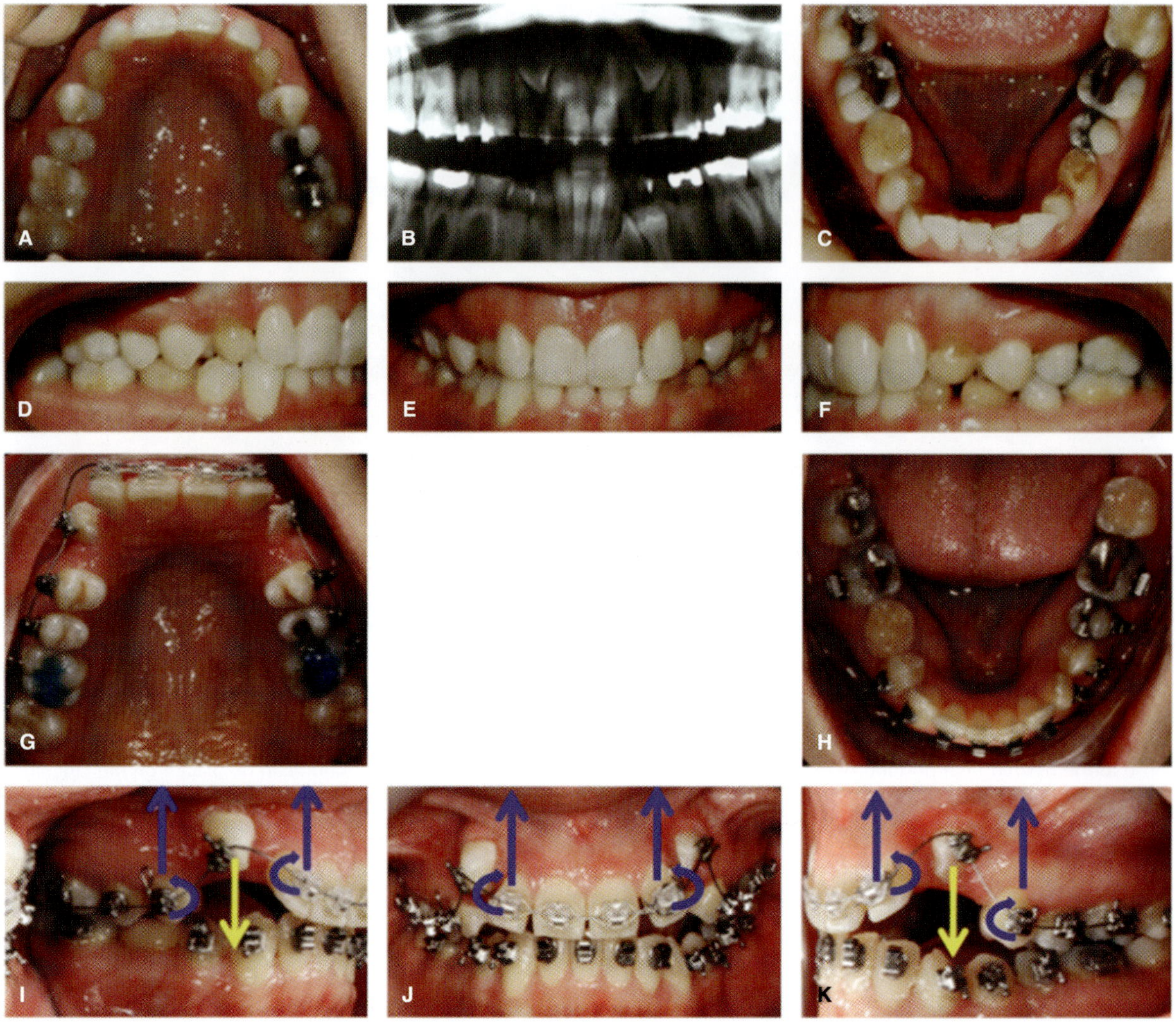

Figure 16.9 Suboptimal mechanics in erupting and aligning impacted canines in a patient with multiple impacted teeth. *A–F*: Pretreatment intraoral photographs and panoramic radiograph of patient with impacted upper canines and lower left canine and first premolar. *G–K*: Treatment progress photographs showing that the use of a continuous NiTi archwire to extrude and align the upper canines (yellow arrows) has resulted in adverse movements of neighboring anchor teeth caused by the intrusive and rotational moments on the incisors and premolars, represented by blue arrows, and adverse changes in the upper arch form.

imply moving the tooth crown and root the shortest distance in 3D. A strategy that can be adapted easily for this purpose is the one couple system, using a segmented approach in which a spring delivers the desired force vector in a controlled and sustained manner (Figure 16.11A,B). The effects of these forces on anchor teeth can be determined easily and their adverse consequences minimized. On the basis of these principles, the authors prefer to use springs made of titanium molybdenum alloy (TMA) wires to deliver 3D pre-determined directions of force that, for

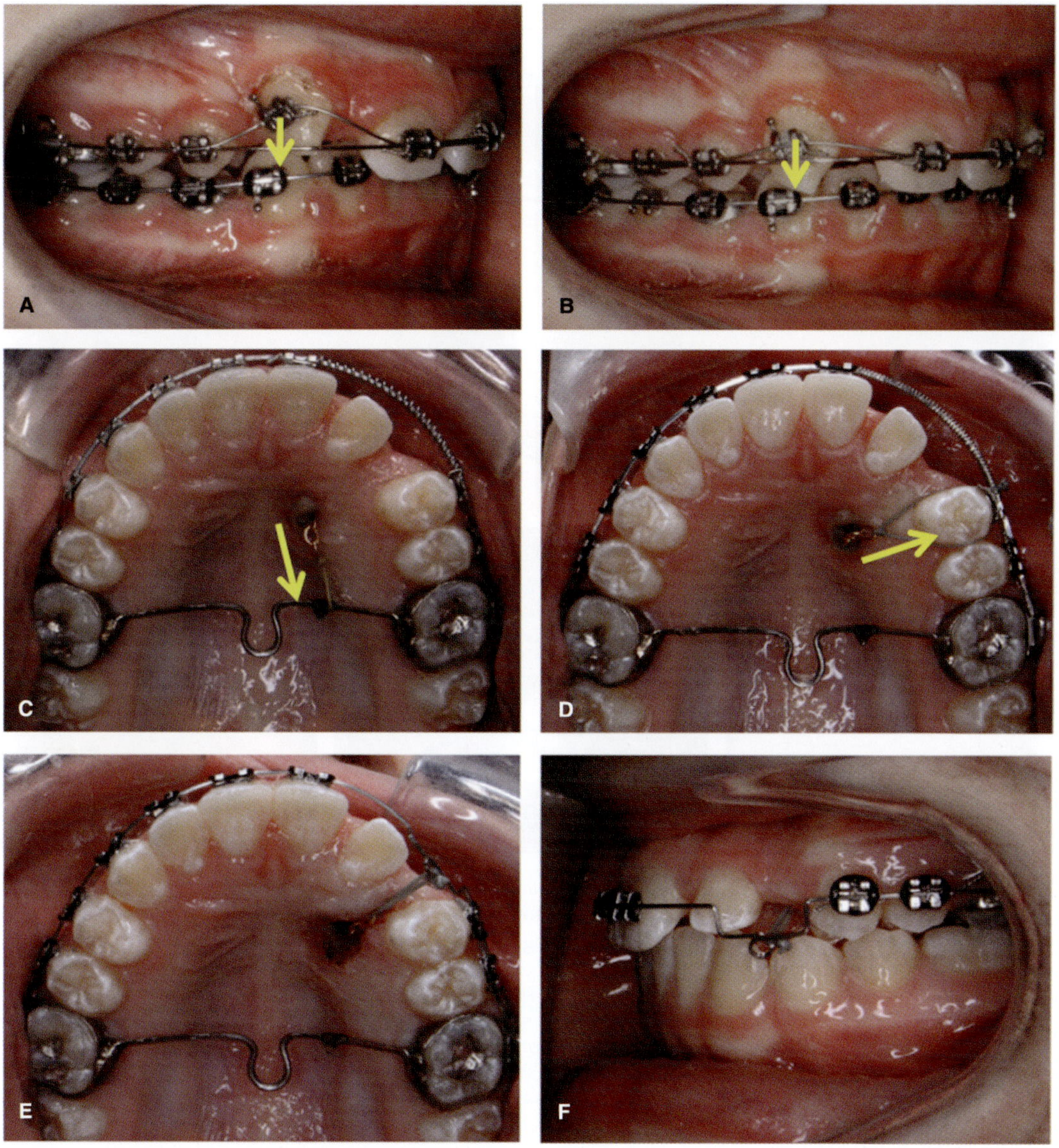

Figure 16.10 Optimizing mechanics to avoid unwanted tooth movement during guided eruption of impacted canines. *A* and *B*: Use of NiTi wire overlay to extrude a buccally impacted tooth with a stainless steel base wire stabilizing adjacent teeth. While this approach may be reasonable for use on mildly malpositioned teeth, its lack of efficiency and control on desired force directions usually make it unsuitable for moderately to severely malpositioned impactions. *C–F*: Guided eruption of a palatally impacted canine by applying an elastomeric thread in different directions during different phases of treatment. *C*: Initial distally directed forces to disengage the canine from the lateral incisor root with the elastomeric thread placed from the chain on the impacted tooth to a soldered stop on a transpalatal arch. *D*: Buccally directed forces with the elastomeric thread tied to the first premolar. *E* and *F*: Buccal and extrusive forces with the elastomeric thread tied to the stainless steel base wire. The force decay in the elastomeric thread and lack of multidimensional control on applied forces likely make this approach inefficient.

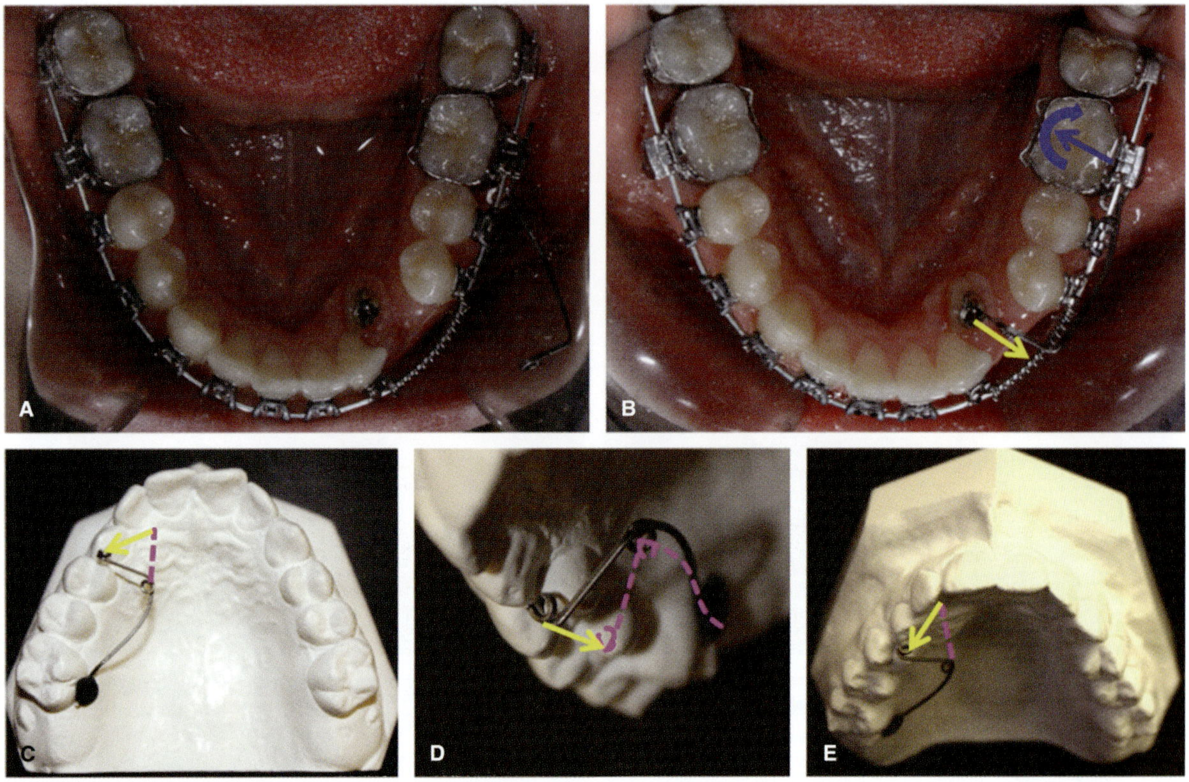

Figure 16.11 Application of optimal force vector to align impacted canines with a TMA spring while maintaining stable anchor units. *A* and *B*: A customized TMA spring is inserted into the auxiliary tube on the first molar to create a one couple asymmetric V-bend system that generates the desired long-acting buccal force vector on the canine (yellow arrow). The adverse movements resulting from lingual force and clockwise moments on the first molar (blue arrows), which serves as the anchor tooth, are minimized by reinforcing anchorage with a stainless steel base continuous archwire engaged in brackets on adjacent teeth. The use of this stiff continuous archwire also enables the simultaneous development of space required for the canine with a NiTi open coil spring. *C–E*: Spring designed to deliver optimal force vector in all three planes of space for extrusion, buccal, and distal movement of a relatively simple canine impaction. The spring is placed into a tube soldered on the lingual side of the upper molar bracket; anchorage on the molar is similar to the case in panels *A* and *B*. The yellow arrow depicts the directions of forces generated by the spring to obtain the desired distal, extrusive, and buccal movement of the canine.

example, may include extrusion, distalization, and buccal movements in the case of a palatally impacted canine. The spring should be customized to each case and placed on the buccal or lingual side of the first molar using auxiliary tubes. Figure 16.11C–F depicts a spring designed to achieve concurrent or sequential distal, buccal, and extrusive tooth movement for a relatively simple impaction that was treated entirely with one spring. More complex cases may require two or more springs, depending on the directions and magnitude of movements required (Figure 16.12, Figure 16.13, Figure 16.14, Figure 16.15, Figure 16.16, and Figure 16.17).

An approximate determination of when the eruption force will need to be redirected after the tooth reaches a certain location in the oral cavity can be planned proactively using CBCT and the springs to facilitate these movements designed accordingly. Thus, as an example for the patient

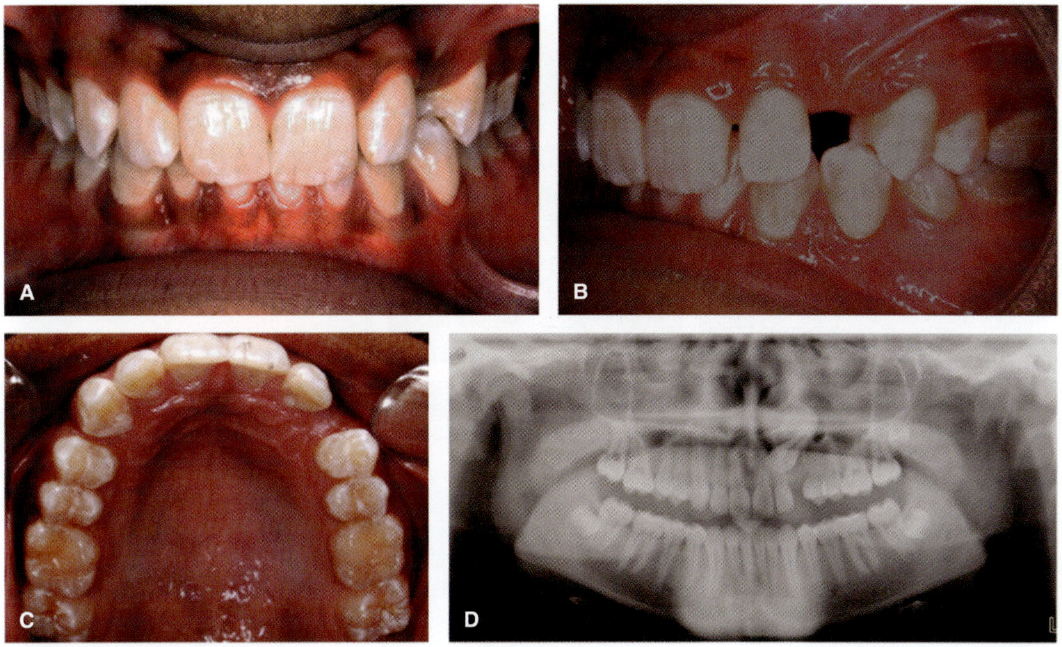

Figure 16.12 Pre-treatment photographs (*A–C*) and panoramic radiograph (*D*) of a 14-year-old patient with a moderately complex impaction of the maxillary left canine as determined from CBCT images shown in Figure 16.13.

shown in Figure 16.12, the CBCT images (Figure 16.13) are used to plan the initial desired distal direction of movement away from the lateral incisor root until the canine crown is in the same sagittal plane as where it will be positioned in the arch. Then the direction of the force can be changed to move the tooth buccally, following which it can be extruded after it has jumped the bite. On the basis of these plans, the springs then are designed and activated to achieve the desired movements as shown in Figure 16.14.

With the knowledge of all the forces placed on the impacted tooth, their adverse effects on the anchor teeth can be determined easily and any undesirable movements minimized by reinforcing the anchorage by incorporating the neighboring teeth as anchor units. Typically, this can be accomplished by placing a rigid base wire through the anchor and neighboring teeth (Figure 16.11A,B). Use of such a wire also enables the development of space using open coil springs concomitantly with traction of the impacted tooth (Figure 16.11A,B and Figure 16.14C,D).

CBCT use in appliance design to avoid or minimize damage to adjacent structures

The case presented in Figure 16.12, Figure 16.13, and Figure 16.14 provides an example of how damage to adjacent structures, most often lateral incisor root resorption and alveolar fenestrations, can be minimized. The strategy involves moving the impacted tooth away from the roots of teeth that it approximates and not engaging teeth in close proximity to the impacted tooth in appliances until the impacted tooth has been moved to some distance from it. This principle is demonstrated in Figure 16.14, where no wire initially is engaged into the lateral incisor bracket and space is developed between the first premolar and lateral incisor. After applying a distalizing force to position the canine at a safe distance from the lateral incisor, the lateral incisor is aligned with an overlay wire to the base wire, following which the bracket is engaged into base wire, which, in turn, facilitates the redistribution of the space between the lateral incisor and first premolar.

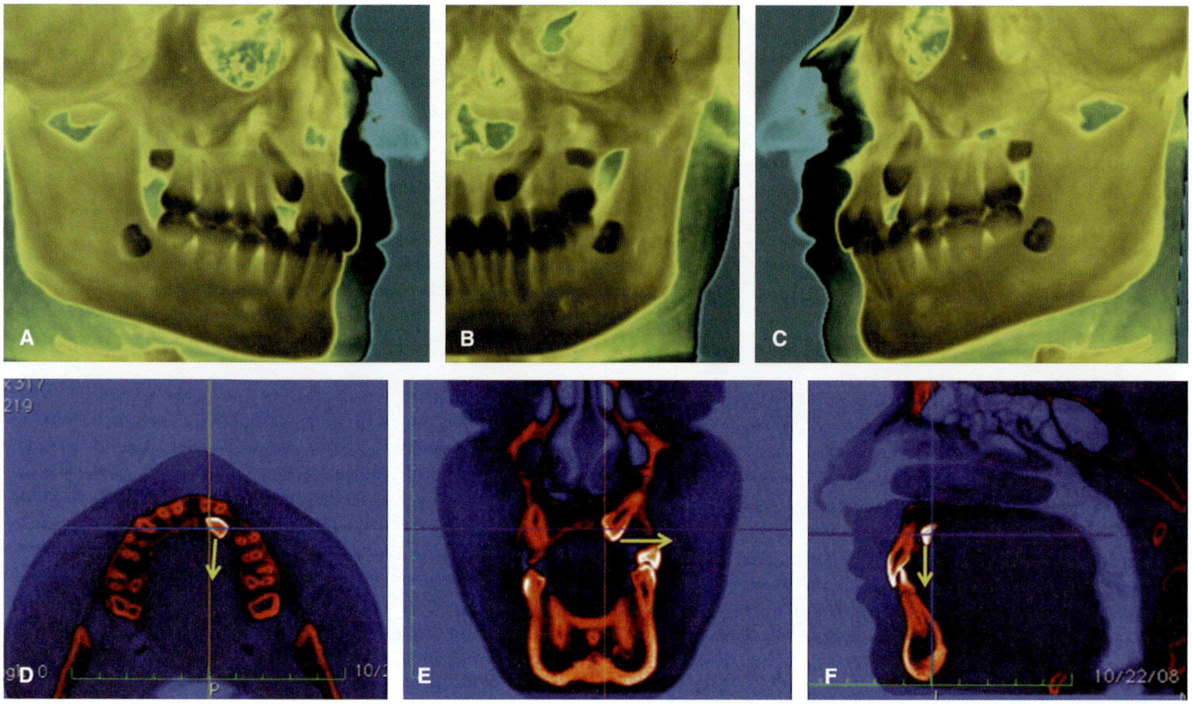

Figure 16.13 3D CBCT volumetric reconstructions (*A–C*) and axial (*D*), coronal (*E*), and sagittal (*F*) sections of patient in Figure 16.12 help to determine the precise spatial position and relationship to neighboring structures of the impacted maxillary left canine. These images enable the clinician to develop proactively a virtual treatment plan to retrieve the canine, which, in this case, would require sequentially applied distal, buccal, and lastly extrusive forces to the tooth represented by yellow arrows in panels *D*, *E*, and *F*, respectively. Because of the proximity of the impacted canine to the lateral incisor root, engaging and moving the lateral incisor should be deferred until after the canine crown has been moved some distance from the root to avoid potential harm. The virtual treatment and biomechanics plan also informs the clinician about the optimal bond position and design of spring(s) to be used, as shown in Figure 16.14.

CBCT application for diagnosis and treatment planning impactions of teeth other than maxillary canines

While impacted maxillary canines present significant challenges to orthodontists in establishing an ideal occlusion, these cases often seem straightforward compared with cases involving impactions of other teeth. Fortunately, the principles of guided eruption that were developed primarily from cases involving impacted maxillary canines are applicable to cases involving other impacted teeth. We present a final case of difficult impactions of lower second premolars that demonstrates the various biomechanical and treatment decisions made from diagnostic records, including CBCT, to retrieve these teeth.

A clinical intraoral examination of the 26-year-old female reveals retained and heavily restored mandibular primary second molars (Figure 16.15). The panoramic projection reconstructed from the CBCT clearly demonstrates that both second premolars are impacted horizontally with the right premolar oriented distally and the left one mesially (Figure 16.16A). If this radiograph was the only one available to the clinician, it would be impossible to determine whether the premolars are buccally or lingually oriented, how close they are to compromising their alveolar boundaries, or how to assess the proximity of their crowns and roots of

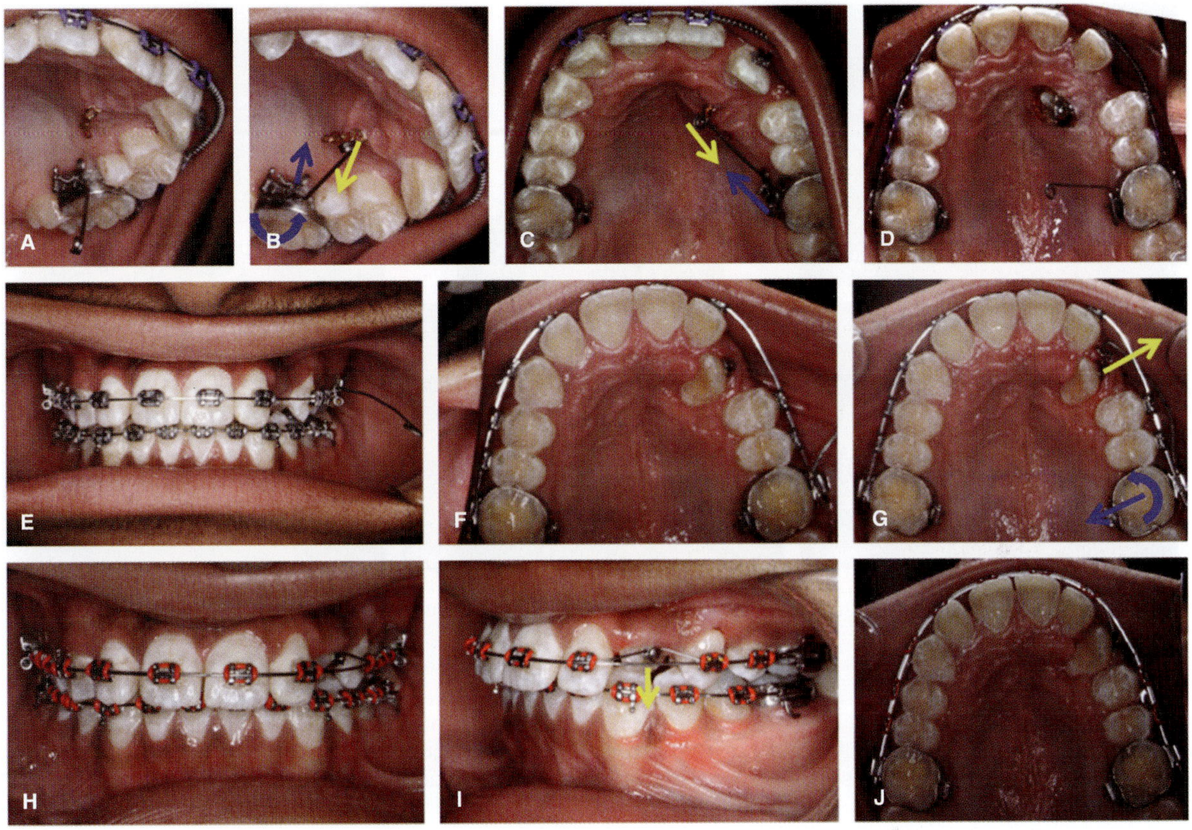

Figure 16.14 In-progress photos of patient shown in Figure 16.12 and Figure 16.13 for which diagnostic information from CBCT and clinical examination was used to derive a virtual treatment plan. *A–C*: The first stage of treatment entailed distal movement with some extrusion of the impacted left canine. During this phase, the lateral incisor was not engaged into the archwire and space was developed between the central incisor and first premolar on a stiff stainless steel wire. *D*: After the canine has been moved away from incisor roots, the lateral incisor can be aligned with an overlay NiTi wire, following which the bracket is engaged into the base wire and space redistributed between lateral and first premolar. *E–G*: The canine is moved bucally during the second stage with minimal extrusion to diminish the need to open the bite to jump the tooth across the lower teeth. Note that adequate space has been developed between the lateral incisor and first premolar. *H–J*: The final stage of treatment involves extrusion of the canine with a NiTi overlay wire and stabilizing stainless steel base wire. Note that the adverse effects of forces and moments on the first molar (blue arrows) in response to forces applied to the canine (yellow arrows) are minimized by engaging the molar and neighboring teeth in a stainless steel wire throughout treatment.

the adjacent teeth. While conventional 2D periapical and occlusal radiographs may be helpful with some of these determinations, developing a sound biomechanics plan on the basis of this information alone that facilitates the eruption of the premolars without damaging adjacent structures still would be challenging. A review of the CBCT images clearly demonstrates the precise 3D spatial position of the premolars, including their unfavorable bucco-lingual orientation across the arch and their relationships to adjacent teeth and to their respective alveolar boundaries, confirming the complexities involved in retrieving these teeth, particularly the right second premolar (Figure 16.16B–F).

The biomechanics plan for this patient must take into account that the premolars are impinging on remarkably thin alveolar boundary bone and the adjacent roots are at risk for resorption if the initial

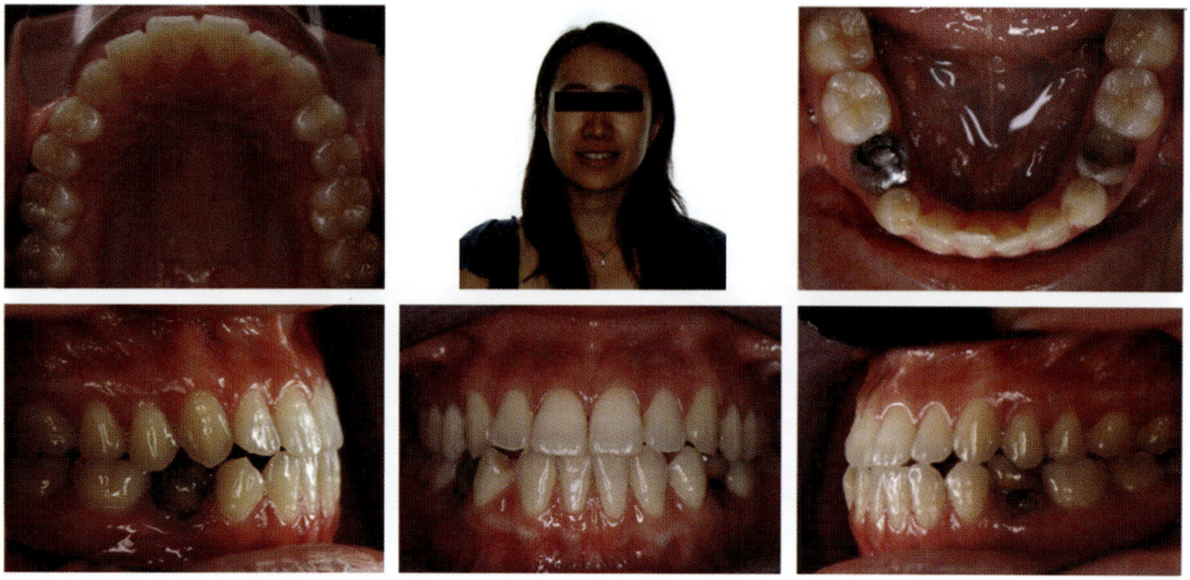

Figure 16.15 Pre-treatment photographs of 26-year-old female presenting with retained mandibular primary second molars and impacted second premolars.

crown eruption vector is directed too far lingually. Indeed, based on the CBCT scans (Figure 16.17), the virtual treatment plan to retrieve the impacted second premolars is split into three stages. In the first stage, springs are designed to move the crowns bucally and roots lingually to disengage the roots from those of the neighboring teeth. This is visualized in the virtual treatment plan by indicating the pre-activation position of each premolar with a dashed line (Figure 16.17A) and its projected post-activation position with a solid line (Figure 16.17B). In the next stage, mesial forces are applied to the right second premolar crown (Figure 16.17C,D), while distal forces are applied to the left premolar crown (Figure 16.17E), causing the teeth to become upright. In the third stage, a different spring was designed to place mesial forces on the right premolar while the left premolar is extruded to finalize its guided eruption (Figure 16.17F–H).

These cases demonstrate the versatility of CBCT for diagnosing and treatment planning of impacted teeth. Perhaps the greatest advantage that CBCT offers to clinicians treating impactions is the ability to visualize clearly the safest directions to move the crown and root of these teeth to enhance the chances of successful retrieval and to minimize damage to adjacent structures.

PRINCIPLES OF 3D DIAGNOSIS AND TREATMENT PLANNING OF TRANSPOSED TEETH

Like impacted teeth, transposed teeth present numerous diagnostic and treatment challenges, many of which can be addressed with CBCT imaging. Treatment of transposed teeth requires consideration of several important diagnostic variables, the most obvious of which is whether or not the patient requires extractions. In such cases, most patients could be treated by extracting one of the two transposed teeth. The decision on which transposed tooth to extract should be based on which tooth is displaced most severely from its normal position, the quality and shape of the teeth, and the location of roots within the alveolar bone. In non-extraction cases, the treatment options include repositioning the teeth into their normal positions (Nishimura *et al.*, 2012) or aligning them into the arch in their transposed positions. In these

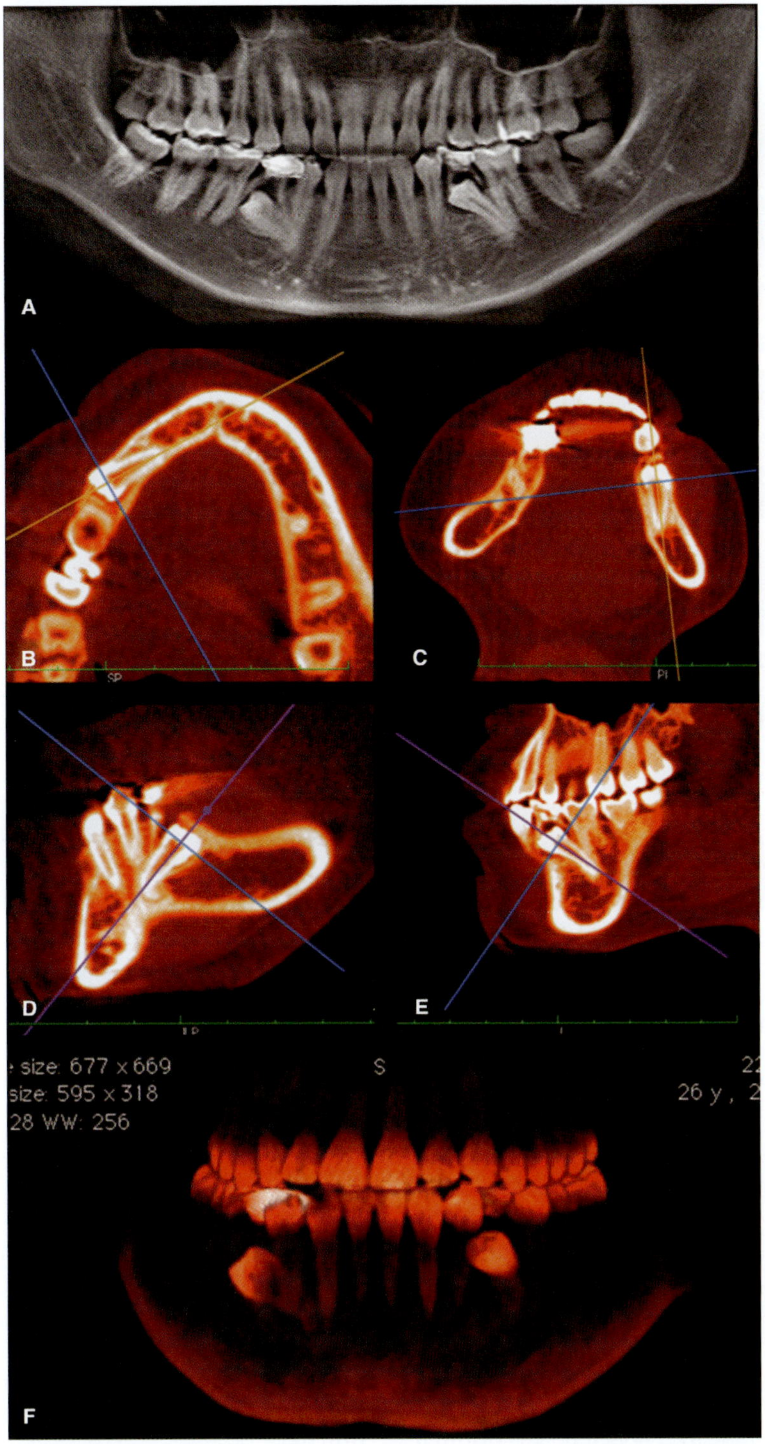

Figure 16.16 Pre-treatment images derived from CBCT of patient in Figure 16.15. *A*: Reconstructed panoramic radiograph shows a distally impacted mandibular right second premolar and mesially impacted mandibular left second premolar. The precise spatial positions of the mandibular second premolars and the relationships to neighboring structures can be determined from axial (*B* and *C*), sagittal (*D* and *E*), and 3D volumetric (*F*) reconstructions to develop a virtual treatment plan.

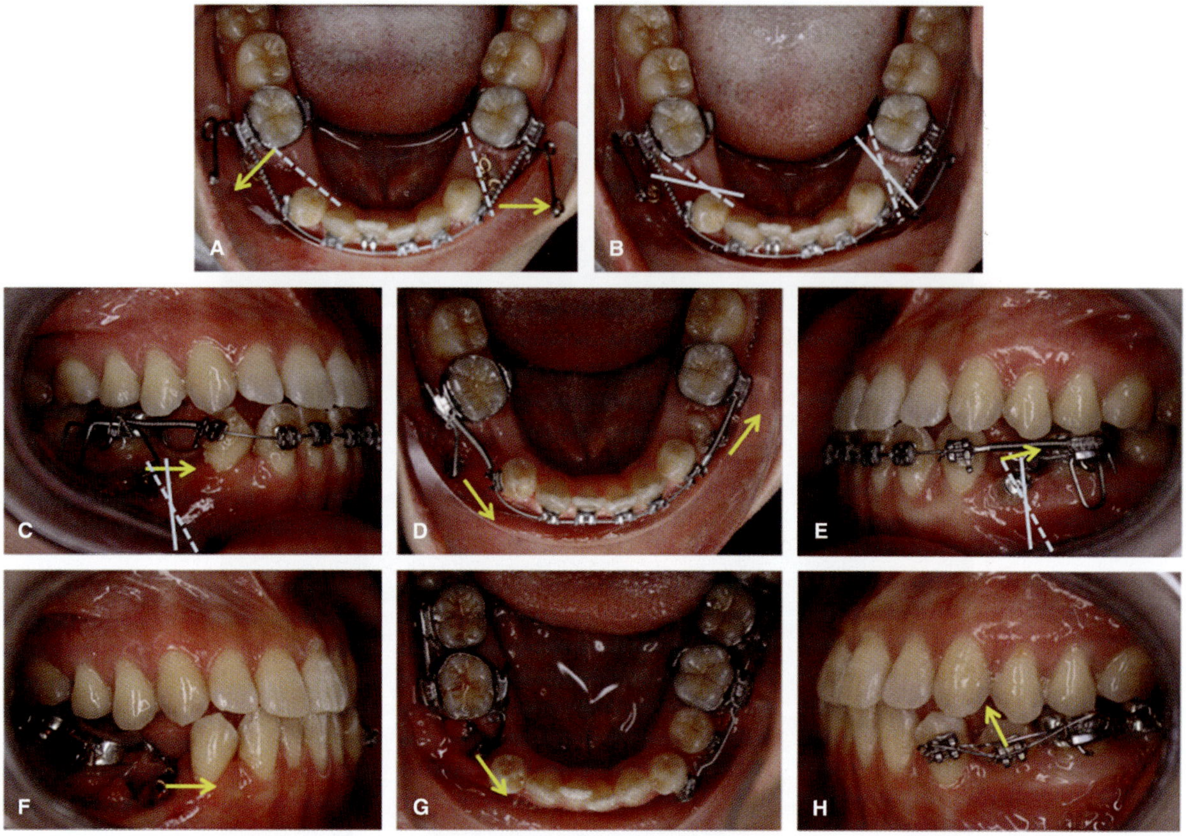

Figure 16.17 Implementation of the virtual treatment plan to retrieve the impacted second premolars of patient in Figure 16.15 and Figure 16.16. The first stage uses springs to move the crowns of the teeth bucally and roots lingually to disengage the crowns and roots from the neighboring teeth shown here prior to (*A*) and after (*B*) activation. In the next stage, mesial forces are applied to the right second premolar crown (*C* and *D*), while distal forces are applied to the left premolar crown (*D* and *E*), causing the teeth to become upright. In the third stage, a different spring is being used to place mesial forces on the right premolar (*F* and *G*), while the left premolar (*G* and *H*) is undergoing extrusion in the final stage of its retrieval. The yellow arrows represent direction of force application. The dashed blue lines in *A–C* and *E* represent the initial tooth positions as determined from the CBCT images. The continuous blue lines represent the desired tooth movement to be accomplished by the springs, which were designed based on the CBCT images.

situations, the treatment of choice typically would depend on the positions of the crowns and roots, whether the transposition is complete or incomplete, the expected duration of treatment, and the quality of the gingivae on the teeth. With the introduction of CBCT, a fourth important variable also should be considered in choosing an optimal approach from these two non-extraction treatment options. This variable is the existing alveolar boundary conditions around the transposed teeth and the potential for or need to move the teeth out of their supporting bone in trying to relocate the teeth into their normal positions (see also Chapter 14). The severity of the transpositions and limitations of the alveolar boundary conditions in turn may define the degree of treatment difficulty and duration and dictate the biomechanics to be utilized.

The case presented in Figure 16.18 demonstrates the value of CBCT imaging in making the decision on how best to treat transposed teeth. The patient presents with bilateral complete transpositions of

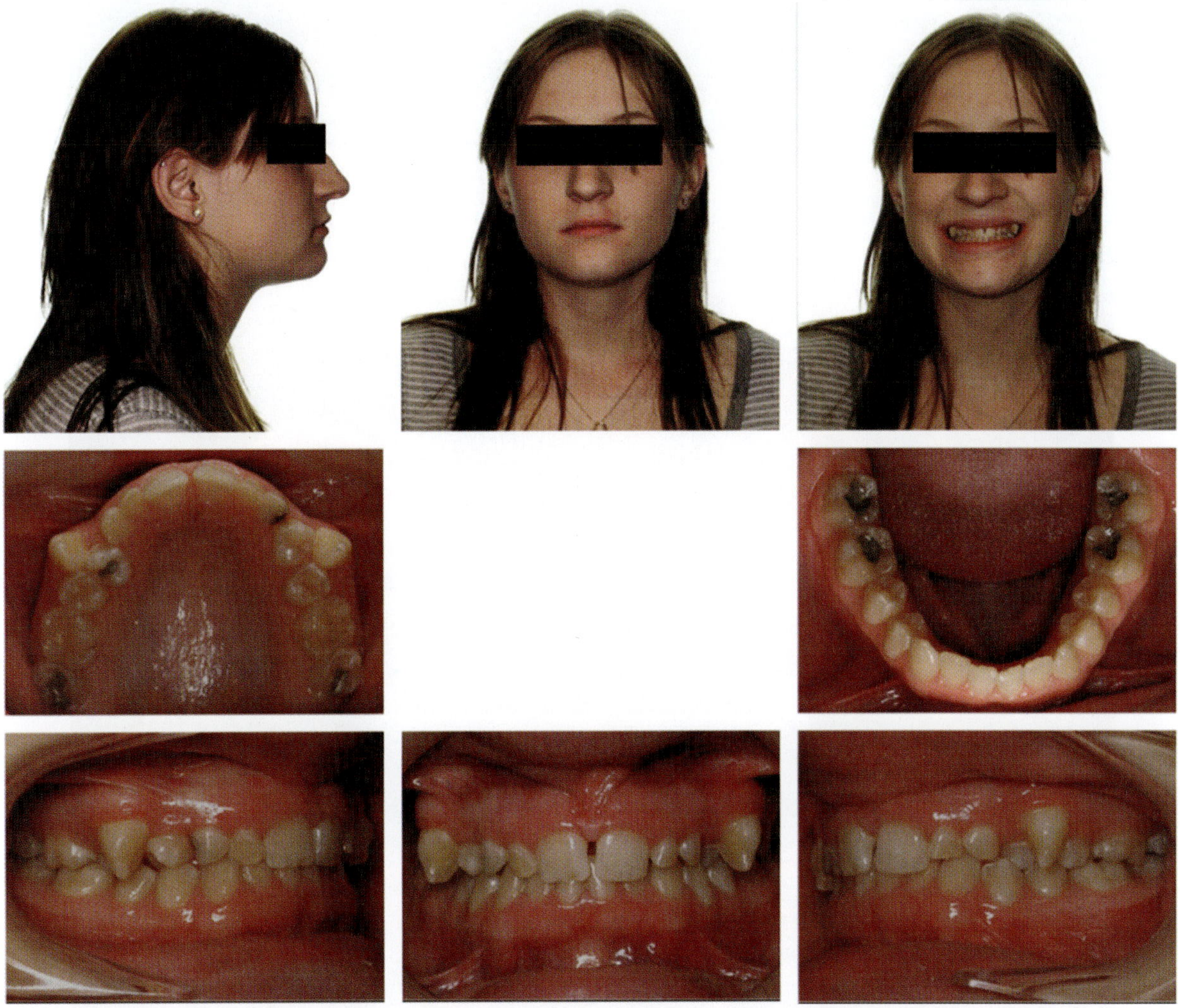

Figure 16.18 Composite of a patient presenting with completely transposed maxillary right and left canines and first premolars, missing permanent lateral incisors, and retained maxillary primary canines and lateral incisors. Extracting any of the transposed teeth is contraindicated in this case due to the patient's flat facial profile and missing lateral incisors.

maxillary canines and first premolars, missing permanent lateral incisors and retained maxillary primary canines and lateral incisors. Extractions of a pair of transposed teeth are contraindicated due to the flat facial profile and missing lateral incisors. Besides confirming the severity of the canine and first premolar root transpositions, the multiplanar and 3D CBCT reconstructions demonstrate the limits of the alveolar boundaries in relocating the canines and premolars to their normal positions (Figure 16.19). Specifically, these images highlight the complexity of the movements required in 3D to ensure that the roots of the teeth are kept within the alveolar boundaries while translocating them past each other, which, in turn, dictates the intricate biomechanics required and the likely long treatment time. Placing the teeth in their normal positions would entail moving the

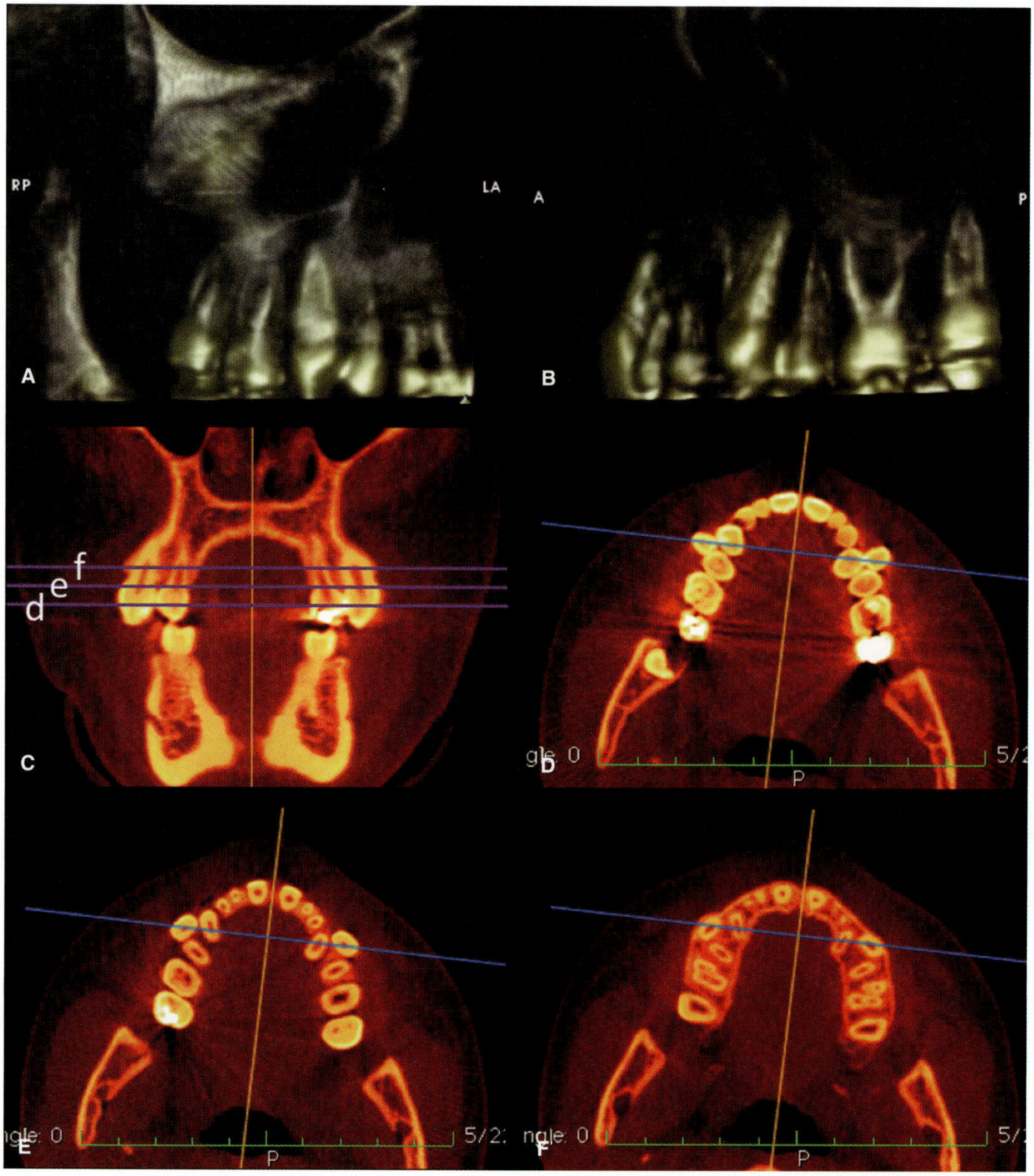

Figure 16.19 Pre-treatment images derived from CBCT of patient in Figure 16.18. 3D volumetric reconstructions of the buccal aspect of the right (*A*) and left (*B*) sides show the complete transposition of the canines and first premolars and detail the spatial positions of the transposed teeth and their relationships to each other and neighboring structures. *C*: Coronal section demonstrating the proximity of the roots of the translocated teeth to each other and to alveolar boundaries. Lines d, e, and f in this panel represent locations at which axial cross-sections of the images, depicted in *D*, *E*, and *F*, respectively, were reconstructed to visualize the relationships of the crowns and roots of the transposed teeth to each other. Axial section at mid-crown (*D*), cemento-enamel junction (*E*), and mid-root (*F*) of the transposed teeth demonstrate details of tooth–tooth and tooth–bone relationships. These images were used to establish the biomechanics plan to mesialize the first premolars and move the canines palatally into the spaces that were developed by mesializing the premolars.

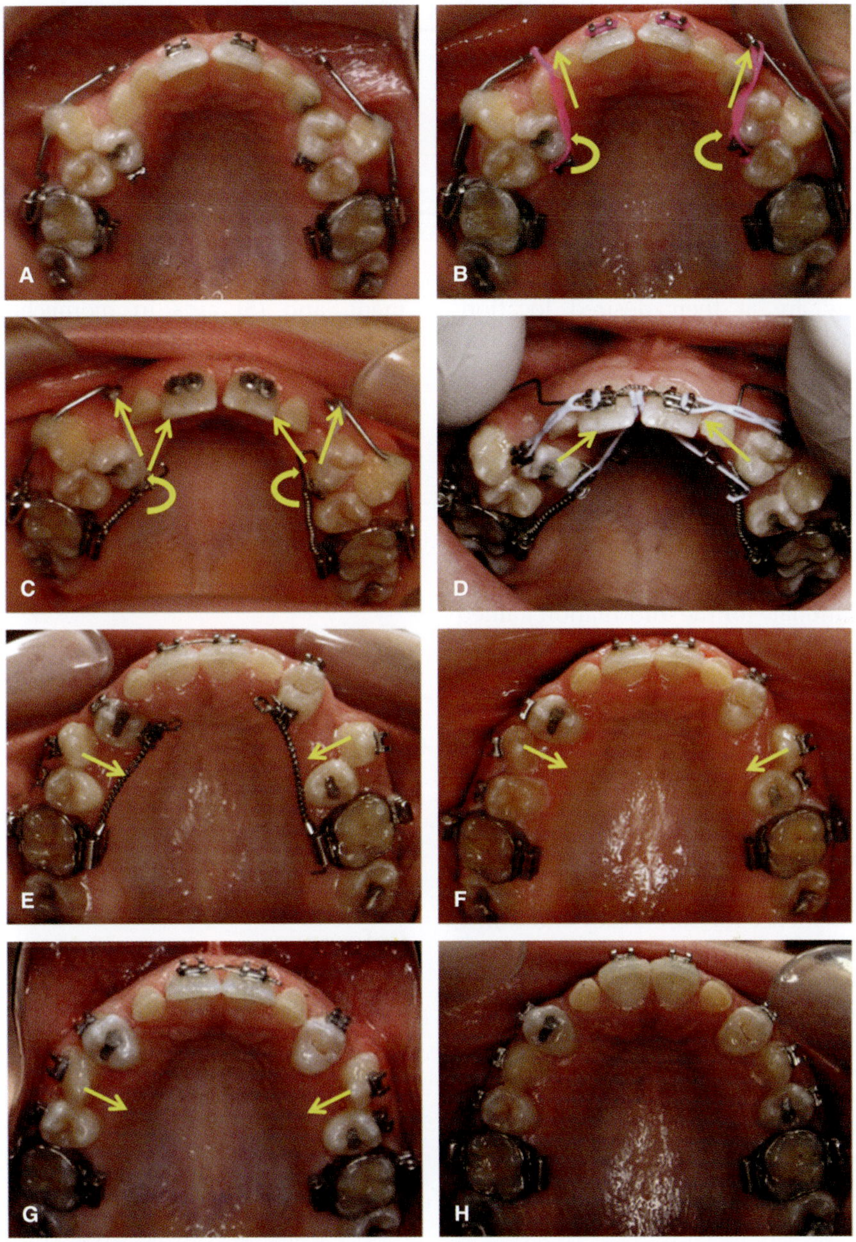

Figure 16.20 Implementation of the biomechanics plan for the patient in Figure 16.18 developed using diagnostic information from the CBCT images shown in Figure 16.19. Due to limitations of alveolar boundary conditions and expected duration of treatment if the transposed teeth were to be relocated to their normal positions, the decision was made to maintain the canines closest to their existing positions. *A* and *B*: A rigid wire on the buccal side was used to engage a power chain to de-rotate the first premolars, enabling the subsequent use of lingual wires and springs to mesialize the first premolars while continuing to de-rotate these teeth (*C*). *D*: Continued mesialization of the first premolars with both the lingual springs and power chains engaged to the incisors, which were anchored with a base wire that is stopped against the molars. *E*: Continued mesialization of the premolars with lingual springs and initiation of lingual movement of canines when adequate spaces had been developed. *F* and *G*: Continued alignment of the canines into the arch. *H*: Achievement of near final position of the first premolars and canines. Yellow arrows depict forces to de-rotate and move the premolars and canines into their respective desired positions. Note that the primary lateral incisors have been retained throughout orthodontic treatment in order to maintain bone for future restorations with implants. The final interdisciplinary component of the treatment entails placement of implants and crowns for the missing lateral incisors, optimally contoured premolar crown restorations on the canines, and minor equilibration of the lingual cusp of the first premolars.

crowns of the first premolars palatally while placing a couple to maintain their roots within bone, as well as torquing and maintaining the canine roots in bone during their mesialization. If the roots of the canines compromise the integrity of the alvelolar bone during their mesial movement, they would need to be torqued back into bone when they are at their desired location. Given these considerations, it would be appropriate to have the patient participate in deciding on the treatment option that he or she would prefer to pursue. In this case, the patient and clinician chose to pursue the option of a shorter treatment time and less complex biomechanics to position the transposed teeth closest to their pre-treatment locations using customized biomechanical approaches (Figure 16.20). Thus, this case highlights the utility and rationale for the information gained using CBCT for selecting the treatment option of choice and determining specific mechanics in achieving the treatment goals.

CONCLUSIONS

This chapter provides foundational information on impacted and transposed teeth, as well as insights into the current evidence for the efficacy and utility of CBCT in diagnosing and treatment of these teeth. As opposed to 2D radiographs that primarily enable the localization of the tooth crown in 2D, CBCT facilitates the determination of the precise 3D spatial position and relationships of impacted and transposed teeth to neighboring structures. Furthermore, relative to 2D radiography, CBCT enhances the detection of root resorption of adjacent teeth, contributes to modifications in treatment plan, and improves the confidence in diagnosis and treatment plans (Walker *et al.*, 2005; Haney *et al.*, 2010; Katheria *et al.*, 2010; Bjerklin & Guitirokh, 2011; Botticelli *et al.*, 2011; Alqerban *et al.*, 2013). This detailed additional information available from CBCT needs to be complemented with precise and sophisticated surgical and biomechanical approaches for the clinician to realize the true promise of the technology in treating impacted and transposed teeth more efficiently and successfully. When used optimally, CBCT (1) provides the ability to enhance diagnosis, (2) aids in identifying existing damage to neighboring teeth and determining the potential risk for additional damage during treatment, (3) helps to define alveolar boundary conditions and their influence on treatment decisions and biomechanics, (4) contributes to refinements and optimization in treatment planning including surgical access and bond placement, and (5) aids in biomechanical planning including the identification of optimal site of force application and tractional pathway(s) in 3D, designing of ideal spring(s), and planning of anchorage. The computerized diagnosis and planning of these cases using CBCT generates a virtual treatment plan that, when applied clinically, should contribute to improved treatment outcomes and efficiencies.

ACKNOWLEDGMENTS

The authors wish to thank their graduate orthodontic residents, Drs. Catherine Cho, Paul Rim, Devin Johnson, Joel Johnson, Adam Donnell, Matthew Lineberger, and Jason Charnley for providing several of the cases included in this chapter.

References

Ahmed, F., Brooks, S.L., & Kapila, S.D. (2012) Efficacy of identifying maxillofacial lesions in cone-beam computed tomographs by orthodontists and orthodontic residents with third-party software. *American Journal of Orthodontics and Dentofacial Orthopedics*, 141 (4), 451–459.

Alqerban, A., Jacobs, R., Souza, P.C., *et al.* (2009a) *In-vitro* comparison of 2 cone-beam computed tomography systems and panoramic imaging for detecting simulated canine impaction-induced external root resorption in maxillary lateral incisors. *American Journal of Orthodontics and Dentofacial Orthopedics*, 136 (6), 764.

Alqerban, A., Jacobs, R., Lambrechts, P., *et al.* (2009b) Root resorption of the maxillary lateral incisor caused by impacted canine: a literature review. *Clinical Oral Investigations*, 13 (3), 247–255.

Alqerban, A., Jacobs, R., Fieuws, S., *et al.* (2011) Comparison of two cone beam computed tomographic systems versus panoramic imaging for localization of impacted maxillary canines and detection of root resorption. *European Journal of Orthodontics*, 33 (1), 93–102.

Alqerban, A., Hedesiu, M., Baciut, M., *et al.* (2013) Presurgical treatment planning of maxillary canine impactions using panoramic *vs* cone beam CT imaging. *Dentomaxillofacial Radiology*, 42 (9), 20130157.

Bedoya, M.M. & Park, J.H. (2009) A review of the diagnosis and management of impacted maxillary canines. *Journal of the American Dental Association*, 140 (12), 1485–1493.

Bertl, K., Benkö, G., Bertl, M.H., *et al.* (2013) A retrospective study on the influence of maxillary canine impaction on premolar root morphology. *Clinical Oral Investigations*, 17 (3), 943–948.

Bjerklin, K. & Guitirokh, C.H. (2011) Maxillary incisor root resorption induced by ectopic canines. *The Angle Orthodontist*, 81 (5), 800–806.

Botticelli, S., Verna, C., Cattaneo, P.M., *et al.* (2011) Two-versus three-dimensional imaging in subjects with unerupted maxillary canines. *European Journal of Orthodontics*, 33 (4), 344–349.

Broadbent, B.H. (1941) Ontogenic development of occlusion. *The Angle Orthodontist*, 11, 223–241.

Caprioglio, A., Siani, L., & Caprioglio, C. (2007) Guided eruption of palatally impacted canines through combined use of 3-dimensional computerized tomography scans and the easy cuspid device. *World Journal of Orthodontics*, 8 (2), 109–121.

Cooke, J. & Wang, H.L. (2006) Canine impactions: incidence and management. *International Journal of Periodontics and Restorative Dentistry*, 26 (5), 483–491.

Coulter, J. & Richardson, A. (1997) Normal eruption of the maxillary canine quantified in three dimensions. *European Journal of Orthodontics*, 19 (2), 171–183.

Dachi, S.F. & Howell, F.V. (1961) A survey of 3,874 routine full-mouth radiographs. II: a study of impacted teeth. *Oral Surgery, Oral Medicine, and Oral Pathology*, 14, 1165–1169.

Ely, N.J., Sherriff, M., & Cobourne, M.T. (2006) Dental transposition as a disorder of genetic origin. *European Journal of Orthodontics*, 28 (2), 145–151.

Ericson, S. & Kurol, J. (1986a) Longitudinal study and analysis of clinical supervision of maxillary canine eruption. *Community Dentistry and Oral Epidemiology*, 14 (3), 172–176.

Ericson, S. & Kurol, J. (1986b) Radiographic assessment of maxillary canine eruption in children with clinical signs of eruption disturbance. *European Journal of Orthodontics*, 8 (3), 133–140.

Ericson, S. & Kurol, J. (1987) Radiographic examination of ectopically erupting maxillary canines. *American Journal of Orthodontics and Dentofacial Orthopedics*, 91 (6), 483–492.

Ericson, S. & Kurol, J. (1988) Early treatment of palatally erupting maxillary canines by extraction of the primary canines. *European Journal of Orthodontics*, 10 (4), 283–295.

Frazier-Bowers, S.A., Puranik, C.P., & Mahaney, M.C. (2010) The etiology of eruption disorders: further evidence of a "genetic paradigm." *Seminars in Orthodontics*, 16 (3), 180–185.

Garib, D.G., Peck, S., & Gomes, S.C. (2009) Increased occurrence of dental anomalies associated with second-premolar agenesis. *The Angle Orthodontist*, 79 (3), 436–441.

Gholston, L.R. & Williams, P.R. (1984) Bilateral transposition of maxillary canines and lateral incisors: a rare condition. *ASDC Journal of Dentistry for Children*, 51 (1), 58–63.

Haney, E., Gansky, S.A., Lee, J.S., *et al.* (2010) Comparative analysis of traditional radiographs and cone-beam computed tomography volumetric images in the diagnosis and treatment planning of maxillary impacted canines. *American Journal of Orthodontics and Dentofacial Orthopedics*, 137 (5), 590–597.

Joshi, M.R. & Bhatt, N.A. (1971) Canine transposition. *Oral Surgery, Oral Medicine, and Oral Pathology*, 31 (1), 49–54.

Kapila, S., Conley, R.S., & Harrell, W.E., Jr. (2011) The current status of cone beam computed tomography imaging in orthodontics. *Dentomaxillofacial Radiology*, 40 (1), 24–34.

Katheria, B.C., Kau, C.H., Tate, R., *et al.* (2010) Effectiveness of impacted and supernumerary tooth diagnosis from traditional radiography versus cone beam computed tomography. *Pediatric Dentistry*, 32 (4), 304–309.

Leonardi, R., Peck, S., Caltabiano, M., *et al.* (2003) Palatally displaced canine anomaly in monozygotic twins. *The Angle Orthodontist*, 73 (4), 466–470.

Manne, R., Gandikota, C., Juvvadi, S.R., *et al.* (2012) Impacted canines: etiology, diagnosis, and orthodontic management. *Journal of Pharmacy and Bioallied Sciences*, 4 (Suppl 2), S234–S238.

Nagpal, A., Pai, K.M., Setty, S., *et al.* (2009) Localization of impacted maxillary canines using panoramic radiography. *Journal of Oral Science*, 51 (1), 37–45.

Ngan, P., Hornbrook, R., & Weaver, B. (2005) Early timely management of ectopically erupting maxillary canines. *Seminars in Orthodontics*, 11, 152–163.

Nishimura, K., Nakao, K., Aoki, T., *et al.* (2012) Orthodontic correction of a transposed maxillary canine and first premolar in the permanent dentition. *American Journal of Orthodontics and Dentofacial Orthopedics*, 142 (4), 524–533.

Novak, H.M., Baccetti, T., Sigler, L.M., *et al.* (2012) A controlled study on diagnostic and prognostic measurements of palatally displaced canines on lateral cephalograms. *Progress in Orthodontics*, 13 (1), 42–48.

Oberoi, S. & Knueppel, S. (2012) Three-dimensional assessment of impacted canines and root resorption using cone beam computed tomography. *Oral Surgery, Oral Medicine, Oral Pathology and Oral Radiology*, 113 (2), 260–267.

Oberoi, S., Gill, P., Chigurupati, R., *et al.* (2010) Three-dimensional assessment of the eruption path of the canine in individuals with bone-grafted alveolar clefts using cone beam computed tomography. *Cleft Palate–Craniofacial Journal*, 47 (5), 507–512.

Parkin, N., Benson, P.E., Thind, B., *et al.* (2008) Open versus closed surgical exposure of canine teeth that are displaced in the roof of the mouth. *Cochrane Database of Systematic Reviews*, (4), CD006966.

Parkin, N., Benson, P.E., Shah, A., *et al.* (2009) Extraction of primary (baby) teeth for unerupted palatally displaced permanent canine teeth in children. *Cochrane Database of Systematic Reviews*, (2), CD004621.

Parkin, N.A., Deery, C., Smith, A.M., *et al.* (2012) No difference in surgical outcomes between open and closed exposure of palatally displaced maxillary canines. *Journal of Oral and Maxillofacial Surgery*, 70 (9), 2026–2034.

Parkin, N.A., Milner, R.S., Deery, C., *et al.* (2013) Periodontal health of palatally displaced canines treated with open or closed surgical technique: a multicenter, randomized controlled trial. *American Journal of Orthodontics and Dentofacial Orthopedics*, 144 (2), 176–184.

Peck, L., Peck, S., & Attia, Y. (1993) Maxillary canine-first premolar transposition, associated dental anomalies and genetic basis. *The Angle Orthodontist*, 63 (2), 99–109.

Peck, S. (1998) On the phenomenon of intraosseous migration of nonerupting teeth. *American Journal of Orthodontics and Dentofacial Orthopedics*, 113 (5), 515–517.

Peck, S. & Peck, L. (1995) Classification of maxillary tooth transpositions. *American Journal of Orthodontics and Dentofacial Orthopedics*, 107 (5), 505–517.

Peck, S. & Peck, L. (1997) Palatal displacement of canine is genetic and related to congenital absence of teeth. *Journal of Dental Research*, 76 (3), 728–729.

Peck, S., Peck, L., & Kataja, M. (1994) The palatally displaced canine as a dental anomaly of genetic origin. *The Angle Orthodontist*, 64 (4), 249–256.

Peck, S., Peck, L., & Kataja, M. (1996a) Prevalence of tooth agenesis and peg-shaped maxillary lateral incisor associated with palatally displaced canine (PDC) anomaly. *American Journal of Orthodontics and Dentofacial Orthopedics*, 110 (4), 441–443.

Peck, S., Peck, L., & Kataja, M. (1996b) Site-specificity of tooth agenesis in subjects with maxillary canine malpositions. *The Angle Orthodontist*, 66 (6), 473–476.

Peck, S., Peck, L., & Kataja, M. (1998) Mandibular lateral incisor-canine transposition, concomittant dental anomalies, and genetic control. *The Angle Orthodontist*, 68 (5), 455–466.

Peck, S., Peck, L., & Kataja, M. (2002) Concomittant occurrence of canine malposition and tooth agenesis: evidence of orofacial genetic fields. *American Journal of Orthodontics and Dentofacial Orthopedics*, 122 (6), 657–660.

Plunkett, D.J., Dysart, P.S., Kardos, T.B., *et al.* (1998) A study of transposed canines in a sample of orthodontic patients. *British Journal of Orthodontics*, 25 (3), 203–208.

Power, S.M. & Short, M.B. (1993) An investigation into the response of palatally displaced canines to removal of deciduous canines and an assessment of factors contributing to favourable eruption. *British Journal of Orthodics*, 20 (3), 215–223.

Quirynen, M., Op Heij, D.G., Adriansens, A., *et al.* (2000) Periodontal health of orthodontically extruded impacted teeth: a split-mouth, long-term clinical evaluation. *Journal of Periodontology*, 71 (11), 1708–1714.

Sajnani, A.K. & King, N.M. (2012) Early prediction of maxillary canine impaction from panoramic radiographs. *American Journal of Orthodontics and Dentofacial Orthopedics*, 142 (1), 45–51.

Schmidt, A.D. & Kokich, V.G. (2007) Periodontal response to early uncovering, autonomous eruption, and orthodontic alignment of palatally impacted maxillary canines. *American Journal of Orthodontics and Dentofacial Orthopedics*, 131 (4), 449–455.

Shalish, M., Peck, S., Wasserstein, A., *et al.* (2002) Malposition of unerupted mandibular second premolar associated with agenesis of its antimere. *American Journal of Orthodontics and Dentofacial Orthopedics*, 121 (1), 53–56.

Shapira, Y. (1980) Transposition of canines. *Journal of the American Dental Association*, 100 (5), 710–712.

Shapira, Y. & Kuftinec, M.M. (2001) Maxillary tooth transpositions: characteristic features and accompanying dental anomalies. *American Journal of Orthodontics and Dentofacial Orthopedics*, 119 (2), 127–134.

Stivaros, N. & Mandall, N.A. (2000) Radiographic factors affecting the management of impacted upper permanent canines. *Journal of Orthodontics*, 27 (2), 169–173.

Strbac, G.D., Foltin, A., Gahleitner, A., *et al.* (2013) The prevalence of root resorption of maxillary incisors caused by impacted maxillary canines. *Clinical Oral Investigations*, 17 (2), 553–564.

Walker, L., Enciso, R., & Mah, J. (2005) Three-dimensional localization of maxillary canines with cone-beam computed tomography. *American Journal of Orthodontics and Dentofacial Orthopedics*, 128 (4), 418–423.

Warford, J.H., Grandhi, R.K., & Tira, D.E. (2003) Prediction of maxillary canine impaction using sectors and angular measurements. *American Journal of Orthodontics and Dentofacial Orthopedics*, 124 (6), 651–655.

Wasserstein, A., Tzur, B., & Brezniak, N. (1997) Incomplete canine transposition and maxillary central incisor impaction: a case report. *American Journal of Orthodontics and Dentofacial Orthopedics*, 111 (6), 635–639.

17 Assessment of Maxillary Transverse Deficiency and Treatment Outcomes by Cone Beam Computed Tomography

Jeanne M. Nervina, DMD, PhD, Sunil D. Kapila, BDS, MS, PhD and Carlos Flores-Mir, DDS, MSc, DSc, FRCD(C)

INTRODUCTION

The maxilla is a complex bone that has fascinated anatomists for centuries. Among the earliest recorded dissections of the maxilla is "A Skull Sectioned" by Leonardo da Vinci from 1489. In a remarkable exhibit presented at the Queen's Gallery at Buckingham Palace in 2012, da Vinci's dissections were paired with volumetric 3D computed tomography (CT) images taken by Dr. Richard Wellings, who sliced the radiographs to mimic the artwork (Figure 17.1). The validation of da Vinci's 15th-century depiction of the maxillofacial skeleton using 21st-century radiographic technology should not be dismissed as a non-scientific curiosity suitable for framing. Indeed, Peter Abrahams, professor of clinical anatomy, Warwick University (United Kingdom), considers da Vinci's work to be 300 years ahead of its time and that 3D radiographs are the only images from the past 524 years that surpass the master's work (Banerji, 2012). Others consider da Vinci's attention to detail a valuable lesson for clinicians in training, whose reliance on state-of-the-art diagnostic tools can lead to misdiagnosis if the machines are considered infallible (Gerrits & Veening, 2012).

In this chapter, the evolution of radiography will be discussed as a critical tool for assessing the maxillary transverse dimension accurately, which is one of the most common contributors to malocclusion. Specifically, topics reviewed will include the role of radiographs in detailing transverse maxillary growth and development, midpalatal sutural changes as we age, and evidence-based conclusions regarding maxillary expansion treatment. The terms rapid maxillary expansion (RME) and rapid palatal expansion (RPE) often are used interchangeably, although they technically refer to two different treatments. Expansion of the entire maxilla, which is performed surgically, traditionally is referred to as RME, while RPE is used to describe expansion of the palate "only" using a tooth- or tooth-tissue-borne palatal expander. However, since the distribution of RPE-generated

Cone Beam Computed Tomography in Orthodontics: Indications, Insights, and Innovations, First Edition. Sunil D. Kapila.

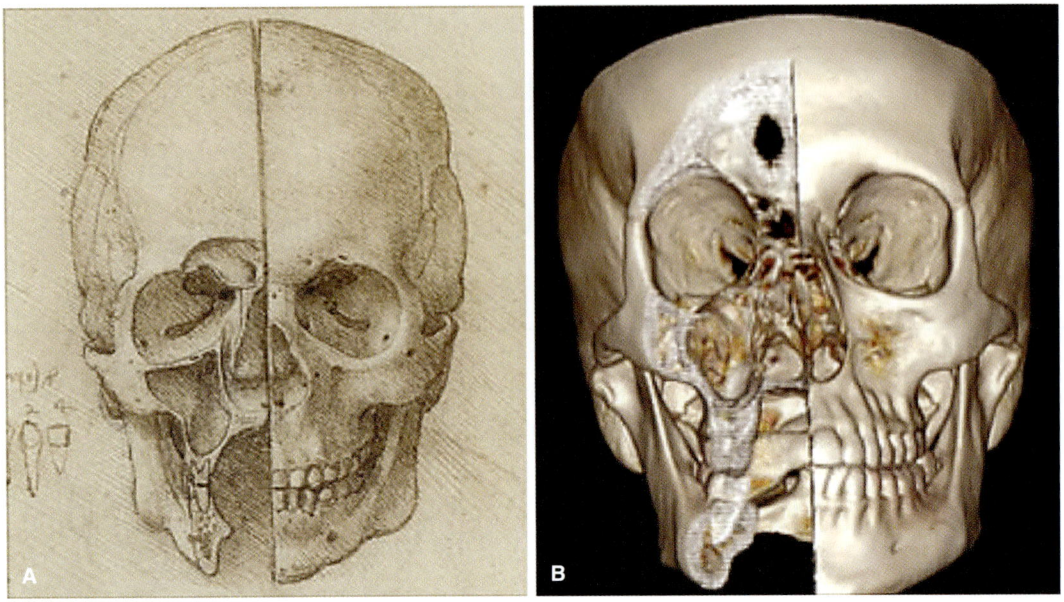

Figure 17.1 Leonardo da Vinci's drawing of the human skull with the right maxilla and mandible sectioned coronally (*A*) compared with a similar rendering of the skull using 3D radiology (*B*). (Panel *A* is reprinted with permission from Royal Collection Trust/© Her Majesty Queen Elizabeth II 2014. Panel *B* is reprinted with permission from Dr. Richard Wellings.)

forces indeed do extend to the entire maxilla and are known to contribute to sutural changes at sites distant from the palate, all expansion treatments will be referred to as RME in this chapter.

ACCURACY OF MAXILLARY WIDTH MEASUREMENTS TAKEN FROM 2D AND 3D RADIOGRAPHS

A critical reader of radiology-based craniofacial morphology studies should understand the technical limitations of the research approach used by the authors. The human skull is unrivaled in its structural complexity, which makes radiographic interpretation of craniofacial morphology especially challenging. Conventional lateral and posterior-anterior (PA) cephalographs suffer from the now well-known litany of problems that arise when a 3D object is projected onto a 2D plane: magnification distortion, geometric distortion, superimposed structures, and inconsistent head position during imaging (Pirttiniemi *et al.*, 1996; Malkoc *et al.*, 2005). While lateral and PA cephalographs are prone to these problems equally, because orthodontists use lateral cephalographs more routinely than PA cephalographs, the accuracy of landmark identification is relatively higher on lateral cephalographs (Hägg *et al.*, 1998). Practitioner inexperience is a major contributor to inaccurate landmark identification on PA cephalographs, which compounds the other technical problems that plague these radiographs (Leonardi *et al.*, 2008). For example, placement of the right and left jugale points ("mx" in Figure 17.2) on a PA cephalograph deviated up to 3 mm horizontally and 7 mm vertically among a group of five clinicians (Athanasiou *et al.*, 1999). Even worse, maxillary molar landmark placement ("um" in Figure 17.2) deviated 4 mm horizontally and up to 8 mm vertically (Athanasiou *et al.*, 1999). It is important to keep these data in mind when assessing studies using conventional 2D PA cephalographs because these two landmarks for the maxillary base and maxillary first molars are used widely to report maxillary width measurements on conventional 2D radiographs.

It also must be noted that there are two approaches to taking PA cephalographs. The

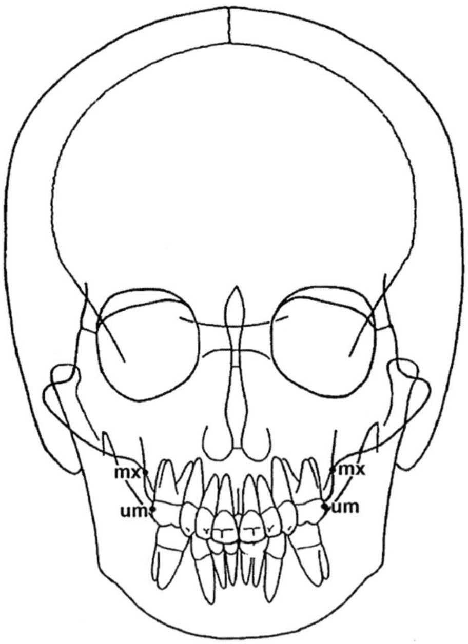

Figure 17.2 Commonly used PA cephalometry landmarks to assess maxillary width. The maxillary base is measured from "mx" to "mx." The intermolar width is measured from "um" to "um." "Mx" also is designated "jugale" or "j" on some tracings. (Modified from Athanasiou *et al.*, 1999.)

standard PA cephalograph is taken with the patient looking straight ahead such that Frankfort horizontal is at 0° with the horizontal plane (Figure 17.3A; Lux *et al.*, 2004b). The depressed PA cephalograph is taken with the patient's head tilted forward such that Frankfort horizontal forms a 35° angle with the horizontal plane (Figure 17.3B). Thus, it is important to recognize that transverse measurements taken from PA cephalographs may be different depending on the imaging technique used. For example, mean maxillary basal widths (bijugale) are larger on standard PA compared with depressed PA cephalographs of children aged 7–16 years (Table 17.1). Yet total transverse growth and overall transverse growth rates are higher on the depressed PA cephalograph relative to the standard PA cephalograph. In this example, it can be argued that the 0.9 mm difference in total transverse growth and the 0.03 mm/year difference in overall growth rate assessed on the different PA projections are not clinically significant, thus making the imaging methodology a moot point. That argument works for comparisons of a small number of studies, but these differences can be magnified if data from a larger number of studies are pooled to perform a meta-analysis. Thus,

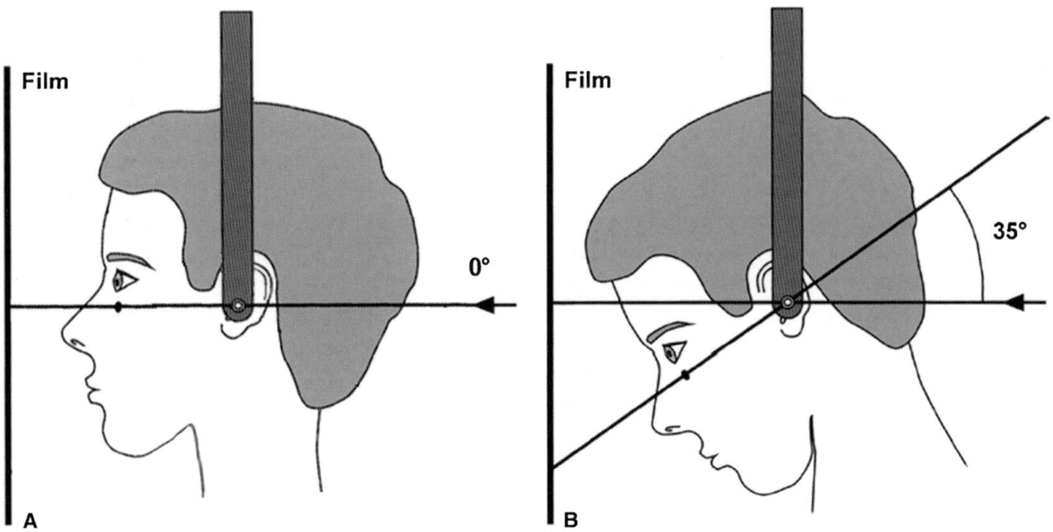

Figure 17.3 Head position for (*A*) standard 2D PA cephalograph with the X-ray beam oriented parallel to the Frankfort horizontal plane and (*B*) depressed 2D PA cephalograph in which the Frankfort horizontal plane is oriented at 35° to the X-ray beam with the head tilted forward. (Modified and reprinted with permission from Lux *et al.*, 2004b.)

Table 17.1 Comparison of maxillary transverse measurements (mean bijugale) and growth rates determined from standard and depressed PA cephalographs. Data demonstrate a consistently smaller yearly bijugale measurement on depressed PA cephalographs, yet the annual growth rate and total growth are higher on these cephalographs compared with the values calculated from the standard PA cephalograph.

Standard PA cephalograph			Depressed PA cephalograph		
Age (years)	Mean bijugale (mm)	Overall maxillary transverse growth rate (mm/year)	Age (years)	Mean bijugale (mm)	Overall maxillary transverse growth rate (mm/year)
7.6	56.24		7	54.04	
10.3	59.26		9	56.11	
12.9	60.59	0.76	11	57.90	0.79
16.5	62.32		13	59.74	
			15	61.11	
Total transverse growth (mm)	6.08			7.07	

Source: Modified from Lux *et al.*, 2004b, and Hesby *et al.*, 2006.

researchers interested in performing such a large-scale analysis must be cautioned to factor the imaging technique used in each study into their derivations and conclusions.

It is clear that landmark placement and measurement accuracies on conventional 2D PA cephalographs suffer from numerous technical problems. In this regard, it is arguable that da Vinci understood maxillary anatomy better than anyone whose primary view of the maxilla comes from conventional 2D radiographs. Fortunately, as demonstrated in Figure 17.1, CT gives today's clinicians an edge over da Vinci's since we can obtain accurate 3D images of the maxilla from *living* people.

There is a sizable literature establishing measurement accuracy including that of maxillary transverse measurements on 3D radiographs (Damstra *et al.*, 2010; Gribel *et al.*, 2011; van Vlijmen *et al.*, 2011). In keeping with the relatively infrequent use of PA cephalographs, it is not surprising that few studies have assessed the accuracy of landmark placement and morphometric measurements specifically on PA (or, more appropriately, coronal) CBCT radiographs (van Vlijmen *et al.*, 2009a, 2009b). In the two latter studies, the investigators radiographed 40 dried human skulls to generate conventional 2D PA cephalographs and constructed CBCT PA radiographs (essentially unsliced coronal CBCT images) and 3D volumetric frontal images of the skulls (Figure 17.4). The reliability of linear and angular measurements was assessed on each image by having the researcher place landmarks and take measurements five times and then calculate the Pearson's correlation coefficient for the replicate measurements. Not surprisingly, each measurement had a higher reliability rating on the CBCT images compared with the conventional 2D PA cephalographs. For example, the average reliability of angular measurements taken from the right and left jugale points was approximately 40% higher on the constructed 3D PA cephalograph and approximately 60% higher on the 3D volumetric frontal image compared with the conventional 2D PA cephalograph. Taken together, data from these studies suggest that although landmark placement and cephalometric assessment of the maxillary transverse dimension are more accurate on 3D than 2D images, orthodontists who choose to assess maxillary width in their diagnostic workup and who are not conversant with related landmarks should heed extra caution in landmark placement on both 2D and 3D PA cephalographs to optimize measurement accuracy.

Although skin decreases the accuracy of landmark placement and measurements on radiographs, human subject–based accuracy studies that

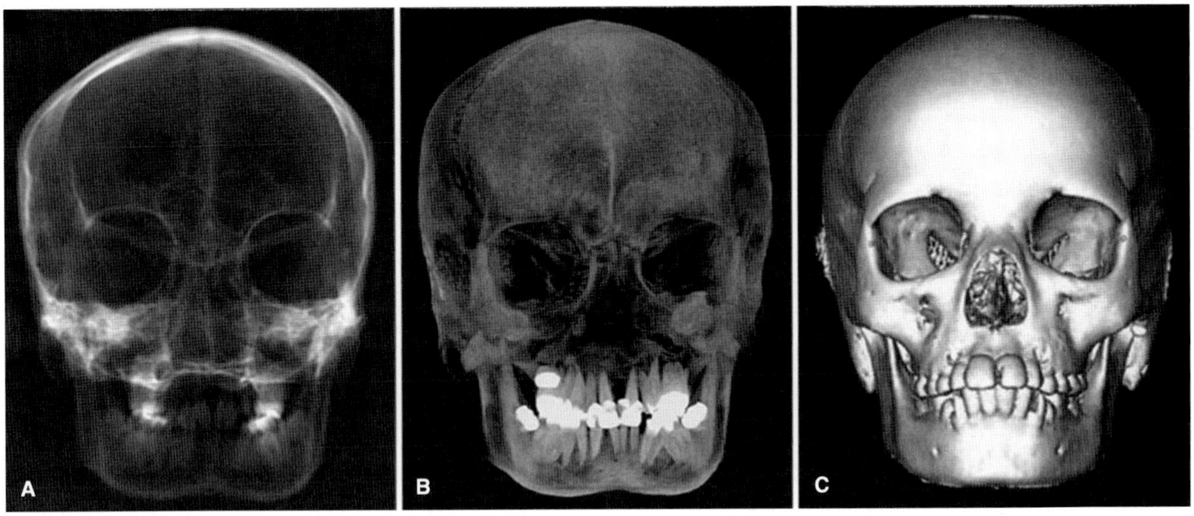

Figure 17.4 Comparison of (*A*) conventional 2D PA cephalograph, (*B*) constructed 2D PA cephalograph constructed from CBCT data, and (*C*) 3D volumetric frontal image derived from CBCT. Landmark placement is most accurate on the images generated by CBCT. (Modified and reprinted with permission from van Vlijmen *et al.*, 2009a, 2009b.)

directly compare transverse measurements taken from 2D and 3D PA cephalographs of patients confirm the reliability of these data, similar to that from the dried skull studies. Transverse measurements taken on volumetric and reconstructed PA cephalographs derived from CBCT data of adults had significantly less variation than measurements taken from conventional 2D PA cephalographs (Kim *et al.*, 2012; Nur *et al.*, 2012). Only one of these studies looked specifically at maxillary width and found a 3.03 mm difference in the measurements taken from the 2D and 3D cephalographs, with the 2D measurement being wider (Nur *et al.*, 2012). This is not likely to be significant clinically given that the mean maxillary width measurements in this study had standard deviations of 4.31 mm on the 2D radiographs and 3.99 mm on the 3D radiographs. From a clinical perspective, therefore, it currently does not appear that CBCT radiographs offer increased precision of transverse measurements that is beneficial diagnostically.

RADIOGRAPHIC ASSESSMENT OF MAXILLARY TRANSVERSE GROWTH

Prior to the now universally accepted "as low as reasonably achievable" (ALARA) principle for prescribing radiographs, 2D lateral and PA cephalographs were taken annually or semi-annually on growing children at several research institutions around the world. These radiographs, which were taken along with dental casts, are the basis for numerous longitudinal growth studies (Cortella *et al.*, 1997; Lux *et al.*, 2004a, 2004b; Wagner & Chung, 2005; Edwards *et al.*, 2007; Vásquez *et al.*, 2009). More often than not, these studies assess sagittal and vertical growth using lateral cephalographs, although there are some that use PA cephalographs to assess transverse growth. As is well known, technical problems with 2D cephalographs, especially PA cephalographs, limit the research questions that can be asked when using these films. While 3D radiographs are not constrained by the technical limitations common to 2D cephalographs, the inability to take annual or semi-annual 3D radiographs for ethical reasons on the same subjects as they grow imposes its own set of restrictions on the research questions that can be asked regarding craniofacial growth. Clinically useful conclusions can be drawn about craniofacial growth from available 2D and 3D cephalograph-based studies that use different children at each time point, provided it is acknowledged that biases may arise due to several factors, such as the impact of the uniqueness of facial growth in individuals in

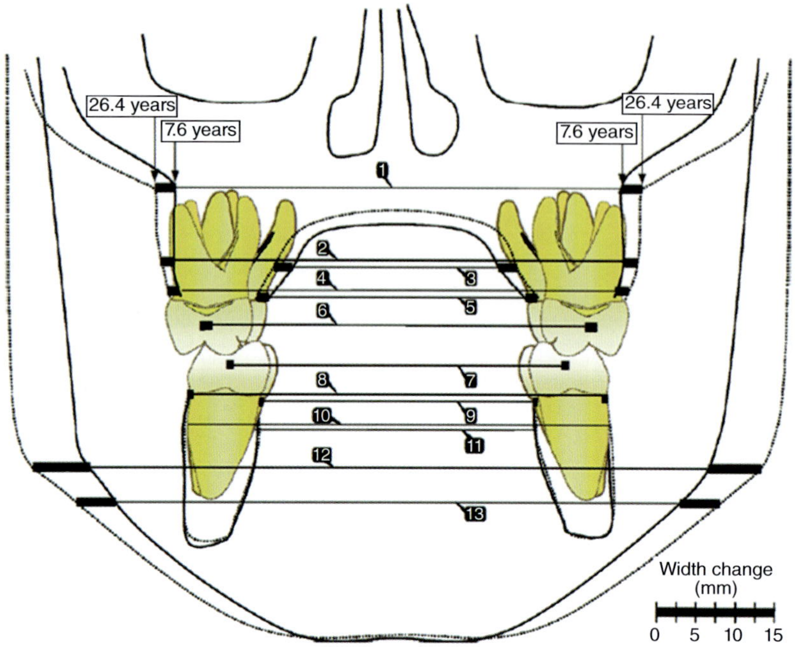

Figure 17.5 Summary of maxillary and mandibular transverse growth between the ages of 7.6 to 26.4 years. Length of black bars indicates the magnitude of growth as per the scale shown on the lower right. Notice the relative stability of the molar cusps compared with the maxillary and mandibular bases, which undergo the greatest increases in transverse growth. (Reprinted with permission from Hesby *et al.*, 2006.)

a small sample size or the lack of untreated controls.

An excellent example of how conventional 2D PA cephalographs could be used to assess normal transverse craniofacial growth was seen in the study by Hesby and colleagues (2006). This group used the Iowa Facial Growth Study PA radiographs to assess transverse maxillary and mandibular growth in untreated Class I subjects aged 7.6–26.4 years (Figure 17.5). Pooled data from 18 girls and 18 boys demonstrated that peak maxillary transverse growth of 0.76 mm/year occurred at 16.5 years. Unlike the maxilla, mandibular transverse growth did not peak during the time course of this study. Instead, mandibular transverse growth increased steadily and rapidly until 16.5 years of age, then increased asymptotically until 26.4 years to give an overall growth rate of 1.24 mm/year. Interestingly, the average transverse growth of the maxillary structures formed an inverted triangle with the greatest transverse growth at the maxillary base (5.37 mm) and the least growth at the maxillary first molars (3.08 mm). Like the maxilla, the mandible also had the greatest transverse growth at its base (14.54 mm), but growth at the alveolar crest and mandibular first molars were nearly identical (1.60 mm and 2.05 mm, respectively). The researchers compared their findings directly with several other longitudinal growth studies and found that the data are consistent across the studies (Hesby *et al.*, 2006, and references therein).

There is generalized clinical agreement that maxillary transverse growth rate in boys and girls peaks early during the pubertal growth spurt and that mandibular transverse growth lags behind maxillary transverse growth (Cortella *et al.*, 1997), not unlike what occurs in maxilla and mandible growth in the sagittal plane. Interestingly, maxillary and mandibular intermolar widths vary little compared with the skeletal base in either jaw, suggesting that transverse occlusal relationships are established and stabilized in early childhood. As will be discussed later, this may contribute to the transverse maxillary patterning that is seen in children with different sagittal and vertical growth patterns.

Related to the timing of the transverse growth spurt, there still is an unresolved controversy regarding when maxillary transverse growth ceases. Some authors conclude that maxillary transverse growth continues asymptotically until adulthood and that the peak transverse growth rate is highest in pre-teens and young teens (13–14 years old; Korn & Baumrind, 1990; Athanasiou *et al.*, 1992; Yavuz *et al.*, 2004; Lux *et al.*, 2004a, 2004b). Conversely, some authors conclude that maxillary transverse growth stops in the early teens (13–14 years) before growth stops in the other planes (Snodell *et al.*, 1993; Wagner & Chung, 2005; Edwards *et al.*, 2007). Resolution of this issue is important because it impacts the related controversy regarding the efficacy of early orthopedic correction of maxillary transverse deficiency (McNamara, 2002). If optimized orthopedic correction is achieved best when treatment begins at the peak growth spurt, then knowing when maxillary transverse growth peaks is critical for developing the appropriate expansion protocol in children with a narrow maxilla.

In addition to providing important insight into craniofacial growth, longitudinal growth studies form the basis for age- and sex-based cephalometric norms used for diagnosing skeletal and dental malocclusions. It is important to note that most of the normative growth studies were performed on Caucasian children with a Class I skeletal relationship. Few PA cephalometric norms for non-Caucasian children are available. In fact, only one study (Al-Azemi & Årtun, 2012) has been published, showing that Kuwaiti adolescents have wider maxillary measurements compared with age-matched Caucasian norms (Ricketts *et al.*, 1982). Interestingly, non-Caucasian adult PA cephalometric norms for Turks (Uysal & Sari, 2005) and Peruvian-Americans (Pérez *et al.*, 2011) do not differ from Ricketts' adult transverse norms. There is a clear need for non-Caucasian PA cephalometric norms, especially in children, to diagnose transverse skeletal malocclusion better in orthodontics patients.

Another important reason to collect normative lateral and PA cephalometric data across ethnic groups, sexes, and ages is to establish sizable databases for future genetic research on craniofacial patterning in human populations (Liu *et al.*, 2012). One of the greatest frustrations of orthodontists is the inability to predict craniofacial growth in children, which greatly hinders orthodontic diagnosis of skeletal malocclusions, which may benefit from early treatment during childhood or adolescence. Determination of the genetic background of individuals with distinct skeletal discrepancies in each plane of space will help in developing a powerful diagnostic tool for predicting growth discrepancies in young children. An initial step toward integrating craniofacial morphology and genetics recently has been made for European adults (Liu *et al.*, 2012).

DIAGNOSING MAXILLARY TRANSVERSE DEFICIENCY USING PA CEPHALOGRAPHS

The clinical need for normative data on maxillary transverse growth is to improve the diagnosis of maxillary transverse discrepancy in children. Early diagnosis offers the best opportunity for orthopedic correction with palatal expansion. Interestingly, maxillary constriction is not always obvious clinically. While a posterior crossbite often is diagnostic for a narrow maxilla, a narrow maxillary intermolar without a crossbite also can indicate the need for maxillary expansion (McNamara, 2002). The absence of a crossbite in a patient with a narrow maxilla possibly results from the stability of intermolar width established early and continues to manifest during maxillary and mandibular transverse growth throughout adolescence. In patients with a narrow maxilla but no posterior crossbite, it is common to find dental compensations such as excessive buccal flaring of the maxillary dentition and a deep Curve of Wilson in the lower dentition that mask the maxillary transverse constriction. CBCT images are invaluable for assessing these dental compensations and the alveolar boundary conditions if addressing crown or root torque is being considered as part of the treatment (see Chapters 11 and 14).

Longitudinal growth studies of children with Class II and Class III skeletal malocclusions demonstrate the value of PA cephalographs in diagnosing a narrow maxilla in young patients. Lux and associates (2003) used conventional 2D PA cephalographs and dental casts to examine growth changes in transverse skeletal and dental measurements in children with four malocclusions: (1) ideal Class I occlusion (19 boys, 18 girls); (2) "good" Class I occlusion with mild crowding (18 boys, 8 girls); (3) Class II, Division 1 (8 boys, 9 girls); and (4) Class II, Division 2 (8 boys, 4 girls). The authors found that Class II, Division 1, boys and girls aged 7–15 had consistently less transverse maxillary growth compared with boys with the three other occlusions. Not surprisingly, the boys and girls with Class II, Division 1 malocclusion had the smallest maxillary intermolar distance throughout growth. Equally important to note is the finding that the boys and girls with a Class II, Division 2 malocclusion had the second smallest maxillary base widths throughout growth. Likewise, 2D PA radiographic analysis of maxillary widths among girls with a Class III malocclusion ($n = 19$) and widths in girls with a Class I occlusion ($n = 20$; Chen *et al.*, 2008) demonstrates that the interjugal maxillary width and the maxillary intermolar distance both were significantly smaller in the Class III subjects at each time point every year between the ages of 10 and 14 years. In summary, both maxillary and/or dental transversal dimensions in Class II and Class III subjects consistently were found to be smaller than in Class I subjects.

Given the inaccuracies associated with conventional 2D PA cephalographs, it would be helpful to know if CBCT images improve diagnosis of maxillary transverse discrepancies in children with different malocclusions. To date, no such studies have been performed, which most likely reflects the limited use of PA cephalographs in clinical practice in general and, by extension, an inadequate understanding on how to use CBCT imaging for diagnosing maxillary transverse deficiency. In addition, current ethical guidelines preclude longitudinal CBCT imaging of subjects for detailed analyses of transversally deficient cases for extracting potential clinically valuable information. Given the latter constraints, at this time, a conventional 2D PA cephalograph—in the hands of an experienced clinician—can serve as a useful tool to diagnose maxillary transverse deficiency in orthodontics patients. Orthodontists must keep in mind that while a posterior crossbite often indicates a narrow maxilla, patients with a Class II or Class III skeletal malocclusion without a posterior crossbite also may have a transverse maxillary deficiency. The only way to diagnose such transverse deficiencies or disharmonies is to take and analyze PA cephalographs accurately. With additional discoveries using CBCT, it is likely that CBCT rather than PA cephalographs will be increasingly utilized for this diagnostic purpose in the future.

RADIOGRAPHIC ASSESSMENT OF MIDPALATAL SUTURE OSSIFICATION

While PA cephalographs are invaluable for diagnosing maxillary transverse deficiency, the choice of maxillary expansion treatment rarely is based on the PA cephalographs. Instead, most orthodontists rely on the maxillary-mandibular intermolar discrepancy and the patient's age to determine the best approach to gain sufficient maxillary width. Patient age is considered an especially important factor for choosing between nonsurgical or surgical approaches to maxillary expansion due to the widespread belief that the midpalatal suture is patent through our early to mid-teens and ossified or interdigitated heavily in late teens and adulthood. A patent midpalatal suture is considered highly responsive to transverse forces, whereas an ossified or interdigitated suture not only is unresponsive to nonsurgical expansion, but also is expanding under these circumstances, potentially is harmful to the alveolar bone and periodontium, and places teeth in potentially unstable buccolingual angulations. Yet there is a surprising lack of consensus on the appropriate approach to maxillary expansion in adults (Handelman, 2011; Northway, 2011). A discussion is needed of how the midpalatal suture changes as we age in order to help clinicians decide which maxillary expansion protocol is suitable for their patients.

Modern anatomists differ from da Vinci primarily in the tools used to perform and analyze their dissections. Where da Vinci was confined to the macroscopic world of organs and tissues, modern anatomists can roam the microscopic world of cells and their subcellular components freely. Modern anatomists studying the maxilla do share one restriction with da Vinci, however: they rely heavily on cadavers for their studies. Fortunately, post-mortem cadavers, if well preserved, are remarkably suitable for performing detailed macroscopic and microscopic anatomical studies and have been used to undertake detailed studies on midpalatal sutures.

Three methods are used to assess midpalatal suture anatomy: histology, 2D radiology, and 3D radiology. Without exception, the most detailed data, hence most accurate, on age-related changes in the midpalatal suture come from histological studies. With improvements in radiographic techniques, it is common to find studies that use both histology and radiology. These studies are valuable especially because they not only provide detailed insights into the sutural growth, but also demonstrate the shortcomings of radiographs as diagnostic tools to assess the degree of sutural ossification in orthodontics patients.

Melsen (1975) pioneered the combined use of detailed histology and microradiology to assess sutural changes in the human palate. Examining post-mortem palates from 33 boys and 27 girls aged 0–18 years, three stages in the midpalatal suture development were described (Figure 17.6). Stage one, the infantile stage, is notable for the wedging of the vomer between the two abutting palatal shelves, which gives the midpalatal suture a Y-shaped configuration when viewed in a coronal section. In stage two, the juvenile stage, the upper portion of the Y flattens out and the vertical portion begins developing curves, effectively increasing the suture's length. Last, stage three, the adolescent stage, is demarcated by the extensive interdigitation that generally is associated with full maturity. This study did not provide specific ages for each stage of sutural maturation, however. Overall, it demonstrated that the lack of excessive interdigitation in younger children is a major reason orthodontists generally agree that nonsurgical maxillary expansion is performed best in younger patients.

Two follow-up studies to Melsen's work on children studied sutural closure in young adults. In the first study, Persson & Thilander (1977) developed the "obliteration index" (OI) to quantify the percentage of ossification in the midpalatal suture. Using post-mortem samples collected from 14 males and 10 females aged 15–35 years, the authors first stained coronal midpalatal suture slices with hematoxylin-eosin. Then they took microphotographs, projected them onto paper, and traced the suture (Figure 17.7). In each tracing, the investigators marked the boundaries of bony bridges, which they then measured to give the total amount of ossification in the suture. The total length of the suture was then measured using a "map-measuring instrument." The OI finally was calculated as the ratio of the total ossification length divided by the total suture length, multiplied by 100. Using this approach, the OI in subjects aged 15–19 years averaged 0.9%. Unfortunately, the mean OI for the older subjects was not calculated. Instead, it was noted that there was a steady increase in OI as the subjects aged. Bony bridges appear most often in the posterior region of the midpalatal suture across the age group studied. Equally important, the findings demonstrated that there is considerable variability in OI between individuals and between different regions of the suture in each individual.

In the second study that followed Melsen's work, Wehrbein & Yildizhan (2001) used post-mortem samples from young adults aged 18–38. This study more closely resembles Melsen's because it uses a combination of radiology and histology to assess midpalatal suture closure. Radiographs were performed so as to mimic clinical occlusal radiographs, which allowed visualization of the midpalatal suture along its length. Three 1-mm-long regions of interest (ROIs) were selected from the anterior, middle, and posterior of the suture, and the sutures were graded as either visible or non-visible. Histological sections then were generated from each of the regions, photographed, and evaluated using computerized morphometric software. The mean suture width and OI were different significantly between the groups with visible versus non-visible sutures. Visible sutures generally were oriented vertically in line with the X-ray beam (Figure 17.8A), had a mean suture width of 231 μm, and a mean OI of 0.45%. Seven of the 10 ROIs in the visible group had an OI of 0%. The morphological features of the non-visible sutures were variable. Some were interdigitated highly (Figure 17.8B), as would be expected

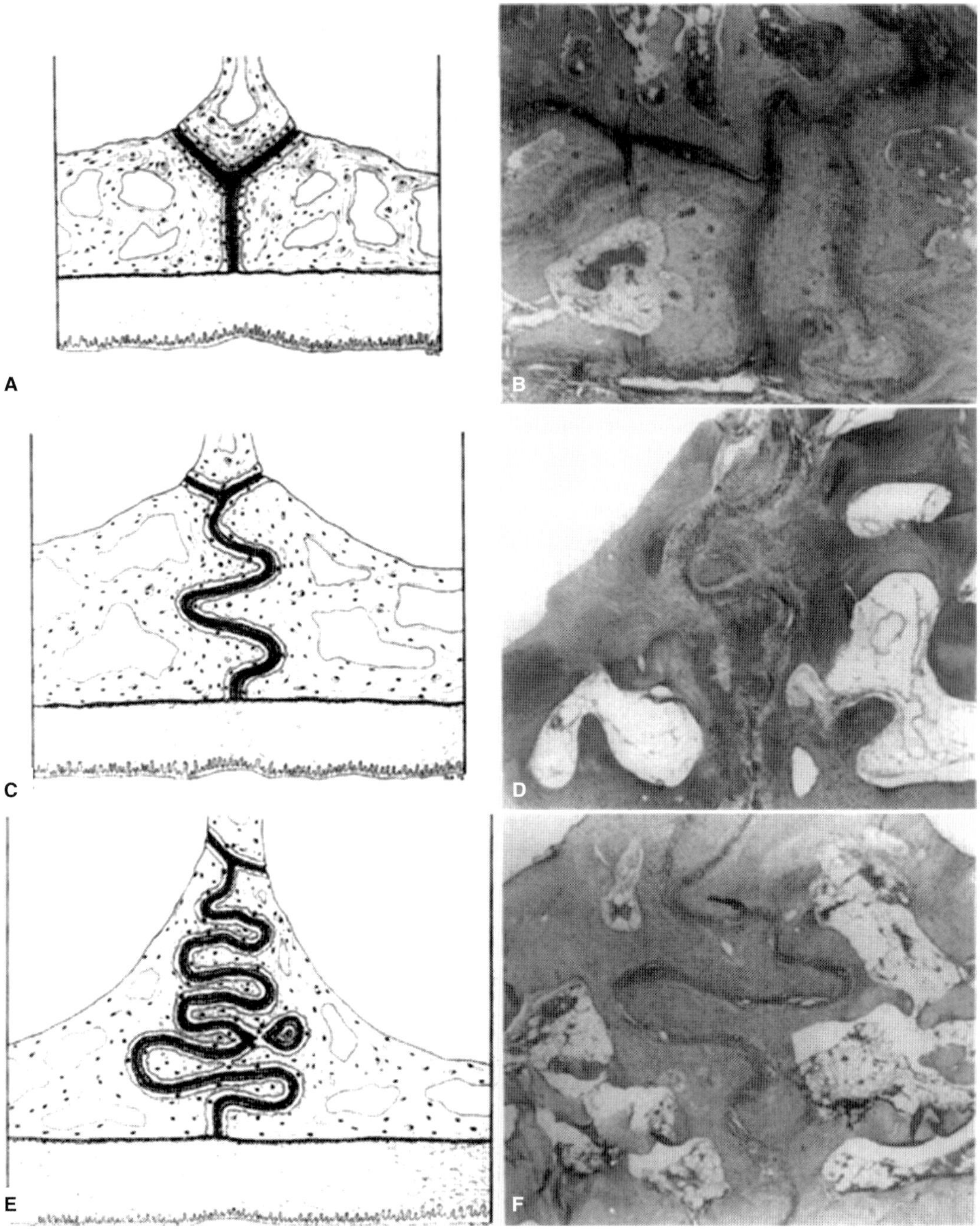

Figure 17.6 Schematic (*A, C, E*) and histological sections (*B, D, F*) of the midpalatal suture configuration during the infantile (*A, B*), juvenile (*C, D*), and adolescent (*E, F*) stages of growth. The vomer and superior portions of the palatal shelves form the upper portion and the midpalatal shelves form the vertical component of the "Y" that demarks the infantile configuration. With age, the upper portion flattens out and the vertical component increases in length as it becomes sinuous. (Reprinted with permission from Melsen, 1975.)

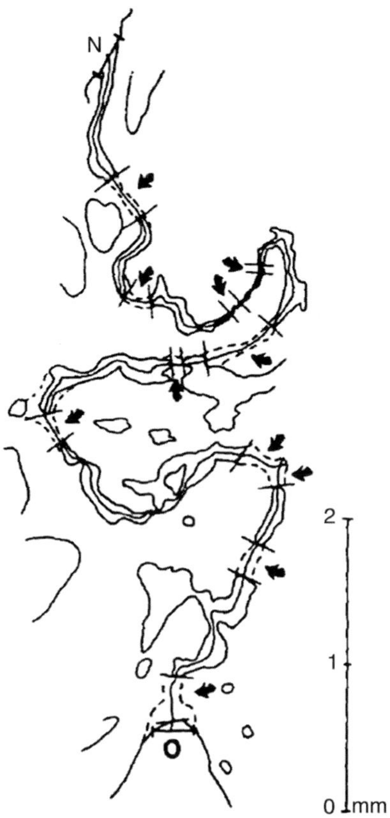

Figure 17.7 Demonstration of midpalatal suture photomicrograph tracing by Persson & Thilander (1977) used to establish the obliteration index (OI) to quantitate the degree of bony fusion along the length of the suture. Solid lines crossing the suture and arrows indicate the extent of individual bony bridges. The total suture length was measured from the nasal (N) to the oral (O) endpoints. OI is calculated as the ratio of the total bony bridge length to the total suture length, multiplied by 100. (Reprinted with permission from Persson and Thilander, 1977.)

in this age group. Others, however, were not highly interdigitated and presented instead with a suture that was oriented obliquely such that the X-ray beam was not parallel to the suture (Figure 17.8C) nor did it retain the Y-shaped configuration of an infantile palate (Figure 17.8D). In the non-visible group, the mean suture width was 201 μm and the mean OI was 1.3%. Eleven of the 20 ROIs in the non-visible group had an OI of 0%.

Two final studies on midpalatal suture closure cover ages 18–63 (Knaup *et al.*, 2004) and 14–71 (Korbmacher *et al.*, 2007). Knaup and coworkers divided their subjects into two groups: ≤25 years old and >25 years old. Using histomorphometry to assess midpalatal suture width and OI, they found that the median sutural width was larger significantly in the younger group compared with the older group (211.2 μm and 161.2 μm, respectively). Similarly, the median OI was less significant in the younger group (0%) compared with the older group (3.11%). This finding especially is remarkable and suggests that the midpalatal suture largely is unossified throughout life. Indeed, Korbmacher and associates arrived at the same conclusion in their histological and radiographic study of midpalatal suture morphology in subjects aged 14–71, who were divided into three groups: ≤25 years old, 25 to <30 years old, and ≥30 years old. The mean OI for each did not vary significantly and each was very low: 0.57%, 1.75%, and 1.67%, respectively.

The study by Korbmacher and associates (2007) also is notable because it is the first time that 3D radiographs were used to assess midpalatal suture morphology. It is important to note that the radiographs in this study are microcomputed tomographs, which have significantly higher resolution than any currently available clinical CBCT machines. Thus, when the coronal slices in the study are viewed, the different sutural configurations are visible (Figure 17.9). These images have sufficiently high resolution to measure the mean OI. Likewise, the axial (Figure 17.10) and sagittal slices provide important information on the aging midpalatal suture. In this study, axial slices were used to measure a new variable, the "interdigitation index" (II; Figure 17.10), which is the ratio of the total midpalatal suture length (measured along the curved pathway of the suture) to the linear distance between the sutural endpoints. As with the OI, the II did not differ among the youngest, middle, and oldest group (1.39, 1.43, and 1.49, respectively). Finally, sagittal slices (Figure 17.11) were used to assess the bone volume to total volume ratio (BV/TV), which is a commonly used index of trabeculation in bone morphometrics. Interestingly, it was mean BV/TV that showed a significant difference among the age groups, with the highest value in the 25- to 30-year-old group (53.2). The youngest and oldest groups had similar mean BV/TV values (47.1 and 43.5, respectively).

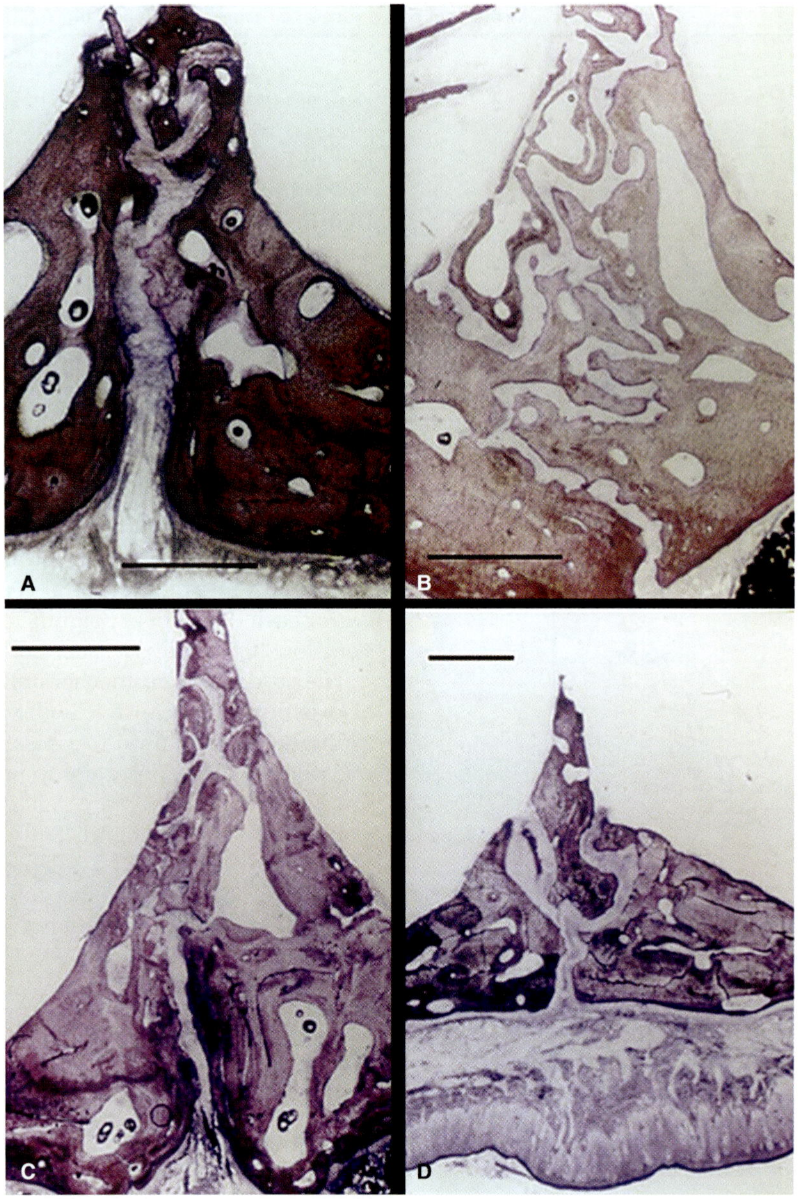

Figure 17.8 Histological sections demonstrating (*A*) a radiographically visible suture that is oriented vertically within the palate and three radiographically obliterated sutures demonstrating (*B*) a high degree of interdigitation, (*C*) a relatively straight but slanting configuration, and (*D*) retention of the infantile "Y" configuration. Note the degree of patency along the length of each suture, taken from (*A*) the anterior palate of a 32-year-old male, (*B*) the midpalate of a 32-year-old male, (*C*) the midpalate of a 25-year-old male, and (*D*) the midpalate of a 20-year-old female. The nasal surface is superior and the oral surface is inferior in each image. (Reprinted with permission from Wehrbein and Yildizhan, 2001.)

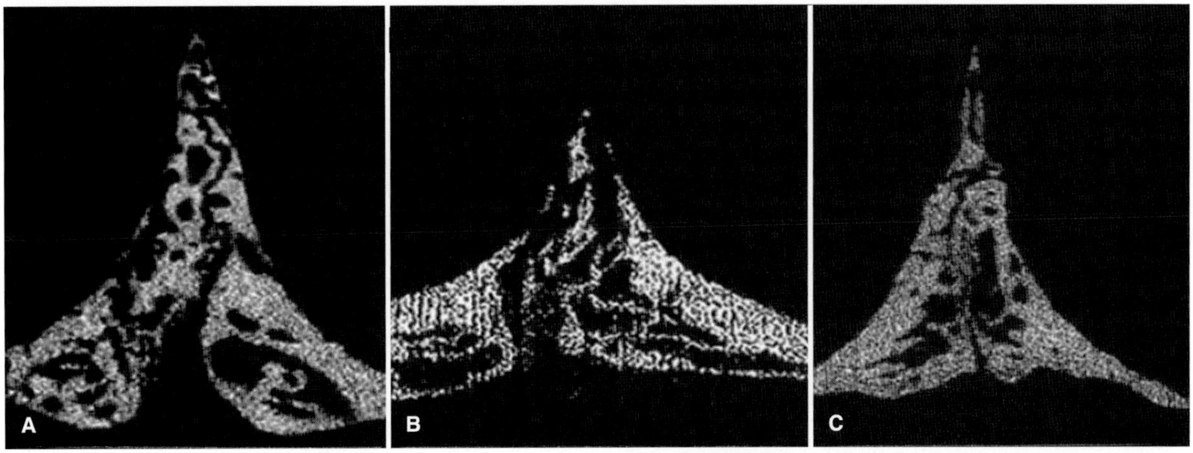

Figure 17.9 Changes in the obliteration index (OI) of the midpalatal suture with age. Coronal microCT images of the midpalate in subjects (*A*) ≤25 years old, (*B*) between 25 and 30 years old, and (*C*) ≥30 years old are used to measure the length of all the bony bridges and the linear distance between the nasal and oral cavity endpoints of the midpalatal suture. These data then are used to determine the mean OI for each group, which is 0.57%, 1.75%, and 1.67%, respectively for subjects in the three age groups. None of these values is significantly different from the others, suggesting that substantial midpalatal suture fusion does not occur with age. (Reprinted with permission from Korbmacher *et al.*, 2007.)

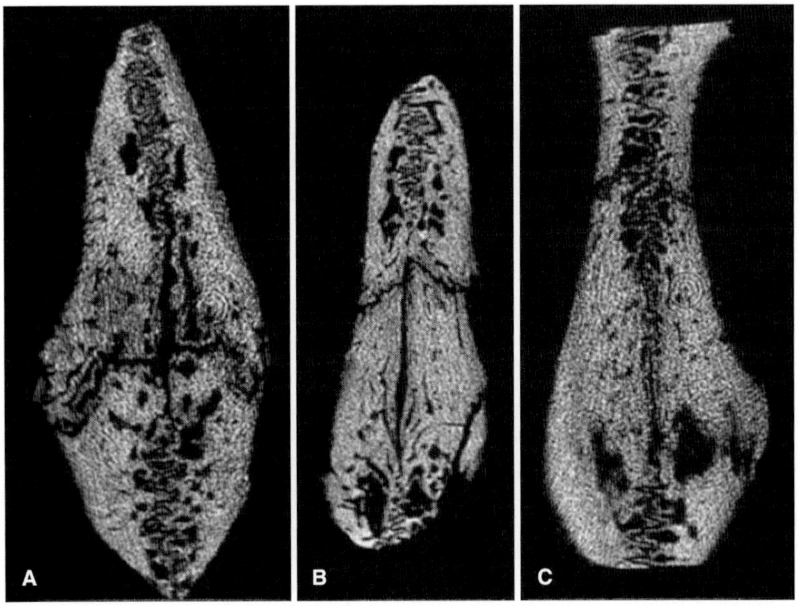

Figure 17.10 Changes in the interdigitation index (II) of the midpalatal suture with age. Axial microCT images of the midpalate in subjects (*A*) ≤25 years old, (*B*) between 25 and 30 years old, and (*C*) ≥30 years old are used to measure the total length of midpalatal suture following the curves of the suture and linear distance between the nasal and oral cavity endpoints of the midpalatal suture. These data then are used to determine the mean II for each group, which is 1.39%, 1.43%, and 1.49%, respectively. None of these values is different significantly from the others, suggesting that midpalatal suture fusion does not occur as we age. (Reprinted with permission from Korbmacher *et al.*, 2007.)

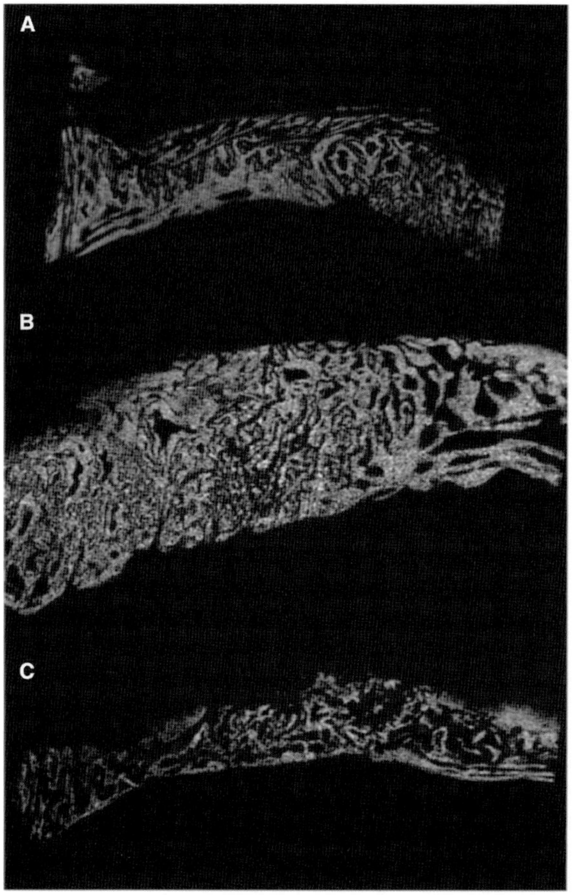

Figure 17.11 Changes in the bone volume/total volume (BV/TV) of the midpalatal suture as we age. Sagittal microCT images of the midpalate in subjects (*A*) ≤25 years old, (*B*) between 25 and 30 years old, and (*C*) ≥30 years old are used to measure the total volume of bony tissue in the total tissue volume captured in the microCT image. These data are then used to determine the mean BV/TV for each group, which is 47.08%, 53.2%, and 43.49%, respectively. The BV/TV value for the 25- to 30-year-old subjects (*B*) is significantly higher than for either of the other age groups. Interestingly, BV/TVs for the youngest (*A*) and oldest (*C*) subjects do not differ. (Reprinted with permission from Korbmacher *et al.*, 2007.)

A higher BV/TV value is indicative of increased bone strength and may offer an explanation for why nonsurgical rapid maxillary expansion (RME) rarely is successful in this age group.

There are four important findings among these studies of midpalatal suture obliteration during aging. First, there is tremendous intrasutural and interindividual variability in the OI. There is no consistent pattern of bony bridge distribution along the length of any given suture. Having stated that, however, if an individual's OI > 0%, then the superior portion of the posterior suture is the most likely region to be ossified. Second, populations of subjects do not have consistent patterns of ossification. Some authors have suggested that this interindividual variation may be related to function (Korbmacher *et al.*, 2007, and references therein). For example, the quality of the diet (hard vs. soft foods) may contribute to the direction and magnitude of force vectors on each half of the maxilla, which results in individual-specific bone remodeling along the midpalatal suture. Recognizing that the midpalatal suture attaches two sites of active remodeling immediately should bring to mind the relationship of the periodontal ligament adjoining alveolar bone and roots. Orthodontic forces stretch and compress the periodontal ligament (PDL), which triggers bone formation and resorption, respectively, in the alveolus. Without bone remodeling, orthodontic tooth movement would be impossible. Similarly, maxillary expansion is possible only because of remodeling of a patent midpalatal suture. Third, it is clear from these studies that the midpalatal suture remains largely unossified throughout life and the amount of ossification present (rarely more than 3% of the total suture) does not seem to offer sufficient resistance to most nonsurgical maxillary expansion protocols. Fourth, these studies also demonstrate the inability to diagnose the degree of sutural closure using clinical radiographs, with the possible exception of an unfused suture that is oriented parallel to the X-ray beam. This is critically important to remember as we consider the evidence regarding clinical outcomes following maxillary expansion treatment in orthodontics patients.

2D AND 3D RADIOGRAPHIC EVALUATION OF MAXILLARY EXPANSION

The most common radiograph used to assess maxillary expansion is the conventional 2D occlusal film (Figure 17.12). These radiographs are

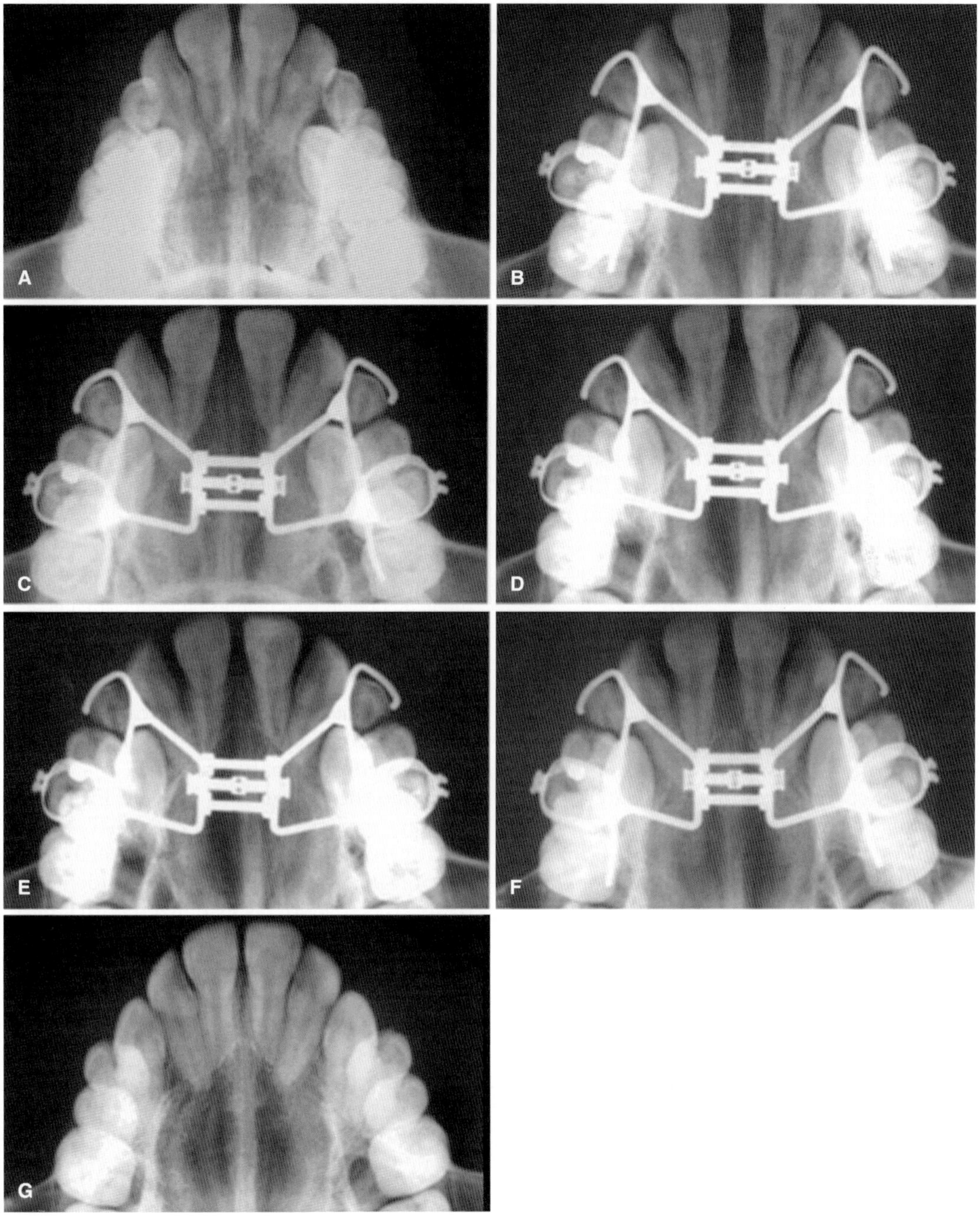

Figure 17.12 Conventional 2D occlusal radiographs demonstrating changes in midpalatal suture following RME in a child. *A*: Pretreatment radiographs showing narrow maxilla during the mixed dentition stage. *B*: Occlusal radiograph at the end of 5 months of activation. *C–F*: Occlusal radiograph at 1, 2, 3, and 4 months post-expansion, respectively. *G*: Radiograph at 23 months after the start of treatment showing increased maxillary width in the permanent dentition stage. (Reprinted with permission from da Silva Filho *et al.*, 2005.)

relatively easy to take and capture nearly the entire palate and maxillary dentition. As shown in Figure 17.12A,B (da Silva Filho *et al.*, 2005), 5 months of RME in a child separates the maxillary bones at the level of the palate, which is visualized as a dramatic increase in the midpalatal suture width and the appearance of a significant diastema between the central incisors. Over the next 4 months (Figure 17.12C–F), the midpalatal suture begins to ossify and the midline diastema closes passively with the maxillary expander in place for retention. The occlusal radiograph that was taken after retention with the palatal expander for 14 months demonstrates continued midpalatal suture ossification, nearly complete diastema closure, and increased maxillary width compared with the initial radiograph (Figure 17.12G).

As is well known, conventional 2D occlusal radiographs cannot be used to diagnose the internal structure of the midpalatal suture. Moreover, like all 2D radiographs, superimposition of structures, geometric distortion, and magnification errors afflict occlusal radiographs equally. The use of 3D radiographs overcomes these problems and provides far more detailed images of post-expansion orthopedic and dental changes. For example, axial slices from 3D scans provide far more precision when measuring the midpalatal suture width compared with conventional 2D occlusal films (Figure 17.13). Moreover, coronal slices allow for evaluation of dental tipping and an additional view of the widened midpalatal suture, which no conventional 2D radiograph can provide (Figure 17.14).

Using 3D radiographs, a much more complete picture of post-treatment effects of RME can be obtained. Specifically, three distinct components of maxillary expansion can be assessed: skeletal expansion, alveolar bending, and dental tipping (Garrett *et al.*, 2008; Ghoneima *et al.*, 2010; Kartalian *et al.*, 2010). In a study of 17 boys and 13 girls (mean age 13.8 ± 1.7 years) treated with RME, Garrett and associates (2008) found that Hyrax expanders produce the most expansion through dental tipping (49%); skeletal expansion (38%) and alveolar bending (13%) account for the remainder of the total expansion in this age group (Figure 17.15). The general consensus in all of the 3D radiograph-based studies is that RME produces more dental tipping than skeletal expansion or alveolar bending, even in younger patients.

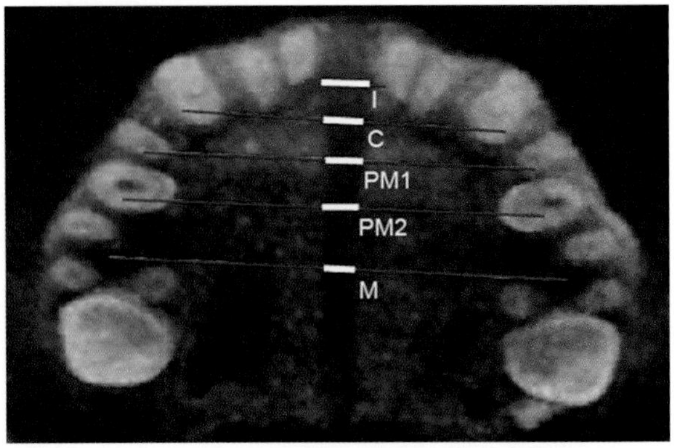

Figure 17.13 Axial CBCT image of midpalatal suture demonstrating sutural expansion at the central incisors (I), canines (C), first premolars (PM1), second premolars (PM2), and permanent first molars (M). Note the well-defined ossified boundaries of the suture, which allow expansion measurements (white bars) to be taken at each reference line (red). (Reprinted with permission from Garrett *et al.*, 2008.)

While the above data provide insights into the average expected changes with RME, they hide the relatively large variability between patients in response to this therapy. This wide variation in responses to RME, as visualized with CBCT, is represented in Figure 17.16, which shows the differences in sutural opening in two same-aged patients with similar initial sutural patency but different initial palatal vault configurations. When observed in the coronal plane, one patient has a narrow V-shaped palate (Figure 17.16A), while the other has a U-shaped palate (Figure 17.16G). Biomechanical principles dictate that RME forces from tooth-borne expanders are distributed primarily through the dentition and alveolar bone, which explains the observation that dental tipping and alveolar bending are major contributors to total maxillary expansion in both these patients (Figure 17.16D,J). It is likely, however, that the geometry of the system will contribute to variations in distribution of the expansion forces and, therefore, to the potential outcomes of the expansion as reflected by the observation that the patient with the narrow,

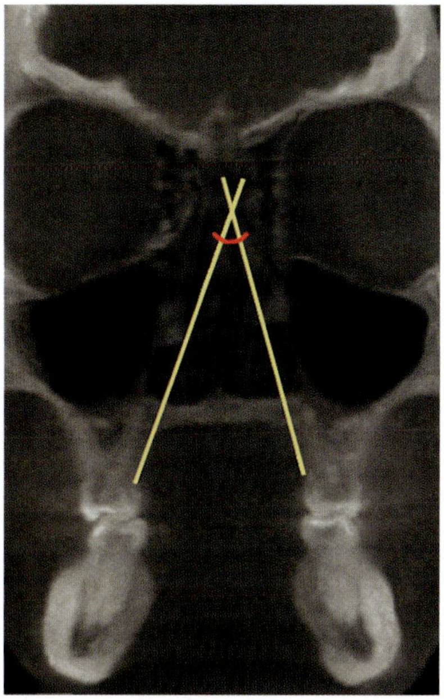

Figure 17.14 Coronal CBCT image demonstrating method for measuring alveolar bending at the first molars following RME. Coronal images are ideal for determining what percentage of total maxillary expansion results from skeletal expansion, alveolar bending, and dental tipping. In this image, alveolar angulation is determined by measuring the angle formed from lines drawn tangent to the palatal alveolar bone at the level of the first molar. (Reprinted and modified with permission from Garrett *et al.*, 2008.)

V-shaped initial palatal vault undergoes significant sutural widening (Figure 17.16E,F) compared with the patient with the U-shaped palatal vault (Figure 17.16K,L). These observations together with the power of 3D radiography enable us now to address similarly complex questions about the possible effects of morphological and sutural phenotypes on the likely outcome of RME treatment.

Assessment of the 3D morphological effects of RME is an especially active area of research because this is one of the most commonly used treatment options for maxillary transverse constriction. Needless to say, RME is not the only treatment option. With numerous expander designs, activation protocols, and surgical options, it should not be surprising that significant research on the efficacies of each approach exists. In fact, this is one of the most commonly reviewed topics in orthodontics. In the next section, the clinical outcomes of the various approaches to treating a constricted maxilla will be discussed.

EVIDENCE-BASED ASSESSMENT OF MAXILLARY EXPANSION TREATMENT

Once the diagnosis of maxillary transverse deficiency is made, the orthodontist must decide how to achieve an ideal, stable maxillary width. For most orthodontists, this decision is based primarily on the patient's age. For children in primary or early mixed dentition, banded continuous wire expanders, such as the quad helix or the W arch, are used most commonly. In older children and teens, banded jackscrew expanders, such as the hyrax or Haas expander, are used most often, with daily or twice daily activation. Adults with a narrow maxilla most often are candidates for surgically assisted RME or for segmental Le Fort I surgery, usually with banded jackscrew expanders. An active area of research has been the assessment the outcomes of each maxillary expansion treatment approach for which the PA cephalograph is an indispensible tool. In this section, we discuss the evidence-based efficacy of maxillary expansion treatment with an emphasis on radiology-based studies including those using CBCT.

Since the early 2000s, a series of systematic reviews (Harrison & Ashby, 2001; Schiffman & Tuncay, 2001; Petrén *et al.*, 2003; Lagravère *et al.*, 2005a, 2005b, 2005c; Gordon *et al.*, 2009; Verstraaten *et al.*, 2010; Baratieri *et al.*, 2011; Zuccati *et al.*, 2013) and traditional reviews (Neeley *et al.*, 2007; Suri & Taneja, 2008; Chrcanovic & Custódio, 2009) have been published in an attempt to consolidate the considerable clinical evidence regarding maxillary expansion and to determine which questions regarding diagnosis and treatment of maxillary transverse deficiency remain unanswered. A summary of key characteristics of the systematic reviews on maxillary expansion is presented in Table 17.2, and the research limitations identified in the available literature are presented in Table 17.3.

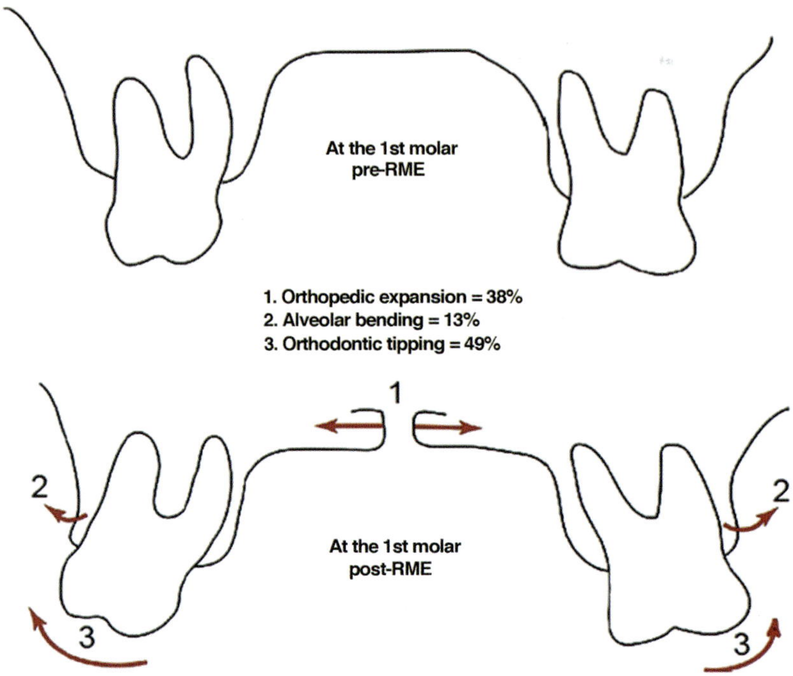

Figure 17.15 Contribution of skeletal expansion, alveolar bending, and dental tipping to total RME. Data such as these can be most accurately collected from coronal CBCT images. Note the significant average contribution of dental tipping to the overall expansion in teenage patients. (Reprinted with permission from Garrett *et al.*, 2008.)

Significant findings of the systematic reviews on maxillary expansion treatment

Spontaneous correction of posterior crossbites is possible in cases where the crossbite is generated by an occlusal interference and not a true skeletal constriction (e.g., when the interfering deciduous tooth is lost during the dentition transition and the mandible is allowed to position itself normally). Because these types of cases are relatively rare, spontaneous correction of posterior crossbites is extremely infrequent. Removal of premature contacts of deciduous teeth, however, is effective in preventing the perpetuation of posterior crossbites in selected cases. This clinical approach does not work when a true maxillary constriction exists, in which case some type of maxillary expansion will be required to correct the posterior crossbite (Harrison & Ashby, 2001).

When active intervention is required for correcting a constricted maxilla, the scientific literature offers no clear answer regarding which treatment approach is most effective. Commonly used approaches (e.g., grinding, expansion plates, quad-helices, and RME devices) are all effective when compared with no treatment, but comparisons between these approaches have not generated a clear best option. As one would expect, the success of expansion plates depends on patient compliance while wearing them, and RME is dependent on the parents to activate the expansion screw. Slow maxillary expansion appears to have less relapse compared with RME, but the difference is questionable clinically. It is noteworthy that the methodological quality of the publications using slow maxillary expansion devices is poorer than the publications using rapid maxillary expanders (Lagravère *et al.*, 2005c), thus it is not clear if slow maxillary expansion has improved long-term stability compared with other approaches.

Most of the studies examined a form of RME that produces a combination of skeletal and dental

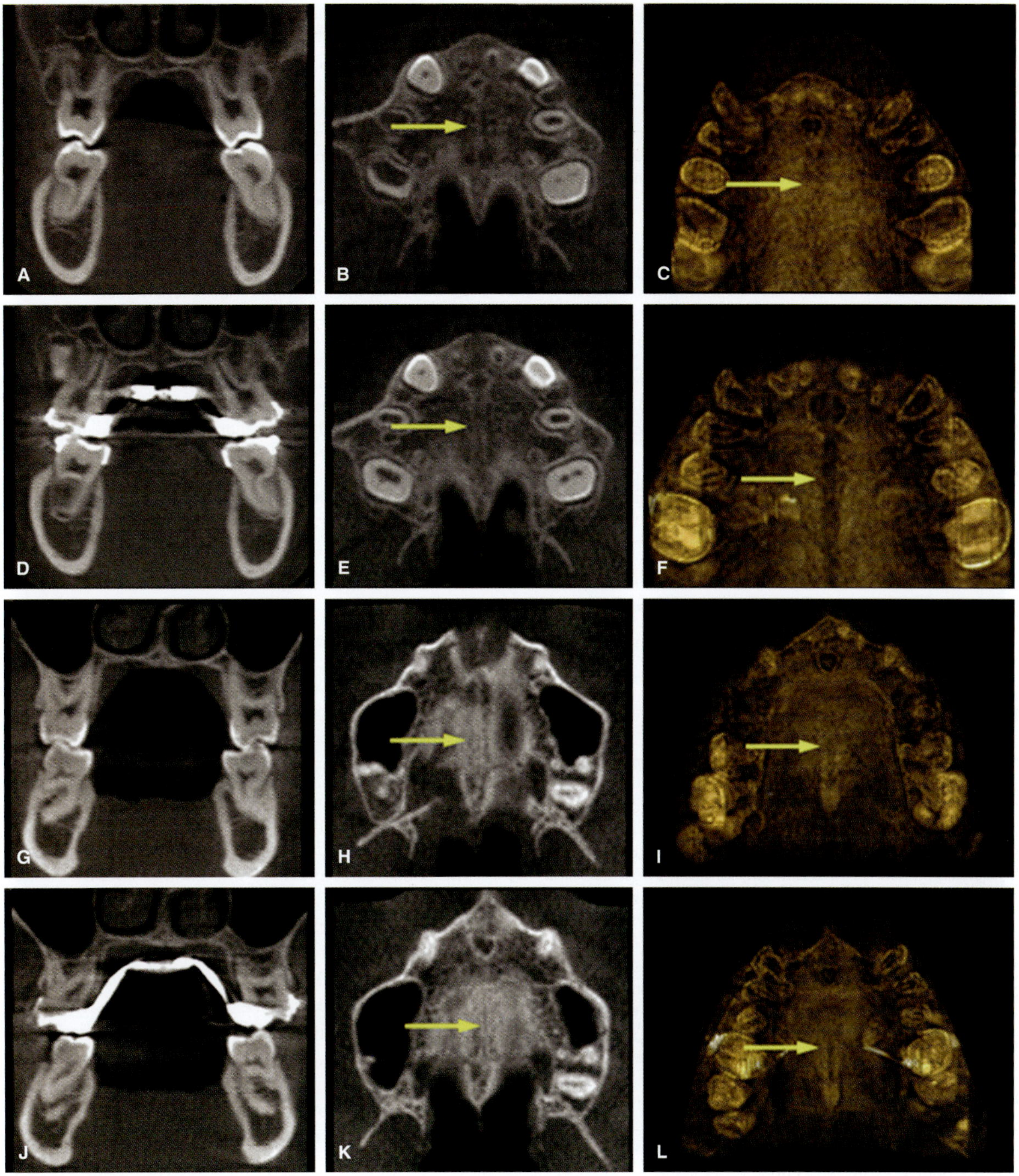

Figure 17.16 Midpalatal suture expansion using tooth-borne palatal expander demonstrates radiographic differences in responses of a patient with a V-shaped palate (*A–F*) compared with one with a U-shaped palate (*G–L*). Pretreatment coronal section, axial section, and 3D volumetric axial reconstruction of CBCT images of a patient with a palate that is V-shaped (*A*, *B*, and *C*, respectively) or U-shaped (*G*, *H*, and *I*, respectively) demonstrating similarity in the radiographic presentation of the intact sutures in both patients (arrows). Post-expansion images show significant dental tipping for both patients in the coronal sections (*D* and *J*). In contrast, the post-treatment axial sections (*E* and *K*) and volumetric axial reconstructions (*F* and *L*) show that while the patient with an initial V-shaped palate has substantial patency of the midpalatal suture, the patient with a U-shaped palate has little apparent suture patency (arrows).

Table 17.2 Snapshot of the included systematic reviews on maxillary expansion.

- Twelve systematic reviews were identified between 2001 and early 2012. Additionally, three conventional reviews were found.
- Based on maxillary expansion appliance type:
  - Five systematic reviews evaluated slow maxillary expansion appliances (quad-helix and expansion plates)
  - Eight assessed rapid maxillary expansion appliances (modified Hass and hyrax designs)
  - Two focused on surgically assisted maxillary expansion appliances (modified hyrax designs)
- None of the systematic reviews included bone-anchored maxillary expanders or archwire expansion.
- The sample sizes evaluated in these systematic reviews varied between 89 and 452 individuals.
- The Cochrane Collaboration group generated only one of the systematic reviews. The University of Alberta group generated the largest number of reviews with five.

Table 17.3 Limitations of the available evidence on maxillary expansion.

- The included studies identified in the systematic reviews almost always have glaring methodological problems, which limits the external validity of their conclusions and, by default, the systematic review conclusions themselves.
- Because patient recall is difficult, long-term post-retention results after maxillary expansion retention have not been conducted. Thus, much of our understanding of RME stability is based on short-term retention periods.
- Fixed orthodontic appliances (brackets and arch wires) usually follow the maxillary expansion after only a few months of retention. Therefore, true maxillary expansion effects assessed after orthodontic treatment represent the effects of RME plus additional orthodontic treatment used to finalize occlusion and esthetics.
- Authors rarely indicate how much expansion is needed in each subject nor do they indicate if the subject's crossbite was corrected. This can bias the conclusions of studies in which subjects with mild and severe maxillary transverse discrepancies are pooled because treatment times and modalities may differ.
- Studies that randomize subjects into a control group who did not receive maxillary expansion treatment until after the conclusion of the study, even though early RME treatment was indicated, are not included in the systematic reviews.

Table 17.4 Summary of the quantified long-term dental and skeletal effects of maxillary expansion.

- An intermolar width increase of 6–8 mm is possible.
- An intercanine width increase of 3–4 mm is possible.
- Only 20% of the total transverse expansion is truly skeletal in nature (based on regular expansion rates, this should be around 2 mm).
- No consistent transverse dental changes were identified.
- No effects on the anteroposterior and/or vertical mandibular position were demonstrable.
- Relapse is significant, with rates between 35% and 50%. This implies that permanent retention is required or a significant overexpansion is needed.
- It needs to be reinforced that these numbers are a reflection of the conventional amounts of maxillary expansion done clinically. In theory, more expansion can be attained, but the concomitant occlusal and facial implications make it unethical to explore.

transverse changes without clinically significant anterior-posterior and vertical changes; the summary of quantifiable changes is shown in Table 17.4. Similar effects have been noted for the other methods of maxillary expansion. Reported differences exist between the two most common RME devices (hyrax and Haas), but they are unlikely to be significant clinically (Harrison & Ashby, 2001; Schiffman & Tuncay, 2001; Petrén *et al.*, 2003; Lagravère *et al.*, 2005a, 2005b, 2005c; Zuccati *et al.*, 2013).

Other approaches to maxillary expansion include surgically assisted RME and bone-anchored RME. The expansion effects with surgically assisted maxillary expansion are similar to those obtained with RME alone, even though the palate and alveolar base are separated surgically from the maxillary complex prior to appliance activation. Moreover, significant relapse still is noticed (Lagravère *et al.*, 2006; Verstraaten *et al.*, 2010; Ribeiro *et al.*, 2012). Bone-anchored maxillary expansion is a relatively new treatment approach (Vyas *et al.*, 2009). Theoretically, this procedure should produce more skeletal than dental expansion effects; initial reports, however, have not shown that these appliances clearly are better than tooth-borne rapid or slow maxillary expansion devices (Lagravère *et al.*, 2010).

Expansion rate does not appear to alter RME outcomes significantly. Turning the expansion screw once every other day or twice per day is a decision that individual clinicians should make based on their experience. No systematic review has evaluated if any difference exists in maxillary expansion between bonding or banding the first premolars. Likewise, there is no review of data on the efficacy of maxillary expanders without premolar attachments.

Skeletal maturation status, more precisely maxillary suture interdigitation, is believed to have significant bearing in the magnitude of changes, although this has not been evaluated yet because, as noted earlier, there is no way to assess sutural maturation precisely in living subjects. Yet it is a commonly held belief that the earlier the maxillary expansion is performed, the greater the effect because the midpalatal suture is patent. Histological studies, however, indicate that this probably is not true (Melsen, 1975; Persson & Thilander, 1977; Wehrbein & Yildizhan, 2001; Knaup *et al.*, 2004; Korbmacher *et al.*, 2007). One biological explanation that may be valid in this regard is that bones in children are less dense and more elastic than bones in adults (Korbmacher *et al.*, 2007). Nonsurgical maxillary expansion may be successful because the expansion force is transmitted throughout the maxillary complex in children, whereas the decreased skeletal flexibility in adults redirects the expansion force along the path of least resistance, which is through the alveolus. This could account for the increased negative side effects of maxillary expansion, especially dehiscences and fenestrations, in adults. For a more detailed look at alveolar boundary condition changes following RME, see Chapter 14.

Two systematic reviews (Gordon *et al.*, 2009; Baratieri *et al.*, 2011) evaluated maxillary expansion effects on upper airway function. Although acoustic rhinometry (rhinomanometry) and CT showed an increase in specific regions of the nasal cavity and reduced nasal airway resistance with a related increase in nasal airflow, the magnitude of changes was not significant clinically. The evaluated outcomes, therefore, do not demonstrate a true change in the respiratory capability that is likely to have a significant effect on the patient's breathing habits. These reviews also noted that inflammatory conditions, exercise, head posture, and emotional and hormonal states could influence the nasal mucosa volume, affecting the measurements made during the study. These potential sampling concerns have clinical implications because it is important to assess individuals in their most decongested state so results can be compared over time or after an intervention. The reader is referred to Chapter 13 for additional details on potential effects of palatal expansion on airway changes.

This section summarized our current knowledge regarding maxillary expansion effects on craniofacial structures based on 2D radiography. It did not take into account the data generated exclusively from clinical or dental cast-based measurements. In the next section, we discuss how 3D radiology is influencing the conclusions drawn from these 2D radiographic studies.

MAXILLARY EXPANSION EFFECTS ASSESSED WITH 3D RADIOGRAPHS

3D radiography allows us to visualize craniofacial structures in a manner that previously was not possible. Medical CT scanners have been available since the early 1980s, and for the patients who required a medical scan of their heads, it allowed us a glimpse of the diagnostic power this technology could offer dental professionals. CBCT technology, specifically geared toward craniofacial applications, has been a valuable innovation for the dental profession. Since the early 2000s, there has been an increased use of CBCT images to diagnose and quantify treatment changes in many fields of dentistry, including orthodontics. An important question is this: how much has 3D imaging changed what we know about the treatment effects of maxillary expansion?

Because this is a relatively new tool, only one of the 12 previously identified systematic reviews (Baratieri *et al.*, 2011) tangentially evaluated 3D studies that were performed to determine the morphologic effects of maxillary expansion. Due to the lack of consolidated summaries, the investigators opted to discuss any clinical studies that used any form of 3D radiography and 3D volumetric changes in the quantification of maxillary expansion effects. A summary of some key descriptive data of the

Table 17.5 Snapshot of the included clinical trials using CT or CBCT.

- Thirty-three clinical trials or case series were identified between 2006 and early 2012. Some 87% were case series and 13% clinical trials.
- Based on expansion appliance type evaluated, 4% evaluated slow maxillary expansion appliances, 67% RME appliances, and 29% surgically assisted maxillary expansion appliances.
- A total of 225 adults and 487 children were examined in these studies.
- Most of the included studies used spiral or medical CT (71%). The remainder (29%) of the included studies used CBCT. This could have significant bearing as medical CTs are taken with the patients lying down. CBCT images may be taken with the patient lying down or sitting. The differences in the two patient positioning options are likely to introduce variability in soft tissues where some cephalometric landmarks are placed due the influences of gravity.
- The studies varied in the amount of expansion prescribed for the subjects. Some 16% of the studies expanded exactly 7 mm, while 84% of the studies expanded as clinically required, including overexpansion for relapse expectation.

included clinical papers can be found in Table 17.5, and important findings are summarized below.

Periodontal and dental effects

One clinical trial (Garib *et al.*, 2006) and three case series (Ballanti *et al.*, 2009; Gauthier *et al.*, 2011; Baysal *et al.*, 2012) were included in our review for this section. Regarding periodontal bone levels (Garib *et al.*, 2006; Ballanti *et al.*, 2009; Gauthier *et al.*, 2011), it appears that the clinical changes provide potentially few detrimental effects in the short term. As expected, bone resorption occurs in the pressure side and apposition in the tension side during this time such that the buccal alveolar bone thickness is reduced 30–60% and the palatal alveolar bone thickness is increased proportionally at the same rate (30–60%; Garib *et al.*, 2006; Ballanti *et al.*, 2009; Gauthier *et al.*, 2011). While the total alveolar width is maintained, however, reduction of buccal bone thickness can be considered to be a potentially important negative consequence of expansion. Therefore, the initial buccal bone thickness and height could be an important consideration in determining whether a patient may undergo adverse changes during expansion. Thus, in such situations, clinicians need to be careful when expanding the arch buccally. Regardless, a partial recovery of bone levels is observed 6 months following expansion. No data exist about the magnitude of this recovery and for how long it occurs.

Regarding dental root volumetric changes following RME (Baysal *et al.*, 2012), significant loss of 8–14% is noted for all evaluated teeth with a large variability between teeth. While some roots on specific teeth are affected more than others, considering the variances, the differences likely are not significant clinically. These studies provide volumetric rather than length measurements; therefore, it is not possible to extrapolate these findings to root length dimensional loss. These are important clinical findings as it is becoming clear that orthodontic treatment, including RME, produces more root resorption than expected (see Chapter 15).

Upper airway effects

Because no clinical trials on airway changes associated with palatal expansion were identified, nine case series on this topic are reviewed (Doruk *et al.*, 2007; Ramires *et al.*, 2008; Tausche *et al.*, 2009; Aras *et al.*, 2010; Deeb *et al.*, 2010; Seeberger *et al.*, 2010; Zhao *et al.*, 2010; Pangrazio-Kulbersh *et al.*, 2012; Ribeiro *et al.*, 2012). There is controversy regarding the area of the largest transverse increase in nasal dimensions following maxillary expansion. Reported nasal volume increase varied between 5% and 20% and is explained by differences between the anterior, middle, and posterior nasal areas. Most studies state that the largest changes occur in the anterior part of the nose. While even a small transverse increase in the posterior nasal area likely will generate a significant volumetric change in the airway, it is not known if this will suffice to overcome the restricted airflow in patients with an uncorrected narrow anterior nasal segment. Acoustic rhinometry also has shown that nasal volume increases after maxillary expansion (Doruk *et al.*, 2007; Aras *et al.*, 2010). Maxillary expansion did not have any effect on the nasal septum, while an increase in maxillary sinus volume was shown in one study (Pangrazio-Kulbersh *et al.*, 2012). Although most studies assume an improvement in nasal breathing concomitant to significant increases in airway dimensions, the reality is that no significant correlation exists between the amount of the transverse dental arch expansion and the increase in nasal volume. Similarly, an increase in nasal volume does not contribute to a clinically significant improvement in nasal breathing. Clinicians, therefore, need to exercise caution in implying that improved breathing is a positive side effect of maxillary expansion. In general, airway changes associated with palatal or maxillary expansion are unpredictable, and we have no exact quantification of how much upper airway flow is needed to detect a clinically significant improvement in breathing.

Although no changes in the nasopharynx were observed after maxillary expansion, oropharyngeal volume did increase, which is important because a narrow oropharyngeal volume is common in maxillary constricted cases (Zhao *et al.*, 2010; Ribeiro *et al.*, 2012). A substantial limitation in these airway studies is the lack of standardized head and tongue positioning while the image is taken, which could significantly affect the reliability of these measurements. Caution is recommended, therefore, in the interpretation of these results for clinical purposes.

Synchondrosis and sutural changes

No clinical trial on changes in synchondrosis and sutures following palatal expansion was identified, but three series of cases on this topic were reviewed (Ghoneima *et al.*, 2010; Leonardi *et al.*, 2010, 2011). Regarding the spheno-occipital synchondrosis (Leonardi *et al.*, 2010), a small widening with palatal expansion was demonstrated (approximately 0.5 mm, or a 20–30% increase), but there was a large variability in the findings. Similar changes have been shown for the circummaxillary sutures (Ghoneima *et al.*, 2010; Leonardi *et al.*, 2011). These studies demonstrate that maxillary expansion forces will most robustly affect sutures that articulate directly with the maxilla and have smaller effects on craniofacial sutures that are more distant from the maxilla. Clinically, the findings in this area need to be considered carefully. The magnitude of the changes is minimal and clearly within measurement error of most 3D radiographic studies. At least two voxels are required to define the interface between tissues and current measurement accuracies ranging from 0.4 to 0.6 mm. Thus, 0.5 mm changes in sutural widening following RME may not be accurate.

CONCLUSIONS

The maxilla has changed little in the more than 500 years since da Vinci drew the human skull with exquisite details of the maxillary sinus, teeth, and alveolar bone (Figure 17.1). Yet it took until the 20th and 21st centuries to develop the technological prowess to surpass what he taught us about the maxilla in the 15th century. As clinicians, we rely heavily on data generated using technological innovations in histology and radiology to advance our understanding of maxillary transverse development and also to improve our diagnostic and treatment capabilities for correction of maxillary constriction.

One of the great paradoxes of science is that with every question is answered, new questions appear. For all of our histological and radiological investigations of maxillary development, few clinicians or developmental biologists would say that we have a complete understanding of the topic. Histological studies have dispelled the idea that the midpalatal suture "fuses" as we age. The remarkable interindividual and intrasutural variability in the obliteration index and interdigitation index revealed by detailed histology raise the questions of "How and when does the suture acquire its morphology?" and "Why is the midpalatal suture's morphology so different along its length and between individuals?" These questions will be answered only when further technological innovations arrive.

3D radiographs have improved our understanding of the maxillary response to expansion therapy vastly, which initially came from conventional 2D PA cephalographs and occlusal radiographs. Yet improvements in the resolution of 3D radiographs still are needed to enable modern anatomists to dissect out the fine details of circummaxillary responses to RME. Even if these improvements arrive soon, the risks of irradiation are much too high to consider 3D radiology as the research tool of choice for assessing maxillary growth and treatment response in living subjects. It is for this reason that researchers are working aggressively to develop new, non-invasive imaging modalities that will give us the image resolution to assess growth and treatment changes fully in our patients. One such promising approach is ultrasound. Sumer and colleagues (2012) used ultrasound to assess the midpalatal suture in patients following surgically assisted RME. Their preliminary study demonstrates that ultrasound produces high-resolution images that are sensitive enough to allow for grading of sutural closure following expansion, which cannot be done with conventional radiographs. This information would be highly valuable for determining the appropriate retention time needed to ensure complete ossification of the newly expanded suture. Clinicians can look forward to major advances in imaging technologies such as ultrasound, which will improve diagnosis and treatment planning of skeletal malocclusions in children and adults.

References

Al-Azemi, R. & Årtun, J. (2012) Posteroanterior cephalometric norms for an adolescent Kuwaiti population. *European Journal of Orthodontics*, 34 (3), 312–317.

Aras, A., Akay, M.C., Cukurova, I., *et al.* (2010) Dimensional changes of the nasal cavity after transpalatal distraction using bone-borne distractor: an acoustic rhinometry and computed tomography evaluation. *Journal of Oral and Maxillofacial Surgery*, 68 (7), 1487–1497.

Athanasiou, A.E., Droschl, H., & Bosch, C. (1992) Data and patterns of transverse dentofacial structure of 6- to 15-year-old children: a posteroanterior cephalometric study. *American Journal of Orthodontics and Dentofacial Orthopedics*, 101 (5), 465–471.

Athanasiou, A.E., Miethke, R.R., & Van Der Meij, A.J. (1999) Random erros in localization of landmarks in postero-anterior cephalograms. *British Journal of Orthodontics*, 26 (4), 273–2834.

Ballanti, F., Lione, R., Fanucci, E., *et al.* (2009) Immediate and post-retention effects of rapid maxillary expansion investigated by computed tomography in growing patients. *The Angle Orthodontist*, 79 (1), 24–29.

Banerji, R. (2012) Leonardo da Vinci: how accurate were his anatomy drawings? *BBC World Service*, May 1, Available at http://www.bbc.co.uk/news/magazine-17907305, accessed May 1, 2012.

Baratieri, C., Alves, M., Jr., De Souza, M.M., *et al.* (2011) Does rapid maxillary expansion have long-term effects on airway dimensions and breathing? *American Journal of Orthodontics and Dentofacial Orthopedics*, 140 (2), 146–156.

Baysal, A., Karadede, I., Hekimoglu, S., *et al.* (2012) Evaluation of root resorption following rapid maxillary expansion using cone-beam computed tomography. *The Angle Orthodontist*, 82 (3), 488–494.

Chen, F., Terada, K., Yang, L., *et al.* (2008) Dental arch widths and mandibular-maxillary base widths in Class III malocclusions from ages 10 to 14. *American Journal of Orthodontics and Dentofacial Orthopedics*, 133 (1), 65–69.

Chrcanovic, B.R. & Custódio, A.L. (2009) Orthodontic or surgically assisted rapid maxillary expansion. *Oral and Maxillofacial Surgery*, 13 (3), 123–137.

Cortella, S., Shofer, F.S., & Ghafari, J. (1997) Transverse development of the jaws: norms for the posteroanterior cephalometric analysis. *American Journal of Orthodontics and Dentofacial Orthopedics*, 112 (5), 519–522.

da Silva Filho, O.G., Lara, T.S., de Almeida, A.M., *et al.* (2005) Evaluation of the midpalatal suture during rapid palatal expansion in children: a CT study. *Journal of Clinical Pediatric Dentistry*, 29 (3), 231–238.

Damstra, J., Fourie, Z., Huddleston Slater, J.J., *et al.* (2010) Accuracy of linear measurements from cone-beam computed tomography-derived surface models of different voxel sizes. *American Journal of Orthodontics and Dentofacial Orthopedics*, 137 (1), 16.e1–16.e6.

Deeb, W., Hansen, L., Hotan, T., *et al.* (2010) Changes in nasal volume after surgically assisted bone-borne rapid maxillary expansion. *American Journal of Orthodontics and Dentofacial Orthopedics*, 137 (6), 782–789.

Doruk, C., Sökücü, O., Biçakçi, A.A., *et al.* (2007) Comparison of nasal volume changes during rapid maxillary expansion using acoustic rhinometry and computed tomography. *European Journal of Orthodontics*, 29 (3), 251–255.

Edwards, C.B., Marshall, S.D., Qian, F., *et al.* (2007) Longitudinal study of facial skeletal growth completion in 3 dimensions. *American Journal of Orthodontics and Dentofacial Orthopedics*, 132 (6), 762–768.

Garib, D.G., Henriques, J.F., Janson, G., *et al.* (2006) Periodontal effects of rapid maxillary expansion with tooth-tissue-borne and tooth-borne expanders: a computed tomography evaluation. *American Journal of Orthodontics and Dentofacial Orthopedics*, 129 (6), 749–758.

Garrett, B.J., Caruso, J.M., Rungcharassaeng, K., *et al.* (2008) Skeletal effects to the maxilla after rapid maxillary expansion assessed with cone-beam computed tomography. *American Journal of Orthodontics and Dentofacial Orthopedics*, 134 (1), 8–9.

Gauthier, C., Voyer, R., Paquette, M., *et al.* (2011) Periodontal effects of surgically assisted rapid palatal expansion evaluated clinically and with cone-beam computerized tomography: 6-month preliminary results. *American Journal of Orthodontics and Dentofacial Orthopedics*, 139 (4 Suppl), S117–S128.

Gerrits, P.O. & Veening, J.G. (2012) Leonardo da Vinci's "A skull sectioned": skull and dental formula revisited. *Clinical Anatomy*, 26 (4), 430–435.

Ghoneima, A., Abdel-Fattah, E., Eraso, F., *et al.* (2010) Skeletal and dental changes after rapid maxillary expansion: a computed tomography study. *Australian Orthodontic Journal*, 26 (2), 141–148.

Gordon, J.M., Rosenblatt, M., Witmans, M., *et al.* (2009) Rapid palatal expansion effects on nasal airway dimensions as measured by acoustic rhinometry: a systematic review. *The Angle Orthodontist*, 79 (5), 1000–1007.

Gribel, B.F., Gribel, M.N., Frazão, D.C., *et al.* (2011) Accuracy and reliability of craniometric measurements on lateral cephalometry and 3D measurements on CBCT scans. *The Angle Orthodontist*, 81 (1), 26–35.

Handelman, C. (2011) Palatal expansion in adults: the nonsurgical approach. *American Journal of Orthodontics and Dentofacial Orthopedics*, 140 (4), 462–466.

Harrison, J.E. & Ashby, D. (2001) Orthodontic treatment for posterior crossbites. *Cochrane Database of Systematic Reviews*, (1), CD000979.

Hägg, U., Cooke, M.S., Chan, T.C., *et al.* (1998) The reproducibility of cephalometric landmarks: an experimental study on skulls. *Australian Orthodontic Journal*, 15 (3), 177–185.

Hesby, R.M., Marshall, S.D., Dawson, D.V., *et al.* (2006) Transverse skeletal and dentoalveolar changes during growth. *American Journal of Orthodontics and Dentofacial Orthopedics*, 130 (6), 721–731.

Kartalian, A., Gohl, E., Adamian, M., *et al.* (2010) Cone-beam computerized tomography evaluation of the maxillary dentoskeletal complex after rapid palatal expansion. *American Journal of Orthodontics and Dentofacial Orthopedics*, 138 (4), 486–492.

Kim, S.J., Park, S.B., Kim, Y.I., *et al.* (2012) The reliability of cone-beam computed tomography (CBCT)-generated frontal cephalograms. *J Craniomaxillofac Surg*, 40 (8), e331–e336.

Knaup, B., Yildizhan, F., & Wehrbein, H. (2004) Age-related changes in the midpalatal suture: a histomorphometric study. *Journal of Orofacial Orthopedics*, 65 (6), 467–474 (in English and German).

Korbmacher, H., Schilling, A., Püschel, K., *et al.* (2007) Age-dependent three-dimensional microcomputed tomography analysis of the human midpalatal suture. *Journal of Orofacial Orthopedics*, 68 (5), 364–376.

Korn, E.L. & Baumrind, S. (1990) Transverse development of the human jaws between the ages of 8.5 and 15.5 years, studied longitudinally with use of implants. *Journal of Dental Research*, 69 (6), 1298–1306.

Lagravère, M.O., Major, P.W., & Flores-Mir, C. (2005a) Long-term dental arch changes after rapid maxillary expansion treatment: a systematic review. *The Angle Orthodontist*, 75 (2), 155–161.

Lagravère, M.O., Major, P.W., & Flores-Mir, C. (2005b) Long-term skeletal changes with rapid maxillary expansion: a systematic review. *The Angle Orthodontist*, 75 (6), 1046–1052.

Lagravère, M.O., Major, P.W., & Flores-Mir, C. (2005c) Skeletal and dental changes with fixed slow maxillary expansion treatment: a systematic review. *Journal of the American Dental Association*, 136 (2), 194–199.

Lagravère, M.O., Major, P.W., & Flores-Mir, C. (2006) Dental and skeletal changes following surgically assisted rapid maxillary expansion. *International Journal of Oral and Maxillofacial Surgery*, 35 (6), 481–487.

Lagravère, M.O., Carey, J., Heo, G., *et al.* (2010) Transverse, vertical, and anteroposterior changes from bone-anchored maxillary expansion vs. traditional rapid maxillary expansion: a randomized clinical trial. *American Journal of Orthodontics and Dentofacial Orthopedics*, 137 (3), 304.e1–304.e12.

Leonardi, R., Annunziata, A., & Caltabiano, M. (2008) Landmark identification error in posteroanterior cephalometric radiography: a systematic review. *The Angle Orthodontist*, 78 (4), 761–765.

Leonardi, R., Cutrera, A., & Barbato, E. (2010) Rapid maxillary expansion affects the spheno-occipital synchondrosis in youngsters: a study with low-dose computed tomography. *The Angle Orthodontist*, 80 (1), 106–110.

Leonardi, R., Sicurezza, E., Cutrera, A., *et al.* (2011) Early post-treatment changes of circumaxillary sutures in young patients treated with rapid maxillary expansion. *The Angle Orthodontist*, 81 (1), 36–41.

Liu, F., van der Lijn, F., Schurmann, C., *et al.* (2012) A genome-wide association study identifies five loci influencing facial morphology in Europeans. *PLoS Genetics*, 8 (9), e1002932.

Lux, C.J., Conradt, C., Burden, D., *et al.* (2003) Dental arch widths and mandibular-maxillary base widths in

Class II malocclusions between early mixed and permanent dentitions. *The Angle Orthodontist*, 73 (6), 674–685.

Lux, C.J., Conradt, C., Burden, D., *et al.* (2004a) Three-dimensional analysis of maxillary and mandibular growth increments. *Cleft Palate Craniofacial Journal*, 41 (3), 304–314.

Lux, C.J., Conradt, C., Burden, D., *et al.* (2004b) Transverse development of the craniofacial skeleton and dentition between 7 and 15 years of age: a longitudinal postero-anterior cephalometric study. *European Journal of Orthodontics*, 26 (1), 31–42.

Malkoc, S., Sari, Z., Usumez, S., *et al.* (2005) The effect of head rotation on cephalometric radiographs. *European Journal of Orthodontics*, 27 (3), 315–321.

McNamara, J.A., Jr. (2002) Early intervention in the transverse dimension: is it worth the effort? *American Journal of Orthodontics and Dentofacial Orthopedics*, 121 (6), 572–574.

Melsen, B. (1975) Palatal growth studied on human autopsy material: a histologic microradiographic study. *American Journal of Orthodontics*, 68 (1), 42–54.

Neeley, W.W., II, Edgin, W.A., & Gonzales, D.A. (2007) A review of the effects of expansion of the nasal base on nasal airflow and resistance. *Journal of Oral and Maxillofacial Surgery*, 65 (6), 1174–1179.

Northway, W. (2011) Palatal expansion in adults: the surgical approach. *American Journal of Orthodontics and Dentofacial Orthopedics*, 140 (4), 463–467.

Nur, M., Kayipmaz, S., Bayram, M., *et al.* (2012) Conventional frontal radiographs compared with frontal radiographs obtained from cone beam computed tomography. *The Angle Orthodontist*, 82 (4), 579–584.

Pangrazio-Kulbersh, V., Wine, P., Haughey, M., *et al.* (2012) Cone beam computed tomography evaluation of changes in the naso-maxillary complex associated with two types of maxillary expanders. *The Angle Orthodontist*, 82 (3), 448–457.

Pérez, I.E., Chávez, A.K., & Ponce, D. (2011) Cephalometric norms from posteroanterior Ricketts' cephalograms from Hispanic Americans Peruvian non-adult patients. *Acta Odontológica Latinoamerica*, 24 (3), 265–271.

Persson, M. & Thilander, B. (1977) Palatal suture closure in man from 15 to 35 years of age. *American Journal of Orthodontics*, 72 (1), 42–52.

Petrén, S., Bondemark, L., & Söderfeldt, B. (2003) A systematic review concerning early orthodontic treatment of unilateral posterior crossbite. *The Angle Orthodontist*, 73 (5), 588–596.

Pirttiniemi, P., Miettinen, J., & Kantomaa, T. (1996) Combined effects of erros in frontal-view asymmetry diagnosis. *European Journal of Orthodontics*, 18 (6), 629–636.

Ramires, T., Maia, R.A., & Barone, J.R. (2008) Nasal cavity changes and the respiratory standard after maxillary expansion. *Brazilian Journal of Otorhinolaryngology*, 74 (5), 763–769.

Ribeiro, A.N., de Paiva, J.B., Rino-Neto, J., *et al.* (2012) Upper airway expansion after rapid maxillary expansion evaluated with cone beam computed tomography. *The Angle Orthodontist*, 82 (3), 458–463.

Ricketts, R.M., Roth, R.H., Chaconas, S.J., *et al.* (1982) *Orthodontic Diagnosis and Planning: Their Roles in Preventive and Rehabilitative Dentistry*. Rocky Mountain Data Systems, Denver, CO.

Schiffman, P.H. & Tuncay, O.C. (2001) Maxillary expansion: a meta analysis. *Clinical Orthodontics and Research*, 4 (2), 86–96.

Seeberger, R., Kater, W., Schulte-Geers, M., *et al.* (2010) Surgically assisted rapid maxillary expansion: effects on the nasal airways and nasal septum. *HNO*, 58 (8), 806–811 (in German).

Snodell, S.F., Nanda, R.S., & Currier, G.F. (1993) A longitudinal cephalometric study of transverse and vertical craniofacial growth. *American Journal of Orthodontics and Dentofacial Orthopedics*, 104 (5), 471–483.

Sumer, A.P., Ozer, M., Sumer, M., *et al.* (2012) Ultrasonography in the evaluation of midpalatal suture in surgically assisted rapid palatal expansion. *Journal of Craniofacial Surgery*, 23 (5), 1375–1377.

Suri, L. & Taneja, P. (2008) Surgically assisted rapid palatal expansion: a literature review. *American Journal of Orthodontics and Dentofacial Orthopedics*, 133 (2), 290–302.

Tausche, E., Deeb, W., Hansen, L., *et al.* (2009) CT analysis of nasal volume changes after surgically-assisted rapid maxillary expansion. *Journal of Orofacial Orthopedics*, 70 (4), 306–317 (in English and German).

Uysal, T. & Sari, Z. (2005) Posteroanterior cephalometric norms in Turkish adults. *American Journal of Orthodontics and Dentofacial Orthopedics*, 127 (3), 324–332.

van Vlijmen, O.J., Bergé, S.J., Swennen, G.R., *et al.* (2009a) A comparison of frontal radiographs obtained from cone beam CT scans and conventional frontal radiographs of human skulls. *International Journal of Oral and Maxillofacial Surgery*, 38, 773–778.

van Vlijmen, O.J., Maal, T.J., Bergé, S.J., *et al.* (2009b) A comparison between two-dimensional and three-dimensional cephalometry on frontal radiographs and on cone beam computed tomography scans of human skulls. *European Journal of Oral Sciences*, 117 (3), 300–305.

van Vlijmen, O.J., Rangel, F.A., Bergé, S.J., *et al.* (2011) Measurements on 3D models of human skulls derived from two different cone beam CT scanners. *Clinical Oral Investigations*, 15 (5), 721–727.

Vásquez, M.J., Baccetti, T., Franchi, L., *et al.* (2009) Dentofacial features of Class II malocclusion associated with maxillary skeletal protrusion: a longitudinal study at the circumpubertal growth period. *American Journal of Orthodontics and Dentofacial Orthopedics*, 135 (5), 568.e1–568.e7.

Verstraaten, J., Kuijpers-Jagtman, A.M., Mommaerts, M.Y., *et al.* (2010) A systematic review of the effects of bone-borne surgical assisted rapid maxillary expansion. *Journal of Craniomaxillofacial Surgery*, 38 (3), 166–174.

Vyas, R.M., Jarrahy, R., Sisodia, M., *et al.* (2009) Bone-borne palatal distraction to correct the constricted cleft maxilla. *Journal of Craniofacial Surgery*, 20 (3), 733–736.

Wagner, D.M. & Chung, C.H. (2005) Transverse growth of the maxilla and mandible in untreated girls with low, average, and high MP-SN angles: a longitudinal study. *American Journal of Orthodontics and Dentofacial Orthopedics*, 128 (6), 716–723.

Wehrbein, H. & Yildizhan, F. (2001) The mid-palatal suture in young adults: a radiological-histological investigation. *European Journal of Orthodontics*, 23 (2), 105–114.

Yavuz, I., Ikbal, A., Baydaş, B., *et al.* (2004) Longitudinal posteroanterior changes in transverse and vertical craniofacial structures between 10 and 14 years of age. *The Angle Orthodontist*, 74 (5), 624–629.

Zhao, Y., Nguyen, M., Gohl, E., *et al.* (2010) Oropharyngeal airway changes after rapid palatal expansion evaluated with cone-beam computed tomography. *American Journal of Orthodontics and Dentofacial Orthopedics*, 137 (4 Suppl), S71–S78.

Zuccati, G., Casci, S., Doldo, T., *et al.* (2013) Expansion of maxillary arches with crossbite: a systematic review of RCTs in the last 12 years. *European Journal of Orthodontics*, 35 (1), 29–37.

18 Planning and Placing Temporary Anchorage Devices with the Aid of Cone Beam Computed Tomography Imaging

Sebastian Baumgaertel, DMD, MSD, FRDC(C)

INTRODUCTION

Advances in medicine usually are driven by new developments in other basic sciences, which then are adapted to medical use. After a new technology has been used successfully in the medical field, it often finds its way into dentistry. Three-dimensional (3D) craniofacial imaging using cone beam computed tomography (CBCT) technology is no exception. Dental implantologists were early adopters of 3D CBCT imaging (Benjamin, 1987; Weinberg, 1993; Cavalcanti *et al.*, 2002). This should come as no surprise, since it can be beneficial to have maximum information on a given implant site to ensure that the implant is placed in the most ideal spatial relationship to the surrounding anatomical structures of relevance with the goal of improving the treatment outcome.

The same rationale can be applied to use of orthodontic miniscrew implants and other endosseous temporary anchorage devices (TADs). However, the simple fact that a certain technology such as CBCT or treatment approaches such as TADs are available does not mean these have to be used on a routine basis. The only way to decide if and when a certain procedure should find application in the diagnosis and treatment of patients is by conducting a diligent risk (cost)-benefit analysis as discussed in Chapters 1 and 6 and as described previously (Pochin, 1982; Zarin & Pauker, 1984; Cassidy *et al.*, 1993). It is the purpose of this chapter to illustrate if and when 3D imaging with CBCT technology should be used for planning and placing endosseous orthodontic TADs, and how best to utilize CBCT-based information for refined diagnosis and treatment planning for TADs.

ADVANTAGES AND DISADVANTAGES OF CBCT IMAGING FOR TAD APPLICATION

This part of the chapter is not intended to be a complete disquisition of the general advantages

Cone Beam Computed Tomography in Orthodontics: Indications, Insights, and Innovations, First Edition. Sunil D. Kapila.

Table 18.1 Anatomical structures that may be at risk during a miniscrew implant insertion.

Jaw	Insertion site	Anatomical structure	Damage risk
Maxilla	Buccal alveolar process	Dental roots	+
		Maxillary sinus	o
		Opposite side cortex	–
	Palatal alveolar process	Dental roots	o
		Maxillary sinus	o
		Opposite side cortex	–
		Greater palatine vein, artery, nerve	–
	Palate	Nasal cavity	o
		Incisive vein, artery, nerve	–
Mandible	Buccal alveolar process	Dental roots	+
		Inferior alveolar vein, artery, nerve	–
	Retromolar area	Inferior alveolar vein, artery, nerve	–

+, high risk; o, moderate risk; –, low risk.

and disadvantages of CBCT imaging, which are discussed elsewhere in this book (Chapters 1 and 6), but is simply a brief overview of the important factors to consider when deciding if image acquisition with this technology is appropriate for placing TADs in the specific case at hand.

Advantages

When placing an endosseous orthodontic TAD, the objective is to anchor the miniscrew securely in the surrounding bone and to avoid any damage to adjacent anatomical structures (Table 18.1). In other words, the miniscrew needs to be navigated through a volume of bone that is restricted by certain anatomical boundaries, which should not be violated by the implant. Depending on the selected insertion site, those spatial restrictions can be more or less pronounced. Some sites, such as the palate, come with only a single boundary in one direction, that is, the floor of the nose in the cranial direction. Other sites, such as the maxillary buccal alveolar process, for example, will come with mesial and distal limitations in terms of dental roots, with a lingual boundary in terms of the lingual cortex of the alveolar process and even cranial and caudal boundaries in terms of the maxillary sinus and dental roots or the alveolar crest, respectively. Obviously, the more boundaries that an insertion site has, the greater the level of precision required for a successful insertion and the greater the degree of difficulty of the insertion.

Without a doubt, it seems beneficial to visualize the different boundaries of a given insertion site, for only if it is known where the obstacle lies can you predictably avoid it. Plain film radiography does not afford that possibility. In the example of the maxillary buccal alveolar insertion site using a periapical or panoramic radiograph, the buccal and lingual surfaces are invisible and the mesial and distal boundaries may be prone to distortion. The same applies for the cranial and caudal boundaries. These limitations arise from the 2D nature of plain film radiography: structures lying in various planes all are depicted on the radiograph as lying in one plane of space (Figure 18.1).

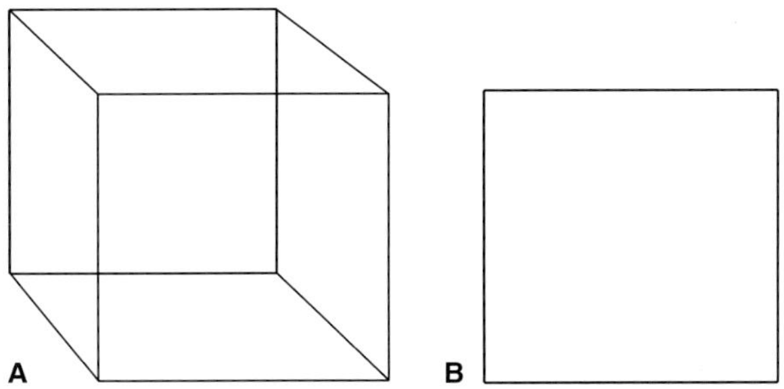

Figure 18.1 Schematic of a complex implant site with six surfaces. *A*: 3D perspective. *B*: Representation on a 2D plain film radiograph (orthogonal projection).

CBCT technology overcomes these limitations. It is possible to view all aspects of the insertion site on the computer screen, virtually, noninvasively, as though you are dissecting your actual patient. Modern software packages generally provide various perspectives that usually are customizable and adjustable based on the clinician's preference. It is possible to view a 3D model (volumetric view) of the entire scanned object or only parts of it or to create tomographic slices in all three planes of space and navigate through the volume in increments of designated thicknesses, which also are customizable (Kau *et al.*, 2005).

Going back to the example of the complex insertion site, CBCT technology allows an exact visual identification of the location, shape, and divergence of the mesial and distal dental roots, the floor of the maxillary sinus, and the buccal and lingual wall of the alveolar process. Qualitative assessments, therefore, can be made with much greater accuracy than on a regular 2D radiograph. Also, in contrast to plain film radiographs, CBCT data can be quantified using the appropriate software packages. Thus distances between two points such as interradicular distance or buccal bone thickness can be measured with considerable accuracy (Timock *et al.*, 2011); angulation between three points can be calculated (e.g., to determine root divergence); and the density of objects including bone can be assessed (Marquezan *et al.*, 2012). This additional information allows for a more detailed approach to planning and placing of the miniscrew implants. The use of this information in placing TADs will be discussed in the following section of this chapter.

Disadvantages

As can be expected, there are few disadvantages of CBCT imaging that relate directly to the planning and placement of an orthodontic miniscrew implant. More information can be helpful if used properly. Besides the general caveats of CBCT imaging noted elsewhere (see Chapters 1 and 6), which require a careful assessment of risk to benefit for each case prior to scanning for TAD placement, the only major disadvantage is that a large amount of information provided by the CBCT can lead to confusion or, even worse, may provide a false sense of security and override the clinical chairside assessment for inexperienced clinicians.

The transfer of the information obtained on the virtual model to the real patient also can be difficult. Imagine a runner that mapped a 5-mile run on his computer using one of the readily available mapping services, but then failed to take the exact route he or she had designed at the runner's computer once the run is begun. The reasons might be plentiful and the deviation could be attributed to distraction, confusion, false landmark identification, or imprecision—but the final result will be the same: the runner potentially either will run too far or will end up short. The same applies to the insertion of a miniscrew implant. Having all the information at the computer still does not guarantee a proper insertion, as many confounding factors can come into play, which can be referred to as the "virtual reality gap." How to mitigate the effect of such confounders will be explained in the section on evaluation of macroanatomical structures of this chapter.

APPROACHES FOR OPTIMAL CLINICAL UTILIZATION OF CBCTS FOR TADS

CBCT imaging protocol for TAD placement

Unless a large field of view (FOV) CBCT scan is needed for other purposes such as in individuals with skeletal discrepancies, asymmetries, or craniofacial anomalies (see Chapters 1 and 8), generally a small FOV, high resolution scan is recommended for placement of TADs. The image then should be utilized preferably in an interactive manner rather than as 2D printouts to define boundary conditions, to determine the location and angulation of insertion, to assess cortical dimensions and quality, and to derive an optimal treatment plan. Typically, a routine radiograph should suffice post-operatively to determine that the TAD has been placed in the desired location and does not impinge on other anatomical structures such as dental roots.

Macro- and microanatomical determinants for successful TAD insertion

We now will focus on the specifics of treatment planning for orthodontic miniscrew implant placement, which includes discussing how CBCT-generated information impacts the utilization of TADs in practice.

In order for an orthodontic miniscrew implant to be stable, it should be placed clear of dental roots and other sensitive anatomical structures, which forms the basis for macroanatomical diagnosis for TADs. Additionally, it needs adequate primary and secondary stability that, in turn, requires intimate contact between the bone and the implant surface immediately upon insertion and over the long-term duration of the miniscrew use, respectively. This stability likely is dependent on the microanatomical bone phenotype.

Evaluation of macroanatomical structures to minimize adverse TAD placement

Several anatomic structures may pose challenges to or limit the placement of TADs. These include dental roots, nasomaxillary cavities, nerves, and blood vessels. The limitations posed by these structures are discussed below together with strategies to minimize potential damage to or encroachment on these structures.

Dental roots

While it theoretically seems necessary to avoid the dental roots during a miniscrew insertion, the long-term sequelae for the roots are less detrimental as might be assumed (Kim & Kim, 2011). However, multiple publications have suggested that in terms of miniscrew stability and success, contact of the implant to the dental root substantially increases the likelihood of failure (Kuroda *et al.*, 2007; Asscherickx *et al.*, 2008; Chen *et al.*, 2008). Contact of the miniscrew and the roots of the adjacent teeth, hence, should be avoided under all circumstances.

Various studies have provided recommendations for suitable interradicular implant sites based on 3D imaging of either dry skulls or live untreated human jaws (Poggio *et al.*, 2006; Hu *et al.*, 2009; Kim *et al.*, 2009; Monnerat *et al.*, 2009). Because of differences in findings of various studies, the contradictory or conflicting conclusions and recommendations can be confusing to the practitioner. A major shortcoming of all these studies is clearly that root morphology can be extremely variable, rendering averages less useful. Also, the majority of miniscrews seem to be placed after the leveling and alignment phase of treatment, where root divergence or convergence can be introduced iatrogenically, creating a situation that has little relationship to the pre-treatment situation. It seems sensible, therefore, to perform pre-insertion imaging of the interradicular implant site to verify its suitability for TAD placement.

Planning an insertion with CBCT technology allows an accurate assessment of the spatial relationship of roots and the bone surface, which should result in a more precise insertion and a reduced probability of implant-to-root contact. In order to interpret the interradicular measurements accurately, however, the question of minimal safety distance or the minimal distance between the implant and a neighboring structure must be determined. For an interradicular insertion, this is the distance between the implant and the periodontal ligament (PDL). The relationship between interradicular distance (*IR*) and safety distance (*SD*) is as follows:

$$IR = 2 \times SD + \text{Implant Diameter}$$

Here, recommendations in the literature once again are variable. Maino and associates (2003) suggest a 2.5–3.0 mm distance between the roots for the use of the Spider Screw implant, which amounts to a safety distance of 0.5–0.75 mm depending on the diameter. On the other end of the spectrum, Liou and colleagues (2004) recommend a safety distance of 2 mm between the implant and the PDL due to their observation that miniscrews may migrate under load. Therefore, the overall recommended interradicular distances according to published sources range from 2.5 to 5.5–6.0 mm depending on the implant diameter. Thus, an example that represents a realistic clinical scenario in the author's practice is that a minimum interradicular distance of 3.6 mm should be present when using a 1.6 mm diameter implant resulting in a desired minimum safety distance of 1.0 mm.

If the interradicular distance is insufficient according to the CBCT-generated measurement, clinicians are advised to establish proper root divergence prior to inserting the miniscrew. This can be achieved through bracket repositioning or adding a root divergence bend to the archwire. Alternatively, a different site can be selected. One site that nearly always offers sufficient interradicular distance for palatal insertion is located between the maxillary second premolar and first molar (Poggio *et al.*, 2006). This is because the maxillary first molar has only a single palatal root offering adequate interradicular distance for TAD insertions (Figure 18.2).

Even an ideal interradicular insertion site such as the one mentioned above leaves, at best, only about 2 mm on either side of the miniscrew. The room for error and imprecision in terms of identifying the precise spot to insert the pin and the most ideal angulation, therefore, is limited. A purchase point located only 1 mm too far distal combined with a few degrees of additional distal angulation surely will lead the implant to be placed too close to the distal limits, namely the mesial edge of the palatal first molar root or mesio-buccal root of first molar, depending on the implant length, of the insertion site. A proper protocol should be in place, therefore, to transfer the information obtained from the CBCT scan to the patient. Two approaches stand out and have been proven effective clinically.

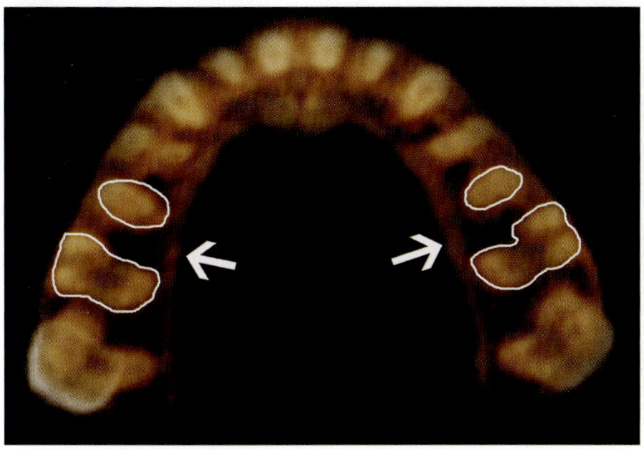

Figure 18.2 The greatest interradicular distance is located between maxillary second premolar and first molar for palatal insertions.

The first, which due to its simplicity, is this author's preferred approach is based on the use of fixed intraoral landmarks that are identified easily on a CBCT scan. The most useful landmark seems to be the interproximal contact of two adjacent teeth and a bracket or the wire. Once the location of the greatest interradicular distance is identified, the perpendicular distance from there to the chosen landmark is measured (Figure 18.3A). This measurement then is transferred easily to the patient using a periodontal probe (Figure 18.3B). The insertion spot is marked with the probe (Figure 18.3C) and the implant is inserted at that site (Figure 18.3D). The dominant shortcoming of this method is the variability in insertion angle, which can be controlled only with proper insertion technique and a steady hand. Novices will have greater difficulty with this technique than experienced clinicians and may choose to diverge roots more aggressively with orthodontic means prior to insertion. For the experienced practitioner, however, this method predictably can lead to successful insertions (Figure 18.3E,F).

The second approach borrows from techniques applied in the dental implant field: the use of laboratory-fabricated surgical stents like the method above allows proper identification of the insertion location and also safeguards the direction of insertion, essentially guiding the implant in 3D. Various techniques for this approach have been described in the literature (Suzuki & Suzuki, 2008; Miyazawa *et al.*, 2010). Most recently, Morea and coworkers (2011) detailed the use and outcome of a stereolithographic surgical guide fabricated from a CBCT scan (Figure 18.4). Using this group's technique, the placement of the TADs

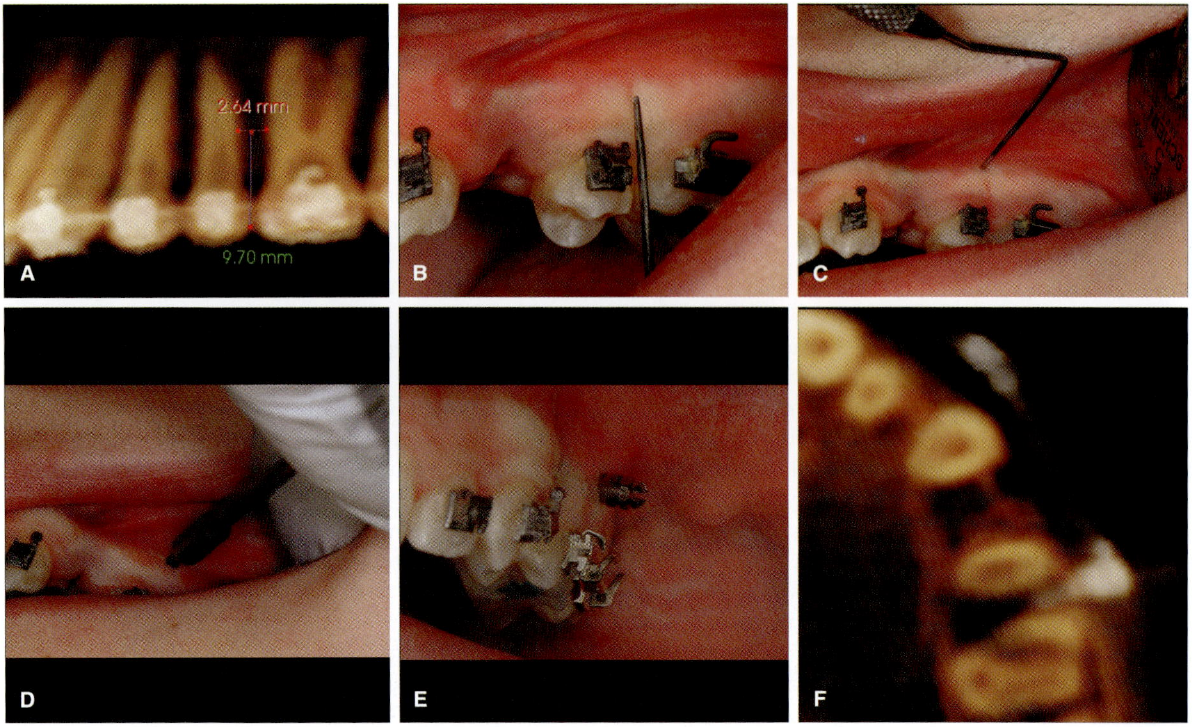

Figure 18.3 Locating and inserting TAD at optimal interradicular site. *A*: Generating measurements on the CBCT to identify the insertion site. *B*: Transfer of the measurements to the patient. *C*: Marking the designated insertion spot. *D*: Transmucosal insertion at the designated insertion spot. *E:* Miniscrew in place (TOMAS Pin, Dentaurum, Ispringen, Germany). *F:* CBCT follow-up to the placement of buccal implant.

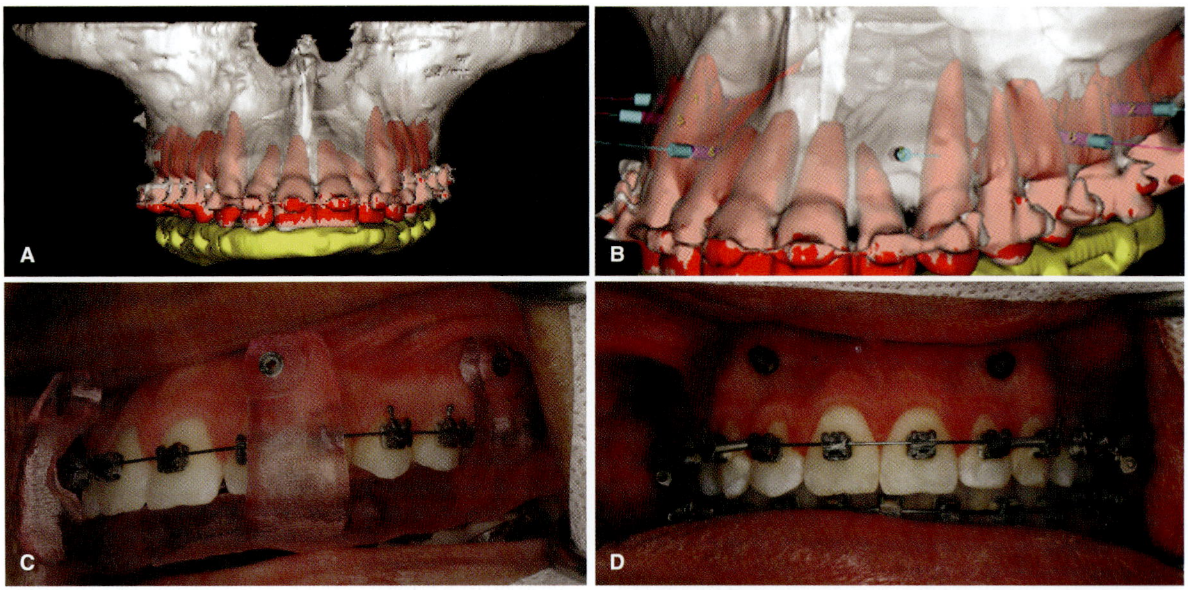

Figure 18.4 *A*: CBCT scan with positioning splint. *B*: CBCT scan with virtual TAD planning. *C*: Stereolithographic surgical guide in place. *D*: TADs placed successfully and accurately. (Images courtesy of Dr. Camillo Morea.)

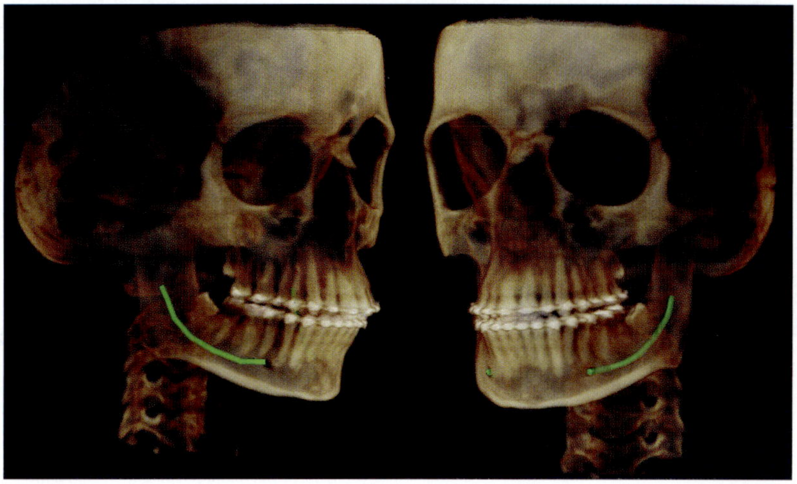

Figure 18.5 Right and left volumetric views with full course of inferior alveolar nerve illustrated (green line).

averaged less than 1 mm displacement and less than 2° variation from its planned position. While this approach comes with good precision and also is implemented easily for inexperienced clinicians, its shortcomings consist of greater cost and increased treatment time because the scan and implant insertion cannot be performed on the same day since guide fabrication is a laboratory procedure that takes time.

An additional aid in preventing or minimizing damage to roots or any other important structures may be the use of a sophisticated software package that allows virtual implant placement simulation. This will be discussed later in greater detail.

Nerves and blood vessels

Table 18.1 illustrates the structures at risk at various insertion sites. Most nerves and vessels can be avoided easily as their course generally is not in areas where miniscrew implants typically are placed. Nevertheless, the use of advanced software packages allows the illustration of the nerves and vessels both on volumetric images (Figure 18.5) and on tomographic images (Figure 18.6). This should make the inserting clinician highly cognizant of the individual course of the nerve of interest and further decrease the probability of violating these structures.

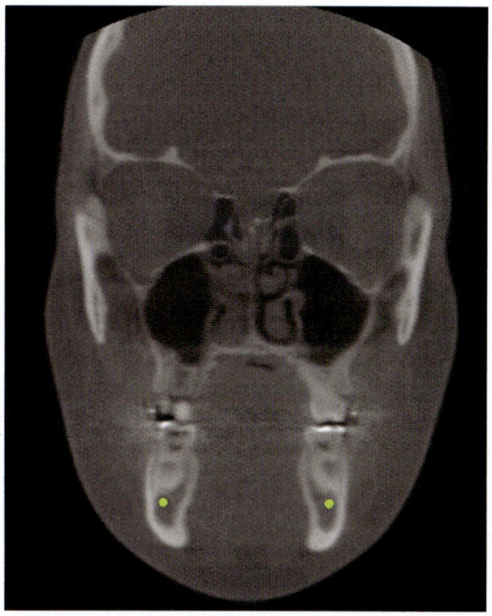

Figure 18.6 Coronal tomographic slice with inferior alveolar nerve illustrated (green dots).

Sinuses and nasal cavity

Three comprehensive anatomical studies (Baumgaertel, 2009, 2011; Baumgaertel & Hans, 2009) have demonstrated that maxillary insertions carry the risk of creating oral-antral perforations

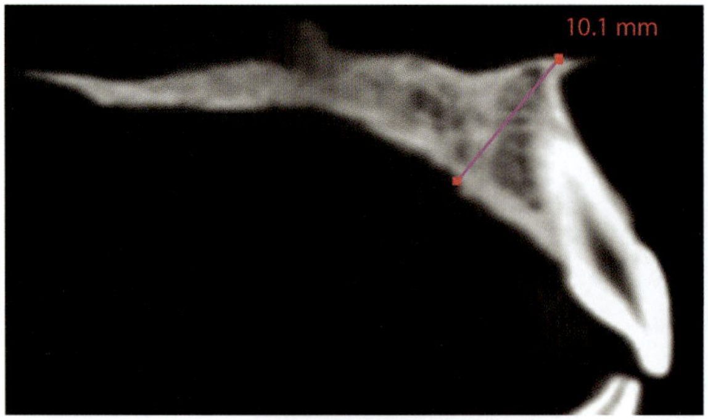

Figure 18.7 Bone depth assessment on a sagittal tomographic slice.

when inserting miniscrew implants. As may be obvious, such perforations can have various risks, including infection, and therefore should be avoided. Other authors have reported greater primary stability with bicortical anchorage and are advocates of targeting the contralateral cortex (Brettin *et al.*, 2008). A diligent risk-benefit assessment does not appear to support this approach in areas where the corresponding cortex forms the boundary of the sinus or other midfacial cavities.

To avoid perforation of the midfacial cavities, the ideal path of insertion can be determined by making a linear measurement from the desired implantation spot on the bone surface at the desired angle to assess the available bone depth. This should be followed by insertion of a miniscrew of appropriate length at the optimal site and angle (Figure 18.7; Baumgaertel & Hans, 2009).

CBCT-based microanatomical analysis for TADs

As pointed out previously, the stability and success of TADs depends on primary stability immediately following TAD placement and the longer-term secondary stability through the duration of its use during orthodontic treatment. Primary stability and its subsequent effect on secondary stability are determined in turn indirectly by insertion torque. These technical aspects of miniscrew implant success and the use of CBCT imaging for their assessment are discussed in greater depth.

Primary stability

Primary stability is defined as the stability of the implant immediately after the insertion (Martinez *et al.*, 2001) and results mainly from the mechanical retention of the implant shank in the bone. It can be measured in many different ways, but the most common assessments of primary stability include insertion torque (Wilmes *et al.*, 2008; Brinley *et al.*, 2009), pullout resistance (Brinley *et al.*, 2009), and resonance frequency analysis (RFA; Su *et al.*, 2009). Various studies have investigated which factors might impact primary stability of miniscrew implants and generally can be divided into three categories, as outlined below.

Implant design

Generally speaking, the greater the implant diameter, the greater the compression of the bone during the insertion and the greater the resulting primary stability (Wilmes *et al.*, 2008). Therefore, conical implants and larger diameter implants present greater initial mechanical retention than cylindrical and small diameter implants (Lim *et al.*, 2008).

Insertion technique

To obtain adequate primary stability, an intimate contact between the implant surface and the bone needs to be established. Therefore, it appears reasonable that the ideal insertion technique should consist of a gentle and steady clockwise rotation with minimal deviation from the ideal path of insertion (Baumgaertel *et al.*, 2008). Additionally, incorporating a pre-drilling procedure will reduce primary stability, simply because it removes a small amount of bone that otherwise would increase mechanical retention. This negative effect on primary stability increases with increasing diameter of the pilot hole (Heidemann *et al.*, 1998).

Microanatomical factors

The dominant anatomical factors that influence primary stability of the miniscrew are the quantity and the quality of the bone at the insertion site. The cortical bone is responsible primarily for the mechanical retention (Dalstra *et al.*, 2004).

Therefore, it is reasonable to presume that the thickness of this layer of bone will determine the primary stability of the miniscrew implant to a large degree. This implies that thick cortical bone will create greater primary stability than thin cortical bone (Wilmes *et al.*, 2006).

The other factor that is becoming an increasing focus of research is the density of the bone. In implant dentistry, this parameter long has been implemented into the planning of a dental implant insertion using medical CT scans (Matteson *et al.*, 1996). It has been demonstrated that increased cortical bone density may have a positive effect on primary stability of miniscrew implants while the overall density at a given insertion site may not (Marquezan *et al.*, 2012). The same working group, however, published a paper only months earlier in which bone density was shown to have no influence on primary stability of miniscrew implants (Marquezan *et al.*, 2011). Thus, at the time of this writing, the jury is still out on how important this factor is regarding miniscrew implant's primary stability and overall success.

Secondary stability

Secondary stability is defined as the stability of the implant at the conclusion of the healing period during which intense bone remodeling can be observed. It can be attributed to "positive remodeling," which constitutes bone formation at the bone-implant interface and the surrounding bone (O'Sullivan *et al.*, 2004; Wilmes *et al.*, 2006). Secondary stability typically is assessed by either RFA or removal torque (O'Sullivan *et al.*, 2004). The latter approach is valid only when used in a live patient or animal model.

While secondary stability also relies on adequate mechanical retention, it is additionally a function of the host response to the implant insertion and results to a large degree from a favorable biologic response. It is secondary stability, not primary stability, that is important for the long-term survival of the miniscrew implant (Baumgaertel, 2010).

Adequate primary stability is a prerequisite for good secondary stability: if the TAD is mobile, (i.e., lacking primary stability after the insertion), it is unrealistic to expect good healing and an intimate adaptation of the bone along the implant surface. Unfortunately, high primary stability does not translate necessarily to good secondary stability. Therefore, it is important to control the host response as much as possible. The most effective way to achieve good primary stability that translates into good secondary stability is by controlling the insertion torque during the placement (Motoyoshi *et al.*, 2006).

Managing insertion torque levels using CBCT

Insertion torque is a proxy measure for the compression of the bone during the insertion and, hence, is a popular measurement for primary stability. It can be measured with various gauges and controlled with certain implant instruments. Low values of this measurement usually mean that poor bone-to-implant contact exists and the mechanical retention of the implant in the bone is insufficient. High values usually mean that the implant is wedged in the bone with the expectation of excellent primary stability. As opposed to inserting a screw into wood, which is an inert material, bone is capable of a biologic response. Herein lies the shortcoming of developing a clinical protocol purely on the results of investigations of primary stability. It long has been demonstrated that excessive compression of the bone carries the risk of substantial damage in terms of microfractures and compression osteonecrosis, which usually will result in resorptive remodeling (Soltesz *et al.*, 1982; Huiskes & Nunamaker, 1984; Ueda *et al.*, 1991). This obviously carries the potential of loosening the miniscrew implant over time (Baumgaertel, 2010). Therefore, the optimum result usually is expected to be at medium torque levels where primary stability is sufficient for high levels of success and bone damage is minimal, allowing for adaptive, depository remodeling and good secondary stability (Motoyoshi *et al.*, 2006).

CBCT technology constitutes a valuable instrument for managing insertion torque. It provides valuable pre-treatment information on the anatomical properties of the implant site including the important microanatomical factors, namely cortical bone thickness and cortical bone density. This imaging thus provides the clinician with the insight necessary to choose the most appropriate implant

Table 18.2 Clinical recommendations for pre-drilling based on cortical bone thickness at the insertion site (Baumgaertel, 2010).

Cortical bone thickness	<0.5 mm	0.5–1.5 mm	1.5–2.5 mm	>2.5 mm
Recommended procedure	Insertion not recommended	No pre-drilling required	Perforate cortical bone only with 1 mm diameter round bur	Perforate cortical bone with 1 mm diameter round bur and then pre-drill with drill bit 1.1 mm diameter, 4 mm length

site and constitutes a powerful aide in determining which implant insertion protocol may be best at any given implant site.

Several studies point to the importance of determining cortical bone quantity and quality in the success of miniscrew implants. Motoyoshi and associates (2006) have shown the importance of medium torque levels for successful miniscrew implant outcomes, while Wilmes and colleagues (2006) demonstrated the influence of cortical bone thickness on insertion torque levels. Heidemann and coworkers (1998) showed that the most effective technique to reduce excessively high insertion torques is the incorporation of a pre-drilling procedure in the insertion protocol. Based on such information and clinical experience, the author has designed an insertion protocol (Table 18.2) contingent on the thickness of the cortical bone and uses it routinely for TAD placement with great success (Baumgaertel, 2010).

A pre-treatment CBCT scan of a patient provides information on the cortical bone thickness at the insertion site, which then delivers a general insertion torque range to be expected. If the cortical bone falls into a range offering the ideal torque, a direct insertion without any further implant site preparation would be the preferred approach to miniscrew implant placement. If the cortical bone is expected to offer excessive torque, pre-drilling can be incorporated into the insertion protocol that will lower the insertion torque into the ideal range and increase the probability for a successful insertion and longevity of the TAD.

VIRTUAL MINISCREW IMPLANT INSERTION

Virtual miniscrew implant insertion can serve as an additional approach to avoid dental roots or other

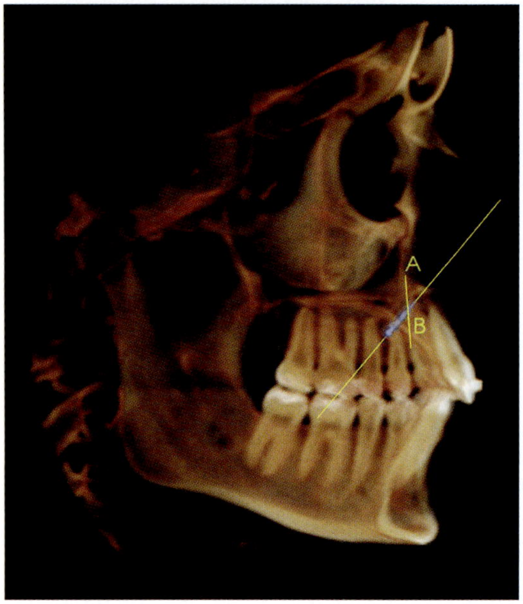

Figure 18.8 Virtually inserted palatal miniscrew. Software: InVivo by Anatomage.

anatomical structures during TAD insertion. This is a powerful tool that essentially constitutes the link between the planning stage and the insertion stage and enables a clinician to undertake a "dry run" prior to the actual insertion of the TAD.

With the use of sophisticated software packages such as InVivo (Anatomage, San Jose, CA) or Dolphin 3D (Dolphin Imaging, Chatsworth, CA), one can customize implant design and dimensions to fit the miniscrew intended for insertion and then position it at the desired location and angulation (Figure 18.8). Visual assessment of the implant's final position allows evaluation of its relationship to adjacent structures, which may lead to modifications of the insertion angle or implant length

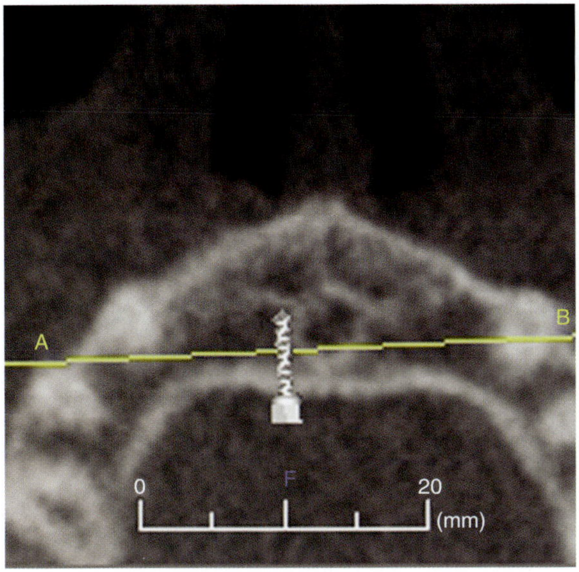

Figure 18.9 Axial tomographic slice of maxillary arch demonstrating anticipated miniscrew position relative to incisive canal.

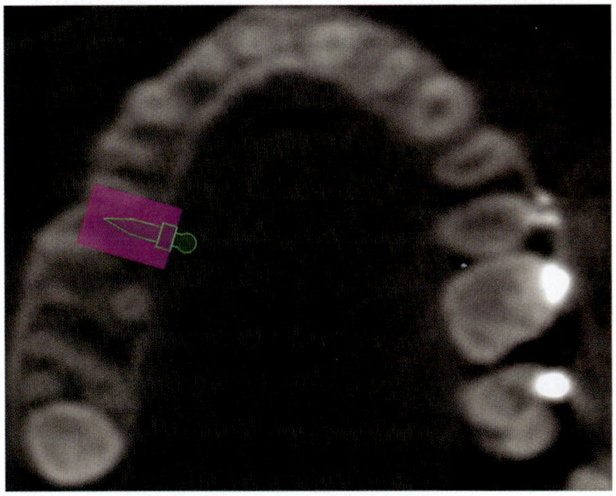

Figure 18.10 Safety distance around miniscrew outlined using Dolphin 3D (Dolphin Imaging software).

during the actual insertion (Figure 18.9). To make the virtual insertion outcome more meaningful and allow visual quantification, Dolphin 3D has a built-in safety distance option that, if selected, projects a halo of a specified radius around the miniscrew (Figure 18.10) and provides the clinician with a sense of the latitude that might exist in the placement of the TAD.

OUTCOMES ASSESSMENT

Outcome of treatments with TADs can be assessed using CBCT technology at two distinct levels: the immediate outcome of TAD placement post-operatively, and comparing the pre- and post-treatment situations to assess and better understand the overall treatment effects.

Post-op insertion evaluation

After treatment planning and placing the miniscrew, the clinician expects a certain outcome. If the virtual insertion option was used, an ideal final result exists already—on the computer screen. However, multiple sources of inaccuracy can cause the real final result to deviate from the planned scenario. It can be beneficial to compare the two for different reasons.

The first reason is quality control. If a patient was anesthetized profoundly for the insertion, most of the adjacent structures will be numbed and the patient will not be able to feel pain until the anesthetic has worn off. In the meanwhile, the practitioner needs to rule out damage to sensitive structures and ensure that the insertion went as planned. Periapical radiographs, while popular and quickly taken, provide only limited information as they are prone to distortion. CBCT imaging allows a much more precise assessment of the treatment outcome. A shortcoming of this technology, however, is that metal objects produce considerable scatter, which later shows screws with greater diameter and length and undefined borders on the scan (Benavides *et al.*, 2012). If a miniscrew was placed close to a structure (e.g., a root), it still will be difficult to determine whether or not the PDL was violated (Figure 18.11).

A modified insertion technique (Baumgaertel Mini-Implant Protocol) can provide some clarity if the anesthesia is performed according to Baumgaertel's "Biofeedback Anesthesia Method" (BAM) such that the PDL of the adjacent roots remains sensitive. A painless insertion here is a guarantee

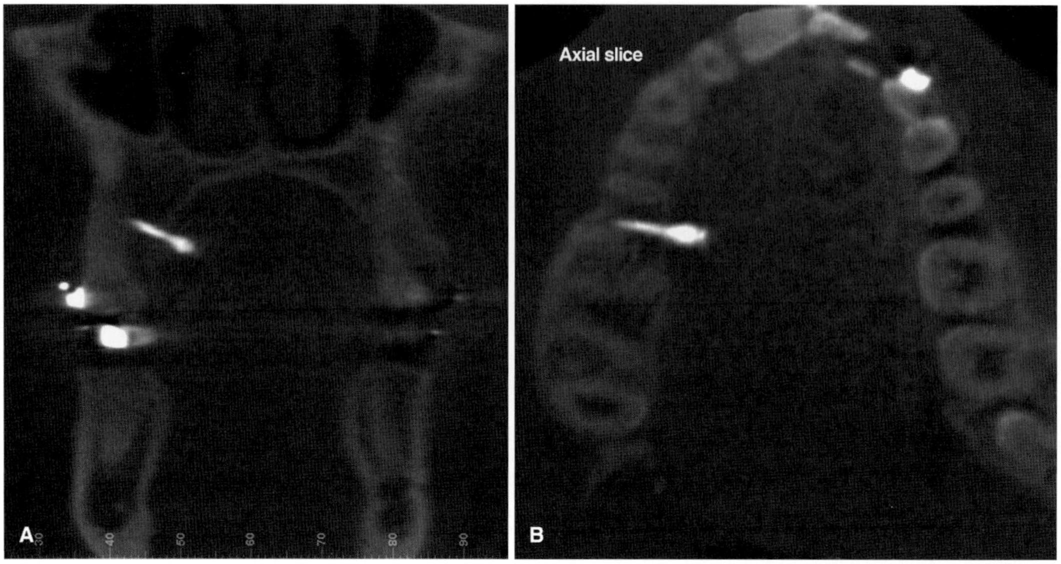

Figure 18.11 Insertion outcome of a miniscrew placed into the palatal alveolar process between second premolar and first molar. *A*: Coronal view. *B*: Axial view.

for an insertion that did not violate any anatomical structures inadvertently. As a matter of fact, post-op imaging to rule out damage to other structures is not necessary when the BAM is used and can help minimize additional radiation (Baumgaertel *et al.*, 2008). This point is exemplified by the case presented in Figure 18.11: the miniscrew appears to be touching the root. However, the patient did not experience any discomfort upon insertion using the BAM. Therefore, it is highly unlikely that actual contact between the screw and the root took place. The misinterpretation of the images can be attributed to scatter radiation and alteration of the screw dimensions on the scan. This is a useful example of how findings from diagnostic imaging should be placed in the perspective of clinical observations.

The second reason for a post-op insertion outcome evaluation is clinician self-assessment. The orthodontist placing miniscrews should evaluate if the implemented clinical protocol led to the desired outcome or at least be aware of how close the final result came to the plannned "ideal insertion." This self-assessment is the primary and important approach to improve future TAD insertions. While a review of the final miniscrew position can be interesting, it is more meaningful if compared with the virtually placed implant (Figure 18.12). Large discrepancies between the two show a need for reduction of the virtual reality gap. This can be achieved either by modifying the protocol to ensure better transfer of the planned miniscrew position to the patient or by improving the practitioner's insertion skills.

Evaluation of treatment outcomes

Radiographic evaluations of orthodontic treatment outcomes are nearly as old as the specialty itself. Most of the traditional approaches have relied on the use of various superimposition techniques of pre- and post-treatment lateral cephalograms (Julius, 1974; McGonagle, 1978). This approach is certainly still an option using CBCT technology, whereby the 3D dataset can be converted to 2D data (cephalogram) and used for comparison. However, it makes little sense to use a technology of the new millennium, whose benefit includes the generation of a great amount of information, and then reduce it purposely to implement an approach that was developed for technology of the

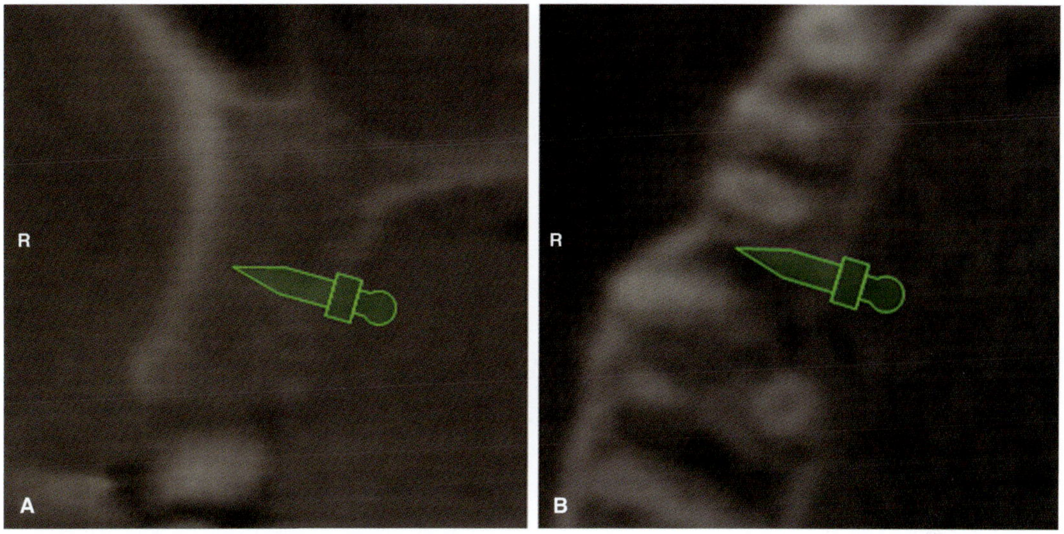

Figure 18.12 Treatment planning for the miniscrew shown in Figure 18.11. *A*: Coronal view of virtual insertion. *B*: Axial view of virtual insertion.

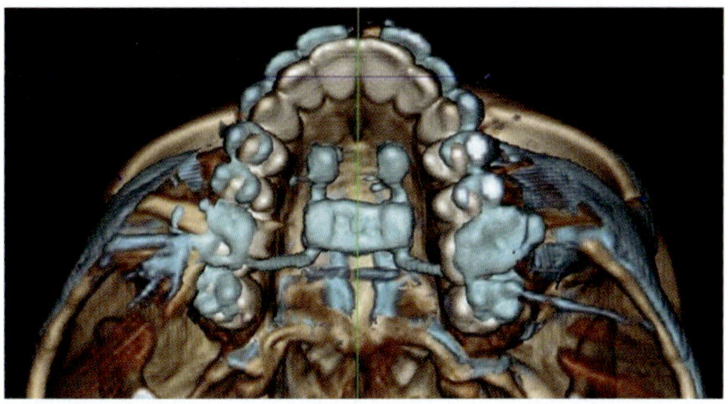

Figure 18.13 3D superimposition of pre-treatment and post-expansion time points using the Hybrid-Hyrax advancer. Tan, pre-expansion; blue, post-expansion. (Reprinted with permission of the *Journal of Clinical Orthodontics*.)

last millennium. Instead, using appropriate software such as Geomagic (Stuttgart, Germany; Ludwig *et al.*, 2010), treatment outcomes with TADs can now be assessed in 3D. This technique utilizes best-fit approach that superimposes images on cranial structures, and then, by choosing appropriate landmarks, both skeletal and dental changes can be evaluated (Figure 18.13). These methods are discussed in greater detail elsewhere in this textbook (see Chapters 19 and 21).

CONCLUSIONS

To date, it has not been proven scientifically that the use of CBCT imaging leads to greater miniscrew success, reduced likelihood of damage to adjacent structures, or superior treatment outcomes in general. This needs to be kept in mind when making the decision on using this technology for the purpose of placing TADs. While the use of CBCT imaging is by no means essential to successfully using TADs, it certainly comes with a number of advantages that can be helpful to both beginners and experienced users of orthodontic miniscrews. This chapter provides a comprehensive, yet critical overview of the potential benefits of using CBCT technology as an adjunct to traditional diagnosis when planning treatment for orthodontic miniscrew implant insertions.

A general rule of thumb should be that CBCT imaging should be considered as a diagnostic tool in cases where questions exist about the intended insertion site. The settings of the apparatus should generate the lowest possible radiation while still delivering diagnostic images (Kwong *et al.*, 2008). This typically implies using the smallest possible FOV unless the CBCT is needed for diagnosis of other conditions or for superimposition analysis, in which case a larger FOV may be preferred.

CBCT imaging currently is not considered the standard of care for TAD insertions. Indeed, the standard of care for imaging or treatment planning procedures required for TADs has not yet been defined. Because of this and until future studies have further addressed several questions posed in this chapter, the type of imaging used to insert miniscrews is likely to depend on the individual practitioner's preference and treatment philosophy.

References

Asscherickx, K., Vande Vannet, B., Wehrbein, H., *et al.* (2008) Success rate of miniscrews relative to their position to adjacent roots. *European Journal of Orthodontics*, 30 (4), 330–335.

Baumgaertel, S. (2009) Quantitative investigation of palatal bone depth and cortical bone thickness for mini-implant placement in adults. *American Journal of Orthodontics and Dentofacial Orthopedics*, 136 (1), 104–108.

Baumgaertel, S. (2010) Pre-drilling of the implant site: is it necessary for orthodontic mini-implants? *American Journal of Orthodontics and Dentofacial Orthopedics*, 137 (6), 825–829.

Baumgaertel, S. (2011) Cortical bone thickness and bone depth of the posterior palatal alveolar process for mini-implant insertion in adults. *American Journal of Orthodontics and Dentofacial Orthopedics*, 140 (6), 806–811.

Baumgaertel, S. & Hans, M.G. (2009) Buccal cortical bone thickness for mini-implant placement. *American Journal of Orthodontics and Dentofacial Orthopedics*, 136 (2), 230–235.

Baumgaertel, S., Razavi, M.R., & Hans, M.G. (2008) Mini-implant anchorage for the orthodontic practitioner. *American Journal of Orthodontics and Dentofacial Orthopedics*, 133 (4), 621–627.

Benavides, E., Rios, H.F., Ganz, S.D., *et al.* (2012) Use of cone beam computed tomography in implant dentistry: the International Congress of Oral Implantologists Consensus Report. *Implant Dentistry*, 21 (2), 78–86.

Benjamin, L.S. (1987) Versatility of the subperiosteal implant utilizing CAD-CAM multiplanar diagnostic imaging. *Journal of Oral Implantology*, 13 (2), 282–296.

Brettin, B.T., Grosland, N.M., Qian, F., *et al.* (2008) Bicortical vs. monocortical orthodontic skeletal anchorage. *American Journal of Orthodontics and Dentofacial Orthopedics*, 134 (5), 625–635.

Brinley, C.L., Behrents, R., Kim, K.B., *et al.* (2009) Pitch and longitudinal fluting effects on the primary stability of miniscrew implants. *Angle Orthodontist*, 79 (6), 1156–1161.

Cassidy, D.W., Jr., Herbosa, E.G., Rotskoff, K.S., *et al.* (1993) A comparison of surgery and orthodontics in "borderline" adults with Class II, division 1 malocclusions. *American Journal of Orthodontics and Dentofacial Orthopedics*, 104 (5), 455–470.

Cavalcanti, M.G., Ruprecht, A., & Vannier, M.W. (2002) 3-D volume rendering using multislice CT for dental implants. *Dentomaxillofacial Radiology*, 31 (4), 218–223.

Chen, Y.H., Chang, H.H., Chen, Y.J., *et al.* (2008) Root contact during insertion of miniscrews for orthodontic anchorage increases the failure rate: an animal study. *Clinical Oral Implants Research*, 19 (1), 99–106.

Dalstra, M., Cattaneo, P.M., & Melsen, B. (2004) Load transfer of miniscrews for orthodontic anchorage. *Orthodontics*, 1, 53–62.

Heidemann, W., Gerlach, K.L., Gröbel, K.H., *et al.* (1998) Influence of different pilot hole sizes on torque measurements and pullout analysis of osteosynthesis screws. *Journal of Craniomaxillofacial Surgery*, 26 (1), 50–55.

Hu, K.S., Kang, M.K., Kim, T.W., *et al.* (2009) Relationships between dental roots and surrounding tissues for orthodontic miniscrew installation. *Angle Orthodontist*, 79 (1), 37–45.

Huiskes, R. & Nunamaker, D. (1984) Local stresses and bone adaptation around orthopedic implants. *Calcified Tissue International*, 36 (Suppl. 1), 110–117.

Julius, R.B. (1974) The reliability of metallic implant and anatomic cephalometric superimposition techniques for the maxilla and mandible. *American Journal of Orthodontics*, 65 (3), 318–319.

Kau, C.H., Richmond, S., Palomo, J.M., *et al.* (2005) Three-dimensional cone beam computerized tomography in orthodontics. *Journal of Orthodontics*, 32 (4), 282–293.

Kim, H. & Kim, T.W. (2011) Histologic evaluation of root-surface healing after root contact or approximation during placement of mini-implants. *American Journal of Orthodontics and Dentofacial Orthopedics*, 139 (6), 752–760.

Kim, S.H., Yoon, H.G., Choi, Y.S., *et al.* (2009) Evaluation of interdental space of the maxillary posterior area for orthodontic mini-implants with cone-beam computed tomography. *American Journal of Orthodontics and Dentofacial Orthopedics*, 135 (5), 635–641.

Kuroda, S., Yamada, K., Deguchi, T., *et al.* (2007) Root proximity is a major factor for screw failure in orthodontic anchorage. *American Journal of Orthodontics and Dentofacial Orthopedics*, 131 (Suppl. 4), S68–S73.

Kwong, J.C., Palomo, J.M., Landers, M.A., *et al.* (2008) Image quality produced by different cone-beam computed tomography settings. *American Journal of Orthodontics and Dentofacial Orthopedics*, 133 (2), 317–327.

Lim, S.A., Cha, J.Y., & Hwang, C.J. (2008) Insertion torque of orthodontic miniscrews according to changes in shape, diameter and length. *Angle Orthodontist*, 78 (2), 234–240.

Liou, E.J., Pai, B.C., & Lin, J.C. (2004) Do miniscrews remain stationary under orthodontic forces? *American Journal of Orthodontics and Dentofacial Orthopedics*, 126 (1), 42–47.

Ludwig, B., Glasl, B., Bowman, S.J., *et al.* (2010) Miniscrew-supported class III treatment with the hybrid RPE advancer. *Journal of Clinical Orthodontics*, 44 (9), 533–539.

Maino, B.G., Bednar, J., Pagin, P., *et al.* (2003) The spider screw for skeletal anchorage. *Journal of Clinical Orthodontics*, 37 (2), 90–97.

Marquezan, M., Souza, M.M., Araújo, M.T., *et al.* (2011) Is miniscrew primary stability influenced by bone density? *Brazilian Oral Research*, 25 (5), 427–432.

Marquezan, M., Lau, T.C., Mattos, C.T., *et al.* (2012) Bone mineral density. *Angle Orthodontist*, 82 (1), 62–66.

Martinez, H., Davarpanah, M., Missika, P., *et al.* (2001) Optimal implant stabilization in low density bone. *Clinical Oral Implants Research*, 12 (5), 423–432.

Matteson, S.R., Deahl, S.T., Alder, M.E., *et al.* (1996) Advanced imaging methods. *Critical Reviews of Oral Biological Medicine*, 7 (4), 346–395.

McGonagle, R.R. (1978) B. Holly Broadbent, Sr. (1894–1977). *American Journal of Orthodontics*, 73 (5), 580–581.

Miyazawa, K., Kawaguchi, M., Tabuchi, M., *et al.* (2010) Accurate pre-surgical determination for self-drilling miniscrew implant placement using surgical guides and cone-beam computed tomography. *European Journal of Orthodontics*, 32 (6), 735–740.

Monnerat, C., Restle, L., & Mucha, J.N. (2009) Tomographic mapping of mandibular interradicular spaces for placement of orthodontic mini-implants. *American Journal of Orthodontics and Dentofacial Orthopedics*, 135 (4), 428.e1–428.e9.

Morea, C., Hayek, J.E., Oleskovicz, C., *et al.* (2011) Precise insertion of orthodontic miniscrews with a stereolithographic surgical guide based on cone beam computed tomography data: a pilot study. *International Journal of Oral and Maxillofacial Implants*, 26 (4), 860–865.

Motoyoshi, M., Hirabashi, M., Uemura, M., *et al.* (2006) Recommended placement torque when tightening an orthodontic mini-implant. *Clinical Oral Implants Research*, 17 (1), 109–114.

O'Sullivan, D., Sennerby, L., & Meredith, N. (2004) Influence of implant taper on the primary and secondary stability of osseointegrated titanium implants. *Clinical Oral Implants Research*, 15 (4), 474–480.

Pochin, E. (1982) Risk and medical ethics. *Journal of Medical Ethics*, 8 (4), 180–184.

Poggio, P.M., Incorvati, C., Velo, S., *et al.* (2006) "Safe zones": a guide for miniscrew positioning in the maxillary and mandibular arch. *Angle Orthodontist*, 76 (2), 191–197.

Soltesz, U., Siegele, D., Riedmüller, J., *et al.* (1982) Stress concentration and bone resorption in the jaw for dental implants with shoulders. In Lee, A.J.C., Albrektsson, T., & Branemark, P.I. (eds.), *Clinical Applications of Biomaterials*. Wiley and Sons, Chichester, pp. 115–122.

Su, Y.Y., Wilmes, B., Hönscheid, R., *et al.* (2009) Application of a wireless resonance frequency transducer to assess primary stability of orthodontic mini-implants: an in vitro study in pig ilia. *International Journal of Oral and Maxillofacial Implants*, 24 (4), 647–654.

Suzuki, E.Y. & Suzuki, B. (2008) Accuracy of miniscrew implant placement with a 3-dimensional surgical guide. *Journal of Oral and Maxillofacial Surgery*, 66 (6), 1245–1252.

Timock, A.M., Cook, V., McDonald, T., *et al.* (2011) Accuracy and reliability of buccal bone height and thickness measurements from cone-beam computed tomography imaging. *American Journal of Orthodontics and Dentofacial Orthopedics*, 140 (5), 734–744.

Ueda, M., Matsuki, M., Jacobsson, M., *et al.* (1991) The relationship between insertion torque and removal torque analyzed in fresh temporal bone. *International Journal of Oral Maxillofacial Implants*, 6 (4), 442–447.

Weinberg, L.A. (1993) CT scan as a radiologic data base for optimum implant orientation. *Journal of Prosthetic Dentistry*, 69 (4), 381–385.

Wilmes, B., Rademacher, C., Olthoff, G., *et al.* (2006) Parameters affecting primary stability of orthodontic mini-implants. *Journal of Orofacial Orthopedics*, 67 (3), 162–174.

Wilmes, B., Su, Y.Y., & Drescher, D. (2008) Insertion angle impact on primary stability of orthodontic mini-implants. *Angle Orthodontist*, 78 (6), 1065–1070.

Zarin, D.A. & Pauker, S.G. (1984) Decision analysis as a basis for medical decision making: the tree of hippocrates. *Journal of Medicine and Philosophy*, 9 (2), 181–213.

19 3D Planning and Treatment Outcomes of Bone Anchored Maxillary Protraction

Tung Nguyen, DMD, MS

INTRODUCTION

Patients with Class III malocclusion account for a small percentage of the population (Proffit *et al.*, 1998) but are among the most difficult to treat. Treatment goals for obtaining positive overjet for these Class III patients are accomplished through a combination of orthopedic correction and dentoalveolar compensation. The current standard for early treatment involves the use of reverse pull headgear (RPHG). This approach has limitations, however, since the forces are applied directly to the teeth, resulting in uncertain skeletal change and often unwanted dentoalveolar effects. Short-term studies on RPHG show limited orthopedic protraction of the maxilla, a clockwise rotation of the mandible, and dentoalveolar compensations, including the proclination of the maxillary incisors and retroclination of the mandibular incisors (Ishii *et al.*, 1987; Baik, 1995; Gallagher *et al.*, 1998; Kim *et al.*, 1999; Macdonald *et al.*, 1999; Kama *et al.*, 2006). In addition, facemask therapy largely has been shown to be successful in the primary or early mixed dentition (Baccetti *et al.*, 2000). Finally, long-term follow-up of maxillary protraction shows that there is an approximate 25–33% chance of relapse to negative overjet once growth is completed (Hagg *et al.*, 2003; Westwood *et al.*, 2003; Baccetti *et al.*, 2004). With the recent increase in use of temporary anchorage devices (TADs) in orthodontic treatment, the concept of maxillary protraction has been revisited and adapted in an attempt to minimize the unwanted dentoalveolar effects while maximizing orthopedic change (Singer *et al.*, 2000; Enacar *et al.*, 2003; Hong *et al.*, 2005; Cornelis *et al.*, 2007; Kircelli & Pektas, 2008). This chapter provides a review of the current status of protocols used for bone anchored maxillary protraction (BAMP) and the treatment outcomes in 3D when using this approach to correct Class III malocclusion.

Cone Beam Computed Tomography in Orthodontics: Indications, Insights, and Innovations, First Edition. Sunil D. Kapila.

TWO-DIMENSIONAL (2D) ANALYSIS OF BAMP

Treatment outcomes of the BAMP protocol until recently have been studied using conventional two-dimensional (2D) imaging. De Clerck and coworkers (2010) compared 21 consecutively treated BAMP patients to 18 untreated Class III patients who were matched with the treatment group based on the severity of malocclusion, age, sex, and duration of observation. The study showed that BAMP produced significant orthopedic maxillary protraction as well as mandibular restraint when compared with untreated Class III controls. The authors also reported a decrease in the mandibular plane angle and decompensation of the lower incisor following BAMP treatment. Additionally, the treatment effects of BAMP using thin-plate spline analysis revealed a marked forward displacement of the maxilla with more moderate favorable changes in the mandible and no change in the vertical dimension (Baccetti *et al.*, 2011).

A subsequent study compared the effectiveness of BAMP versus conventional Class III therapy that utilized face mask (FM) combined with rapid maxillary expansion (RME/FM) in treating Class III malocclusion (Cevidanes *et al.*, 2010). The BAMP protocol produced significantly larger maxillary advancement than RME/FM therapy. Vertical changes were controlled better with BAMP than with RME/FM therapy. Finally, relative to the RME/FM treatment, BAMP treatment resulted in no counterclockwise rotation of the mandible, lack of retroclination of the lower incisors, and a greater improvement in the sagittal intermaxillary relationships.

RATIONALE FOR USING 3D IMAGING IN ASSESSING TREATMENT EFFECTS

For the last half-century, the lateral cephalometric head film has been the standard radiographic image used to aid in diagnosis and treatment planning of orthodontic malocclusions. Recent advances of three-dimensional (3D) radiographic imaging in dentistry have made it possible to gain substantially greater information than conventional 2D imaging. There is no doubt that accurate images of the craniofacial region are critical for the development of a good diagnosis and treatment plan. However, there are some limitations with standard 2D imaging that particularly impact on the ability to achieve a comprehensive understanding of treatment outcomes. Until recently, diagnosis, treatment planning, and assessment of change over time have been based on the use of 2D landmarks. Angular and linear measurements between landmarks provide useful information about change over time in the anteroposterior and vertical planes of space, but even then, the assessment is based on change that occurred at discrete points placed on a 2D rendering of a 3D object. An inherent limitation in this approach is the inability to assess how entire surfaces, rather than discrete points, changed. Furthermore, the lateral cephalogram provides no information with regard to the transverse plane of space, while the postero-anterior (PA) cephalogram is of only limited value for assessing change in this dimension. It seems clear that the greater amount of information acquired with 3D imaging techniques has the potential to allow for more thorough diagnosis, treatment planning, and assessment of changes in anatomy and position of facial structures over time.

Although the introduction of conventional computed tomography (CT) enhanced the potential to derive high quality, accurate 3D images of any anatomic region, the associated expense and high ionizing radiation has limited its use in dentistry. The recent advances in 3D dental radiographic imaging, including the introduction of cone beam computed tomography (CBCT; Kapila & Farman, 2003; Ludlow *et al.*, 2006), provide a lower cost and lower radiation alternative to view maxillofacial region in 3D via a digital representation of the patient's anatomy as it exists in nature. This imaging approach represents a definite advantage over traditional 2D views whose caveats include rotational, geometric, and head positioning errors (Lou *et al.*, 2007). These errors may lead to inaccurate representation of anatomic landmarks, poor visualization of some structures, or inaccurate recording of growth and/or treatment changes (Park *et al.*, 2006). In addition, the problem of necessary image calibration for magnification of the 2D projection also is eliminated with CBCT data. Traditional 2D imaging always yields some level of projection error due to the fact that the anatomic area of interest is some distance from the film onto which the image is being projected. CBCT projections are orthogonal, which implies that the X-ray beams are parallel to one another, and the source-to-object distance is small, resulting in little projection error. The small amount of projection error that exists is corrected by the CBCT scanner's software, resulting in one-to-one data (Mah & Hatcher, 2004). Thus, the use of this imaging modality offers advantages to the detailed study of the effects of BAMP on changes in maxillary and mandibular anatomy and position in correction of Class III malocclusions.

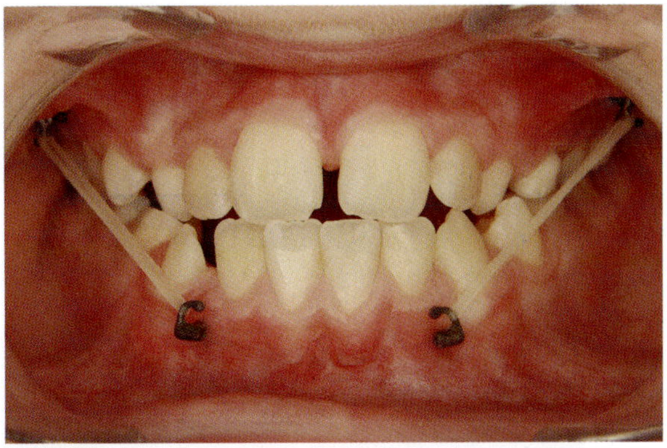

Figure 19.1 Hooks on bone anchors inserted into the underlying bone for engaging intermaxillary elastics to deliver forces to the maxilla and mandible.

CLINICAL METHODOLOGY AND PROTOCOLS

In recent years, titanium miniplates (or bone anchors) have been modified for orthodontic use. They offer certain advantages over miniscrews, including increased stability, rigid fixation, and placement at sites away from the roots (Cornelis *et al.*, 2007). At the 2003 European Orthodontic Society meeting, De Clerck presented treated cases that introduced the idea of BAMP as a means to obtain orthopedic correction in young Class III patients as outlined below.

Surgical and orthopedic protocol

In the original protocol, four Bollard miniplates were placed in each patient—two in each infrazygomatic crest of the maxilla and two in the anterior mandible between the lateral incisor and canine. Surgical flaps were reflected at these sites and the plates were secured with titanium screws (2.3 mm diameter and length of 5–7 mm; Cornelis *et al.*, 2008). The titanium miniplates were modified to include an extension arm that emerges in attached gingiva at or near the mucogingival junction. In addition, the miniplates contained hooks for the application of interarch elastics (Figure 19.1).

The miniplates were loaded 3 weeks after surgery. Class III vector elastics were applied between the hooks of the miniplates with an initial loading force of approximately 150 g to each side and gradually increased to 250 g (Figure 19.1). Patients were instructed to wear the elastics 24 hours per day with instructions to replace the elastics at least once per day. The duration of treatment was approximately 12 months when adequate positive overjet was achieved (De Clerck *et al.*, 2009). In many of the cases, an ovecorrection of the overjet was achieved.

Imaging protocol

To analyze the treatment changes in 3D, CBCT scans were taken after placement of the miniplates and after approximately 1 year of treatment. The scans were acquired with an iCat machine (Imaging Sciences International, Hatfield, PA) with a 40-second scan and a 16 cm × 22 cm field of view (FOV). Image analysis of each CBCT was processed using the methods described by Cevidanes and colleagues (2009). Briefly, the native Digital Imaging and Communications in Medicine (DICOM) format files were compressed to a 0.5 mm voxel isotropic Guys Image Processing Lab (GIPL) volume file to prepare for the segmentation of the models. Segmentation is the process of outlining the 3D surface of anatomic structures from each cross-sectional slice of the CBCT data (axial, coronal, and sagittal; Figure 19.2). This semi-automatic process is performed using ITK-SNAP (Yushkevich *et al.*, 2006) and employs an algorithm that expands a

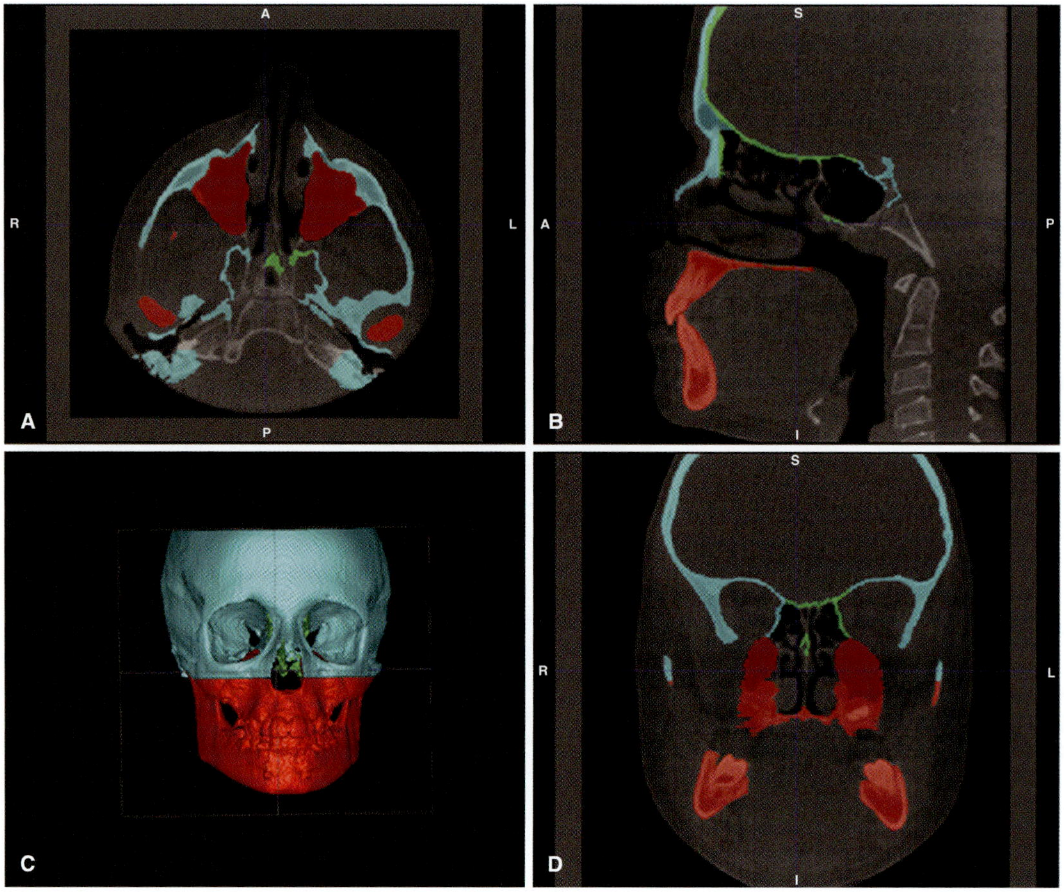

Figure 19.2 The 3D segmented model in ITK-SNP in axial (*A*), sagittal (*B*), and coronal (*D*) multiplanar reconstructions and in 3D (*C*). Regions of interest such as the cranial base, maxilla, mandible, and teeth can be labeled with different colors for visualization and analysis.

deformable bubble until it reaches the predefined anatomic border. The borders themselves are set by either threshold intensity or edge surfaces. While the process is fairly accurate for anatomic regions with dense bone or regions where the neighboring borders have distinct differences in grayscale levels, it tends to fail in regions with thin cortical bone such as the glenoid fossa and pterygoid plates or when anatomic borders are not demarcated well (Periago *et al.*, 2008). For these regions, manual segmentation is necessary.

To access growth and treatment changes, the longitudinal models first must be registered on a stable nongrowing region. For the purposes of assessing treatment outcomes with BAMP, the anterior cranial fossa, specifically the endocranial surfaces of the cribiform plate region of the ethmoid bone and the internal surface of the frontal bone regions, were chosen because of their early completion of growth (Figure 19.3; Cevidanes *et al.*, 2009). This registration step was performed on the grayscale volumes rather than the segmented models and utilizes a sequence of fully automated voxel-wise rigid registration using the Imagine software, developed by the National Alliance of Medical Imaging Computing. This process is computing-intensive but is necessary to eliminate operator bias and avoid segmentation errors that can

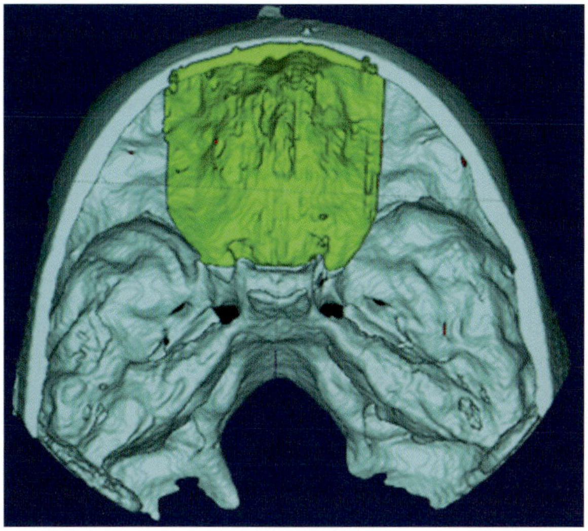

Figure 19.3 Masked 3D image showing the stable region of cranial base registration in green.

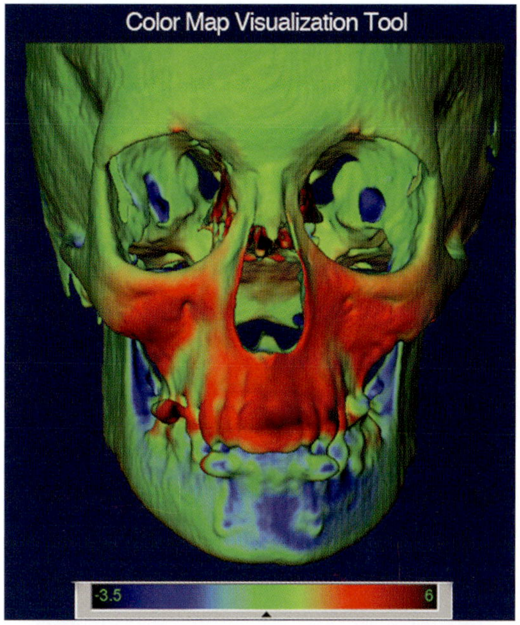

Figure 19.4 3D superimposition color map visualization tools. With the color map tool, areas in red represent surface distances with outward movement from T1 to T2 models. Areas in blue represent surfaces with inward movement between the two time points, while areas that are green have little or no change in surface distance between the T1 and T2 models. The color scale bar at the bottom depicts the range of the magnitude of changes from −3.5 mm inward movement mainly localized to the mandible to 6 mm outward movement primarily observed in the maxilla and maxillary teeth.

produce registration and superimposition errors. To verify the accuracy of the registration, the registered T1 and T2 CBCTs were superimposed and the grayscale volumes of the anterior cranial fossa were viewed slice by slice to determine an accurate fit. In addition, surface models of the registered and superimposed anterior cranial fossa were generated and measured to validate the accuracy of the registration. The steps for measurements between superimposed models are described below.

After the registration process, the T1 and T2 models were superimposed to assess treatment change in 3D. The visualization software used in these cases was CMFApp (developed by the Institute for Surgical Technology and Biomechanics, Bern, Switzerland; Chapuis *et al.*, 2007). The treatment changes were expressed via color maps that represent the closest-point surface distance from the final model to the initial one. Areas on the red end of the spectrum have positive mean surface-distance values and represent outward movement. Areas on the blue end of the spectrum have negative mean surface-distance values and represent inward movement. Areas that are green depict little or no change in surface distance between the initial and final models (Figure 19.4). For additional quantitative assessment of the changes between the T1 and T2 models, the isoline tool was used (Heymann *et al.*, 2010). It allows the user to define a surface-distance value that then is expressed as a contour line (isoline) that corresponds to regions having a surface distance equal to or greater than the defined value. The color map allows for both visual and quantitative assessments of treatment changes. An alternative way of illustrating the treatment change is to superimpose both 3D models, modifying the final model to be semi-transparent or in mesh-like surface so that the underlying initial model can be visualized (Figure 19.5). This tool provides a qualitative assessment of the areas and magnitudes of change.

The reliability of the 3D superimpositions was tested by three examiners, each of whom created

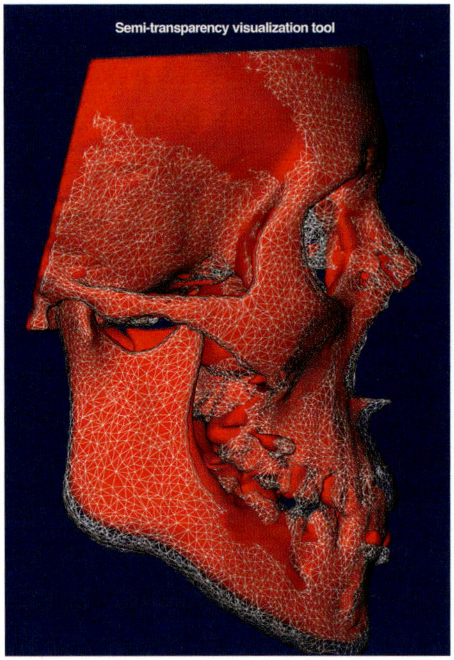

Figure 19.5 Alternative method to determine treatment changes utilizing a 3D superimposition semi-transparency tool. The T1 model is shown in solid red, while the superimposed T2 model is displayed as a semitransparent white mesh to allow qualitative assessment of treatment change.

models from T1 and T2 for the first three patients. Minimum surface-distance changes in several anatomic regions were compared across examiners for each patient. The values were all less than or equal to the 0.5 mm voxel resolution of the CBCT volume. That is, in each case, the differences in measurements were equal to or smaller than the resolution of the image.

OUTCOMES ASSESSMENT OF BAMP TREATMENT IN 3D

Several studies subsequently have provided information of the effects of BAMP treatment on pertinent maxillary and mandibular anatomic regions. These include the anterior surface of the maxilla in the region around Point A, anterior surface of the zygomatic bone, anterior surface of the maxillary incisors, anterior mandible in the region of pogonion, posterior surface of the ramus, anterior and posterior surfaces of the condyles, and the glenoid fossae, as summarized below.

The midface

All patients showed a positive (outward) movement in the maxilla, zygomatic region, and maxillary incisors (Nguyen *et al.*, 2011). The average forward displacement in the maxilla was approximately 3.7 mm with a range from 1.5 mm to as high as 8.5 mm. One explanation for the high variations in treatment response between patients might be due to the diversity of the original malocclusions. Other reasons include compliance with elastics, age, and maturation of the cranial sutures at the onset of treatment. Some of the Class III patients presented with a severe −5.0 mm overjet, while others manifested a mild edge-to-edge incisor relationship. Other reasons for the high variation on treatment response include compliance with elastics, age, skeletal malocclusion (maxillary deficiency vs. mandibular prognathism), and maturation of the cranial sutures at the start of treatment. The zygomas also showed a forward displacement of approximately 3.7 mm, while the incisors had a slightly higher displacement of 4.3 mm.

Statistical analysis of these data showed a high correlation between the anterior movement of the maxilla, zygoma, and incisors, suggesting that BAMP treatment produced a uniform forward displacement of the midface. To explain this phenomenon, the circumaxillary sutures were examined. Separation of the zygomatico-frontal, zygomatico-temporal, palatino-maxillary, and, to a lesser extent, zygomatico-maxillary sutures were observed in a number of subjects (Figure 19.6). It may be plausible that a constant force from the elastics effectively produced distraction of these sutures, resulting in the forward displacement of the entire midface. Recent animal studies have shown that continuous force application is more effective at expanding the sutures when compared with intermittent forces (Liu *et al.*, 2010). Interestingly,

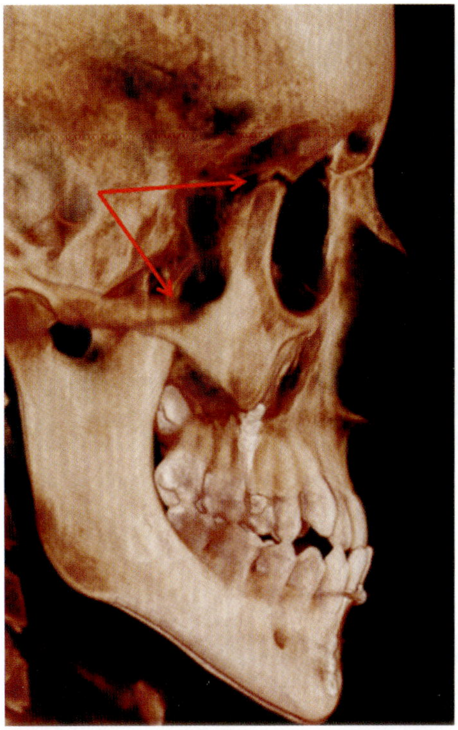

Figure 19.6 3D volume rendering at T2 showing distraction of the zygomatico-frontal and zygomatico-temporal sutures during BAMP therapy.

forward displacement of the maxilla was observed without disarticulation of the cranial sutures advocated by Liou (2005; Wang *et al.*, 2009). A recent 3D study by Ghoneima and associates (2011) reported that rapid maxillary expansion (RME) produced separation of multiple sutures surrounding the maxilla but did not affect the zygomatico-frontal, zygomatico-temporal, zygomatico-maxillary, or palatino-maxillary sutures. These findings further support Vaughn and coworkers' (2005) study, which showed that rapid expansion to loosen the sutures may not be needed to protract the maxilla effectively.

The mandible and temporomandibular joint (TMJ)

The changes in the anterior mandibular region were more variable in both magnitude and direction than that of the maxilla. Many subjects exhibited a distal displacement of the chin, while some continued to grow in the expected normal forward direction (De Clerck *et al.*, 2012). While the anterior position of the chin remained in relatively the same position throughout the course of treatment (−0.1 mm), this was significantly different from the mean forward growth of 2.2 mm in matched untreated Class III subjects during the same time interval (De Clerck *et al.*, 2010). It also is interesting that BAMP and untreated Class III subjects showed nearly identical growth changes in corpus of the mandible (gonion to gnathion) and ramus (condylion to gonion), suggesting that the BAMP protocol did not restrain endochondral growth of the mandible. So how was BAMP able to restrict the anterior-posterior (AP) displacement of the chin if it did not affect AP or vertical growth of the mandible? The answer lies in the posterior gonial region. All subjects showed distal displacement of the posterior surface of the ramus along with a closure of the gonial angle (Figure 19.7). This combined effect maintains the mandibular plane angle while producing a compensatory restraint of the chin. In addition, there was small mean posterior displacement of the condyles accompanied by an adaptive remodeling of the glenoid fossa (Figure 19.8). Long-term studies are needed to evaluate the stability of this compensatory mechanism as well as the health of the TMJ complex.

CONCLUSIONS

This chapter provided insights into the effectiveness and modality of action of BAMP treatment as determined in 3D by CBCT imaging. 3D imaging of subjects who underwent BAMP treatment showed changes in maxillary and mandibular structures that otherwise would be impossible to depict using 2D imaging methods. Specifically, the findings showed that BAMP resulted in correction of Class III malocclusion by producing significant maxillary protraction and maintaining mandibular position. The findings indicate the utility of this approach in the skeletal and dental correction of Class III malocclusions in the growing patient.

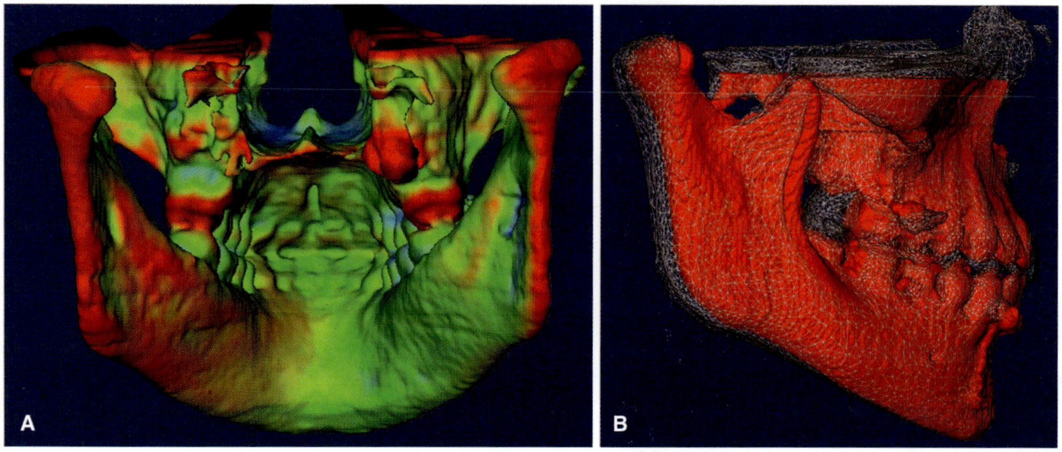

Figure 19.7 Color map (*A*) and semi-transparency (*B*) of the mandible and maxilla to demonstrate mandibular treatment changes. The posterior surface of the ramus showed distal displacement with closure of the gonial angle, thereby maintaining the mandibular plane angle.

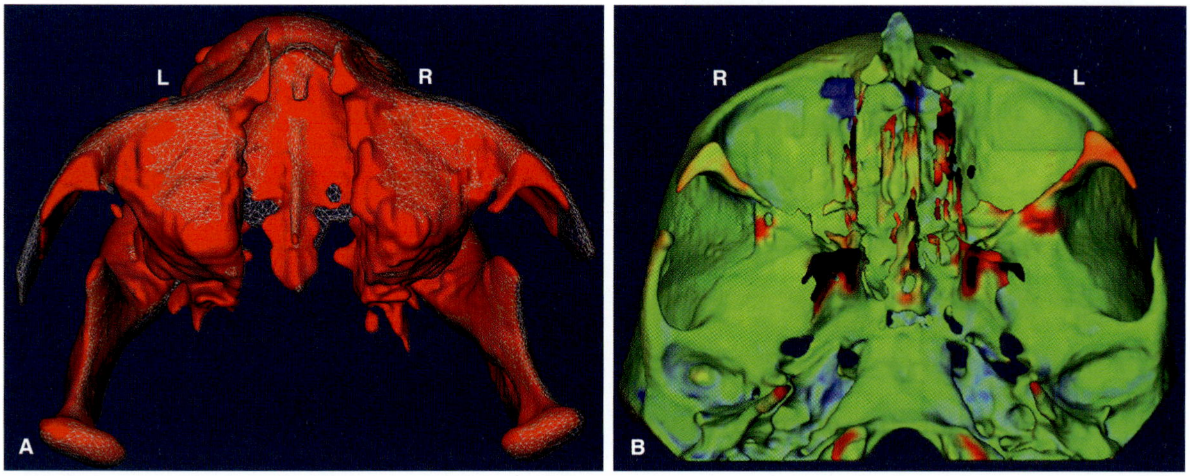

Figure 19.8 Color map of the inferior view of the cranial base (*A*) and semi-transparency of the superior view of the condyles (*B*) to demonstrate treatment changes in the condyles and glenoid fossa, respectively. The condyles showed a slight posterior displacement, and the glenoid fossa exhibited adaptive remodeling.

References

Baccetti, T., Franchi, L., & McNamara, J.A. Jr. (2000) Treatment and post-treatment craniofacial changes after rapid maxillary expansion and facemask therapy. *American Journal of Orthodontics and Dentofacial Orthopedics*, 118 (4), 404–413.

Baccetti, T., Franchi, L., & McNamara, J.A. Jr. (2004) Cephalometric variables predicting the long-term success or failure of combined rapid maxillary expansion and facial mask therapy. *American Journal of Orthodontics and Dentofacial Orthopedics*, 126 (1), 16–22.

Baccetti, T., De Clerck, H.J., Cevidanes, L.H., *et al.* (2011) Morphometric analysis of treatment effects of bone-anchored maxillary protraction in growing Class III patients. *European Journal of Orthodontics*, 33 (2), 121–125.

Baik, H.S. (1995) Clinical results of the maxillary protraction in Korean children. *American Journal of Orthodontics and Dentofacial Orthopedics*, 108 (6), 583–592.

Cevidanes, L.H.S., Heymann, G., Cornelis, M.A., *et al.* (2009) Superimposition of 3-dimensional cone-beam computed tomography models of growing patients. *American Journal of Orthodontics and Dentofacial Orthopedics*, 136 (1), 94–99.

Cevidanes, L., Baccetti, T., Franchi, L., *et al.* (2010) Comparison of two protocols for maxillary protraction: bone anchors versus face mask with rapid maxillary expansion. *The Angle Orthodontist*, 80 (5), 799–806.

Chapuis, J., Schramm, A., Pappas, I., *et al.* (2007) A new system for computer-aided preoperative planning and intraoperative navigation during corrective jaw surgery. *IEEE Transactions on Information Technology in Biomedicine*, 11, 274–287.

Cornelis, M.A., Scheffler, N.R., De Clerck, H.J., *et al.* (2007) Systematic review of the experimental use of temporary skeletal anchorage devices in orthodontics. *American Journal of Orthodontics and Dentofacial Orthopedics*, 131 (Suppl 4), S52–S58.

Cornelis, M.A., Scheffler, N.R., Mahy, P., *et al.* (2008) Modified miniplates for temporary skeletal anchorage in orthodontics: placement and removal surgeries. *Journal of Oral Maxillofacial Surgery*, 66 (7), 1439–1445.

De Clerck, H.J., Cornelis, M.A., Cevidanes, L.H., *et al.* (2009) Orthopedic traction of the maxilla with miniplates: a new perspective for treatment of midface deficiency. *Journal of Oral Maxillofacial Surgery*, 67 (10), 2123–2129.

De Clerck, H., Cevidanes, L., & Baccetti, T. (2010) Dentofacial effects of bone-anchored maxillary protraction: a controlled study of consecutively treated Class III patients. *American Journal of Orthodontics and Dentofacial Orthopedics*, 138 (5), 577–581.

De Clerck, H.J., Nguyen, T., de Paula, L.K., *et al.* (2012) Mandibular and glenoid fossa changes in 3D following bone anchored Class III intermaxillary traction. *American Journal of Orthodontics and Dentofacial Orthopedics*, 142 (1), 25–31.

Enacar, A., Giray, B., Pehlivanoglu, M., *et al.* (2003) Facemask therapy with rigid anchorage in a patient with maxillary hypoplasia and severe oligodontia. *American Journal of Orthodontics and Dentofacial Orthopedics*, 123 (5), 571–577.

Gallagher, R.W., Miranda, F., & Buschang, P.H. (1998) Maxillary protraction: treatment and posttreatment effects. *American Journal of Orthodontics and Dentofacial Orthopedics*, 113 (6), 612–619.

Ghoneima, A., Abdel-Fattah, E., Hartsfield, J., *et al.* (2011) Effects of rapid maxillary expansion on the cranial and circummaxillary sutures. *American Journal of Orthodontics and Dentofacial Orthopedics*, 140 (4), 510–519.

Hagg, U., Tse, A., Bendeus, M., *et al.* (2003) Long-term follow-up of early treatment with reverse headgear. *European Journal of Orthodontics*, 25 (1), 95–102.

Heymann, G.C., Cevidanes, L., Cornelis, M., *et al.* (2010) Three-dimensional analysis of maxillary protraction with intermaxillary elastics to miniplates. *American Journal of Orthodontics and Dentofacial Orthopedics*, 137 (2), 274–284.

Hong, H., Ngan, P., Han, G., *et al.* (2005) Use of onplants as stable anchorage for facemask treatment: a case report. *The Angle Orthodontist*, 75 (3), 453–460.

Ishii, H., Morita, S., Takeuchi, Y., *et al.* (1987) Treatment effect of combined maxillary protraction and chincap appliance in severe skeletal Class III cases. *American Journal of Orthodontics and Dentofacial Orthopedics*, 92 (4), 304–312.

Kama, J.D., Ozer, T., & Baran, S. (2006) Orthodontic and orthopaedic changes associated with treatment in subjects with Class III malocclusions. *European Journal of Orthodontics*, 28 (5), 496–502.

Kapila, S. & Farman, A.G. (eds.) (2003) *Craniofacial Imaging in the 21st Century: Proceedings of Conferences on Orthodontic Advances in Science and Technology Foundation. Orthodontics and Craniofacial Research, Copenhagen, Denmark.* Munksgard Press, Copenhagen. Vol. 6 (Suppl. 1).

Kim, J.H., Viana, M.A., Graber, T.M., *et al.* (1999) The effectiveness of protraction face mask therapy: a meta-analysis. *American Journal of Orthodontics and Dentofacial Orthopedics*, 115 (6), 675–685.

Kircelli, B.H. & Pektas, Z.O. (2008) Midfacial protraction with skeletally anchored face mask therapy: a novel approach and preliminary results. *American Journal of Orthodontics and Dentofacial Orthopedics*, 133 (3), 440–449.

Liou, E.J. (2005) Effective maxillary orthopedic protraction for growing Class III patients: a clinical application simulates distraction osteogenesis. *Progress in Orthodontics*, 6 (2), 154–171.

Liu, S., Kyung, H., & Buschang, P. (2010) Continuous forces are more effective than intermittent forces in expanding sutures. *European Journal of Orthodontics*, 32, 371–380.

Lou, L., Lagravère, M.O., Compton, S., *et al.* (2007) Accuracy of measurements and reliability of landmark identification with computed tomography (CT) techniques in the maxillofacial area: a systematic review.

Oral Surgery, Oral Medicine, Oral Pathology, Oral Radiology and Endodontology, 104 (3), 402–411.

Ludlow, J.B., Davies-Ludlow, L.E., Brooks, S.L., *et al.* (2006) Dosimetry of 3 CBCT devices for oral and maxillofacial radiology: CB Mercuray, NewTom 3G and i-CAT. *Dentomaxillofacial Radiology*, 35 (4), 219–226.

Macdonald, K.E., Kapust, A.J., & Turley, P.K. (1999) Cephalometric changes after the correction of class III malocclusion with maxillary expansion/facemask therapy. *American Journal of Orthodontics and Dentofacial Orthopedics*, 116 (1), 13–24.

Mah, J. & Hatcher, D. (2004) Three-dimensional craniofacial imaging. *American Journal of Orthodontics and Dentofacial Orthopedics*, 126 (3), 308–309.

Nguyen, T., Cevidanes, L.H.S., Cornelis, M., *et al.* (2011) Three-dimensional assessment of changes associated with bone anchored maxillary protraction. *American Journal of Orthodontics and Dentofacial Orthopedics*, 140 (6), 790–798.

Park, S.H., Yu, H.S., Kim, K.D., *et al.* (2006) A proposal for a new analysis of craniofacial morphology by 3-dimensional computed tomography. *American Journal of Orthodontics and Dentofacial Orthopedics*, 129 (5), 600.e23–600.e34.

Periago, D., Scarfe, W., Moshiri, M., *et al.* (2008) Linear accuracy and reliability of cone beam CT derived 3-dimensional images constructed using an orthodontic volumetric rendering program. *The Angle Orthodontist*, 78 (3), 387–395.

Proffit, W.R., Fields, H.W. Jr., & Moray, L.J. (1998) Prevalence of malocclusion and orthodontic treatment need in the United States: estimates from the NHANES III survey. *International Journal of Adult Orthodontics & Orthognathic Surgery*, 13 (2), 97–106.

Singer, S.L., Henry, P.J., & Rosenberg, I. (2000) Osseointegrated implants as an adjunct to facemask therapy: a case report. *The Angle Orthodontist*, 70 (3), 253–262.

Vaughn, G., Mason, A., Moon, H., *et al.* (2005) The effects of maxillary protraction therapy with or without rapid palatal expansion: a prospective, randomized clinical trial. *American Journal of Orthodontics and Dentofacial Orthopedics*, 128 (3), 299–309.

Wang, Y.C., Chang, P.M., & Liou, E.J. (2009) Opening of circumaxillary sutures by alternate rapid maxillary expansions and constrictions. *The Angle Orthodontist*, 79 (2), 230–234.

Westwood, P.V., McNamara, J.A. Jr., Baccetti, T., *et al.* (2003) Long-term effects of Class III treatment with rapid maxillary expansion and facemask therapy followed by fixed appliances. *American Journal of Orthodontics and Dentofacial Orthopedics*, 123 (3), 306–320.

Yushkevich, P.A., Piven, J., Hazlett, H.C., *et al.* (2006) User-guided 3D active contour segmentation of anatomical structures: significantly improved efficiency and reliability. *NeuroImage*, 31 (3), 1116–1128.

20 Applications of Cone Beam Computed Tomography to Orthognathic Surgery Treatment Planning

Sean P. Edwards, DDS, MD, FRCD(C), and R. Scott Conley, DMD

INTRODUCTION

Cone-beam computed tomography (CBCT) has created the potential for several advancements in orthognathic surgery. As opposed to two-dimensional (2D) radiography, three-dimensional (3D) CBCT imaging offers improved analysis of craniofacial deformities, improved quality control with enhanced post-operative assessment of surgical results, and the potential to improve and streamline the process by which orthognathic surgical planning is transferred to the operating room. The objective of this chapter is to present evolving concepts on the utilization and efficacy of CBCT in enhancing diagnosis and treatment outcomes in orthognathic surgery.

ADVANTAGES OF IN-OFFICE CT SCANNING

CBCT scanning generally is inferior to conventional multi-slice CT (MSCT) scanning in image quality. In spite of this, its popularity has grown exponentially in dental specialties because of the increase in diagnostic quality and three-dimensionality of the images compared with conventional dental radiographic imaging. CBCT also offers significant advantages in dosimetry and, since most CBCT units are located in dental offices, provides greater patient and provider convenience than medical imaging. The ability to locate CBCT units in dental offices is facilitated by virtue of their small footprint (which often is no greater than an orthopantomogram unit), lack of need for special electrical installations, and affordability. A second important advantage of in-office CBCT is that splints and other dentally relevant markers can be made in an onsite dental lab and used during the scan for registration and diagnosis. Furthermore, most CBCT scans taken in a dental office typically are performed by a dental assistant who is familiar with concepts of capturing the condyles and having the patient's lips in resting posture with the mandible in centric relation. This contrasts with medical radiologists undertaking MSCT in hospitals who

Cone Beam Computed Tomography in Orthodontics: Indications, Insights, and Innovations, First Edition. Sunil D. Kapila.

typically are not cognizant of or acquainted with these important concepts of dental imaging and therefore are likely to overlook them.

EVOLUTION FROM 2D TO 3D RADIOGRAPHY FOR ORTHOGNATHIC SURGERY

Cephalometric analysis is a hallmark in the proper diagnosis and treatment planning for patients with severe malocclusion. A myriad of analyses are available (Wylie *et al.*, 1987), some preferred by orthodontists and others by surgeons. Most of the more popular cephalometric analyses for orthodontists utilize several angular measurements that are excellent for evaluating tooth position, but are less precise in assessing jaw position (Steiner, 1953; Ricketts, 1981). In addition, nearly all lateral cephalometric analyses use intracranial reference marks that are difficult to identify and, rather than using operator-assisted natural head position (NHP), use reference planes such as the Frankfort Horizontal Plane that are more appropriate for anthropology (Broca, 1862). Finally, angular measurements are difficult to translate to planning and implementing surgical changes. To overcome these deficiencies, a cephalometric analysis was developed (Burstone *et al.*, 1978; Legan & Burstone, 1980) that uses mostly millimetric linear measurements made in the NHP that correspond to the various types of surgical movements the surgeon can accomplish during orthognathic surgery and are transferable directly to the operating room.

Even with the improved lateral cephalometric analysis, the third dimension in the transverse or coronal plane largely has been overlooked. Subsequently, two significant papers were published to highlight the importance of the transverse dimension in surgical orthodontic treatment planning (Grummons & Kappeyne van de Coppello, 1987; Betts *et al.*, 1995). Unfortunately, the only tool available at the time for transverse analysis was the postero-anterior (PA) cephalogram, which is fraught with exposure and tracing errors. These errors result from small rotations in head position during exposure that lead to inaccurate diagnosis of asymmetry, and the substantial superimposition artifacts make the PA cephalogram difficult to read and interpret and consistently identify landmarks (Major *et al.*, 1994, 1996).

The deficiencies of both the lateral and the PA cephalometric analyses can be overcome with CBCT. Not only do CBCT data enable the accurate creation of 2D radiographs (Bholsithi *et al.*, 2009; van Vlijmen *et al.*, 2010; Pape *et al.*, 2012; Zamora *et al.*, 2012), but by navigating slice by slice through the dataset to avoid superimposition artifacts, the scans also permit much more accurate measurement of the recommended PA cephalometric dimensions than do PA cephalograms. However, while utilizing traditional cephalometric analysis on 2D images derived from CBCT is a step in the right direction, this methodology does not harness the full power and capabilities of this imaging technology. Currently, attempts are being made to perform true 3D structure analysis with CBCT. The methods are in their infancy and many still need to be validated (Fuhrmann *et al.*, 1996; Olszewski *et al.*, 2006; Noguchi *et al.*, 2007; Chenin, 2010), but a true 3D cephalometric analysis that complements the 3D clinical and facial exam and utilizes the same terminology that surgeons use will be a tremendous asset for more accurate diagnosis of and treatment planning for the surgical patient, particularly the asymmetric patient.

From the surgeon's perspective, 3D imaging offers multiple advantages when preparing for and evaluating the results of an orthognathic surgery case. Pre-operative assessment of bone support of the dentition and interdental spacing for interdental osteotomies ideally is performed with CBCT imaging (Figure 20.1). For example, this 3D

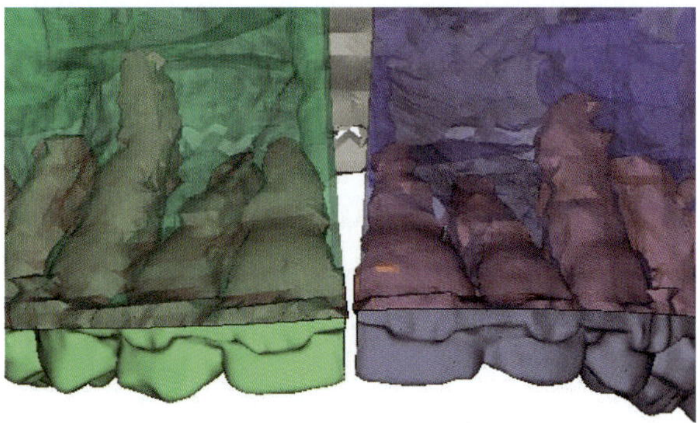

Figure 20.1 Visualization of interdental spacing and root anatomy for an interdental osteotomy from CBCT.

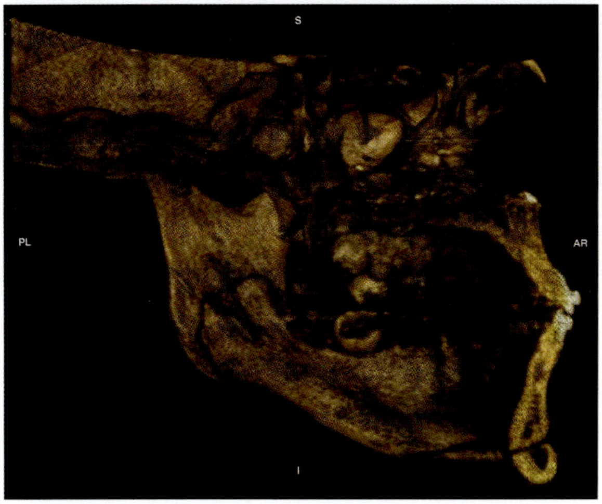

Figure 20.2 3D volumetric rendering to demonstrate post-operative appearance of the Hunsuck modification to the bilateral sagittal split osteotomy (BSSO).

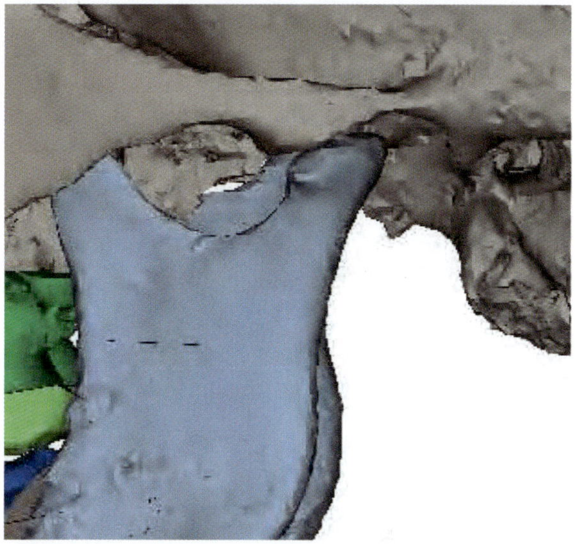

Figure 20.3 Pre-operative imaging in a patient with a significant Class II malocclusion shows an anterior position of the condyle. The patient's habitual mandibular protrusion made it difficult to obtain centric relation. The CBCT image enabled this postural relationship of the condyle to be recognized pre-operatively, thus facilitating enhanced surgical planning and sequencing.

assessment helps to eliminate parallax errors, visualize variations in root anatomy such as dilacerations, and determine the pre-operative position and course of the inferior alveolar nerve, which can be useful for planning slight variations in the position of the sagittal split osteotomy to help minimize injury to the nerve.

Post-operative assessment with 3D imaging allows a high-resolution determination of osteotomies and fixation that are essential in implementing continuous quality improvement processes. These include enabling surgeons to appraise their results critically, thereby helping to avoid making the same mistakes and facilitating evolution in their techniques. For example, CBCT enables (1) the documentation of the incidence and position of pterygoid plate fractures and of deflected septums after LeFort osteotomies; (2) good visualization of the position of the Hunsuck fracture in the bilateral sagittal split osteotomy (Figure 20.2); (3) visualization and documentation of pre-surgical centric relation (Figure 20.3) and post-operative alterations in condylar anatomy, condylar position, as well as errors in achieving centric relation (Figure 20.4); and (4) pre- and post-surgical superimpositions to be performed to document condylar changes and to elucidate the precision in achieving pre-operative plans (Figure 20.5).

Another example where CBCT offers distinct advantages over 2D imaging is in the diagnosis, treatment planning, and correction of facial asymmetries in which the CBCT dataset can be segmented to better visualize, localize, assess, and quantify a patient's asymmetry. Once segmented, the surgeon can use the mirroring technique to plan the surgical procedures virtually in substantial detail for subsequent delivery of treatment in the operating room (Peck & Peck, 1970; Figure 20.6; see also Chapter 21).

COMPUTER-ASSISTED ORTHOGNATHIC SURGERY (CAOS)

Orthognathic surgery constitutes a powerful combination of orthodontic and surgical techniques that permit the 3D repositioning and reconstruction of the facial skeleton, offering significant functional, esthetic, and psychological benefits to

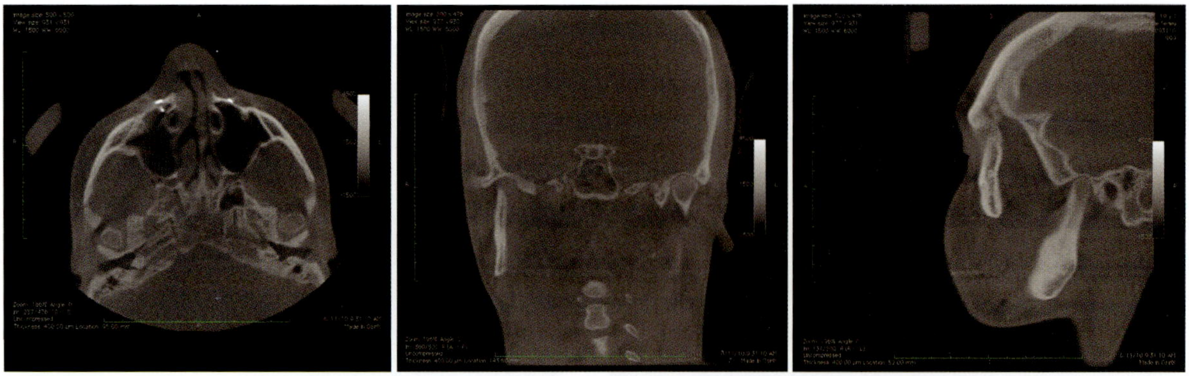

Figure 20.4 Multiplanar reconstructions of a patient following mandibular surgery demonstrating optimal condylar positioning in the fossa with a normal lateral and rotational location within the fossa with the teeth in occlusion.

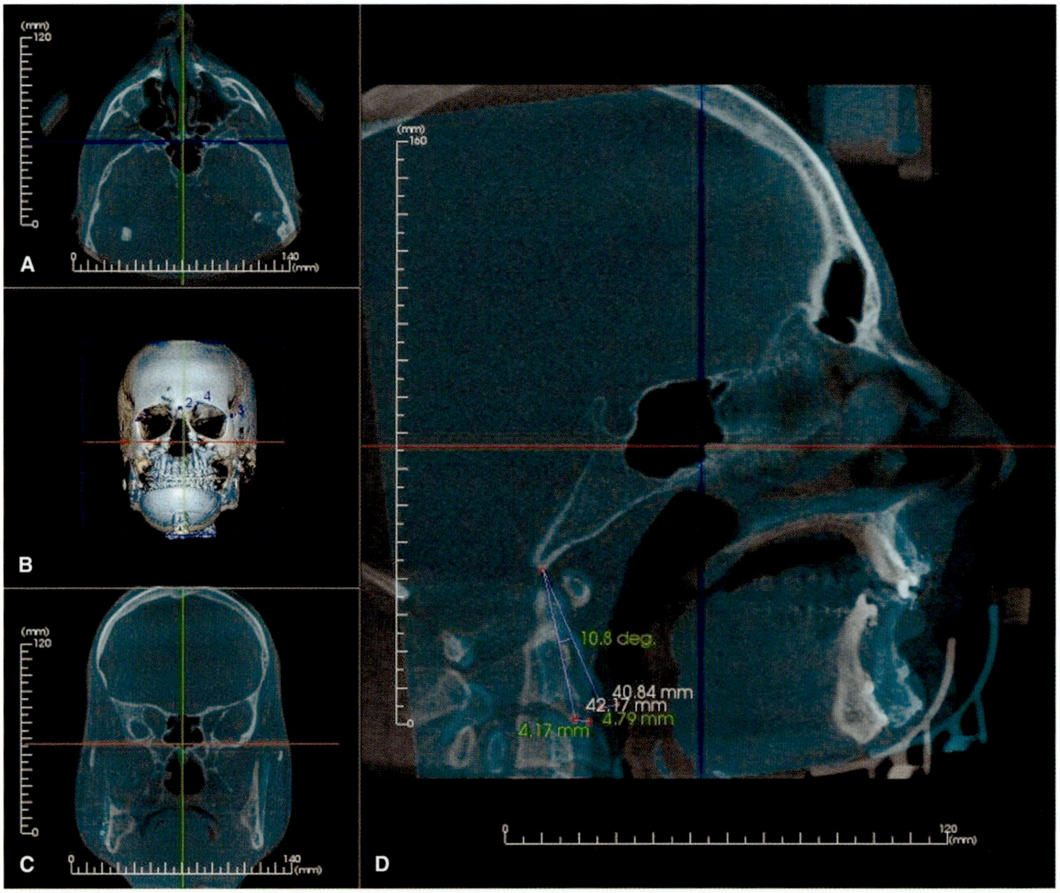

Figure 20.5 Pre-operative (white) and post-operative (green) superimpositions of CBCT images in multiplanar reconstuctions (*A*, *C*, and *D*) and volumetric rendering (*B*) to demonstrate changes resulting from maxillary and mandibular advancements.

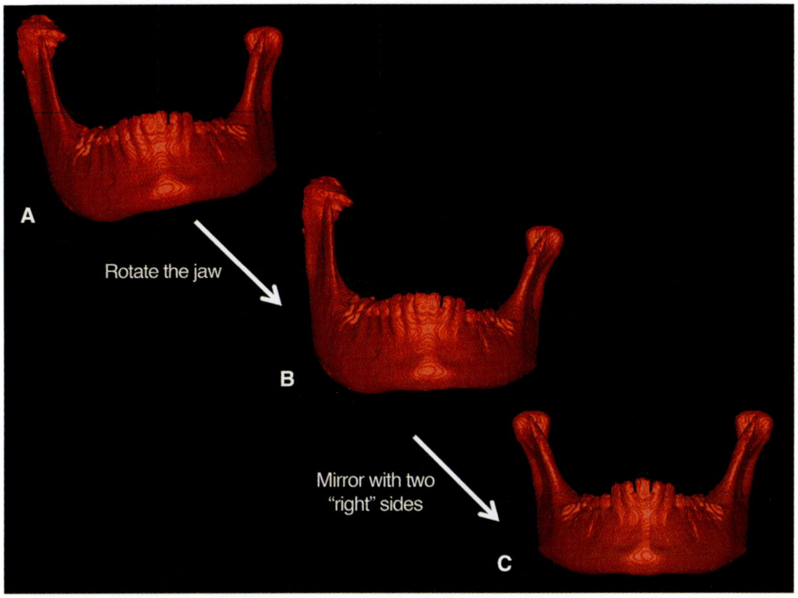

Figure 20.6 When using the mirroring technique to simulate an asymmetric surgical correction, the original 3D image (*A*) first must be rotated into the proper orientation (*B*). The normal side, which in this case is the left half of the mandible, is "mirrored" on the contralateral side using the midsagittal reference plane to simulate the desired symmetric mandible (*C*). Some software packages allow the additional step of overlaying the normal onto the abnormal side, which provides the surgeon with more precise information regarding how much bone must be removed from the hyperplastic side, added to the hypoplastic side, or a combination of the two.

patients with moderate to severe skeletal discrepancies. Over the past few decades, the process by which these cases are prepared, planned, and effected has evolved to be relatively precise but labor-intensive and time-consuming. Many of the steps involved in the delivery of care to these patients cannot be delegated and, as such, are surgeon-intensive. For example, most surgeons will take their own facebow and centric relation records, while impressions may be delegated to an assistant. Model surgery and splint fabrication also are performed by the surgeon. The asymmetric face, whose details and specifics cannot be captured completely or measured precisely both clinically and with conventional 2D cephalometrics, poses additional diagnostic problems. These hurdles, along with concerns about declining reimbursement rates for orthognathic surgery, have led to a decline in surgeons' willingness to offer orthognathic surgery as a service to their patients. 3D imaging including CBCT offers substantial promise in overcoming many of these hurdles of traditional approaches and steps in undertaking orthognathic therapy. These include refined 3D diagnosis, virtual treatment planning, and computer-assisted algorithms for deriving optimal approaches to pre-planning and delivery of intraoperative procedures. The practicality of performing each of these steps has been advanced greatly with the advent of in-office CBCT technology. The integration of advanced imaging and planning software will continue to improve our understanding of a deformity, allow creation of better surgical plans, and improve the efficiency of the process of transferring this planning to the operating room. The entire process, often referred to as Computer-Assisted Orthognathic Surgery (CAOS), is readily adoptable by the oral and maxillofacial surgeon because its end product, the occlusal surgical splint, is identical to that produced in conventional planning methods, to which the surgeons already are well accustomed.

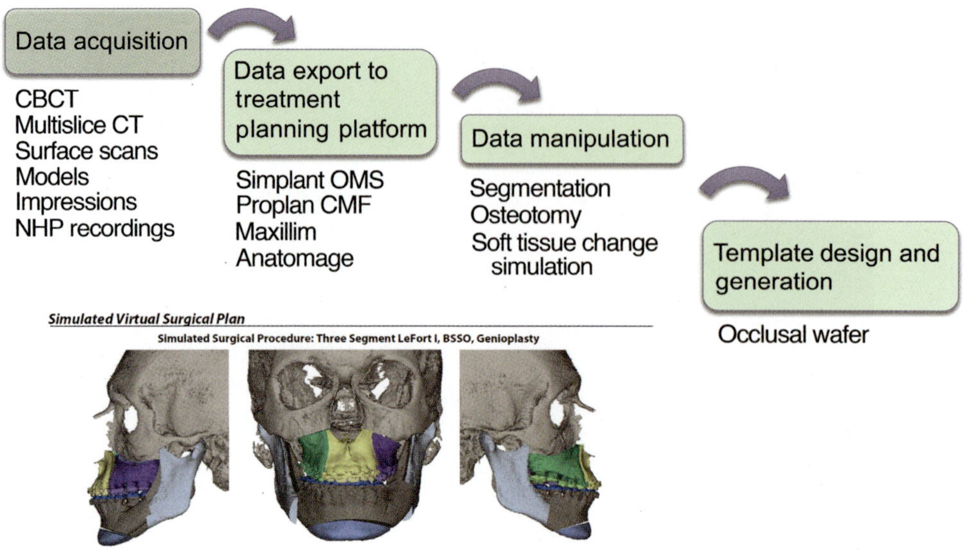

Figure 20.7 Workflow for CAOS in which data are acquired from one or more sources, exported to a treatment planning software, and manipulated to plan the surgery (as shown in the bottom panel) and to visualize changes in soft and hard tissues. The virtual surgical plan is used to derive a virtual occlusal wafer, which is then fabricated using stereolithography (SLA) or selective laser sintering (SLS). NHP, natural head position.

The general workflow of CAOS is shown in Figure 20.7. At its simplest, CT or CBCT images and dental models are merged to create a virtual model of a patient's skull and occlusion. These data are manipulated virtually to simulate the desired surgical plan. Once these simulations are complete to the satisfaction of the surgeon, the data are exported to rapid prototyping hardware to generate templates that will guide the operation. If the process is accurate and the templates are effective, then the operation and its results will match the virtual plan. Thus, CAOS is dependent on specialized software that permits analysis, surgical simulation, and design and fabrication of surgical splints.

There has been recent commercial interest in developing software to facilitate orthognathic surgery diagnosis, treatment planning, and splint fabrication. The two most commonly used software platforms are Simplant OMS (Materialise NV, Leuven, Belgium) and Maxilim (Medicim, Mechelen, Belgium); the former is used most commonly in North America. Splints can be manufactured using a variety of rapid prototyping techniques, such as stereolithography (SLA) and selective laser sintering (SLS).

Simulating orthognatic surgery in the virtual environment requires the same exigencies as conventional cephalometrics and model surgery. When understanding this new process, it is helpful first to compare it with the more familiar traditional paradigm. With the computer-assisted plan, the CT or CBCT images serve as the semi-adjustable articulator with mounted models. For this to be precise, the scan must be acquired in centric relation and a clear view of the occlusion obtained. Orthodontic appliances pose a substantial problem in this regard because of the considerable artifact created around the dentition during CBCT/CT scanning. This precludes a CBCT/CT scan from being a reliable source of optimal occlusal detail. Large dental restorations would have a similar impact on the optimal representation of occlusal and dental anatomy. The CBCT/CT imaging artifact is circumvented best by using scanned dental models that can be surface-imaged using a laser or CBCT or CT scanner. The data from the stone models will be clear and then can be superimposed

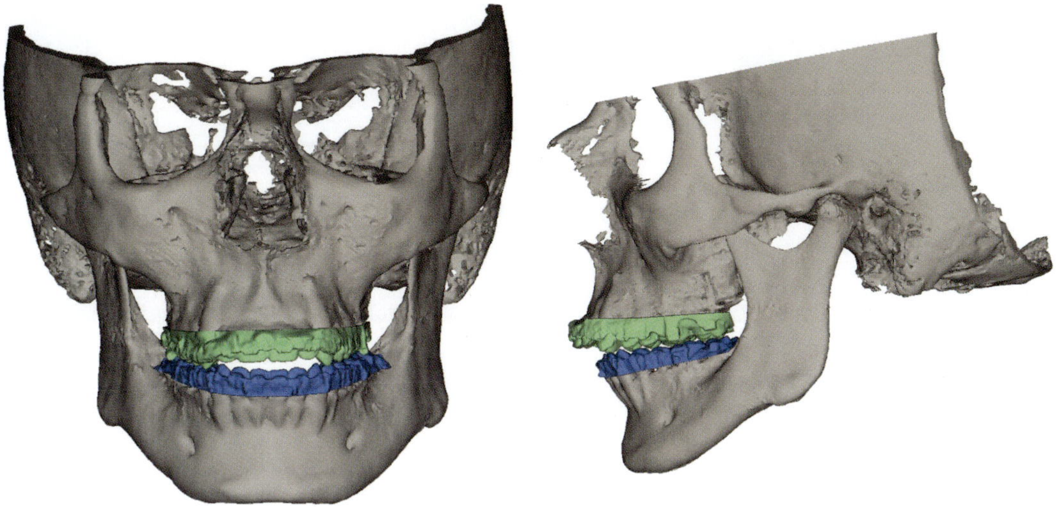

Figure 20.8 Construction of a 3D virtual model by fusing data from CBCT (gray) and surface scans of dental stone casts (green and blue).

on the teeth in the virtual environment (Figure 20.8; see also Chapter 4). This image fusion can be performed manually or by using an automated process that achieves optimal superimposition of the images using fiducials, with both of these approaches having been shown to be accurate (Miller *et al.*, 2003; Xia *et al.*, 2009; Chang *et al.*, 2010; Plooij *et al.*, 2011).

Since surgical movements that are not possible clinically may be accomplished in the virtual environment, an additional hurdle of CAOS stems from the need to establish a final virtual occlusion that truly is achievable in the operating room. Detection of collisions, which is a function of the software platform wherein two 3D objects are not permitted to pass through each other, is not possible in most virtual treatment planning platforms. As such, occlusal interferences, easily detected when articulating casts by hand, would not be discernible during the virtual surgical procedure. Several approaches have been developed to overcome this hurdle, ranging from automated occlusal designs to spring-coil systems that approximate ideal occlusal contact points. At this point, none of these approaches is as practical as articulating the casts by hand, establishing the desired occlusion, and then taking a bite registration of this interocclusal relationship. Articulating casts by hand is an approach with which surgeons are comfortable and permits rapid identification of occlusal interferences and instabilities that can be corrected with enameloplasty, segmental osteotomies, or further orthodontic preparation. This interocclusal registration then is scanned and incorporated into the virtual model built for treatment simulation by superimposing the scanned maxilla over the native maxilla. In the case of a segmented maxilla, the incisors serve as the primary point of registration.

The treatment algorithm used in the author's practice is based on the considerable work of Xia and coworkers (2005) and Hsu and associates (2013). A centric relation record is obtained with a rigid impression material using a specialized jig (Figure 20.9) prior to the CBCT scan. The CBCT scan then is acquired with the centric relation (CR) record in place, ensuring the desired mandibular position is maintained during image acquisition. A virtual facebow with fiducial markers also can be attached to the jig, facilitating the subsequent image fusion process (Figure 20.9C). Last, a gyroscope is attached to the CR record and is used to acquire an NHP recording. The NHP is recorded three times after instructing the patient to relax and look toward the horizon. This last step is key to the development of an external reference system for 3D cephalometric analysis.

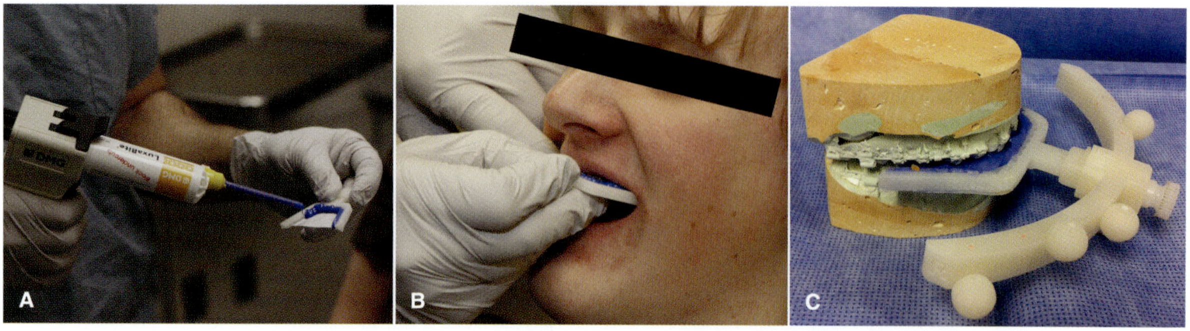

Figure 20.9 *A* and *B*: Centric relation record taken prior to CBCT scanning. Ideally, the record should be as thin as possible so as not to distort the patient's vertical dimension, and the impression material should be rigid. *C*: Stone models placed in centric relation record with virtual facebow in place, which has fiducial markers contained within the spheres attached to the jig that facilitate the transfer of the centric relation to the virtual patient.

3D IMAGE CEPHALOMETRICS FOR SURGICAL PLANNING

The development of an external reference system–based cephalometric analysis has been one of the most significant advances in surgical planning (Gateno *et al.* 2011). To understand this system and its significance, it is useful to compare it with the more conventional internal reference systems with which surgeons and orthodontists are familiar. In this paradigm, when a portion of the face is described in terms of size and/or position, it is done in reference to another portion of the face, which constitutes the internal reference. For example, the position of the maxilla and mandible often are described relative to the skull base, typically either the Sella-Nasion line (SNA and SNB, respectively) or the Frankfort Horizontal Plane (A and B point to Nasion perpendicular, respectively). Use of an internal reference for assessing other parts of the face assumes that the portion of the face/skull being used as a reference is normal. This assumption is the biggest limitation of the internal reference system because it is rare for an asymmetry to be localized to one part of the face.

Although determination of the vertical proportions of the face and the sagittal position of the jaws is accomplished well with the lateral cephalogram, asymmetries are not characterized well with the PA cephalogram. This particularly affects determinations of two types of asymmetries in the frontal plane, classified as cant and yaw deformities. A cant is simply a tip in the occlusal plane when comparing the left and right sides. This can be characterized in millimeters, but it can be difficult to measure in an asymmetric face where other facial features also may be asymmetric. To further illustrate the point, consider a maxillary cant, which can be measured accurately if there is a normal horizontal plane such as that constructed using orbitale and porion (Frankfort Horizontal Plane). In patients in whom the ears and/or orbits are not symmetric, an accurate internal reference plane cannot be developed from which a cant can be measured. Thus if the ear and/or orbits are not symmetric bilaterally, it will not be possible to construct a symmetric 3D Frankfort Horizontal, making it impossible to measure a cant relative to this internal reference system. A yaw deformity is a rotational asymmetry in the occlusion. Clinically, this presents as asymmetries in buccal corridor widths and a more anterior presentation of one side of the dentition. This asymmetry too is not measured well either clinically or with traditional cephalograms.

In contrast to the internal reference, an external reference system does not rely on the face to characterize and measure a deformity. This has an important advantage in the asymmetric face since deformities rarely are limited to one part of the face; therefore, no valid internal reference system will exist in these types of cases. An external reference system is akin to a plumb line where a weight is hung from a string and allowed to hang freely.

This defines the vertical reference as determined by gravity. When this external reference is superimposed on the face and placed on nasion, it can serve as a mid-sagittal reference axis. Next, the face is superimposed with a horizontal that is perpendicular to the mid-sagittal reference axis to create the horizontal plane. Finally, a coronal plane is constructed at 90° to both of these planes. The three planes generate a Cartesian coordinate system that is external to and independent of the face. The Cartesian coordinate system then is superimposed on the face with the vertical centered on nasion, such that the mid-sagittal plane defines the midline of the face when the head is in NHP.

Using the CBCT scan and the CAOS algorithm proposed by Xia and coworkers (2011), a gyroscope is used to capture NHP, permitting an external reference system to be superimposed on the face. This recording is related back to the CBCT data by attaching the recording to the CR record. When this Cartesian system is superimposed over the patient's skull, virtually any portion of a patient's deformity can be quantified orthogonal to one of these planes. A yaw deformity now can be quantified relative to tooth position from the mid-sagittal plane and/or its distance from a coronal plane. Heretofore, this was a nonexistent capability in any orthognathic surgery treatment algorithm. A cant now can be quantified based on the horizon and no longer is susceptible to errors from orbital and auricular asymmetries. These and other differences between derivations from internal and external reference systems are highlighted in Table 20.1.

An external reference system is not without limitations. First, the relative positions of different facial parts are important and must be considered in treatment planning. This is a fundamental component of balance of proportions. Second, while the external reference system is an excellent way to obviate the influence of facial asymmetries on deformity correction, there are instances when correcting a face to this plan would be incorrect since the derivations are based on the position of the head relative to the external reference. Examples of these include patients with habitual altered head postures, cervical spine abnormalities, and torticollis. In such situations, the surgeon must select the most appropriate compromise that represents that best correction for a given patient.

Table 20.1 Comparison of internal and external reference systems used in cephalometrics.

Cephalometrics	
Internal reference system	External reference system
Skeletal and soft tissue landmarks	Face characterized in reference to orthogonal planes not part of the face/head
Subject to errors introduced by facial asymmetries	Obviates errors derived from skeletal asymmetries
Independent of head position	Dependent on head position
Closest paradigm to traditional cephalometrics	

SURGICAL SIMULATION

The virtual surgical simulation in 3D is a highly valuable tool for the surgeon that provides novel perspectives for diagnosis as well as planning and execution of surgery not offered with conventional model surgery and 2D prediction tracings. The virtual simulation begins with the 3D model built where there is a full view of the facial skeleton oriented into NHP; the mandible is in centric relation; and there is an artifact-free occlusion that can be used for visualization of the deformity and the production of surgical splints.

At this point, the scanned and final occlusion is superimposed on the un-operated maxilla. In cases where the maxilla is to be segmented, a best-fit approximation is used. Small errors in this process are acceptable because the final position of the maxilla will be optimized according to an external reference system. Generally, midlines are corrected first, followed by implementation of the planned anterior-posterior and vertical movements of the maxilla. Next, any yaw deformities in the occlusion are corrected. Further, yaw deformities still may be apparent at this stage at the ramus level in cases undergoing mandibular osteotomies. If these skeletal yaw deformities still are present, in general, the author prefers not to correct them because this would require changing the final position of the occlusion. Instead, the preferred treatment involves adjusting these skeletal disharmonies with osteoplasty while maintaining the occlusion in the most ideal position for the desired smile esthetics and interocclusal relationships. Finally, intentional occlusal plane angle changes are incorporated. Cant correction also can be individualized in this setting. Cants rarely are even in their magnitude and, therefore, typically require some approximation. With a 3D treatment algorithm and an orthogonal plane, the cant can be quantified at each tooth such that an informed decision can be made about how much correction should be made and where it should take place. A decision then is made on surgery sequencing and splint design. The splints are manufactured with rapid prototyping hardware such as selective laser sintering or stereolithograthy.

This surgical planning and splint fabrication process is streamlined considerably and is efficient relatively compared with traditional model surgery schemes. An informal comparison of the time required to generate a splint for a two-jaw orthognathic surgery case involving a multisegment maxilla was performed at the University of Michigan Oral and Maxillofacial Surgery Department by determining the time taken from the beginning of record completion until splints were ready. While there was considerable variation between residents and each resident improved his or her timing with experience, the computer-assisted scheme took 1–2 hours, while the duration for conventional planning ranged from 6 to 9 hours. This demonstrates a significant time savings between the two approaches, which contributes to an immediate benefit for the surgeon.

As opposed to the traditional model surgery treatment planning paradigm, the 3D process allows the surgeon to visualize what will happen to the skeleton with greater accuracy. This allows the surgeon to predict and plan an operation better and also provides an intra-operative checkpoint (i.e., if the intra-operative appearance of the realigned bony segments does not match the computer-based plan, then an explanation must be sought). Model surgery on an articulator can show reliably what happens at the tooth level but does not reveal much about the concomitant skeletal changes. The additional information on 3D skeletal changes accompanying the achievement of specific occlusal goals is useful in that treatment planning now can incorporate the skeletal changes reliably, whereas these were predicted but never visualizable previously. For example, being able to visualize residual skeletal asymmetries after the occlusion has been corrected is helpful for surgical planning (Figure 20.10). Quantifying and planning for correcting such residual deformities can be performed virtually and implemented during the surgical procedure.

Case study

An asymmetric two-jaw correction with a genioplasty will be used to illustrate further the potential of the virtual 3D treatment planning process and demonstrate the steps applied. From a practical standpoint, the surgeon can complete the entire process with access to rapid prototyping facilities, though efficiency may be maximized by working with a third-party service such as Medical Modelling (Golden, CO). Treatment planning then is completed with an online conference, splints fabricated by the third party, and then sent *via* courier to the surgeon in advance of surgery.

Once the CBCT data have been acquired, they first are converted from DICOM file format to .stl format. DICOM is the international standard for radiologic data acquisition and .stl is used for rapid prototyping. These .stl files are 3D objects comprised only of surface data, and this conversion involves the loss of data of internal data components of a CBCT scan. Laser scans of stone models then can be superimposed on the CBCT scan data for an artifact-free 3D model of the patient. Figure 20.11 demonstrates the virtual model created for an adolescent patient with a hypoplastic left condyle and resultant Class II open bite deformity. The desired vertical and sagittal movements are determined based on clinical impression and cephalometric analysis. The latter can be performed with traditional 2D cephalometrics because of the surgeon's current familiarity and comfort with this paradigm. Subsequent refinements of the treatment plan will occur in the 3D environment, particularly as it relates to midline, cant, and yaw

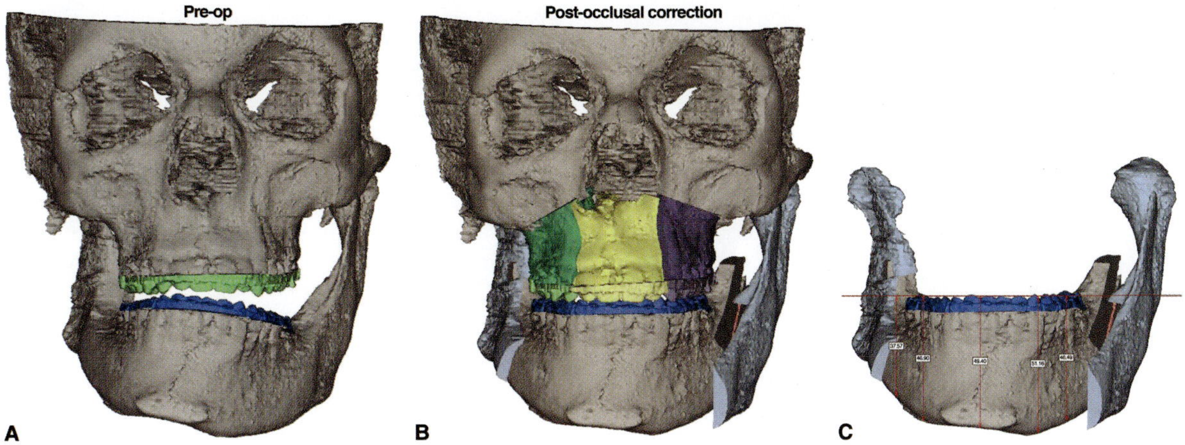

Figure 20.10 Patient with severe facial asymmetry where virtual treatment planning is used to determine treatment needs. *A*: Pre-surgical rendering of skeletal structures (gray) fused with images from dental casts (colored) demonstrate the severity of the deformity. *B*: The virtual surgery following correction of occlusal asymmetries demonstrates that considerable residual mandibular skeletal deformity remains. The need for additional osteoplasty and grafting now is obvious and easily planned in advance. *C*: Correction of this residual deformity can be quantified and a virtual treatment plan determined. In this case, the differences in the heights of the mandibular corpus, determined relative to an external reference system, indicate a treatment approach involving bone resection and grafting.

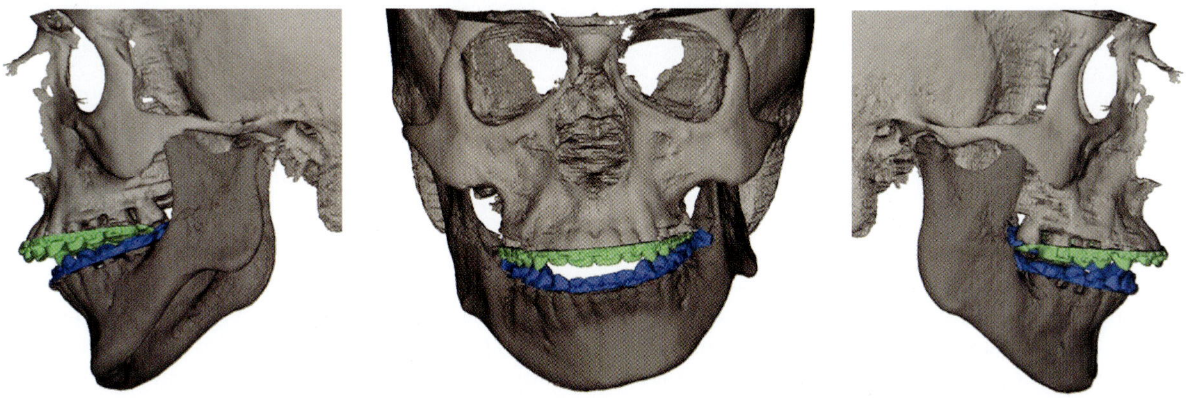

Figure 20.11 Virtual model created for a patient with unilateral condylar hypoplasia and associated skeletal deformities after DICOM file conversion to .stl and fusion with images of the teeth derived from stone casts.

corrections. Figure 20.12 and Figure 20.13 demonstrate the steps in correcting the deformity with a three-piece LeFort I maxillary osteotomy, a bilateral sagittal split osteotomy, and asymmetric genioplasty. Figure 20.14 demonstrates the magnitude of anticipated bony changes in the maxilla that can serve as a roadmap intraoperatively. If, for example, the intraoperative situation does not match the planned appearance of the osteotomy, this should cue the surgeon to explain the variance so as to avoid systematic errors in correcting a patient's deformity. The genioplasty then is planned and the magnitude of vertical correction determined relative to the new horizontal of the corrected

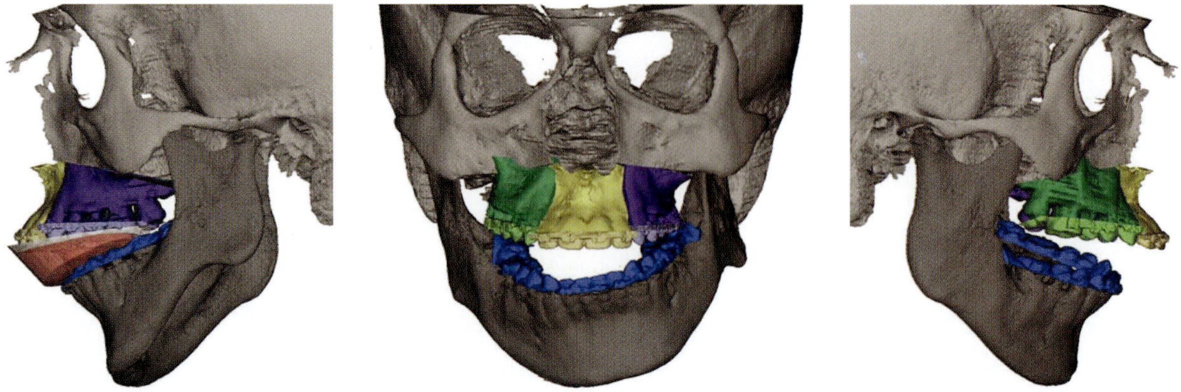

Figure 20.12 Demonstration of the virtual treatment plan in repositioning and correcting the maxilla.

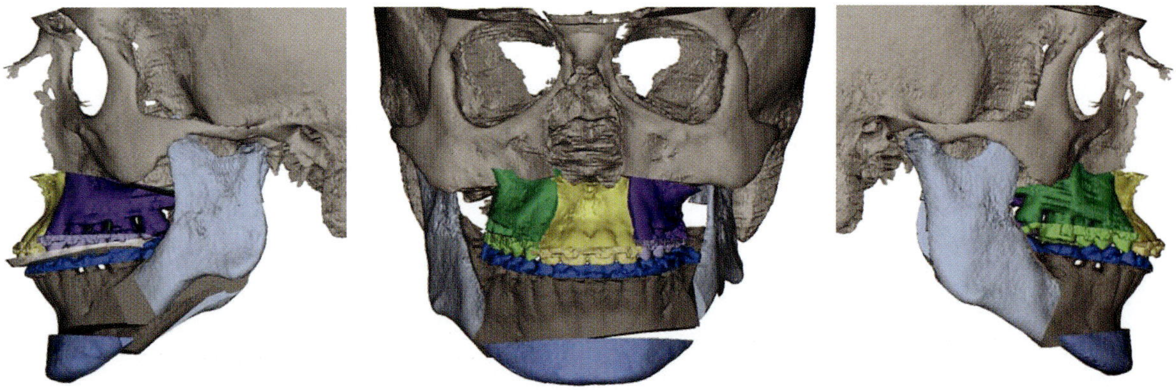

Figure 20.13 Virtual treatment for mandibular correction demonstrating the outcomes of a mandibular osteotomy. This involves incorporating 7 mm of cant correction at the first molars but only 3 mm cant correction at the canines.

occlusion (Figure 20.15A). In this case, a correction of 7 mm differential in height is required for correcting the residual mandibular chin asymmetry. This information is transferred easily to the case wherein a 3.5 mm wedge of bone can be resected from one side of the chin and then interposed on the opposite side as a bone graft, as demonstrated intraoperatively (Figure 20.15B,C). Figure 20.16 demonstrates the evaluation of the proximal segments after completion of the desired movements. Following the achievement of the desired surgical goals with the virtual treatment plan, traditional splints are designed and rapidly prototyped. Initial concerns that the manufacturing process would result in splints that do not fit have not been realized. Splint fit has been consistent and reliable in more than 100 cases, with superior indexing of piggyback splints when used. Figure 20.17 demonstrates that accuracy of the splint fit. With the end result of the process being a surgical splint that is the same as in the traditional model surgery paradigm, there really are few changes incorporated in the operating room. Only the improved 3D visualization of the treatment plan is incorporated to the case, making it easy for most surgeons to transition to and adopt this new paradigm.

Technique appraisal

CBCT technology has provided surgeons with a valuable tool for diagnosing facial deformities and

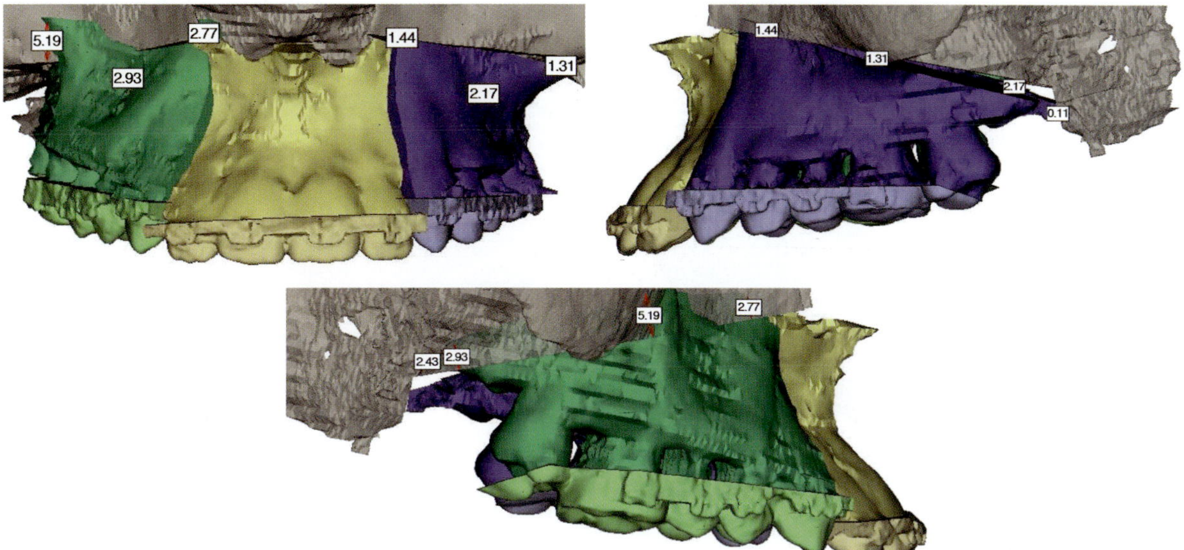

Figure 20.14 A roadmap of the planned skeletal changes and magnitudes of desired movements is created and may be referred to intraoperatively. This example demonstrates such a roadmap for the planned maxillary movements.

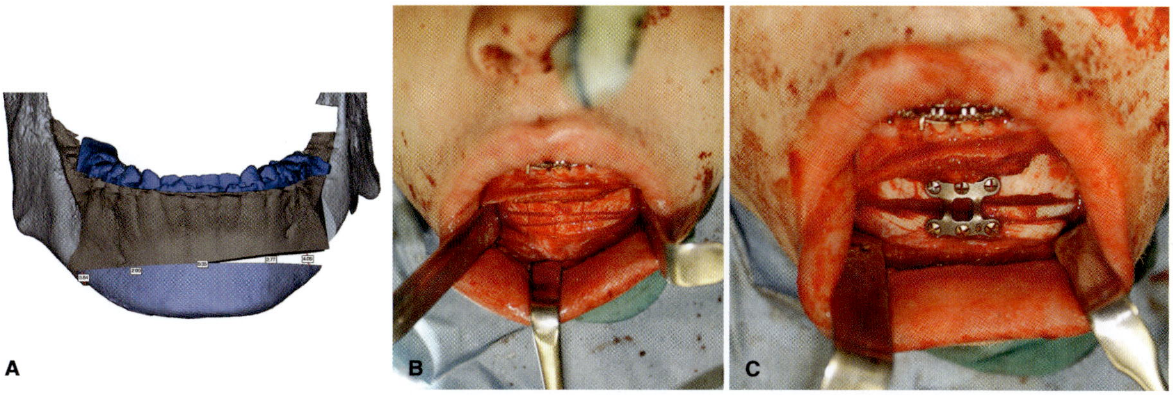

Figure 20.15 Virtual treatment planning of the genioplasty to correct the residual chin asymmetry (*A*) and the intraoperative implementation of this plan (*B* and *C*).

planning their correction. The virtual planning is transferred easily to the operating room. This process introduces significant improvements in the efficiency of treatment planning, which potentially can save the surgeon several hours of work for each case. Facial asymmetries clearly are evaluated better using this process as compared with the traditional 2D cephalometrics combined with model surgery. Previously estimated components of a facial deformity now are measured easily and reliably and built into the surgical correction. Xia and colleagues (2007) completed an initial appraisal of the accuracy of the computer-assisted process and found linear deviations between the plan and the result to be 0.9 mm and angular variances of 1.7°. A follow-up multicenter study of 65 patients

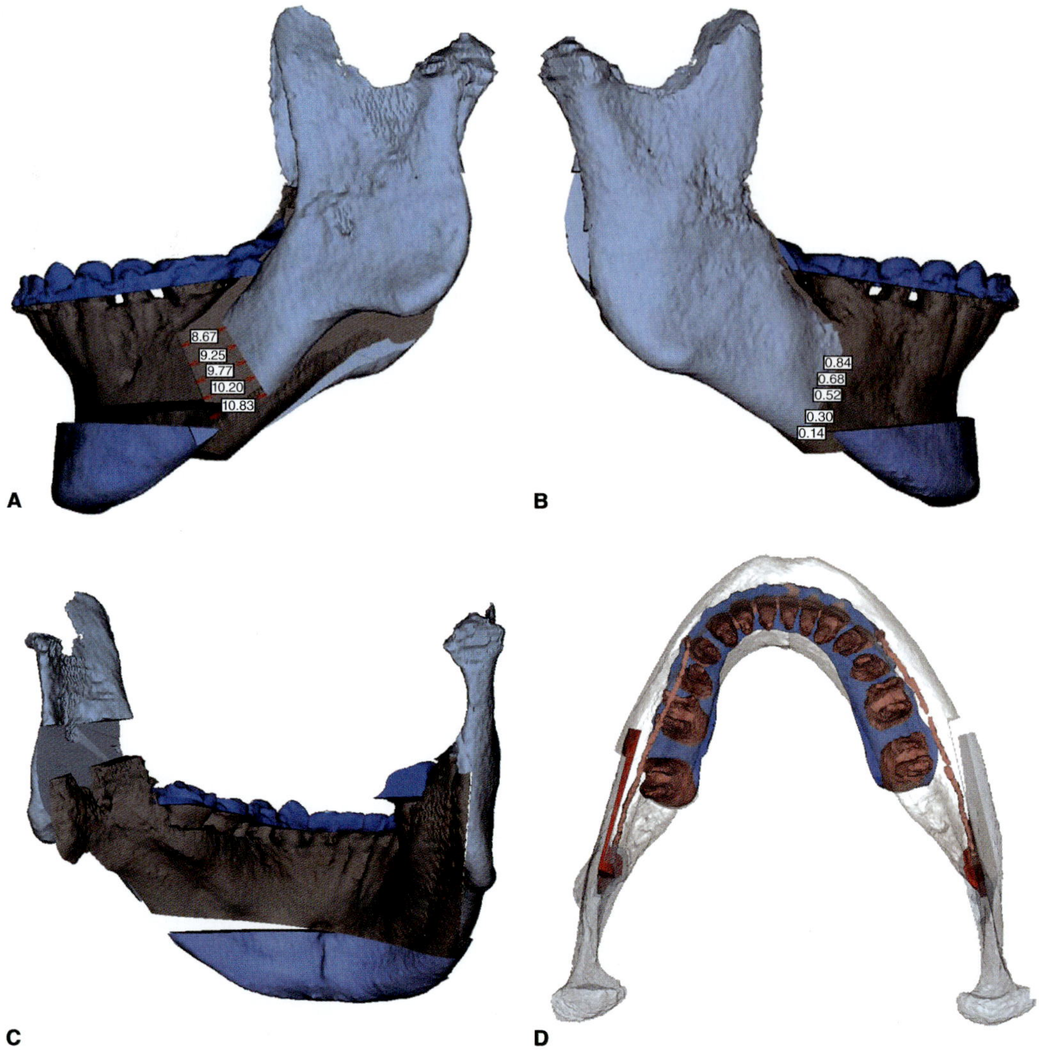

Figure 20.16 *A–C*: Evaluation of proximal segments to determine the presence of interferences and to proactively plan for their correction intraoperatively. Care also is taken to not lengthen the pterygomasseteric sling to ensure improved surgical stability. Any skeletal movements that would result in lengthening of the pterygomasseteric sling can be visualized and minimized during this virtual treatment planning step. *D*: When a proximal segment collision is detected, as in this case, the surgeon may choose to correct this intraoperatively with osteoplasty of the proximal and distal segments for passive adaptation of the two segments or, in rare instances, to change the yaw of the occlusion.

confirmed this accuracy with similar variances (Hsu *et al.*, 2013), which are highly desirable outcomes. The accuracy, efficiency, and facility of the process have led to the rapid adoption of the system by a growing number of surgeons. Future advances in the virtual treatment planning and splint fabrication processes will evolve with improvements in software interfaces and as new methods of NHP recording become integrated into the process.

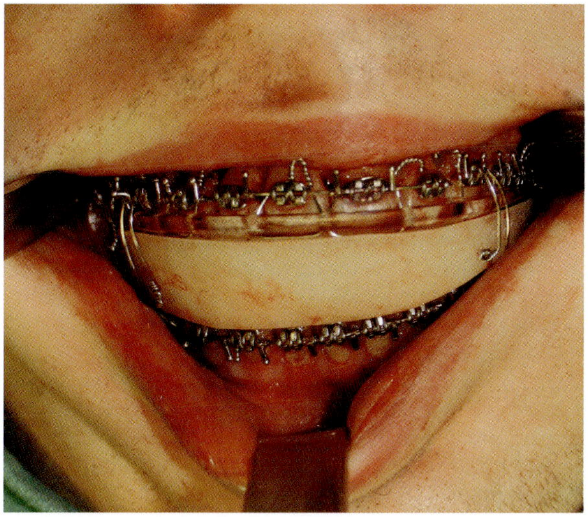

Figure 20.17 Excellent indexing of piggyback splints demonstrated during intraoperative use.

CONCLUSIONS

CBCT technology has contributed to significant advances in orthognathic surgery diagnostics and treatment. It has enabled the advent of 3D cephalometrics that increasingly is becoming commonplace in the profession. The precision and efficiency of orthognathic surgery has improved as a result of the technology and due to continued enhancements in software being developed to take advantage of CBCT data. Finally, surgeons now have a tool to evaluate their results fully and critically and to advance the art and science of the discipline.

References

Betts, N.J., Vanarsdall, R.L., Barber, H.D., *et al.* (1995) Diagnosis and treatment of transverse maxillary deficiency. *International Journal of Adult Orthodontics and Orthognathic Surgery*, 10 (2), 75–96.

Bholsithi, W., Tharanon, W., Chintakanon, K., *et al.* (2009) 3D vs. 2D cephalometric analysis comparisons with repeated measurements from 20 Thai males and 20 Thai females. *Biomedical Imaging and Intervention Journal*, 5 (4), e21.

Broca, M. (1862) Sur les projections de la tete et sur un noveau procede de cephalometrie. *Bulletins de la Société d'Anthropologie de Paris*, 3, 514–545 (in French).

Burstone, C.J., James, R.B., Legan, H., *et al.* (1978) Cephalometrics for orthognathic surgery. *Journal of Oral Surgery*, 36 (4), 269–277.

Chang, Y.B., Xia, J.J., Gateno, J., *et al.* (2010) An automatic and robust algorithm of reestablishment of a digital dental occlusion. *IEEE Transactions on Medical Imaging*, 29 (9), 1652–1663.

Chenin, D.L. (2010) 3D cephalometrics: the new norm. *Alpha Omegan*, 103 (2), 51–56.

Fuhrmann, R., Feifel, H., Schnappauf, A., *et al.* (1996) Integration of three-dimensional cephalometry and 3D-skull models in combined orthodontic/surgical treatment planning. *Journal of Orofacial Orthopedics*, 57 (1), 32–45.

Gateno, J., Xia, J.J., & Teichgraber, J.F. (2011) New 3-dimensional cephalometric analysis for orthognathic surgery. *Journal of Oral and Maxillofacial Surgery*, 69 (3), 606–622.

Grummons, D.C. & Kappeyne van de Coppello, M.A. (1987) A frontal asymmetry analysis. *Journal of Clinical Orthodontics*, 21 (7), 448–465.

Hsu, S.S., Gateno, J., Bell, R.B., *et al.* (2013) Accuracy of a computer-aided surgical simulation protocol for orthognathic surgery: a prospective multicenter study. *Journal of Oral and Maxillofacial Surgery*, 71 (1), 128–142.

Legan, H.L. & Burstone, C.J. (1980) Soft tissue cephalometric analysis for orthognathic surgery. *Journal of Oral Surgery*, 38 (10), 744–751.

Major, P.W., Johnson, D.E., Hesse, K.L., *et al.* (1994) Landmark identification error in posterior anterior cephalometrics. *The Angle Orthodontist*, 64 (6), 447–454.

Major, P.W., Johnson, D.E., Hesse, K.L., *et al.* (1996) Effect of head orientation on posterior anterior cephalometric landmark identification. *The Angle Orthodontist*, 66 (1), 51–60.

Miller, R.J., Kuo, E., & Choi, W. (2003) Validation of Align Technologies Treat III digital model superimposition tool and its case application. *Orthodontics & Craniofacial Research*, 6 (Suppl 1), 143–149.

Noguchi, N., Tsuji, M., Shigematsu, M., *et al.* (2007) An orthognathic simulation system integrating teeth, jaw and face data using 3D cephalometry. *International Journal of Oral and Maxillofacial Surgery*, 36 (7), 640–645.

Olszewski, R., Cosnard, G., Macq, B., *et al.* (2006) 3D CT-based cephalometric analysis: 3D cephalometric theoretical concept and software. *Neuroradiology*, 48 (11), 853–862.

Pape, R., Pizelle, C., & Foucart, J.M. (2012) Measurement errors in 3D cephalometrics: about the buccal cranio-facial analysis. *L'Orthodontie Française*, 83 (1), 37–44 (in French).

Peck, H. & Peck, S. (1970) A concept of facial esthetics. *The Angle Orthodontist*, 40 (4), 284–318.

Plooij, J.M., Maal, T.J., Haers, P., *et al.* (2011) Digital three-dimensional image fusion processes for planning and evaluating orthodontics and orthognathic surgery: a systematic review. *International Journal of Oral and Maxillofacial Surgery*, 40 (4), 341–352.

Ricketts, R.M. (1981) Perspectives in the clinical application of cephalometrics: the first fifty years. *The Angle Orthodontist*, 51 (2), 115–150.

Steiner, C. (1953) Cephalometrics for you and me. *American Journal of Orthodontics*, 39 (10), 729–755.

van Vlijmen, O.J., Maal, T., Berge, S.J., *et al.* (2010) A comparison between 2D and 3D cephalometry on CBCT scans of human skulls. *International Journal of Oral and Maxillofacial Surgery*, 39 (2), 156–160.

Wylie, G.A., Fish, L.C., & Epker, B.N. (1987) Cephalometrics: a comparison of five analyses currently used in the diagnosis of dentofacial deformities. *International Journal of Adult Orthodontics and Orthognathic Surgery*, 2 (1), 15–36.

Xia, J.J., Gateno, J., & Teichgraber, J.F. (2005) Three-dimensional computer-aided surgical simulation for maxillofacial surgery. *Atlas of the Oral and Maxillofacial Surgery Clinics of North America*, 13 (1), 25–39.

Xia, J.J., Gateno, J., Teichgraber, J.F., *et al.* (2007) Accuracy of the computer-aided surgical simulation (CASS) system in the treatment of patients with complex craniomaxillofacial deformity: a pilot study. *Journal of Oral and Maxillofacial Surgery*, 65 (2), 248–254.

Xia, J.J., Gateno, J., & Teichgraber, J.F. (2009) New clinical protocol to evaluate craniomaxillofacial deformity and plan surgical correction. *Journal of Oral and Maxillofacial Surgery*, 67 (10), 2093–2106.

Xia, J.J., McGrory, J.K., Gateno, J., *et al.* (2011) A new method to orient 3-dimensional computed tomography models to the natural head position: a clinical feasibility study. *Journal of Oral and Maxillofacial Surgery*, 69 (3), 584–591.

Zamora, N., Llamas, J.M., Cibrian, R., *et al.* (2012) A study on the reproducibility of cephalometric landmarks when undertaking a three-dimensional (3D) cephalometric analysis. *Medicina Oral, Patologia Oral, y Cirugia Bucal*, 17 (4), e678–e688.

21 3D Diagnosis and Management of Facial Asymmetries

Abeer AlHadidi, DDS, MS, Dipl ABOMR, Lucia H.S. Cevidanes, DDS, MS, PhD, and Beatriz Paniagua, PhD

INTRODUCTION

Craniofacial deformities occur in around 5% of the U.S. population. Of these individuals, 2% have facial asymmetry severe enough to be disabling and stigmatizing. Facial asymmetry includes a spectrum of malformations that result from maxillary and/or mandibular hypoplasia or hyperplasia on the affected side of the face (Severt & Proffit, 1997; Proffit *et al.*, 1998). Because of challenges in identifying the precise location and magnitude of the asymmetric structures in the face, this entity often poses a challenge in diagnosis and treatment planning. Also due to the wide variability in the etiology and presentation of the disorders, the proper assessment and quantification of the differences between the right and left sides is crucial for optimized diagnosis, treatment planning, and follow-up of these patients.

Although cephalometric radiography has been and probably will continue to be the routine radiographic examination for many patients seeking orthodontic treatment with or without orthognathic surgery, the "inappropriateness of conventional cephalometrics" for these purposes had been recognized as early as 1979 (Moyers & Bookstein, 1979). These two-dimensional (2D) radiographs are problematic particularly when rotational or asymmetrical correction is required, since the clinical presentation of these disorders and their surgical correction are inherently three-dimensional (3D; Sandor *et al.*, 2007).

The use of cone beam computed tomography (CBCT) or spiral computer tomography (CT) provides the 3D imaging data necessary to generate precise knowledge of the location and the magnitude of specific features contributing to the asymmetry, which are essential for the diagnosis of facial deformities and planning of corrective procedures. Even though the clinician may be able to visualize facial asymmetry in 3D surface models, this does not imply necessarily that he or she has the capability to quantify and precisely locate sites of the asymmetry. For optimized diagnosis and

Cone Beam Computed Tomography in Orthodontics: Indications, Insights, and Innovations, First Edition. Sunil D. Kapila.

treatment planning of asymmetric patients, the clinician must have the ability to perform a detailed analysis of the positional and morphological discrepancies between the normal and affected sides of the face. An increasing number of studies have demonstrated that computer-aided surgical simulation (CASS) can predict possible surgical complications and lower material costs while decreasing the duration of surgery, with comparable or better surgical outcomes (Xia *et al.*, 2000a, 2000b; Hassfeld & Muhling, 2001; Troulis *et al.*, 2002; Gateno *et al.*, 2003, 2007). These approaches could prove highly valuable in the diagnosis and treatment of facial asymmetries.

3D imaging and associated image analysis methods developed recently have the potential for additional advancements that will contribute to enhancing and quantifying the diagnosis of facial asymmetries. The use of relatively low radiation dose CBCT scanners in dental practices facilitates the examination of anatomical structures in a multiplanar view. It also provides a rich data source for the application of different image analysis techniques to further extract diagnostic information from available volumes. Creation of 3D virtual surface models from CBCT volumes, registration of these models, and measurements of the surface distances between different models is a well-documented approach used to study growth, treatment changes, and the stability of those changes (Chapter 19; Cevidanes *et al.*, 2005a, 2005b, 2005c, 2006, 2007). This chapter provides the necessary and essential background in novel methods for 3D assessment and management of mandibular asymmetry that take advantage of the promising advancements in 3D hardware and software technologies. These approaches described for mandibular asymmetries have applications to asymmetries affecting other parts of the face.

MIDLINE DETERMINATION AND MIRRORING TECHNIQUES

Various approaches have been described in the literature in an attempt to use 3D imaging for the detection and quantification of craniofacial asymmetry (Katsumata *et al.*, 2005; Maeda *et al.*, 2006; Park *et al.*, 2006). Most of these techniques depend on landmark identification and manual identification of a straight "midsagittal plane," both of which are challenging and prone to operator error.

Prima and colleagues (2002) presented a method to define the midsagittal plane of the brain automatically in 2D cross-sectional slices; however, the accurate definition of the mid-sagittal plane in the maxillofacial area as proposed in this study remains a challenge because the plane is a curved surface in faces that have a chin deviation. In 2005, an alternative method for determining a plane of symmetry that mirrors the mandible in any arbitrary plane with rigid registration of the mirrored mandible to the original image was proposed (Glerup, 2005). However, this procedure did not take into consideration the morphological relationships of the mandible to the maxilla and the cranial base. A modification of this approach that first mirrors the entire image including the mandible and then registers it on the cranial base can provide information on the entire facial structure rather than just the mandible (Cevidanes *et al.*, 2006).

AlHadidi and colleagues (2011) compared these two previously proposed methods of assessing mandibular asymmetry (Glerup, 2005; Cevidanes *et al.*, 2006). The first method uses mirroring of the mandible in the mid-sagittal plane (Figure 21.1); the second uses mirroring of the mandible and registration on the cranial base (Figure 21.2). For the first approach, a mid-sagittal plane was defined for each of 22 randomly selected asymmetric patients as the plane passing through nasion (Na), anterior nasal spine (ANS), and basion (Ba). This mid-sagittal plane and the degree of asymmetry were determined five times from this patient cohort. Differences between repeated assessments of asymmetry served as a measure of reproducibility of mid-sagittal plane identification. Additionally, mirror images for both halves of the mandible were created.

The second approach consisted of mirroring the image volume by flipping the left and right sides and then registering the mirrored image onto the cranial base using a mutual information maximization method. Both mirroring techniques provided similar quantification of mandibular asymmetry in the patient cohort studied; however, neither approach could be applied indiscriminately to any patient. The findings showed that mirroring using

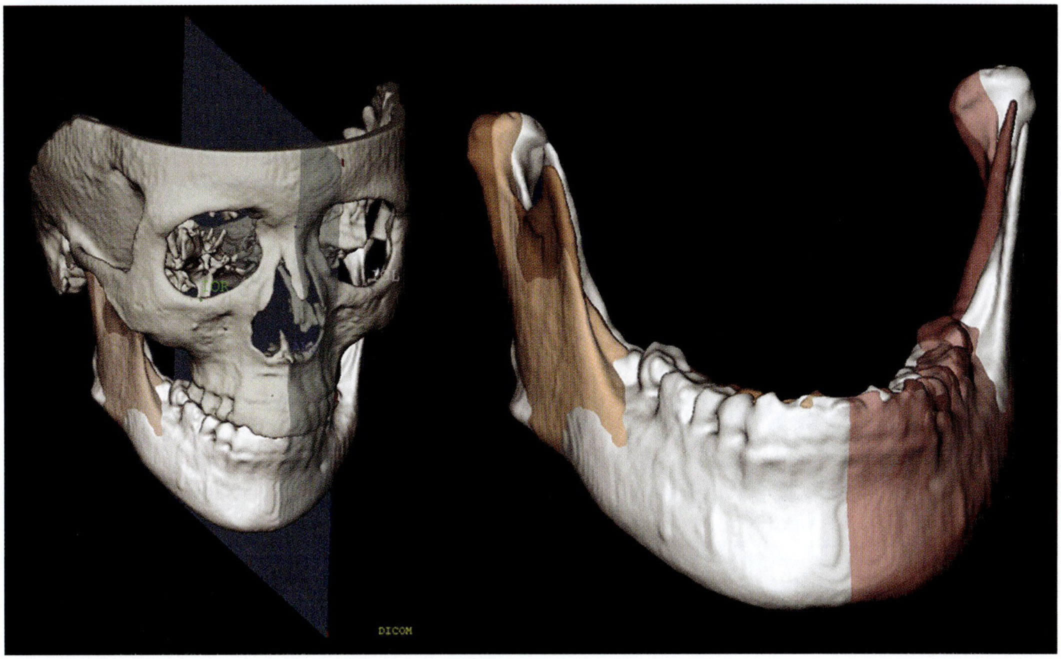

Figure 21.1 Mirroring on a mid-sagittal plane for quantitation of mandibular asymmetry. A mid-sagittal plane was defined for this patient based on Na, Ba, and ANS. The left ramus was mirrored onto the right side using this plane. The other side also was mirrored based on the same mid-sagittal plane. Asymmetry was defined by the difference between one half of the mandible and the mirror of the contralateral side. White, original mandible; color, mirrors.

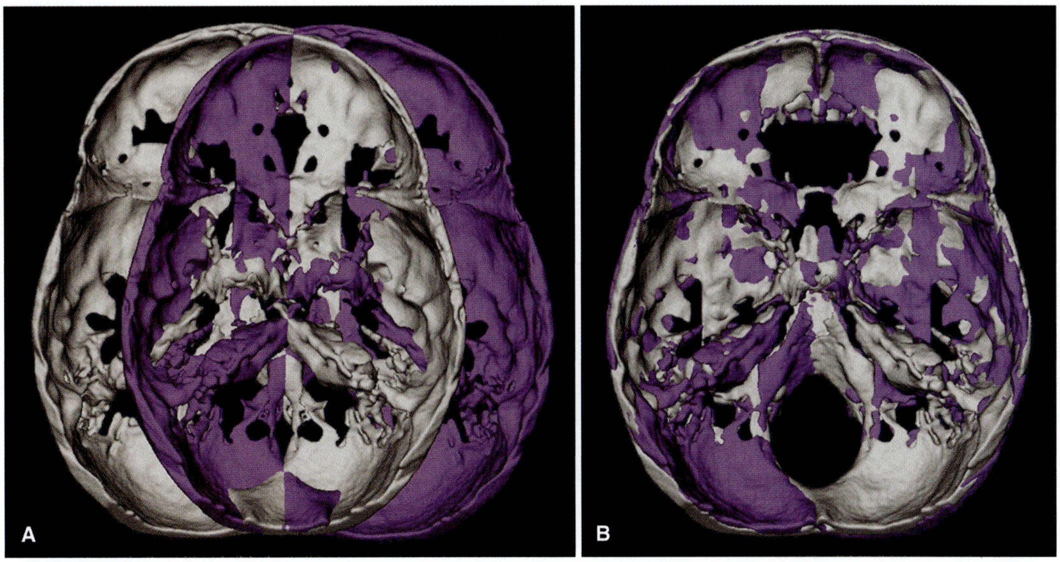

Figure 21.2 Arbitrary plane mirroring followed by cranial base registration approach for assessment of mandibular asymmetry. Symmetric cranial base in nongrowing patients is considered a stable registration area to fit the original volume and the mirror in the same reference plane. *A*: Cranial base virtual surface model for a patient (white) and arbitrarily mirrored image model (purple). *B*: Original model and arbitrary mirror matching on the cranial base as a result of a voxel-based registration.

the mid-sagittal plane generates inaccurate and clinically irrelevant results for patients such as those with cleft palate who present with facial features that affect the midline position of the points (NA, ANS, Ba) used to define this plane. Similarly, in patients with asymmetries involving the cranial base, registration on the cranial base also results in suboptimal results. This implies that patient-specific methods may be indicated for optimal localization and quantification of mandibular asymmetries.

SEGMENTATION AND SURFACE DISTANCE COMPUTATION

Using 3D imaging analysis, mandibular asymmetry has been quantified as the surface distances between the affected side of the mandible and the mirror image of the opposite side. Surface models of mandibles need to be segmented out of the original volumes for surface distance measurements.

Segmentation involves outlining the shape of structures visible in the cross-sections of a volumetric dataset in the CBCT-3D images. Segmentation of anatomic structures can be performed using ITK-SNAP, which is an open-source software (http://www.itksnap.org; Yushkevich *et al.*, 2006). 3D virtual models then are built for each patient from a set of approximately 300 axial cross-sectional slices for each image with the image voxels reformatted for an isotropic resolution of 0.5 mm × 0.5 mm × 0.5 mm. This resolution is used because higher spatial resolution with smaller slice thickness results in a large image file size that requires greater computational power and user interaction time. After segmentation with ITK-SNAP tool, a 3D graphic rendering of the volumetric object allows navigation between voxels in the volumetric image and the 3D graphic representation with zooming, rotating, and panning (Figure 21.3).

Most commercially available and academic software that are able to compute color-coded surface distance maps use closest point algorithm to obtain surface distances. Closest point is a brute force algorithm that calculates a vertex-to-vertex Euclidean closest point distance (Besl & McKay, 1992; De Momi *et al.*, 2006). This method does not map corresponding surfaces based on anatomical geometry, and, thus, it usually underestimates rotational and large translational movements.

The application of conventional closest point distances for mirror images in mandibles of patients with rudimentary condyles, severe cants, or a rotated mandible represents not the difference between corresponding anatomical locations, but rather differences based on the minimal distances between any point in the original and mirrored models. These clinical situations (Figure 21.4) mandate the use of more "anatomy sensitive" shape analysis techniques such as shape correspondence.

Shape correspondence is a promising alternative to overcome the shortcomings of the commonly used closest point algorithm. It is one of the currently used statistical shape analysis techniques that allows measuring the surface distance between an area on one model to the corresponding anatomical area in the other model regardless of the alignment of those models. The main challenges to shape correspondence involve the representation of a population by means of correspondent point-based models (Figure 21.5). Surface representation could be accomplished by several different options, including matching of template surface geometry (curvature and location; Meyer *et al.*, 2002), entropy-based particle systems (Oguz, 2009), or spherical harmonic representation (SPHARM; Gerig *et al.*, 2001). In SPHARM, the surface model gets mapped in a sphere, and correspondence point-based models are computed after finding the spherical harmonic basis that best fits the model (Styner *et al.*, 2006). After surface mapping is achieved, correspondence could be based on different frameworks depending on the clinical problem on hand.

SPHARM-PDM (point distribution models) allows for comprehensive statistical evaluations for the models developed with this approach to be computed for the correspondent models as a whole or for specific regions of interest within these models. For the assessment and future treatment planning of asymmetries, an individual-based approach is preferred to one that is based on group analysis (AlHadidi *et al.*, 2012b). Group analysis usually is used to examine general trends and cross-sectional tendencies, both of which have limited utility to patient-specific treatment planning.

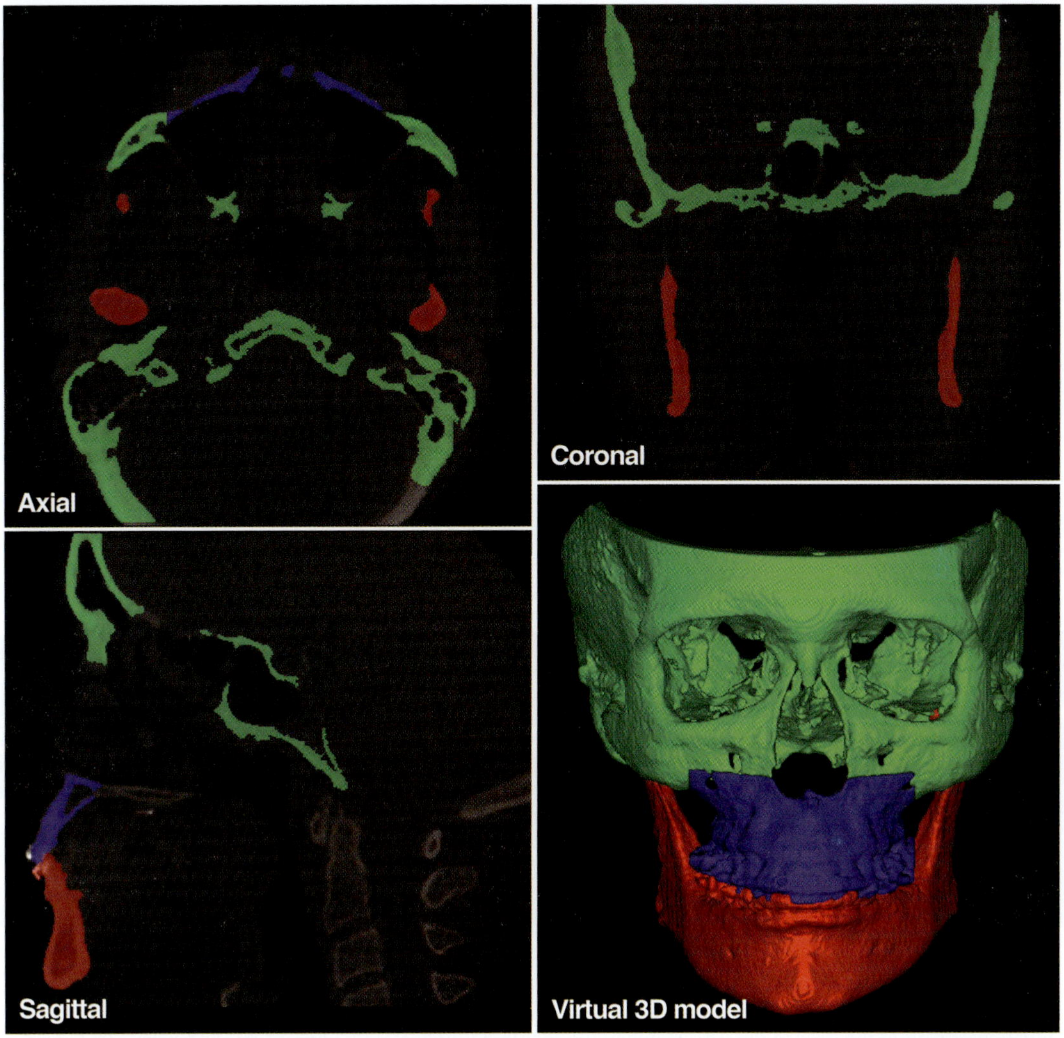

Figure 21.3 Image segmentation. CBCT images are imported as DICOM files into ITK-SNAP. In a process known as semi-automatic segmentation, anatomical areas of interest are identified and delineated. Manual editing is performed to ensure accuracy of the segmentations. The images can be viewed in 3D and as axial, coronal, and sagittal multiplanar slices of each image.

The subtraction of mirrored and original asymmetric mandible models provides color-coded corresponding distance maps and maps of vectors of differences between these models. The distance maps measure the magnitude of the differences between the point-based models, while the vector maps offer directionality. To maximize the usefulness of the extensive data that SPHARM-PDM can provide, regions of interest that correspond to surgical segments could be analyzed separately. This quantitative asymmetry measure could be either communicated to the surgeon or used as an input for surgical simulation software, as explained later.

Procrustes can be used to capture translational and rotational differences between each hemimandible and the mirror of the contralateral side in the three planes of space. The six degrees of freedom of the differences can be calculated using

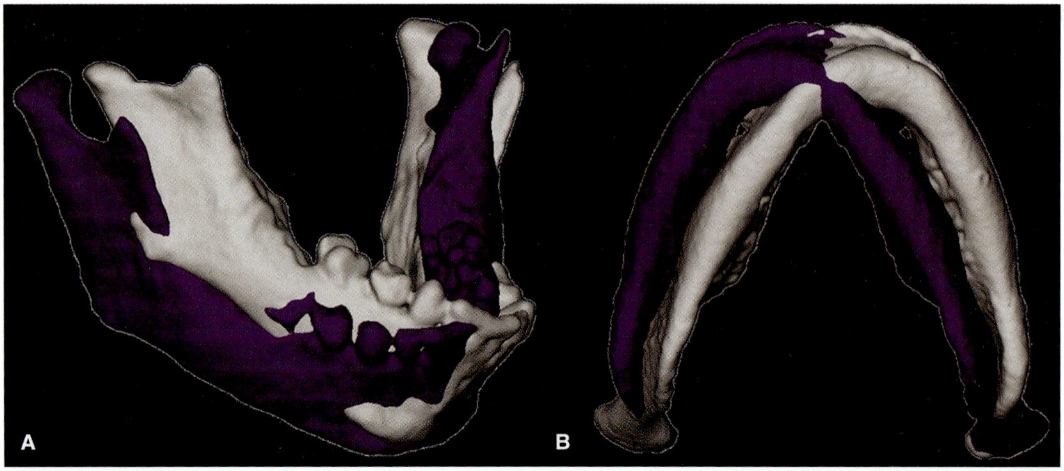

Figure 21.4 Examples of patients with challenging asymmetries for quantification. Severe cant (*A*) and rotation (*B*) are hard to quantify using closest point algorithm. White, original mandible; violet, mirrored mandible.

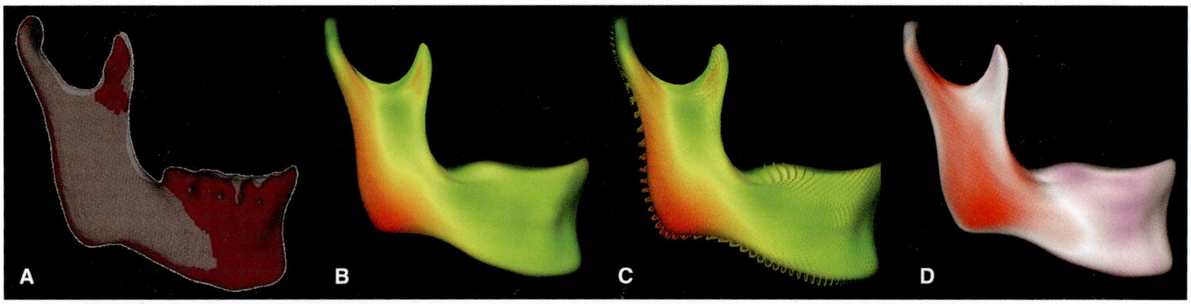

Figure 21.5 Quantification of mandibular asymmetry for a patient using shape correspondence. *A*: Original model (gray) and left hemi-mandible arbitrary mirror matching on the cranial base (maroon). *B*: Surface distance map showing the difference between those two models. *C*: Shape correspondence can be used to quantify the right and left differences as represented in this vectorial color map of the surface distance between the registered original and arbitrary mirror models. *D*: Signed color maps showing the directionality of the differences.

rigid Procrustes alignment, which is the geometric transformation that best maps and measures positional changes between point-based correspondent models.

SURGICAL SIMULATION AND OUTCOME DESIGN

Facial asymmetry is a complex clinical entity that comprises two main components: a shape and a positional component. During growth, the shape discrepancies lead to compensatory positional differences that contribute to disturbances in the harmony of the maxillofacial complex. Clinicians need to diagnose both shape and positional components of the asymmetry prior to the design and execution of the corrective surgery. In the past, the inability to appreciate the interplay between maxillo-mandibular roll and yaw was a missing link in classification and diagnosis of asymmetries. When one sees a major midline shift, a Class II

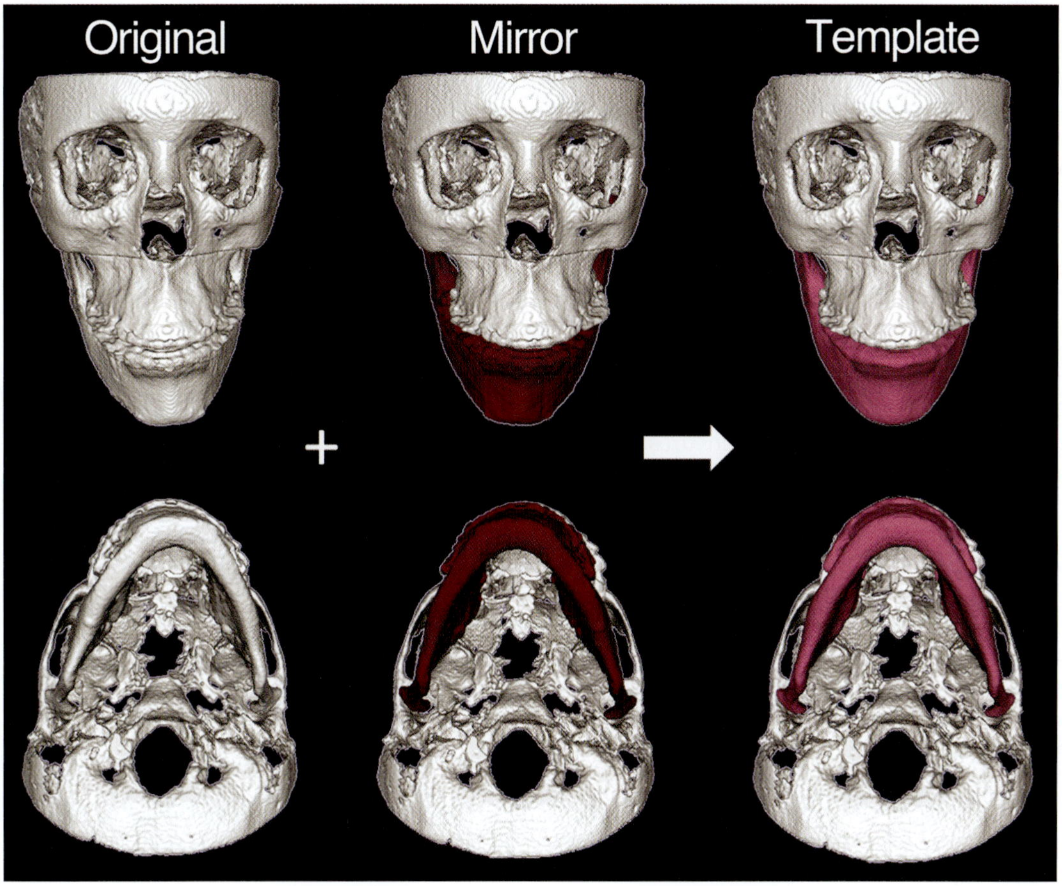

Figure 21.6 Atlas formation. The original mandible (white) and its registered mirror (maroon) are both used to compute an atlas (pink) that will serve subsequently as a template for surgical simulation.

subdivision, a Class III molar relationship, or a true unilateral crossbite, quantification of the mandibular roll and yaw is essential before the actual left and right differences can be quantified correctly. The extent of asymmetric yaw is a major determinant in whether treatment is limited to asymmetric mechanics or might extend to asymmetric extractions, unilateral bone anchors, or surgery (Ackerman *et al.*, 2007). For surgeons to reach a "symmetric" result in the patient, positional asymmetries in the roll and yaw need to be corrected first, following which the 3D shape asymmetry can be assessed properly and addressed. The use of conventional mirror images does not guide surgeons adequately on the correction of facial asymmetries because it does not compensate for the positional component.

Because of the limitations of current methods to evaluate and quantify asymmetries, a patient-specific atlas has been proposed for use as a template for corrective surgeries for patients with mandibular asymmetry (AlHadidi *et al.*, 2012a). In this approach, surface models for both the diseased mandible of each patient and its registered mirror are used to compute an atlas using deformable fluid registration. For the pilot study, templates were computed for three patients with histories of favorable clinical outcomes of the correction of their mandibular asymmetry. A favorable outcome was based on post-operative clinical exam, post-operative dental casts, and photos. Virtual corrective surgery was simulated using the atlas computed for each patient as a template, and the outcome was compared with the real surgical outcome. The detected differences between the virtual simulated outcome and the actual surgical outcome, as characterized in six degrees of freedom, were smaller than 2 mm of translation and 5° of rotation. This indicates that the location of the synthesized template is similar to the desired clinical outcome.

The use of the patient's own anatomy for the computation of the custom-made template accommodates the large variability in the clinical presentation of mandibular asymmetry. It ensures that the outcome virtual template has the basic features (condylar position, relative size), while maintaining the harmony between the mandible and the rest of the maxillofacial area (Figure 21.6). This approach also helps to eliminate the need to identify the "healthy" (normal) side for the mandible to use as a template for mirroring, especially because conceptually an asymmetric mandible is not likely to have a "healthy" side due to the inherent physiological compensation processes that occur during asymmetric growth.

FUTURE PERSPECTIVES

Unfolding the details of how the soft tissue interplays with the underlying hard tissue to mask or exacerbate existing asymmetries, how it behaves on correction of asymmetry, and how it affects the stability of corrective surgeries of those patients is a rich area for future research and has substantial clinical implications. At this point, however, the theories of how soft tissue behaves or our tools to measure morphological features of soft tissue have not yielded sufficient evidence for clinical application.

Although the above-mentioned image analysis techniques have been validated and applied on cross-sectional data, future randomized clinical studies are needed to assess true outcome changes and the stability of those changes attributable to the use of 3D image analysis techniques utilized in the assessment and treatment planning of facial asymmetry patients.

References

Ackerman, J., Proffit, W., Sarver, D., *et al.* (2007) Pitch, roll, and yaw: describing the spatial orientation of dentofacial traits. *American Journal of Orthodontics and Dentofacial Orthopedics*, 131 (3), 305–310.

AlHadidi, A., Cevidanes, L.H., Mol, A., *et al.* (2011) Comparison of two methods for quantitative assessment of mandibular asymmetry using cone beam computed tomography image volumes. *Dentomaxillofacial Radiology*, 40 (6), 351–357.

AlHadidi, A., Cevidanes, L.H., Cook, R., *et al.* (2012a) The use of a custom made atlas as a template for corrective surgeries of asymmetric patients. *Proceedings of SPIE. Volume 8317, 83171Y*. Available at http://dx.doi.org.libproxy.lib.unc.edu/10.1117/12.911048, accessed April 15, 2012.

AlHadidi, A., Cevidanes, L.H., Paniagua, B., *et al.* (2012b) 3D quantification of mandibular asymmetry using the SPHARM-PDM tool box. *International Journal of Computer Assisted Radiology and Surgery*, 7 (2), 265–271.

Besl, P.J. & McKay, N.D. (1992) A method for registration of 3-D shapes. *IEEE Transactions on Pattern Analysis and Machine Intelligence*, 14 (2), 239–256.

Cevidanes, L.H., Franco, A.A., Gerig, G., *et al.* (2005a) Assessment of mandibular growth and response to orthopedic treatment with 3-dimensional magnetic resonance images. *American Journal of Orthodontics and Dentofacial Orthopedics*, 128 (1), 16–26.

Cevidanes, L.H., Franco, A.A., Gerig, G., *et al.* (2005b) Comparison of relative mandibular growth vectors with high-resolution 3-dimensional imaging. *American Journal of Orthodontics and Dentofacial Orthopedics*, 128 (1), 27–34.

Cevidanes, L.H., Bailey, L.J., Tucker, Jr., G.R., *et al.* (2005c) Superimposition of 3D cone-beam CT models of orthognathic surgery patients. *Dentomaxillofacial Radiology*, 34 (6), 369–375.

Cevidanes, L.H., Styner, M.A., & Proffit, W.R. (2006) Image analysis and superimposition of 3-dimensional cone-beam computed tomography models. *American Journal of Orthodontics and Dentofacial Orthopedics*, 129 (5), 611–618.

Cevidanes, L.H., Bailey, L.J., Tucker, S.F., *et al.* (2007) Three-dimensional cone-beam computed tomography for assessment of mandibular changes after orthognathic surgery. *American Journal of Orthodontics and Dentofacial Orthopedics*, 131 (1), 44–50.

De Momi, E., Chapuis, J., Pappas, I., *et al.* (2006) Automatic extraction of the mid-facial plane for cranio-maxillofacial surgery planning. *International Journal of Oral Maxillofacial Surgery*, 35 (7), 636–642.

Gateno, J., Teichgraeber, J.F., & Xia, J.J. (2003) Three-dimensional surgical planning for maxillary and midface distraction ostogenesis. *Journal of Craniofacial Surgery*, 14 (6), 833–839.

Gateno, J., Xia, J.J., Teichgraeber, J.F., *et al.* (2007) Clinical feasibility of computer-aided surgical simulation (CASS) in the treatment of complex cranio-maxillofacial deformities. *Journal of Oral and Maxillofacial Surgery*, 65 (4), 728–734.

Gerig, G., Styner, M., Jones, D., *et al.* (2001) Shape analysis of brain ventricles using SPHARM. *Proceedings IEEE Workshop on Mathematical Methods in Biomedical Image Analysis MMBIA 2001*. IEEE Computer Society, 171–178.

Glerup, N. (2005) Asymmetry measures in medical image analysis. PhD thesis, University of Copenhagen.

Hassfeld, S. & Muhling, J. (2001) Computer assisted oral and maxillofacial surgery: a review and an assessment of technology. *International Journal of Oral and Maxillofacial Surgery*, 30 (1), 2–13.

Katsumata, A., Fujishita, M., Maeda, M., *et al.* (2005) 3D-CT evaluation of facial asymmetry. *Oral Surgery, Oral Medicine, Oral Pathology, Oral Radiology and Endodontology*, 99 (2), 212–220.

Maeda, M., Katsumata, A., Ariji, Y., *et al.* (2006) 3D-CT evaluation of facial asymmetry in patients with maxillofacial deformities. *Oral Surgery, Oral Medicine, Oral Pathology, Oral Radiology and Endodontology*, 102 (3), 382–390.

Meyer, M., Desbrun, M., Schröder, P., *et al.* (2002) Discrete differential-geometry operators for triangulated 2-manifolds. *Proceedings of Visualization and Mathematics*, 3 (7), 34–57.

Moyers, R.E. & Bookstein, F.L. (1979) The inappropriateness of conventional cephalometrics. *American Journal of Orthodontics*, 75 (6), 599–617.

Oguz, I. (2009) Groupwise shape correspondence with local features. PhD thesis, University of North Carolina at Chapel Hill.

Park, S.H., Yu, H.S., Kim, K.D., *et al.* (2006) A proposal for a new analysis of craniofacial morphology by 3-dimensional computed tomography. *American Journal of Orthodontics and Dentofacial Orthopedics*, 129 (5), 600.e23–600.e34.

Prima, S., Ourselin, S., & Ayache, N. (2002) Computation of the mid-sagittal plane in 3D images of the brain. *IEEE Transactions of Medical Imaging*, 21 (2), 122–138.

Proffit, W.R., Fields Jr, H.W., & Moray, L.J. (1998) Prevalence of malocclusion and orthodontic treatment need in the United States: estimates from the NHANES III survey. *International Journal of Adult Orthodontics and Orthognathic Surgery*, 13 (2), 97–106.

Sandor, G.K., McGuire, T.P., Ylikontiola, L.P., *et al.* (2007) Management of facial asymmetry. *Oral and Maxillofacial Surgery Clinics of North America*, 19 (3), 395–422.

Severt, T.R. & Proffit, W.R. (1997) The prevalence of facial asymmetry in the dentofacial deformities population at the University of North Carolina. *International Journal of Adult Orthodontics and Orthognathic Surgery*, 12 (3), 171–176.

Styner, M., Oguz, I., Xu, S., *et al.* (2006) Framework for the statistical shape analysis of brain structures using SPHARM-PDM. *The Insight Journal*, 1071, 242–250.

Troulis, M.J., Everett, P., Seldin, E.B., *et al.* (2002) Development of a three-dimensional treatment planning system based on computer tomographic data. *International Journal of Oral and Maxillofacial Surgery*, 31 (4), 349–357.

Xia, J., Ip, H.H., Samman, N., *et al.* (2000a) Computer-assisted three-dimensional surgical planning and simulation: 3D virtual osteotomy. *International Journal of Oral and Maxillofacial Surgery*, 29 (1), 11–17.

Xia, J., Samman, N., Yeung, R.W., *et al.* (2000b) Three-dimensional virtual reality surgical planning and simulation workbench for orthognathic surgery. *International Journal of Adult Orthodontics and Orthognathic Surgery*, 15 (4), 265–282.

Yushkevich, P.A., Piven, J., Hazlett, H.C., *et al.* (2006) User-guided 3D active contour segmentation of anatomical structures: significantly improved efficiency and reliability. *NeuroImage*, 31 (3), 1116–1128.

22 3D Assessment of Orthognathic Surgical Outcomes

Yoon-Ji R. Kim, DDS, MSD, PhD, Yang-Ho Park, DDS, MSD, PhD, Leonardo Koerich de Paula, MS, DDS, and R. Scott Conley, DMD

INTRODUCTION

Assessment of treatment outcomes that typically are made relative to the pre-treatment presentation or the planned treatment objectives is performed best through a careful evaluation of post-treatment records that include radiographs. Radiographic imaging allows the orthodontist and surgeon to visualize and quantify clearly the dental, skeletal, and soft tissue changes resulting from treatment. Critical post-treatment analysis forces clinicians to assess objectively whether the treatment provided met the established pre-treatment goals; continual assessment wherein clinicians reproduce the successful and abandon the unsuccessful treatment modalities eventually improves treatment outcomes. It is hoped that by analyzing the final state of a patient's craniofacial anatomy, clinicians also will be able to assess the factors that may be associated with relapse more fully in order to better predict long-term stability for future patients (Plooij *et al.*, 2009; Kim *et al.*, 2011).

This chapter describes some of the limitations of determining treatment outcomes by two-dimensional (2D) orthognathic surgery imaging. It also highlights how three-dimensional (3D) imaging with CBCT may provide greater insight to the purported dental and skeletal components associated with relapse and post-treatment functional deficiencies.

HISTORY AND BACKGROUND OF ORTHOGNATHIC SURGERY

Surgery on the jaws initially was performed as early as the 1840s, even before the invention and routine use of radiography (Hullihen, 1849). At that time, there were multiple limitations to successful treatment, including lack of adequate anesthesia, difficulty controlling bleeding, incomplete knowledge of surgical anatomy, lack of understanding of the biological basis for successful surgery, and inability to control infection. While

Cone Beam Computed Tomography in Orthodontics: Indications, Insights, and Innovations, First Edition. Sunil D. Kapila.

improving the patient's condition was the stated primary goal, living through the ordeal without experiencing significant complications often was the more practical goal. As an example, Cheever in the first reported LeFort I maxillary osteotomy exposed and removed a nasopharyngeal carcinoma (Moloney & Worthington, 1981). The operation was a success and the carcinoma was removed; however, the patient died about 3 days later.

In the 1930s, Wassmund and others began to revisit surgery on the jaws (Wassmund, 1935). At this time, surgery to correct severe jaw deformities concentrated almost exclusively on the mandible for correction of mandibular prognathism (Blair, 1906; Limberg, 1928; Sowray & Haskell, 1968). Outcome studies were limited and largely relied on isolated case reports or case series using extraoral facial analysis, since lateral cephalometry had not begun to be used routinely yet.

Mandibular surgery was revolutionized by Trauner & Obwegeser (1957) when they reported a novel technique, the sagittal split ramus osteotomy (SSRO), to alter mandibular position. Their technique represented the first intraoral approach to retract the mandible bodily that later was adopted also to advance the mandible. The intraoral approach was made possible with the advent of antibiotics shortly after World War II, which enabled the surgeon to control infections caused by the intraoral flora. Post-surgical relapse and normalization of function remained a shortcoming with the procedure; however, due to wire osteosynthesis, trismus following the 6–8 weeks of intermaxillary fixation, and the unsatisfactory and unpredictable control of the proximal and distal segments, post-surgical relapse and normalization of function remained a shortcoming with the procedure (Isaacson *et al.*, 1978). No new types of osteotomies have been introduced to the field since 1957; rather, various modifications to the original surgical technique have been made (Dal Pont, 1961; Hunsuck, 1968; Epker & Wylie, 1986). Each of these modifications has focused on the goal of enhancing surgical stability, predictability, and return to pre-operative functional levels for which, until recently, the outcomes largely have been assessed by 2D radiography.

Maxillary surgery did not become routine until the late 1970s and early 1980s following the classic microangiography study on monkeys (Bell, 1973), which established the biological rationale for the LeFort I osteotomy. This work, combined with the advent of rigid internal fixation in the 1980s (Reitzik *et al.*, 1981; Barer *et al.*, 1987; Ellis *et al.*, 1988), led to the routine use of orthognathic surgery in coordination with orthodontic treatment in appropriate cases, the subsequent outcome studies for which were performed again mostly by 2D analyses.

2D MANDIBULAR ORTHOGNATHIC SURGERY STUDIES

Until recently, most studies examining the stability of orthognathic surgery have been performed using analyses from the lateral view. These studies include evaluation of proximal and distal segment rotation (Isaacson *et al.*, 1978), surgical stability (Proffit *et al.*, 1991; Bailey *et al.*, 2008), and the relationship of soft tissue to skeletal tissue changes (Scheideman *et al.*, 1981; Mansour *et al.*, 1983; Stella *et al.*, 1989). For example, Legan & Anderton (1991) compared relapse attributable to changes in the orientations of the proximal and distal segments with two surgical techniques, the SSRO and the intraoral vertical ramus osteotomy (IVRO), following mandibular setback surgery in Class III patients. Since SSRO and IVRO have different osteotomy lines, it is expected that the resultant orientation and approximation of the proximal and distal segments also would be different and could be an influencing factor on skeletal stability. The investigators found that when adverse proximal segment rotation occurs in the rigidly fixated SSRO group, it resulted in a direct negative effect on the position of pogonion resulting in up to 42% relapse. In contrast, in the nonrigid fixation IVRO group, the teeth and pogonion remain stable while the pterygomasseteric sling and the hyoid musculature act to "reseat" the proximal segment to a physiologic position. Since physiological proximal segment seating can compensate for unfavorable and unanticipated intra-operative surgical positioning of the proximal segment, some surgeons advocate IVRO as the preferred technique for mandibular setback procedures.

In Class II patients, SSRO is the primary surgical option, since IVRO does not allow for the requisite bony overlap of the proximal and distal segments without an interpositional bone graft. Historically, alternative mandibular surgery techniques such as the "inverted L" and the "C" osteotomies were used for mandibular advancement, but they have been abandoned due to inferior results attributed to muscular influences on the proximal and distal segment orientation. In comparing stability of mandibular advancement surgery with wire osteosynthesis versus rigid internal fixation with SSRO surgery, Dolce and coworkers (2000) found that while the occlusal results remained stable with both fixation methods, the two approaches had different patterns of relapse: rigid fixation patients had more dental relapse, while wire fixation patients underwent greater skeletal changes.

This overview of previous surgical stability studies performed with 2D analyses implicates several variables in surgical relapse, including proximal segment positioning, type of fixation, and muscular influences. However, these studies examined patients only in the lateral plane of space, potentially missing information on other sources of relapse (e.g., condylar remodeling) or extracting additional details on known factors already associated with relapse that might be discernible only with CBCT.

Several studies also have assessed post-surgical changes in soft tissue, many of which have focused on correlating the changes in soft tissue anatomy to its corresponding skeletal landmarks in 2D. In general, these studies show variable soft tissue changes with one-jaw surgery. Thus, soft tissue changes range from 40 to 80% of skeletal change following maxillary advancement surgery. For mandibular advancement surgery, greater consistency is observed with nearly universal 90–100% change in soft tissue to change in corresponding skeletal tissue landmarks. In contrast, changes in soft tissue relative to skeletal tissues are unpredictable in mandibular setback surgery. Overall, these results must be viewed with caution since tremendous inter-patient variability exists: some patients exhibit high magnitudes of change, while others undergo mild changes. While these lateral cephalometric data offer helpful insights on post-surgical changes in soft tissue profiles, this type of analysis is limited by the lack of 3D structural information of the face. Consequently, it is difficult to identify some of the landmarks that are located on both sides of the face and often are observed as double images on 2D analyses. Therefore, 3D information of the shape and true volumetric surgical changes is preferred because this would provide the clinician with accurate data of the whole face and not just that of landmarks located in the midline of the face (e.g., nose tip and chin).

Although cephalometric radiography has been used for post-surgical outcome assessment for many years, this technique has several caveats, including magnification and distortion, superimposition of structures, and the fact that creating a 2D image of a 3D object inherently loses information (Baumrind & Frantz, 1971). In addition, some areas such as the temporomandibular joint (TMJ) cannot be visualized adequately with plane 2D radiography. Even Broadbent's (1931) attempt to use two orthogonal radiographs to create a 3D view of the subject had limited success. Although these studies were steps in the right direction, extrapolation of two 2D images to reconstruct a "3D" image simply does not generate a true 3D image. While these reconstructions may be adequate for analysis of sagittal and vertical extraoral soft tissue and skeletal changes, they are insufficient to answer a myriad of other questions such as intraoral soft tissue changes, possible surgical effects on airway, and assessment of true condylar position and its potential impact on surgical orthodontics treatment stability.

EVOLVING METHODS FOR USING 3D IMAGING FOR SURGICAL OUTCOMES ASSESSMENT

Until recently, surgical skeletal changes in 2D typically were analyzed by using anatomic landmarks on lateral and frontal cephalograms. Anteroposterior (AP) and vertical movements of the maxilla and mandible were analyzed using vectors on a 2D coordinate system; angular changes of cephalometric planes such as palatal plane and mandibular plane were investigated to understand rotations of the maxilla and the mandible. With the availability of medical computed tomography (CT), it became possible to obtain 3D images for pre-surgical diagnosis and treatment planning.

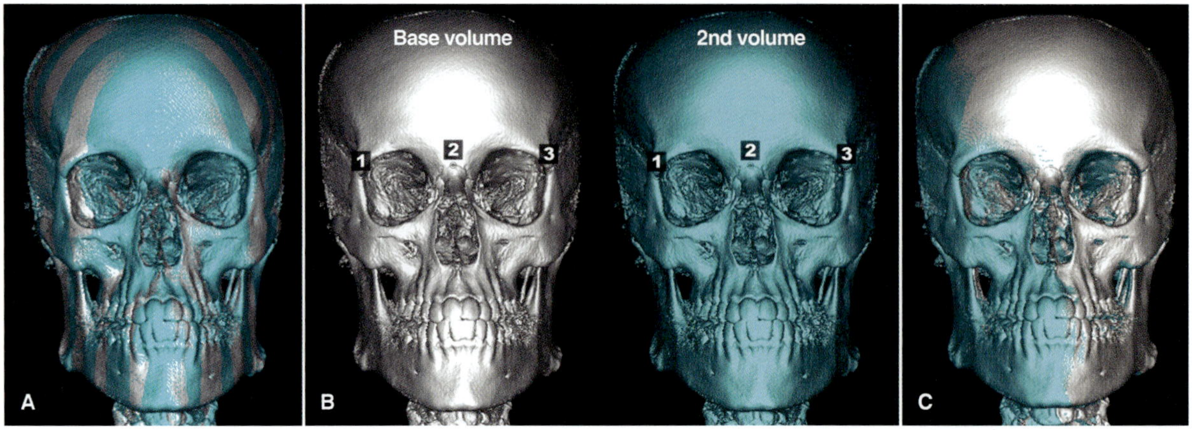

Figure 22.1 Landmark-based method for superimposition. *A*: To test in a perfect superimposition example, the same CBCT was opened as base volume and second volume depicted in silver and aqua color, respectively. *B*: Three landmarks (labeled 1, 2, and 3) were selected in areas that are easy to reproduce in both volumes. *C*: The two volumes superimposed using these landmarks resulted in substantial lack of agreement of the two volumes, thereby showing that this method of superimposition is not reliable.

However, because of cost and high radiation exposure, the risks of using CT in more routine orthognathic surgery cases outweigh its benefits. Therefore, CTs were used rarely and performed primarily in cases with large asymmetries, severe deformities, or craniofacial defects. The introduction of cone beam CT (CBCT; Mozzo *et al.*, 1998) has provided substantial advances and advantages in overcoming the caveats of costs and high radiation of CTs, while providing images that truly are 3D, are free of structural superimposition errors, and have no magnification. Recent studies (Hilgers *et al.*, 2005) also have shown good accuracy in condylar measurements made from CBCT, but not with 2D images even when the 2D images were reconstructed from a CBCT. Other studies (Berco *et al.*, 2009; Kamburoglu *et al.*, 2011) show good reliability of craniofacial measurements made from 3D cross-sections relative to those from the imaged dry skull. While these findings subsequently have fostered increasing numbers of CBCT studies, an important question of how best to transition the methodologies and approaches used in 2D to 3D remains to be addressed. Of these, the two key issues related to data analysis with CBCT are: (1) how best to superimpose structures in serial CBCT volumes and (2) how to devise methods to derive standardized measurements. These issues have been addressed by various approaches in several contemporary studies performed to evaluate surgical orthodontic treatment outcomes.

Superimpositions of 2D cephalograms traditionally have utilized landmarks in stable areas unaffected by the surgery and growth (Melsen, 1974; Bjork & Skieller, 1983; Nielsen, 1989; Cook *et al.*, 1994). Today, some commercially available software programs allow the operator to perform a similar type of superimposition in 3D using an analogous approach requiring superimposition on three or more landmarks (Figure 22.1). Because this approach is not reliable, however, clinical outcome studies have not utilized this 3D superimposition technique. A second method performs a fully automated, operator-independent registration of scans from two time points using the gray scale intensity voxel by voxel for the cranial base region of non-growing patients (Cevidanes *et al.*, 2005; Figure 22.2). This technique has a high level of reliability and reproducibility (Cevidanes *et al.*, 2010), and several recently published surgical orthodontic studies have used this superimposition technique to demonstrate treatment outcomes (Cevidanes *et al.*, 2007; Carvalho Fde *et al.*, 2010; Almeida *et al.*, 2011; Motta *et al.*, 2011; see also Chapter 21).

In terms of standardizing and making measurements for 3D analysis, three main methods have

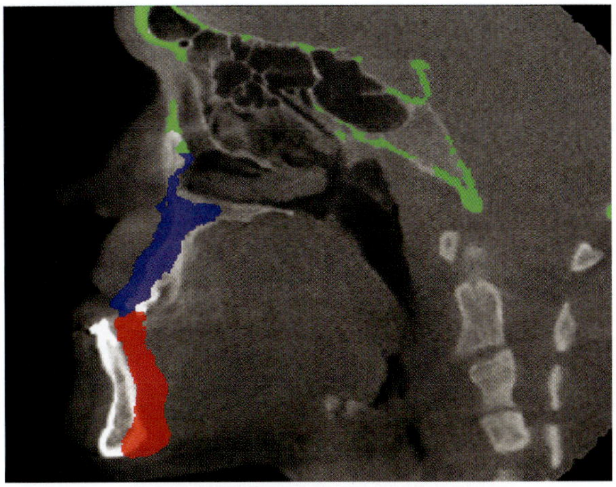

Figure 22.2 Cranial base superimposition with a voxel-wise method. Software display showing grayscale of a two-jaw surgery patient before surgery, and the segmentation (colored structures) of the same patient after surgery. Notice that the red (mandible) and blue (maxilla) colors do not match the grayscale; however, the cranial base (green) does match, thereby demonstrating that changes depicted using this method are related to the cranial base.

been utilized. One is based on linear and angular measurements (Jung *et al.*, 2009; Kim *et al.*, 2010, 2011; Park *et al.*, 2012a) that apply the concepts used routinely in 2D cephalometry to 3D images. The second method is based on the use of iterative closest point algorithms (Cevidanes *et al.*, 2007; Carvalho Fde *et al.*, 2010; Almeida *et al.*, 2011; Motta *et al.*, 2011) that analyze the smallest displacements between two structures but do not take into account the shape being measured. The third and most recent method is called shape correspondence (Figure 22.3). This method correlates the displacement of the same landmark from two or more time points and, through color-coded maps and vectors, depicts the magnitude and directionality of the movement, respectively. Paniagua and colleagues (2010) showed the shape correspondence technique to be a reliable approach for orthognathic surgery simulations.

Another key area of interest in assessing post-surgical changes is the pharyngeal airway. The pharyngeal airway is a tubular-shaped space that is filled with air, surrounded by the muscles, mucosa, and a network of lymphatic tissues. Its complex morphology varies greatly depending on the facial skeletal pattern, age, head posture, obesity, and presence of respiratory diseases (e.g., acute tonsillitis). In the past, lateral headfilms were used to screen for pharyngeal airway constrictions that often are caused by adenoid and tonsillar hypertrophy, tongue position, and other abnormalities such as velopharyngeal incompetence. Quantitative analyses for these studies often has included determination of airway widths measured at different levels using reference landmarks such as cervical bones and adenoids and calculations of areas of the adenoids, as well as of different subregions of airways. However, much anatomic information is lost when the 3D airway is represented in a 2D lateral cephalogram, and, as a result, linear and angular measurements alone do not provide adequate information about the structure.

With CBCT, it now is possible to analyze both cross-sectional areas of the airway in all three planes and volumetric measurements of the pharyngeal airway, making it possible to analyze the complex airway anatomy with great accuracy. Recent studies (Ozbek *et al.*, 1998; Aboudara *et al.*, 2009; see also Chapter 13) have confirmed that the cross-sectional area and volumetric measurements have much greater variability than linear and angular measurement of the airway, indicating that these, rather than 2D measurements, likely better represent the normal variations in airway anatomy.

CLASS III SURGICAL EVALUATIONS

Despite the vast amount of research concerning surgical evaluation and its long-term effects on post-operative stability and function, most of these studies have been performed using 2D lateral and/or frontal cephalograms with limited evaluation of changes in lengths and areas. CBCT technology has expanded diagnostic capabilities by making it possible to visualize craniofacial anatomy accurately and to perform volumetric analysis, such as that of the changes in relationship of skeletal structures, facial soft tissues, and the pharyngeal airway. This fast-paced and constant evolution of imaging and evaluation techniques can be illustrated using the following examples.

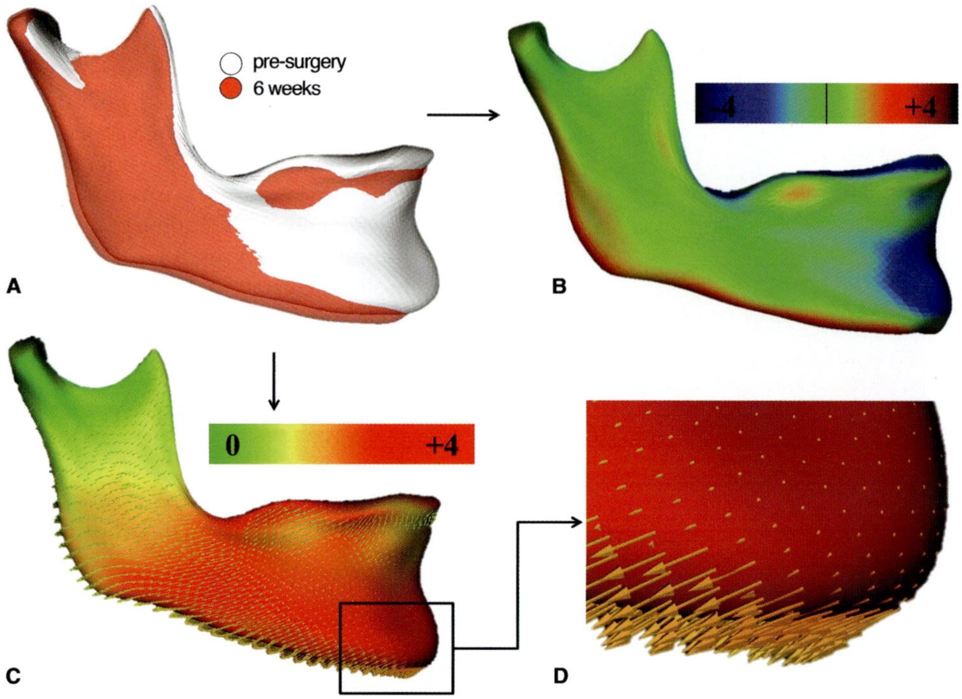

Figure 22.3 Evaluation of post-surgical changes in 3D following superimpositions on the cranial base. Changes at the mandible for the same patient are shown with different methods. *A*: Visual assessment can be performed easily with semi-transparency superimposition; however, the surgical changes cannot be quantified. *B*: Color-coded map of the closest point method where blue represents inward and red outward changes with the magnitude of change shown in the accompanying color scale. *C*: Outcomes assessment with the shape correspondence method depicts a color-coded map and vectors that provide the direction and magnitude of the displacement. *D*: A zoomed-in image of the chin to demonstrate the vectors in greater detail.

Maxillomandibular changes

Cevidanes and associates (2011) used a combination of cranial base superimpositions and the shape correspondence approach to examine surgical orthodontic treatment results of 50 Class III patients. Patients were distributed equally into two groups; the first consisted of maxillary advancement (LeFort I) only, and the second received combined maxillary advancement with concomitant mandibular set back (LeFort I + SSRO). Both groups received rigid internal fixation. CBCT scans were taken pre-surgery, 6 weeks after surgery at splint removal, and 1 year after surgery. Comparisons were performed between pre-surgery and 6-week splint removal representing the surgical displacement, as well as from splint removal to 1 year after surgery representing post-surgical adaptations.

The study demonstrated that the average surgical displacement of the maxilla was similar for both the one- and two-jaw surgery groups, as were the resulting post-surgical changes. However, there was no consistent direction of post-surgical change; some cases demonstrated primarily vertical changes while others exhibited primarily sagittal changes (Figure 22.4).

For both groups of patients, the condyles were displaced in a postero-superior direction, though the magnitude of this movement varied between individuals. Additionally, condylar rotation was observed in the two-jaw surgery group, likely resulting from a combination of torquing due to

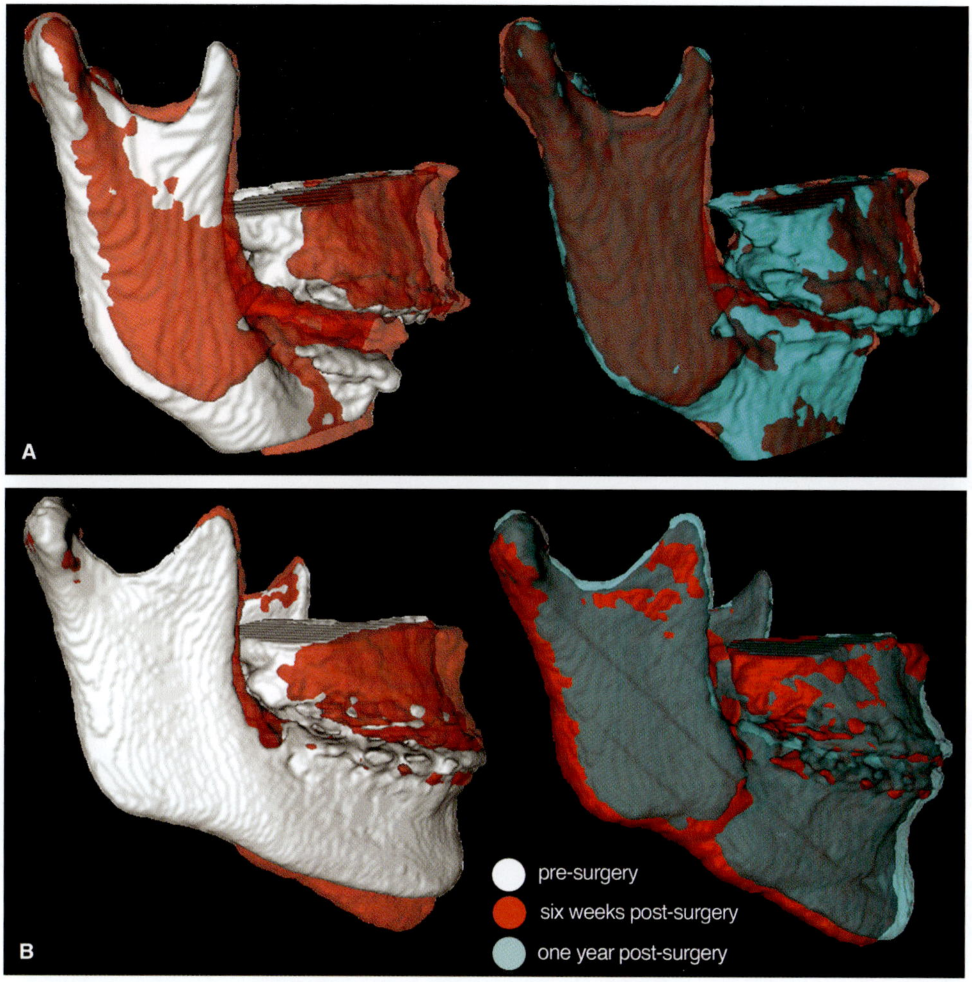

Figure 22.4 Two cases depicting different types of post-surgical maxillary changes. *A*: Superimposition 6 weeks after surgery (left panel) shows that the maxilla was advanced. One-year follow-up shows a post-surgical change in a horizontal direction (right panel). *B*: Superimposition 6 weeks after surgery shows that the maxilla was advanced and moved down (left panel). The pattern of post-surgical change in this case was different with vertical component and counterclockwise rotation of the maxilla noticed from the incisors coming up and forward and anterior nasal moving backward (right panel).

the proximal/distal segment fixation and the rotation due to a wider portion of the mandible being articulated against the ascending ramus due to the setback. Post-surgical condylar adaptations were in the opposite direction of the displacement that occurred immediately following surgery in both groups. Thus, the condyles tended to move antero-inferiorly in both groups and rotational adaptation occurred within the two-jaw surgery group as early as 6 weeks post-surgery (Figure 22.5).

The two study groups also demonstrated differences in surgical changes in the ramus. For the LeFort I-only group, the changes were associated directly with the surgical displacement and post-surgical changes of the maxilla such that the ramus adapted with either clockwise or counterclockwise rotation, depending on the surgical movement of

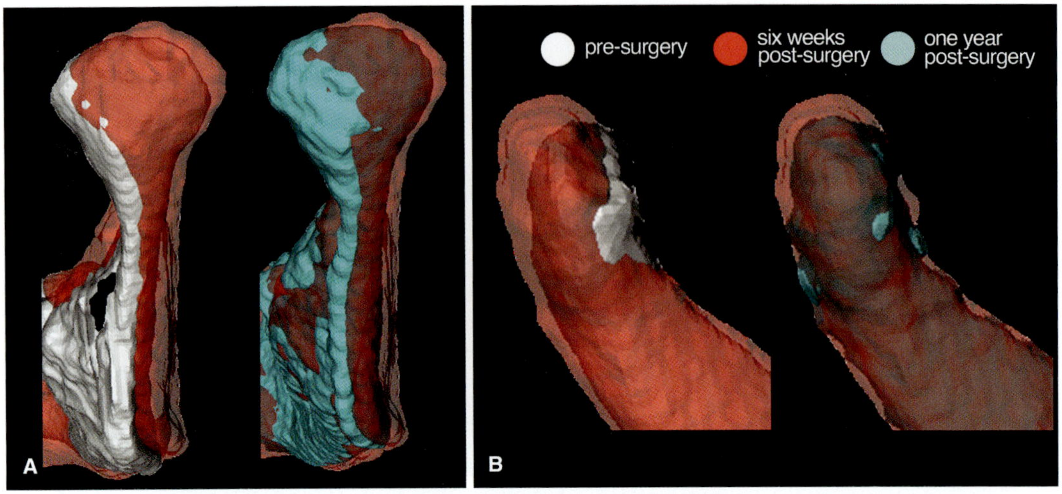

Figure 22.5 Condyle changes 6 weeks and 1 year after surgery in a patient following two-jaw surgery involving LeFort I with mandibular setback using SRRO procedure. *A*: Posterior view of the condyle showing its rotation and a noticeable rotation of the ramus in both the first 6 weeks (left panel) and 1 year (right panel) following surgery. *B*: Lateral view showing the postero-superior condyle changes at 6 weeks after surgery (left panel) and its adaptation toward the original position 1 year after surgery (right panel).

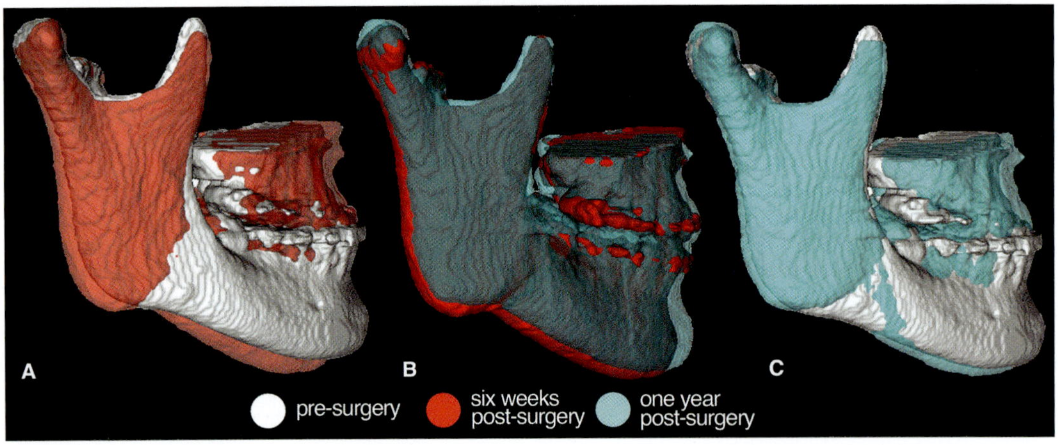

Figure 22.6 Changes in the ramus and chin 6 weeks and 1 year after surgery in a patient following two-jaw surgery involving LeFort I with mandibular setback using SRRO procedure. *A*: Surgical changes 6 weeks after surgery showing posterior displacement of the gonial angle. *B*: Post-surgical adaptation of ramus and chin moving forward between 6 weeks and 1 year following surgery. *C*: Pre-surgery to 1 year post-surgery changes showing the net amounts of surgical changes that were maintained for both the maxilla and mandible.

the maxilla. Changes in the ramus in the two-jaw surgery group not only followed the same pattern as that in the maxillary surgery-only group, but also demonstrated lateral rotation of the condyle and a greater anterior ramus displacement when compared with the maxilla-only group (Figure 22.6). This may be the result of the previously reported anterior relapse following surgical mandibular setback reported in studies using 2D analyses, but also could represent a condylar malpositioning that 3D imaging now is able to detect more precisely.

Not surprisingly, displacement of the chin in the LeFort I–only group was due primarily to the amount of vertical displacement of the maxilla. Therefore, the clockwise (maxillary inferior positioning) or counterclockwise (maxillary superior reposition of the mandible) rotation resulted in a corresponding downward and backward or upward and forward displacement of the chin, respectively. In addition to the rotation from an altered maxillary position, the two-jaw surgery group demonstrated a greater posterior displacement of the chin due to the sectioning of the mandible and the posterior positioning of the distal segment. These results led to different post-surgical changes of the chin; the LeFort I-only group exhibited small primarily rotational changes and the two-jaw group demonstrated both posterior displacement and rotation.

Soft tissue changes

Because facial appearance is an important factor in human interrelationships and affects social and psychological development, orthognathic surgery must have the objective of correcting skeletal discrepancies as well as altering facial balance to achieve esthetic results in patients with severe disharmony of the jaws (Soncul & Bamber, 2004; Baik & Kim, 2010). The ideal positioning of the jaws through orthognathic surgery does not always result in an ideal soft tissue appearance because the patient's facial soft tissue does not respond to movement of the underlying skeletal tissues in a 1:1 ratio (Lim *et al.*, 2010; Ryckman *et al.*, 2010). Therefore, surgical treatment objectives must focus on the desired soft tissue outcome (Sarver, 1998), rather than on the correction of skeletal discrepancies only.

For the lower third of the face, including chin and lower lip, one- or two-jaw surgeries generally result in similar soft tissue changes, particularly for those with advancement surgery. There is a greater variation in responses within the middle third of the face, however, depending on the type of surgery. The changes in soft tissue anatomy following surgery for Class III correction utilizing landmarks described in Table 22.1 are summarized below.

Lower third of the face

The soft tissue response of the chin and lower lip area is similar after one- or two-jaw surgery for Class III correction. This involves posterior movement of the soft tissue B point and the soft tissue pogonion and retraction of the lower lip.

Middle third of the face

There are significant differences in the soft tissue changes following one- and two-jaw surgery in the upper lip and landmarks of the nose and cheeks. Even with isolated mandibular setback, the upper lip moves backward (Hershey & Smith, 1974; Suckiel & Kohn, 1978; Sung *et al.*, 2000; Lim *et al.*, 2010; Kim *et al.*, 2012) because both the upper and lower lips are influenced by the protruded mandibular incisors. With the posterior positioning of the mandible, the maxillary incisors rather than the mandibular incisors begin to provide the main support for the upper lip, resulting in an overall reduction in the sagittal projection of the upper lip (Lim *et al.*, 2010). In contrast, due to the LeFort I advancement in two-jaw surgery, the upper lip moves forward (Jensen *et al.*, 1992; Kim *et al.*, 2012). This change can be augmented or attenuated by occlusal plane rotations providing increased or decreased support, respectively, in the upper incisor region.

After both one- and two-jaw orthognathic surgery, the right and left corners of the mouth (cheilion) move backward. It should be noted that cheilion moves backward after two-jaw surgery, despite the forward movement of the upper lip (Kim *et al.*, 2012). This suggests that cheilion is affected by the AP position of the mandible, whereas the central portion of the upper lip is influenced primarily by the maxillary position.

Both one- and two-jaw orthognathic surgeries for Class III correction result in forward and upward movement of the nasal tip (Jung *et al.*, 2009; Lim *et al.*, 2010; Park *et al.*, 2012a) that results from remodeling of the perioral musculature (Jung *et al.*, 2009). The other primary change in nasal esthetics after two-jaw surgery results from

Table 22.1 Soft tissue landmarks of the face.

Soft tissue landmarks		Definition
Lip measurements	Rt.Cu (right Cupid's bow)	Most prominent point of vermilion border of right Cupid's bow of upper lip
	Lt.Cu (left Cupid's bow)	Most prominent point of vermilion border of left Cupid's bow of upper lip
	Rt.Ch (right cheilion)	Most lateral extent of outline of lip in right side
	Lt.Ch (left cheilion)	Most lateral extent of outline of lip in left side
	LL (lower lip)	Most prominent point of vermilion border of Cupid's bow of lower lip
Cheek measurements	Rt.Ck (right cheek)	Most prominent point of cheek in right side
	Lt.Ck (left cheek)	Most prominent point of cheek in left side
Chin measurements	Pog′ (soft tissue pogonion)	Most anterior point in chin
	B′ (soft tissue B point)	Most concave point on curve between LL and Pog′
Nasal measurements	Pn (pronasale)	Most anterior point in nose
	Rt.Al (right alar base)	Most lateral point in curved base line of alar in right side, indicating facial insertion of nasal wing base
	Lt.Al (left alar base)	Most lateral point in curved base line of alar in left side, indicating facial insertion of nasal wing base
	Sn (subnasale)	Point at which columella merges with upper lip in sagittal plane

widening of the nasal base, the nares, and forward rotation of the nasal tip (Park *et al.*, 2012b). Adjunctive procedures such as alar cinch suture and V-Y closure may be performed respectively to prevent these unfavorable changes, but their effects are not always satisfactory (Park *et al.*, 2012a). Because the alar width increase also occurs during the surgical treatment of skeletal Class II, Class III, and openbite regardless of the amount and direction maxillary movement (Honrado *et al.*, 2006), some have asserted that the unfavorable change is the result of the maxillary surgical incision rather than actual repositioning of the maxilla (Altman & Oeltjen, 2007). This is supported further by the fact that patients undergoing isolated mandibular setback surgery show minimal changes of the alar base area.

The paranasal area around the cheeks moves forward after both isolated mandibular setback and two-jaw maxillary advancement or posterior impaction with mandibular setback (McCance *et al.*, 1992; Soncul & Bamber, 2004; Kim *et al.*, 2012). The amount of change after two-jaw surgery is significantly greater than that observed after one-jaw surgery (Kim *et al.*, 2012). Therefore, two-jaw surgery with maxillary advancement or posterior impaction would be effective in augmenting the midfacial area and would significantly improve the patient's facial profile.

Correlations between hard and soft tissue movement

Soft tissue changes after orthognathic surgery are predictable more in the lower third than in the middle third of the face because changes in lower part of the face are correlated highly with the amount of mandibular setback (Kim *et al.*, 2012). In contrast, soft tissue changes in the maxillary region are more difficult to predict than those associated with the mandible because the former are affected by soft tissue manipulation during maxillary surgery, resulting in larger variations in the ratio of soft- to hard-tissue displacement in the middle third of the face (Cho & Yang, 1996). Thus, the location of the incision and type of suture affect the soft tissue changes more than the maxillary movement itself (Betts *et al.*, 1993). This is due to the differences in anatomical relationships within the maxilla and the mandible because the soft tissue of the mandible and the underlying jaw are related closely to each other, whereas the soft tissue of the maxilla is connected strongly to the nasal cavity as well as to the upper jaw (Cho & Yang, 1996).

Condylar positions and post-surgical stability

Post-surgical stability of orthognathic surgery is a major concern for oral and maxillofacial surgeons as well as orthodontists. Major factors related to surgical relapse include post-operative occlusion and positional change of the condyle (Landes & Sterz, 2003). Good occlusion that is achieved through optimal pre- and post-operative orthodontics ensures the stability of bony segments after surgery. However, condylar position is difficult to control during and after surgery and its contributions to relapse (post-operative positional changes) have been difficult to determine precisely in the past due to the limitations of 2D imaging. Post-operative condylar position is affected by many factors such as rotational movement of the proximal segment, tensional balance of the surrounding muscles, fixation method, and the surgeon's experience (Lee & Park, 2002). The several suggested methods for avoiding condylar displacement and guiding post-operative position of the condyle include monitoring by sonography, using guiding splints and special devices, and intra-operative awakening (Helm & Stepke, 1997; Landes & Sterz, 2003; Renzi *et al.*, 2003; Landes, 2004; Politi *et al.*, 2007). Because there is substantial evidence of the effects of condylar positioning after SSRO on post-operative stability (Gu *et al.*, 2000; Mucedero *et al.*, 2008; Baek *et al.*, 2009; Jakobsone *et al.*, 2011), accurate positional assessment of the condyle during and immediately following orthognathic surgery is vital to maximize surgical stability for achieving predictable and favorable treatment outcomes.

CBCT with its 3D views can enhance diagnostic abilities and add to our understanding of the spatial relationship of the bony segments. Condylar rotations and displacements, which occur as a result of orthognathic surgery, now can be assessed using multiplanar reconstruction and by measuring surface distances. Both the position and angulation of the condyles can be measured in axial, frontal, and sagittal slices with dimensional accuracy (Cevidanes *et al.*, 2006). Superimpositions of 3D reconstructed images of the craniofacial complex combined with surface distance analysis and color-mapping techniques have enabled users to assess the surgical displacements visually as well as to quantify the skeletal changes resulting from orthognathic surgery (Cevidanes *et al.*, 2005; Figure 22.5 and Figure 22.6).

Linear and angular changes

Linear and angular changes of the condyles after orthognathic surgery can be measured in 2D reformatted views. This method minimizes potential measurement errors that could occur from locating landmarks on curved 3D reconstructed surfaces (Grauer *et al.*, 2009). For this purpose, precise construction of horizontal and vertical reference planes is crucial because it provides the reference to which linear and angular measurements are made (Figure 22.7).

Changes in the axial plane

Condyles tend to rotate medially as a result of mandibular setback surgery either with or without maxillary surgery (Lee & Park, 2002; Baek *et al.*, 2006; Kim *et al.*, 2013). The V-shaped mandibular morphology and the location of the osteotomy line contribute to the inward rotation of the condylar head as the proximal segments are fixated to the narrower distal segment.

Changes in the sagittal plane

Anterior rotation of the condyle in the sagittal view typically is observed following two-jaw surgery

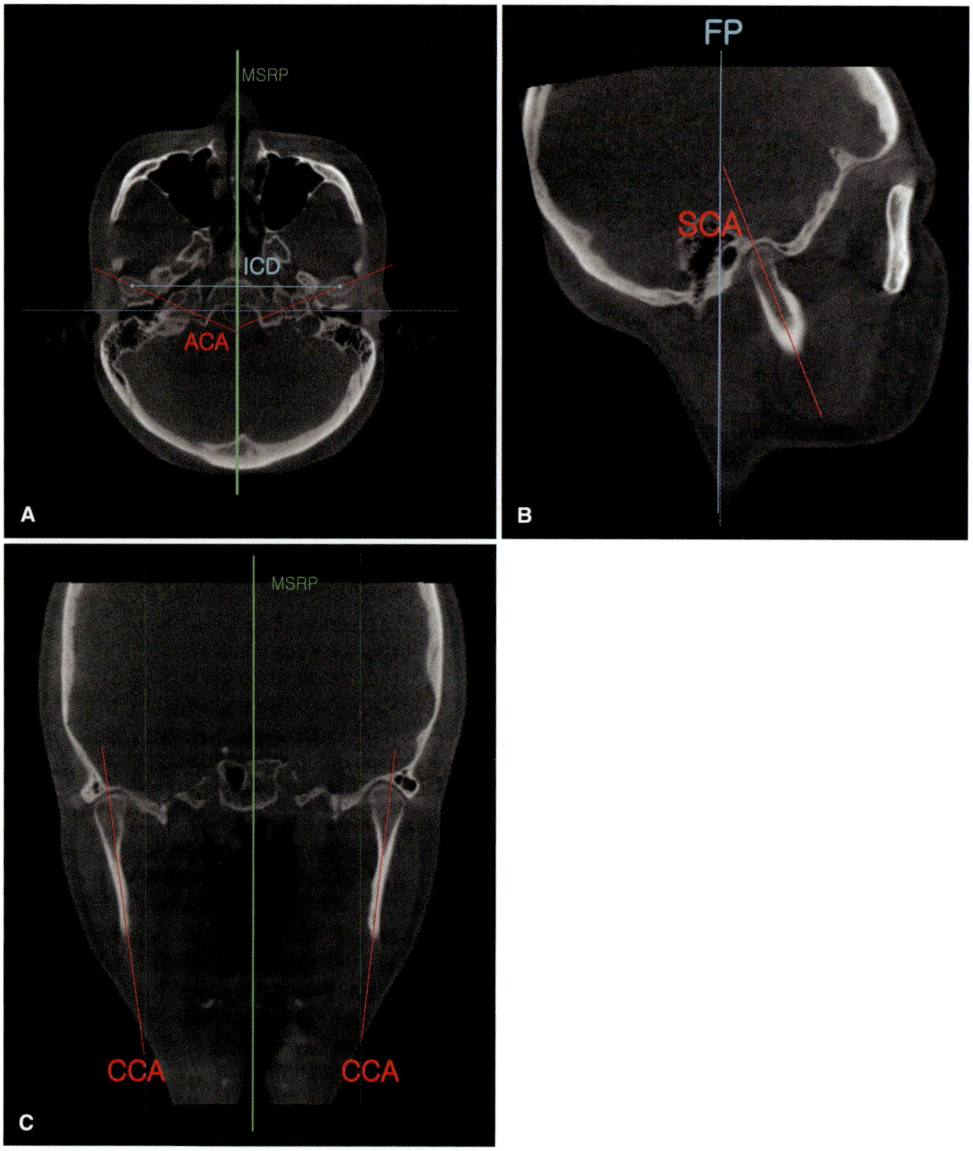

Figure 22.7 Linear and angular measurements to assess condylar position and post-surgical changes. *A*: Condylar angulation can be determined by measuring the condyle angle in the axial plane (ACA) formed by a line connecting the medial and lateral pole of the condylar head with the midsagittal reference plane (MSRP). Intercondylar distance (ICD) can be measured from midpoints of the right and left condylar heads. *B*: Condylar angulations in the sagittal plane (SCA) can be measured from a line bisecting the anterior and posterior border of the condylar head to the frontal plane (FP) that is perpendicular to the Frankfort horizontal plane. *C*: Condylar angulation in the coronal plane (CCA) can be determined by measuring angles formed by lines bisecting the medial and lateral pole of the condylar heads to the MSRP (Kim *et al.*, 2012).

involving posterior impaction or advancement of the maxilla and mandibular setback, while the condyle remains stable after a one-jaw mandibular setback procedure (Kim *et al.*, 2013). When there are no changes in the proximal segment, surgical stability is anticipated. Although previous reports have concluded that isolated mandibular setback is an unstable procedure, the lack of stability associated with this procedure likely is related to the surgical technique (Proffit *et al.*, 2000; Busby *et al.*, 2002; Cevidanes *et al.*, 2007). Thus, if the position of the proximal segment is controlled poorly, it can be displaced as the distal segment is set back. Following rigid fixation, the displaced proximal segment then can "rebound" to its original position bringing the chin with it (Proffit *et al.*, 2007). In the double-jaw surgery group, although condylar angulations in the sagittal plane show significant changes, the direction of the condylar rotation is forward instead of backward, resulting in minimal effects on the forward horizontal relapse of the chin.

Changes in the coronal plane

Generally, condylar angulations in the coronal plane remain constant after both one- and two-jaw surgery. This observation is consistent with the minimal change of the intercondylar distance and intercondylar angles (Draenert *et al.*, 2010; Kim *et al.*, 2013). Intercondylar relationship may be influenced by factors such as fixation method and surgical techniques.

Surface distance analysis

Condylar displacements can be calculated by reconstructing and superimposing pre- and post-operative 3D models to visualize surface distances of the positional changes resulting from surgery. This type of analysis is accurate with intra- and inter-observer variability as low as 0.02–0.05 mm (Cevidanes *et al.*, 2009; Nada *et al.*, 2011). The amount of condylar displacements in frontal, sagittal, and axial planes range from 0.03 mm to 0.53 mm; no differences exist in these displacements between one- and two-jaw surgery (Lee & Park, 2002; Baek *et al.*, 2006; Cevidanes *et al.*, 2007). Although condylar displacements vary between patients, these generally are less than 2 mm and, therefore, are considered to be insignificant clinically. Post-surgical changes in condylar displacements do not demonstrate a normal distribution and only a few patients show considerable changes (Proffit *et al.*, 2007). Regarding long-term changes of the condylar positions, the condyles move backward immediately post-surgery, and then return to their original position during the retention period (Kim *et al.*, 2010). Last, there is no specific relationship between the amount of mandibular setback and the amount of condylar changes (Magalhaes *et al.*, 1995; Lee & Park, 2002; Baek *et al.*, 2006).

Pharyngeal airway

The effects of respiratory function on craniofacial development have been studied for decades, and most clinicians now understand that respiratory function is highly relevant to orthodontic diagnosis and treatment planning (Linder-Aronson, 1979; Woodside *et al.*, 1991; Aboudara *et al.*, 2009). Similarly, it is important to understand the effects that orthognathic surgery has on positional changes of the maxillomandibular complex and its consequences on structural alterations in the pharyngeal airway. These airway changes following mandibular setback surgery are important because of their potential impact on normal respiration and because changes in the associated soft tissues and muscles are an etiologic factor in skeletal relapse (Joss & Vassalli, 2009).

As stated above and in Chapter 13, 2D airway analysis using lateral head films is not reliable because the 2D measurements of airway lack much of the structural information of this 3D structure (Aboudara *et al.*, 2009). Using CBCT, it is possible to visualize the airway and extract volumetric measurements on a 1:1 ratio with high-dimensional accuracy (Lagravère *et al.*, 2008). When assessing pharyngeal airway, patient positioning and head orientation are critical because the cross-sectional area of the pharynx decreases with a change from the upright to the supine position (Fouke & Strohl, 1987) and because changes in head posture affect upper airway size due to its postural effects on the tongue (Pirila-Parkkinen *et al.*, 2012) as well as the suprahyoid musculature.

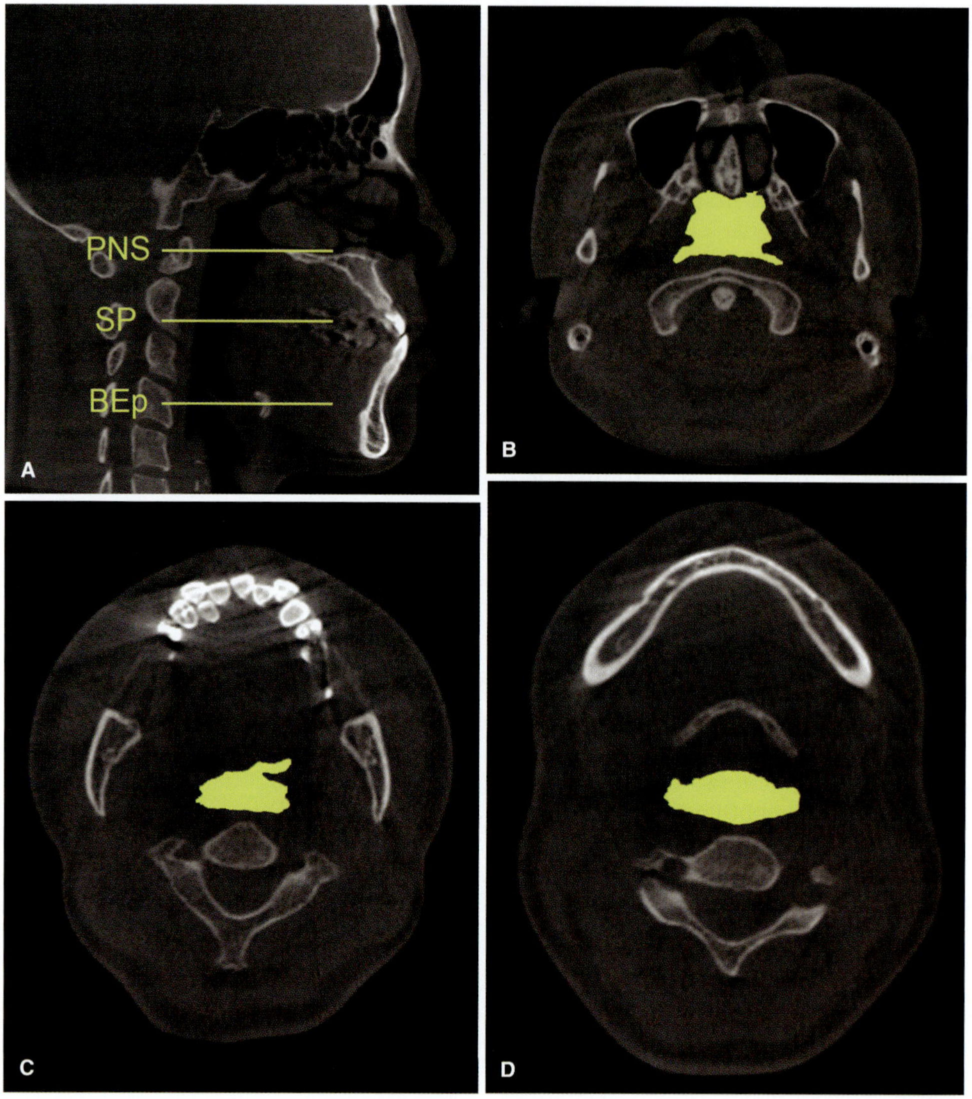

Figure 22.8 Anatomic landmarks in the midsagittal section can be used to locate planes for assessing cross-sections of the airway. *A*: After orientation of the sagittal view using the Frankfort horizontal plane as a horizontal reference plane, axial planes passing through posterior nasal spine (PNS), most inferior point of the soft palate (SP), and base of epiglottis (BEp) are used for cross-sectional analysis of the nasopharynx (*B*), oropharynx (*C*), and hypopharynx (*D*).

Cross-sectional dimensions and airway length

When assessing the airway, anatomic landmarks such as posterior nasal spine (PNS), soft palate, and epiglottis can be used to define cross-sectional planes of all portions of the upper airway, namely the nasopharynx, oropharynx, and hypopharynx (Figure 22.8). While isolated portions of the airway may not change, several AP dimensions and cross-sectional area changes occur within the airway following one- and two-jaw surgery (Wickwire *et al.*, 1972; Tselnik & Pogrel, 2000; Hong *et al.*, 2011). After mandibular setback surgery, the sagittal cross-section at the soft palate and epiglottis decreases significantly while the cross-section at PNS shows minimal changes. Following two-jaw surgery involving maxillary advancement and mandibular setback, the airway cross-section at the soft palate and epiglottis may remain unchanged, while the AP cross-sectional area at PNS increases; the latter results primarily due to the maxillary advancement. The length of the pharyngeal airway can decrease significantly after two-jaw surgery if the posterior maxilla is impacted or can increase if the maxilla is positioned inferiorly, whereas no significant change occurs in this pharyngeal dimension after one-jaw surgery (Hong *et al.*, 2011).

Airway volume

The post-operative pharyngeal airway space decreases either after isolated mandibular setback or combined maxillary advancement and mandibular setback; however, the effect of a narrowed airway on post-operative orthognathic stability and sleep apnea is unclear. Though both procedures affect the airway dimension, two-jaw surgery tends to demonstrate comparatively less narrowing of the airway (Samman *et al.*, 1992; Chen *et al.*, 2007; Degerliyurt *et al.*, 2008; Hong *et al.*, 2011). For this reason, the two-jaw surgical approach may be preferred over the mandibular setback procedure in correcting mandibular prognathism in at-risk patients (Wickwire *et al.*, 1972; Hong *et al.*, 2011). With this approach, the patient also will have a diminished likelihood of developing respiratory problems since the widening of the pharyngeal airway at the level of the PNS will compensate partly for the constriction of lower part of the airway resulting from the posterior displacement of the mandible.

SURGERY FOR CLASS II CORRECTION

In addition to the topics already discussed for Class III orthognathic surgery, CBCT can be used to evaluate other critical aspects of changes associated with bilateral SSRO for Class II patients. One important aspect of the surgical procedure is the shape and form of the fracture resulting from the mandibular osteotomy, which can have a significant impact on stability and cannot be assessed adequately with 2D radiographs. Plooij and associates (2009) used CBCT to evaluate the fracture pattern obtained during bilateral SSRO for mandibular advancement, particularly the amount of "Hunsuck," which is the propagation of the controlled fracture of the lingual cortex as the initial ramus cuts are pried or teased apart (Figure 22.9). This prospective 3D study utilized CBCT scans performed on 40 consecutive patients with skeletal mandibular deficiency. The surgical goal included obtaining a consistent "Hunsuck" approach to reduce the muscle pull on the proximal and distal segments. Though the surgeon and surgical technique were consistent, only about half of the fracture lines propagated along the line originally were described by Hunsuck. The authors concluded that the enhanced imaging technique was suitable for analyzing surgical outcome and "has the potential to provide substantial data on the position of the proximal segments as a result of the lingual fracture line." However, it is not possible yet to state whether the variation in fracture pattern will result in different levels of post-surgical stability. It is hoped that the authors will be able to follow the patients over a longer period of time to help answer this question.

In a more recent two-patient case report, Lloyd and colleagues (2011) suggested that CBCT may be useful in the management of unfavorable fractures during mandibular surgery. Following unfavorable surgical outcome, the authors used CBCT to attempt to determine if there were any anatomic or surgical explanations for the propagation of an unfavorable surgical split. While limited in scope, difficult to generalize to a broad surgical population, and insufficient to draw cause and effect conclusions, the paper presents a logical suggestion that given a large enough pool of data, the findings eventually could be used pre-operatively to prevent negative surgical outcomes.

CONCLUSIONS

This chapter described recent work with CBCT to assess surgical orthodontics treatment outcomes that represents some of the latest advances in the field. Initial results with CBCT imaging in surgical cases show its promise in addressing some of the

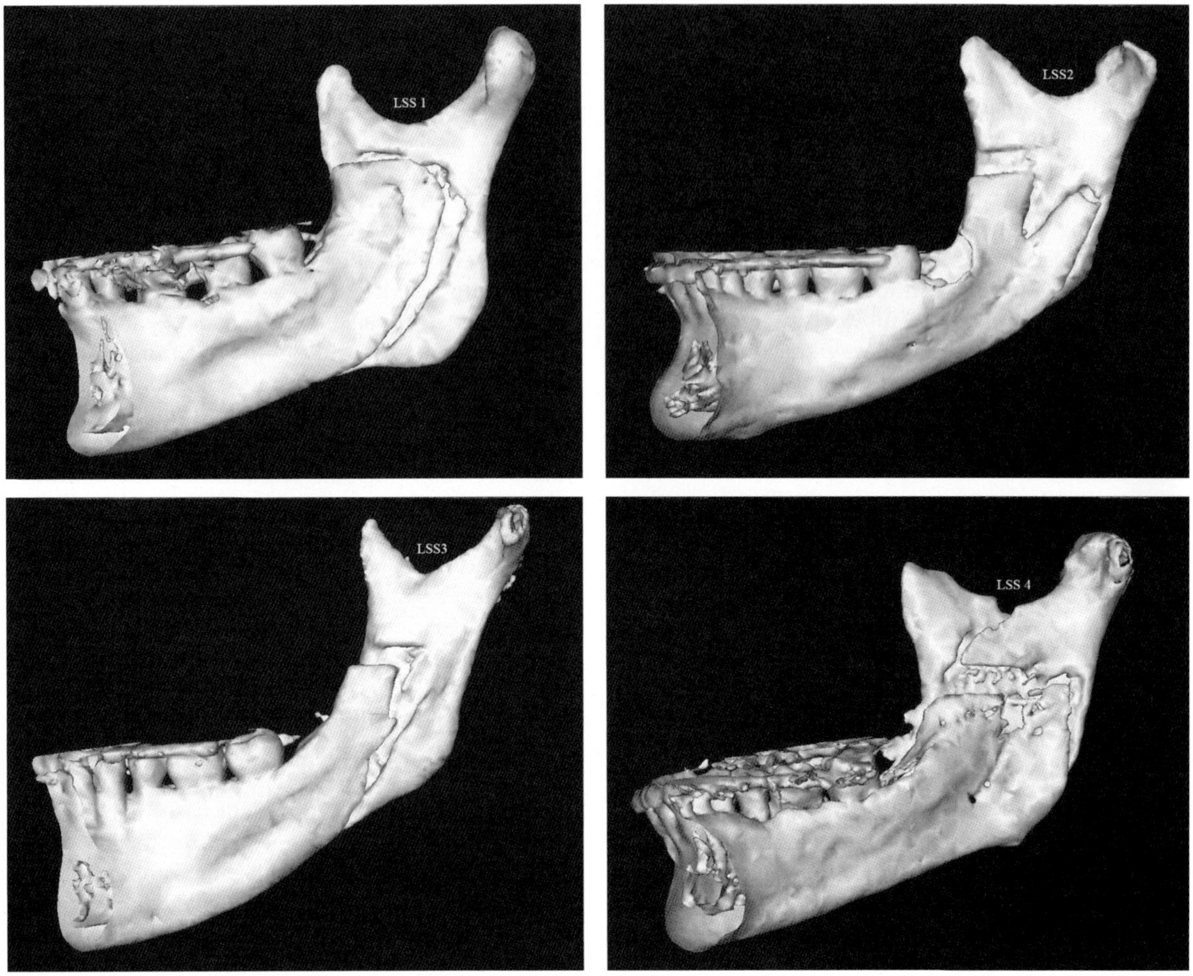

Figure 22.9 The lingual fracture pattern for a sagittal split ramus osteotomy is considered to be one of the factors associated with relapse. With conventional 2D imaging techniques, it is not possible to observe the fracture pattern, which now can be visualized clearly with CBCT. This additional information is being used to evaluate why the outcomes of surgery are not as expected in cases with poor treatment results with the hope that this information will minimize future negative outcomes. (Reprinted with permission from Plooij *et al.*, 2009.)

questions the profession has struggled to answer previously with 2D methods. CBCT technology has contributed to a better understanding of the spatial relationships of the bony segments resulting from surgery by providing 3D superimposition and analysis tools such as surface-distance analysis and shape-correspondence technique. It also allows clinicians to assess the overall changes of the craniofacial structures qualitatively using tools such as color maps and vectors. In addition, not only can changes in the conventional 2D cephalometric landmarks be analyzed, but any point on a patient's craniofacial anatomy including jaw bones, dentition, and soft tissues can be assessed quantitatively and observed from all directions.

CBCT studies that are longer term, utilize large study populations, and focus more closely on the TMJ will be necessary to investigate more fully and achieve an understanding of variables previously implicated as sources of surgical instability. For now, previous studies (Proffit *et al.*, 2007) that reported the hierarchy of surgical stability remain the hallmark for the profession. With continued investigations using 3D imaging, these findings may be supported by even stronger evidence or may need to be reviewed and revised given the newer information derived from 3D data. This information, in turn, will aid in modifying treatment protocols to the benefit of patients undergoing surgery. Thus, assessment of orthodontic surgery patients with CBCT brings new, exciting, and potentially highly relevant information for further enhancing treatment outcomes in the future.

References

Aboudara, C., Nielsen, I., Huang, J.C. *et al.* (2009) Comparison of airway space with conventional lateral headfilms and 3-dimensional reconstruction from cone-beam computed tomography. *American Journal of Orthodontics and Dentofacial Orthopedics*, 135 (4), 468–479.

Almeida, R.C., Cevidanes, L.H., & Carvalho, F.A. (2011) Soft tissue response to mandibular advancement using 3D CBCT scanning. *International Journal of Oral and Maxillofacial Surgery*, 40 (4), 353–359.

Altman, J.I. & Oeltjen, J.C. (2007) Nasal deformities associated with orthognathic surgery: analysis, prevention, and correction. *Journal of Craniofacial Surgery*, 18 (4), 734–739.

Baek, S.H., Kim, T.K., & Kim, M.J. (2006) Is there any difference in the condylar position and angulation after asymmetric mandibular setback? *Oral Surgery, Oral Medicine, Oral Pathology, Oral Radiology and Endodontics*, 101 (2), 155–163.

Baek, S.H., Kim, K., & Choi, J.Y. (2009) Evaluation of treatment modality for skeletal class III malocclusion with labioversed upper incisors and/or protrusive maxilla: surgical movement and stability of rotational maxillary setback procedure. *Journal of Craniofacial Surgery*, 20 (6), 2049–2054.

Baik, H.S. & Kim, S.Y. (2010) Facial soft-tissue changes in skeletal Class III orthognathic surgery patients analyzed with 3-dimensional laser scanning. *American Journal of Orthodontics and Dentofacial Orthopedics*, 138 (2), 167–178.

Bailey, L.J., Phillips, C., & Proffit, W.R. (2008) Long-term outcome of surgical Class III correction as a function of age at surgery. *American Journal of Orthodontics and Dentofacial Orthopedics*, 133 (3), 365–370.

Barer, P.G., Wallen, T.R., McNeill, R.W., *et al.* (1987) Stability of mandibular advancement osteotomy using rigid internal fixation. *American Journal of Orthodontics and Dentofacial Orthopedics*, 92 (5), 403–411.

Baumrind, S. & Frantz, R.C. (1971) The reliability of head film measurements. 1: Landmark identification. *American Journal of Orthodontics*, 60 (2), 111–127.

Bell, W.H. (1973) Biologic basis for maxillary osteotomies. *American Journal of Physical Anthropology*, 38 (2), 279–289.

Berco, M., Rigalli, P.H. Jr., Miner, R.M., *et al.* (2009) Accuracy and reliability of linear cephalometric measurements from cone-beam computed tomography scans of a dry human skull. *American Journal of Orthodontics and Dentofacial Orthopedics*, 136 (1), 17, e1–e9.

Betts, N.J., Vig, K.W., Vig, P., *et al.* (1993) Changes in the nasal and labial soft tissues after surgical repositioning of the maxilla. *International Journal of Adult Orthodontics and Orthognathic Surgery*, 8 (1), 7–23.

Bjork, A. & Skieller, V. (1983) Normal and abnormal growth of the mandible: a synthesis of longitudinal cephalometric implant studies over a period of 25 years. *European Journal of Orthodontics*, 5 (1), 1–46.

Blair, V. (1906) Report of a case of double resection for the correction of protrusion of the mandible. *The Dental Cosmos*, 48, 817–820.

Broadbent, B.H. (1931) A new X-ray technique and its application to orthodontia. *The Angle Orthodontist*, 1 (2), 45–66.

Busby, B.R., Bailey, L.J., Proffit, W.R., *et al.* (2002) Long-term stability of surgical class III treatment: a study of 5-year postsurgical results. *International Journal of Adult Orthodontics and Orthognathic Surgery*, 17 (3), 159–170.

Carvalho Fde, A., Almeida, R.C., Almeida, M.A., *et al.* (2010) Efficiency of light-emitting diode and halogen units in reducing residual monomers. *American Journal of Orthodontics and Dentofacial Orthopedics*, 138 (5), 617–622.

Cevidanes, L.H., Bailey, L.J., Tucker, G.R. Jr., *et al.* (2005) Superimposition of 3D cone-beam CT models of orthognathic surgery patients. *Dentomaxillofacial Radiology*, 34 (6), 369–375.

Cevidanes, L.H., Styner, M.A., & Proffit, W.R. (2006) Image analysis and superimposition of 3-dimensional cone-beam computed tomography models. *American Journal of Orthodontics and Dentofacial Orthopedics*, 129 (5), 611–618.

Cevidanes, L.H., Bailey, L.J., Tucker, S.F., *et al.* (2007) Three-dimensional cone-beam computed tomography for assessment of mandibular changes after orthognathic surgery. *American Journal of Orthodontics and Dentofacial Orthopedics*, 131 (1), 44–50.

Cevidanes, L.H., Heymann, G., Cornelis, M.A., *et al.* (2009) Superimposition of 3-dimensional cone-beam computed tomography models of growing patients. *American Journal of Orthodontics and Dentofacial Orthopedics*, 136 (1), 94–99.

Cevidanes, L.H., Motta, A., Proffit, W.R., *et al.* (2010) Cranial base superimposition for 3-dimensional evaluation of soft-tissue changes. *American Journal of Orthodontics and Dentofacial Orthopedics*, 137 (4 Suppl), S120–S129.

Cevidanes, L.H.S, Paniagua, B., de Paula, L.K., *et al.* (2011) One year assessment of surgical outcomes using shape correspondence. Available at http://iadr.confex.com/iadr/2011sandiego/webprogramschedule/Paper149662.html, accessed December 20, 2012.

Chen, F., Terada, K., Hua, Y., *et al.* (2007) Effects of bimaxillary surgery and mandibular setback surgery on pharyngeal airway measurements in patients with Class III skeletal deformities. *American Journal of Orthodontics and Dentofacial Orthopedics*, 131 (3), 372–377.

Cho, E.J. & Yang, W.S. (1996) Soft tissue changes after double jaw surgery in skeletal Class III malocclusion. *Korean Journal of Orthodontics*, 26, 1–16. Available at http://www.koreamed.org/SearchBasic.php?RID=0123KJOD/1996.26.1.1&DT=1, accessed January 8, 2013.

Cook, A.H., Sellke, T.A., & Begole, E.A. (1994) The variability and reliability of two maxillary and mandibular superimposition techniques. Part II. *American Journal of Orthodontics and Dentofacial Orthopedics*, 106 (5), 463–471.

Dal Pont, G. (1961) Retromolar osteotomy for the correction of prognathism. *Journal of Oral Surgery, Anesthesia, and Hospital Dental Service*, 19, 42–47.

Degerliyurt, K., Ueki, K., Hashiba, Y., *et al.* (2008) A comparative CT evaluation of pharyngeal airway changes in class III patients receiving bimaxillary surgery or mandibular setback surgery. *Oral Surgery, Oral Medicine, Oral Pathology, Oral Radiology and Endodontics*, 105 (4), 495–502.

Dolce, C., Van Sickels, J.E., Bays, R.A., *et al.* (2000) Skeletal stability after mandibular advancement with rigid versus wire fixation. *Journal of Oral and Maxillofacial Surgery*, 58 (11), 1219–1227.

Draenert, F.G., Erbe, C., Zenglein, V., *et al.* (2010) 3D analysis of condylar position after sagittal split osteotomy of the mandible in mono- and bimaxillary orthognathic surgery: a methodology study in 18 patients. *Journal of Orofacial Orthopedics*, 71 (6), 421–429.

Ellis, E. III, Reynolds, S., & Carlson, D.S. (1988) Stability of the mandible following advancement: a comparison of three postsurgical fixation techniques. *American Journal of Orthodontics and Dentofacial Orthopedics*, 94 (1), 38–49.

Epker, B.N. & Wylie, G.A. (1986) Control of the condylar-proximal mandibular segments after sagittal split osteotomies to advance the mandible. *Oral Surgery, Oral Medicine, and Oral Pathology*, 62 (6), 613–617.

Fouke, J.M. & Strohl, K.P. (1987) Effect of position and lung volume on upper airway geometry. *Journal of Applied Physiology*, 63 (1), 375–380.

Grauer, D., Cevidanes, L.S., & Proffit, W.R. (2009) Working with DICOM craniofacial images. *American Journal of Orthodontics and Dentofacial Orthopedics*, 136 (3), 460–470.

Gu, G., Gu, G., Nagata, J., *et al.* (2000) Hyoid position, pharyngeal airway and head posture in relation to relapse after the mandibular setback in skeletal Class III. *Clinical Orthodontics and Research*, 3 (3), 67–77.

Helm, G. & Stepke, M.T. (1997) Maintenance of the preoperative condyle position in orthognathic surgery. *Journal of Craniomaxillofacial Surgery*, 25 (1), 34–38.

Hershey, H.G. & Smith, L.H. (1974) Soft-tissue profile change associated with surgical correction of the prognathic mandible. *American Journal of Orthodontics*, 65 (5), 483–502.

Hilgers, M.L., Scarfe, W.C., Scheetz, J.P., *et al.* (2005) Accuracy of linear temporomandibular joint measurements with cone beam computed tomography and digital cephalometric radiography. *American Journal of Orthodontics and Dentofacial Orthopedics*, 128 (6), 803–811.

Hong, J.S., Park, Y.H., Kim, Y.J., *et al.* (2011) Three-dimensional changes in pharyngeal airway in skeletal Class III patients undergoing orthognathic surgery. *Journal of Oral and Maxillofacial Surgery*, 69 (11), e401–e408.

Honrado, C.P., Lee, S., Bloomquist, D.S., *et al.* (2006) Quantitative assessment of nasal changes after maxillomandibular surgery using a 3-dimensional digital imaging system. *Archives of Facial Plastic Surgery*, 8 (1), 26–35.

Hullihen, S. (1849) Case of elongation of the under jaw and distortion of the face and neck caused by a burn, successfully treated. *American Journal of Dental Science*, 9, 157–165.

Hunsuck, E.E. (1968) A modified intraoral sagittal splitting technic for correction of mandibular prognathism. *Journal of Oral Surgery*, 26 (4), 250–253.

Isaacson, R.J., Kopytov, O.S., Bevis, R.R., *et al.* (1978) Movement of the proximal and distal segments after mandibular ramus osteotomies. *Journal of Oral Surgery*, 36 (4), 263–268.

Jakobsone, G., Stenvik, A., Sandvik, L., *et al.* (2011) Three-year follow-up of bimaxillary surgery to correct skeletal Class III malocclusion: stability and risk factors for relapse. *American Journal of Orthodontics and Dentofacial Orthopedics*, 139 (1), 80–89.

Jensen, A.C., Sinclair, P.M., & Wolford, L.M. (1992) Soft tissue changes associated with double jaw surgery. *American Journal of Orthodontics and Dentofacial Orthopedics*, 101 (3), 266–275.

Joss, C.U. & Vassalli, I.M. (2009) Stability after bilateral sagittal split osteotomy advancement surgery with rigid internal fixation: a systematic review. *Journal of Oral and Maxillofacial Surgery*, 67 (2), 301–313.

Jung, Y.J., Kim, M.J., & Baek, S.H. (2009) Hard and soft tissue changes after correction of mandibular prognathism and facial asymmetry by mandibular setback surgery: three-dimensional analysis using computerized tomography. *Oral Surgery, Oral Medicine, Oral Pathology, Oral Radiology and Endodontics*, 107 (6), 763–771.

Kamburoglu, K., Kolsuz, E., Kurt, H., *et al.* (2011) Accuracy of CBCT measurements of a human skull. *Journal of Digital Imaging*, 24 (5), 787–793.

Kim, B.R., Oh, K.M., Cevidanes, L.H., *et al.* (2013) Analysis of 3D soft tissue changes after 1- and 2-jaw orthognathic surgery in mandibular prognathism patients. *Journal of Oral and Maxillofacial Surgery*, 71, 151–161.

Kim, Y.I., Jung, Y.H., Cho, B.H., *et al.* (2010) The assessment of the short and long-term changes in the condylar position following sagittal split ramus osteotomy (SSRO) with rigid fixation. *Journal of Oral Rehabilitation*, 37 (4), 262–270.

Kim, Y.I., Cho, B.H., Jung, Y.H., *et al.* (2011) Cone-beam computerized tomography evaluation of condylar changes and stability following two-jaw surgery: Le Fort I osteotomy and mandibular setback surgery with rigid fixation. *Oral Surgery, Oral Medicine, Oral Pathology, Oral Radiology and Endodontics*, 111 (6), 681–687.

Kim, Y.J., Oh, K.M., Hong, J.S., *et al.* (2012) Do patients treated with bimaxillary surgery have more stable condylar positions than those who have undergone single-jaw surgery? *Journal of Oral and Maxillofacial Surgery*, 70, 2143–2152.

Lagravère, M.O., Carey, J., Toogood, R.W., *et al.* (2008) Three-dimensional accuracy of measurements made with software on cone-beam computed tomography images. *American Journal of Orthodontics and Dentofacial Orthopedics*, 134 (1), 112–116.

Landes, C.A. (2004) Proximal segment positioning in bilateral sagittal split osteotomy: intraoperative dynamic positioning and monitoring by sonography. *Journal of Oral and Maxillofacial Surgery*, 62 (1), 22–28.

Landes, C.A. & Sterz, M. (2003) Proximal segment positioning in bilateral sagittal split osteotomy: intraoperative controlled positioning by a positioning splint. *Journal of Oral and Maxillofacial Surgery*, 61 (12), 1423–1431.

Lee, W. & Park, J.U. (2002) Three-dimensional evaluation of positional change of the condyle after mandibular setback by means of bilateral sagittal split ramus osteotomy. *Oral Surgery, Oral Medicine, Oral Pathology, Oral Radiology and Endodontics*, 94 (3), 305–309.

Legan, H. & Anderton, K. (1991) A retrospective analysis of mandibular setback surgery comparing two techniques. IADR Abstract #2147.

Lim, Y.K., Chu, E.H., Lee, D.Y., *et al.* (2010) Three-dimensional evaluation of soft tissue change gradients after mandibular setback surgery in skeletal Class III malocclusion. *The Angle Orthodontist*, 80 (5), 896–903.

Limberg, A. (1928) New method of plastic lengthening of the mandible in unilateral microgenia and asymmetric face. *Journal of the American Dental Association*, 15, 851–871.

Linder-Aronson, S. (1979) Respiratory function in relation to facial morphology and the dentition. *British Journal of Orthodontics*, 6 (2), 59–71.

Lloyd, T., Drage, N., & Cronin, A. (2011) The role of cone-beam computed tomography in the management of unfavourable fractures following sagittal split mandibular osteotomy. *Journal of Orthodontics*, 38 (1), 48–54.

Magalhaes, A.E., Stella, J.P., & Tahasuri, T.H. (1995) Changes in condylar position following bilateral sagittal split ramus osteotomy with setback. *International Journal of Adult Orthodontics and Orthognathic Surgery*, 10 (2), 137–145.

Mansour, S., Burstone, C., & Legan, H. (1983) An evaluation of soft-tissue changes resulting from Le Fort I maxillary surgery. *American Journal of Orthodontics*, 84 (1), 37–47.

McCance, A.M., Moss, J.P., Fright, W.R., *et al.* (1992) A three dimensional analysis of soft and hard tissue changes following bimaxillary orthognathic surgery in skeletal III patients. *British Journal of Oral and Maxillofacial Surgery*, 30 (5), 305–312.

Melsen, B. (1974) The cranial base. *Acta Odontologica Scandinavica*, 32 (Suppl 62), 9–111.

Moloney, F. & Worthington, P. (1981) The origin of the Le Fort I maxillary osteotomy: Cheever's operation. *Journal of Oral Surgery*, 39 (10), 731–734.

Motta, A.T., Cevidanes, L.H., Carvalho, L.H., *et al.* (2011) Three-dimensional regional displacements after mandibular advancement surgery: one year of follow-up. *Journal of Oral and Maxillofacial Surgery*, 69 (5), 1447–1457.

Mozzo, P., Procacci, C., Tacconi, A., *et al.* (1998) A new volumetric CT machine for dental imaging based on the cone-beam technique: preliminary results. *European Radiology*, 8 (9), 1558–1564.

Mucedero, M., Coviello, A., Baccetti, T., *et al.* (2008) Stability factors after double-jaw surgery in Class III malocclusion: a systematic review. *The Angle Orthodontist*, 78 (6), 1141–1152.

Nada, R.M., Maal, T.J., Breuning, K.H., *et al.* (2011) Accuracy and reproducibility of voxel based superimposition of cone beam computed tomography models on the anterior cranial base and the zygomatic arches. *PLoS One*, 6 (2), e16520.

Nielsen, I.L. (1989) Maxillary superimposition: a comparison of three methods for cephalometric evaluation of growth and treatment change. *American Journal of Orthodontics and Dentofacial Orthopedics*, 95 (5), 422–431.

Ozbek, M.M., Memikoglu, T.U., Gögen, H., *et al.* (1998) Oropharyngeal airway dimensions and functional-orthopedic treatment in skeletal Class II cases. *The Angle Orthodontist*, 68 (4), 327–336.

Paniagua, B., Cevidanes, L., Zhu, H., *et al.* (2010) Outcome quantification using SPHARM-PDM toolbox in orthognathic surgery. *International Journal of Computer Assisted Radiology and Surgery*, 6 (5), 617–626.

Park, S.B., Yang, Y.M., Kim, Y.I., *et al.* (2012a) Effect of bimaxillary surgery on adaptive condylar head remodeling: metric analysis and image interpretation using cone-beam computed tomography volume superimposition. *Journal of Oral and Maxillofacial Surgery*, 70, 1951–1959..

Park, S.B., Yoon, J.K., Kim, Y.I., *et al.* (2012b) The evaluation of the nasal morphologic changes after bimaxillary surgery in skeletal Class III maloccusion by using the superimposition of cone-beam computed tomography (CBCT) volumes. *Journal of Craniomaxillofacial Surgery*, 40 (4), e87–e92.

Pirila-Parkkinen, K., Pirttiniemi, P., Paakko, E., *et al.* (2012) Pharyngeal airway in children with sleep-disordered breathing in relation to head posture. *Sleep & Breathing*, 16, 737–746..

Plooij, J.M., Naphausen, M.T., Maal, T.J., *et al.* (2009) 3D evaluation of the lingual fracture line after a bilateral sagittal split osteotomy of the mandible. *International Journal of Oral and Maxillofacial Surgery*, 38 (12), 1244–1249.

Politi, M., Toro, C., Costa, F., *et al.* (2007) Intraoperative awakening of the patient during orthognathic surgery: a method to prevent the condylar sag. *Journal of Oral and Maxillofacial Surgery*, 65 (1), 109–114.

Proffit, W.R., Phillips, C., Dann, C.T., *et al.* (1991) Stability after surgical-orthodontic correction of skeletal Class III malocclusion. I: mandibular setback. *International Journal of Adult Orthodontics and Orthognathic Surgery*, 6 (1), 7–18.

Proffit, W.R., Bailey, L.J., Phillips, C., *et al.* (2000) Long-term stability of surgical open-bite correction by Le Fort I osteotomy. *The Angle Orthodontist*, 70 (2), 112–117.

Proffit, W.R., Turvey, T.A., & Phillips, C. (2007) The hierarchy of stability and predictability in orthognathic surgery with rigid fixation: an update and extension. *Head & Face Medicine*, 3, 21.

Reitzik, M., Lowe, A., & Schmidt, E. (1981) Stability following mandibular advancement using rigid internal fixation. *International Journal of Oral Surgery*, 10 (Suppl 1), 276–280.

Renzi, G., Becelli, E., Di Paolo, C., *et al.* (2003) Indications to the use of condylar repositioning devices in the surgical treatment of dental-skeletal class III. *Journal of Oral and Maxillofacial Surgery*, 61 (3), 304–309.

Ryckman, M.S., Harrison, S., Oliver, D., *et al.* (2010) Soft-tissue changes after maxillomandibular advancement surgery assessed with cone-beam computed tomography. *American Journal of Orthodontics and Dentofacial Orthopedics*, 137 (Suppl 4), S86–S93.

Samman, N., Tong, A.C., Cheung, D.L., *et al.* (1992) Analysis of 300 dentofacial deformities in Hong Kong. *International Journal of Adult Orthodontics and Orthognathic Surgery*, 7 (3), 181–185.

Sarver, D.M. (1998) *Esthetic Orthodontics and Orthognathic Surgery*. Mosby, St. Louis, MO.

Scheideman, G.B., Legan, H.L., & Bell, W.H. (1981) Soft tissue changes with combined mandibular setback and advancement genioplasty. *Journal of Oral Surgery*, 39 (7), 505–509.

Soncul, M. & Bamber, M.A. (2004) Evaluation of facial soft tissue changes with optical surface scan after surgical correction of Class III deformities. *Journal of Oral and Maxillofacial Surgery*, 62 (11), 1331–1340.

Sowray, J.H. & Haskell, R. (1968) Ostectomy at the mandibular symphysis. *British Journal of Oral Surgery*, 6 (2), 97–102.

Stella, J.P., Streater, M.R., Epker, B.N., *et al.* (1989) Predictability of upper lip soft tissue changes with maxillary advancement. *Journal of Oral and Maxillofacial Surgery*, 47 (7), 697–703.

Suckiel, J.M. & Kohn, M.W. (1978) Soft-tissue changes related to the surgical management of mandibular prognathism. *American Journal of Orthodontics*, 73 (6), 676–680.

Sung, S.J., Park, H.D., Kim, J.S., *et al.* (2000) Changes in soft tissue profile after surgical correction of prognathic mandible. *Korea Journal of Orthodontics*, 30, 355–365. Available at http://koreamed.org/SearchBasic.php?RID=0123KJOD%2F2000.30.3.355&DT=1&QY=%22Korean+J+Orthod%22+%5BJTI%5D++AND+2000+%5BDPY%5D+AND+Jun+%5BDPM%5D, accessed January 8, 2013.

Trauner, R. & Obwegeser, H. (1957) The surgical correction of mandibular prognathism and retrognathia with consideration of genioplasty. I: surgical procedures to correct mandibular prognathism and reshaping of the chin. *Oral Surgery, Oral Medicine, and Oral Pathology*, 10 (7), 677–689.

Tselnik, M. & Pogrel, M.A. (2000) Assessment of the pharyngeal airway space after mandibular setback surgery. *Journal of Oral and Maxillofacial Surgery*, 58 (3), 282–285.

Wassmund, M. (1935) *Lehrbuch der Praktischen Chirurgie des Mundes und der Kiefer*. 1, 260–282..

Wickwire, N.A., White, R.P. Jr., & Profitt, W.R. (1972) The effect of mandibular osteotomy on tongue position. *Journal of Oral Surgery*, 30 (3), 184–190.

Woodside, D.G., Linder-Aronson, S., Lundstrom, A., *et al.* (1991) Mandibular and maxillary growth after changed mode of breathing. *American Journal of Orthodontics and Dentofacial Orthopedics*, 100 (1), 1–18.

23 3D Imaging in Diagnosis and Treatment Planning of Craniofacial Anomalies

Snehlata Oberoi, DDS, MDS, Jeanne M. Nervina, DMD, PhD, and Karin Vargervik, DDS

INTRODUCTION

The goals of diagnosis and orthodontic treatment planning for patients with craniofacial anomalies (CFA) are no different from those for any patient. These objectives are to establish (1) an ideal, stable occlusion, (2) an esthetically pleasing smile, and (3) ideal facial proportions. What differs between craniofacial and non-craniofacial patients is the initial severity of the discrepancy in CFA patients from these ideals and the magnitude of change required to achieve relatively normal anatomy and relationships. Because of the magnitude of correction required in these patients, the maxim that orthodontics is a 6-millimeter profession lays bare the challenge faced by orthodontists in addressing skeletal and dental discrepancies that substantially exceed this magnitude often in all three planes of space. For this reason, orthodontists and surgeons who treat CFA patients readily adopt technological advances that improve the quality of care they can provide their patients. It is not surprising that these technologies subsequently find their way into everyday practice to the benefit of all orthodontic patients. Three-dimensional (3D) radiographic imaging is one of these technologies, of which cone beam computed tomography (CBCT) is used most widely in orthodontics.

CBCT provides 3D imaging that greatly improves the diagnosis, treatment planning, and assessment of treatment progress and outcomes for all orthodontic patients (Kapila *et al.*, 2011). Moreover, CBCT imaging joins the rapidly expanding armamentaria of digital photography, radiography, and dental cast imaging that are replacing traditional film-based photographs and cephalometric, panoramic and intraoral radiographs and plaster models.

Clearly, there are many advantages to digital records. They can be viewed immediately to ensure they are taken properly and provide the needed information, and can be retaken immediately if needed. Backup copies can be made for storage, and the images can be printed immediately or sent

Cone Beam Computed Tomography in Orthodontics: Indications, Insights, and Innovations, First Edition. Sunil D. Kapila.

electronically for communication with patients, parents, and other clinicians. In this chapter, we present the current uses of radiographic and non-radiographic 3D imaging in the treatment of patients with common and rare CFAs and syndromes, with a focus on how these technologies are improving diagnosis, treatment planning, and outcomes assessment for individuals with these disorders. We also discuss the importance of integrating 3D imaging data with accurate genetic testing to understand the array of craniofacial anomalies fully and to develop advanced treatments for these patients.

3D IMAGING MODALATIES FOR CRANIOFACIAL PATIENTS

Multislice computed tomography

Multislice computed tomography (MSCT) scans produce excellent details of skeletal morphology, skeletal pathology, patency of sutures, and temporomandibular joint (TMJ) anatomy and ankylosis. While computed tomography (CT) scans are good for imaging mineralized tissues in particular, they also capture soft tissue anatomy. This is valuable for CFA patients who can present with anomalous soft tissue structures, such as soft palate clefting or velopharyngeal insufficiency.

Cone beam computed tomography (CBCT)

CBCT has become a useful tool in diagnosis of and treatment planning for CFA patients. There are several advantages of CBCT imaging over other forms of radiography. The effective radiation dose from CBCT is dependent on the field of view (FOV) and can be as low as 20% of traditional MSCT. Another important advantage of CBCT imaging with CFA patients is the increased anatomic detail and measurement accuracy, which is critical for orthodontic and surgical treatment planning. Digital 3D images can be used to map the distances and directions of dental and skeletal movements precisely that are needed to optimize the treatment outcome (Kapila *et al.*, 2011). In addition, CBCT is invaluable for assessing unerupted tooth position and identifying root resorption caused by unerupted teeth, which are common in CFA patients. As ever-growing numbers of graduate orthodontic programs and private practice orthodontists use CBCT and other forms of 3D imaging for diagnosis and treatment planning, the demand for user-friendly software packages for managing and analyzing Digital Imaging and Communications in Medicine (DICOM) images is increasing. In response to this demand, clinicians now have a wide selection of programs that ease the transition from conventional two-dimensional (2D) to 3D radiography. For both CBCT and MSCT the available software permits multiplanar reconstruction to view the craniofacial skeleton and soft tissues in all three planes of space. Furthermore, 3D models generated from CT scans allow clinicians to appreciate the extent of a patient's craniofacial anomaly fully and can optimize treatment planning and sequencing among the craniofacial team members.

Magnetic resonance imaging (MRI)

MRI produces precise images of intracranial soft tissue structures without radiation. In the craniofacial region, it is used extensively in diagnosing brain and spinal pathology. For example, MRI has been used to study brain morphology in patients with Van der Woude Syndrome and cleft lip and palate (CL/P; Nopoulos *et al.*, 2007, 2010). MRI also is the imaging modality of choice for diagnosing TMJ abnormalities, especially disc displacement (Hamada *et al.*, 2000; see also Chapter 12). Interestingly, MRI use is expanding into prenatal diagnosis (Munch *et al.*, 2009). One limitation of MRI is that it cannot be used on patients with orthodontic appliances in place because the metal in the appliances interferes with the powerful magnetic field needed to generate the images. However, improvements in MRI technology are reducing this limitation (Proffit *et al.*, 2003).

3D photography

3D photography records soft tissue surfaces of craniofacial structures without any radiation.

Although useful, its accuracy still may not be adequate to diagnose craniofacial anomalies (Plooij *et al.*, 2011). However, it can add to the assessment of surgical outcomes such as cleft lip repair and has been used to evaluate variations and phenotypes of syndromes such as trisomy 21. 3D virtual models and shape changes in the noses of CL/P patients after secondary repair have been studied using 3D stereophotogrammetry (van Loon *et al.*, 2010; Sforza *et al.*, 2012). Furthermore, 3D color maps have been used to provide an objective assessment of craniofacial treatment changes (Jayaratne *et al.*, 2010).

3D motion analysis systems historically were developed for gait analysis and now are being adapted for facial motion capture, as represented by the 3dMD Face Dynamic Imaging System (Lubbers *et al.*, 2010). This technology recently has been used for studying facial movements in cleft and non-cleft children (Trotman, 2011).

3D dental models

Dental impressions or casts can be laser-scanned or intraoral scans taken to recreate 3D digitized dental models. The 3D images have the advantage of allowing viewing by rotating on a 2D screen, which also allows for accurate measurements. Physical casts can be produced from the digital data through a computer-aided design/computer-aided manufacturing (CAD/CAM) system (Figure 23.1) and also can be merged with CBCT data (see also Chapter 4).

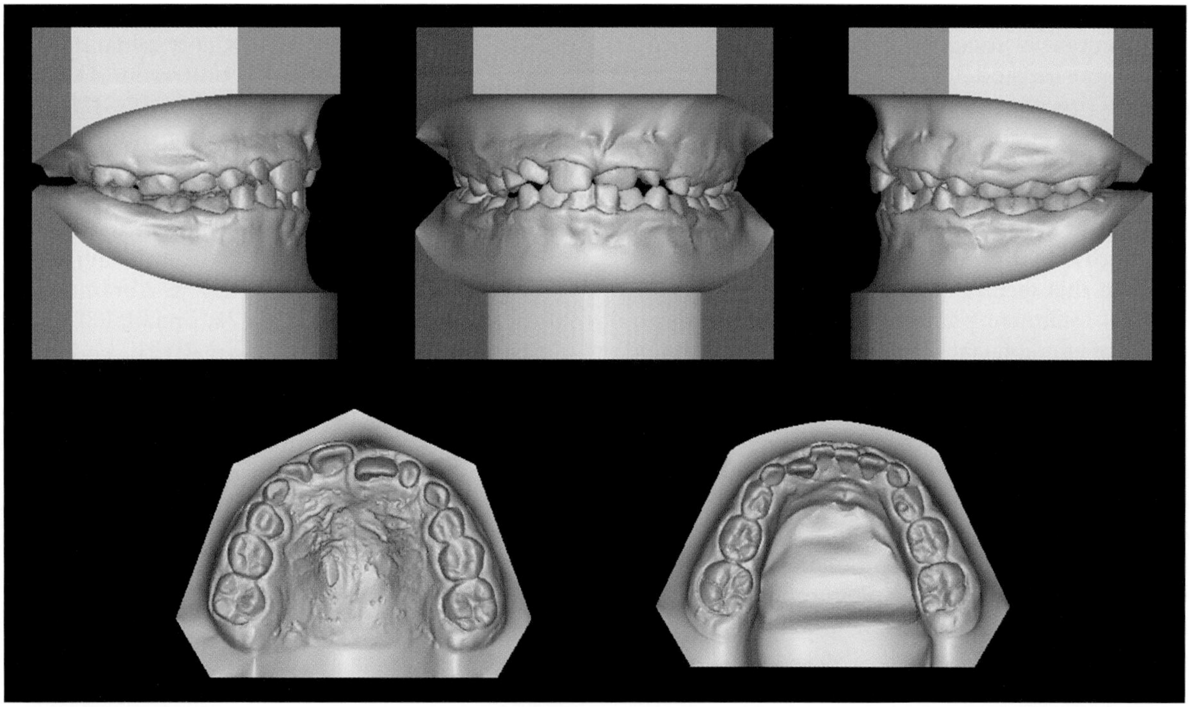

Figure 23.1 E-models of a 7-year-old girl with unilateral CL/P. 3D imaging of the dentition provides virtual casts that can be manipulated to assess the efficacy of different treatment plans. In complex cases, such as CL/P, this feature is valuable especially when it is paired with CBCT images that demonstrate the location of teeth that are likely to erupt into the cleft site. The orthodontist and surgeon also can use the merged images to determine the ideal graft volume needed to accommodate the permanent teeth or implant.

3D surgical simulation models

Treatment planning for CFA patients can be difficult when relying on conventional 2D lateral and frontal cephalograms because 3D structures are superimposed within two dimensions. This complicates estimations of actual size and shape of anomalies and consequently introduces a higher potential for discrepancy between surgical planning and surgical outcome. While surgical simulation models greatly improve surgical outcomes in CFA patients, these models traditionally have been developed from conventional 2D radiographs. 3D surgical simulation models overcome many of the limitations associated with traditional model surgery, most notably the simultaneous access to information on the patient's skeletal anatomy during the planning process (Swennen *et al.*, 2009; see also Chapters 4, 20, and 21). Concomitant with improved 3D imaging is the rapidly increasing availability of computer software that is designed to mitigate these problems by combining craniofacial imaging modalities to produce a 3D composite model that can be used to simulate surgical procedures. While the imaging techniques used to generate 3D models vary, they typically employ a combination of CT imaging, soft-tissue surface scanning, and digitized tooth molds (see Chapter 4). Simulation software is used to plan individual procedures and assess outcomes. Because this technology allows more predictable surgical treatment planning for complex manipulation of craniofacial structures, it is well suited for use in craniofacial anomalies (Xia *et al.*, 2007). In fact, recent studies indicate that such fusion techniques can predict actual post-operative results more precisely than single treatment planning approaches alone (Gateno *et al.*, 2007; Plooij *et al.*, 2011). These studies indicate that mean linear differences between simulation and surgical results in patients with complex craniofacial deformities were a mere 0.85 mm, with only 1.7° angular discrepancy (Donatsky *et al.*, 1997; Xia *et al.*, 2007). Considering previous data suggesting that differences up to 2.0 mm and 4.0° are insignificant clinically, it is clear that the 3D image analyses and manipulation by the software contribute to the highly predictable results in these cases (Donatsky *et al.*, 1997).

APPLICATION OF 3D IMAGING IN CRANIOFACIAL ANOMALIES

Prenatal diagnosis

Advances in fetal ultrasound and MRI have increased the range and diagnostic accuracy of fetal anomalies. This is valuable because the presence of a structural anomaly in the fetus greatly increases the likelihood of a syndrome or abnormal karyotype (Estroff, 2012). Genetic testing then can be performed to verify the ultrasound or MRI findings.

Ultrasound is used widely to diagnose clefts prenatally and, not surprisingly, 3D ultrasound is superior to 2D ultrasound in detecting cleft lip accurately (Chen *et al.*, 2001). The 3D reverse face view allows a relatively straightforward view of the fetal palate, enabling accurate diagnosis of cleft palate (Campbell *et al.*, 2005). During the past two decades, 3D/4D ultrasound has expanded diagnostic abilities, especially in the prenatal diagnosis of facial clefts, brain anomalies, and spinal defects. In contrast to conventional 2D ultrasound, which allows imaging only of single planes, 3D/4D ultrasound offers a precise demonstration of the normal and abnormal anatomy of the fetus, displaying anatomy in ways not possible with 2D imaging. Digital storage of volumes permits virtual examinations by reloading of volumes and navigating through them at any time (Merz & Abramowicz, 2012). In a study to detect CL/P, prenatal 3D axial ultrasound showed 100% sensitivity and 90% specificity (Baumler *et al.*, 2011).

While ultrasound is excellent for assessing prenatal craniofacial morphology, the views can be limited by shadowing from ossified bone. Thus, MRI is being used increasingly to overcome this problem and to supplement ultrasound. In fact, MRI provides better detection and classification of facial clefts than does ultrasound alone (Mailath-Pokorny *et al.*, 2010). While MRI shows excellent soft tissue contrast with no radiation dose, it is not used routinely in 3D reconstruction due to long scan times, motion artifacts, and poor contrast in anatomically complex regions (Rathnayaka *et al.*, 2013). Motion artifacts particularly are problematic, as they distort 3D reconstruction from the scan data (Rathnayaka *et al.*, 2012).

Research is ongoing in the prenatal detection of craniosynostosis by using 3D ultrasonography. A case report that compared 2D and 3D ultrasound showed that while craniosynostosis was diagnosed with 2D ultrasound and positional molding with 3D ultrasound, the patient indeed had positional molding as confirmed by neonatal radiographs (Krakow *et al.*, 2001). 3D ultrasound enables the visualization of the full length of the cranial suture, which is not possible with conventional 2D ultrasound. Ultrasonography also can be useful in detecting bony abnormalities associated with the syndrome-related causes of craniosynostosis. While a detailed account of prenatal detection of various anomalies is beyond the scope of this chapter, interested readers are referred to several case reports that used both 3D ultrasound and MRI to improve prenatal diagnosis of craniofacial anomalies (Robson & Barnewolt, 2004; Elia *et al.*, 2008; Ginsberg *et al.*, 2011; Luedders *et al.*, 2011; Beegun *et al.*, 2012).

Craniosynostosis and craniosynostosis syndromes

Craniosynostosis is characterized by early closure of one or more cranial sutures. Early diagnosis and treatment are essential to release synostosed sutures and allow for skull expansion as the brain grows (Parisi *et al.*, 1989). 3D CT, particularly maximum intensity projection (MIP), permits clinicians to view the degree of cranial suture closure and deformity due to its ability to separate imaging of blood vessels from soft tissue (see "Vascular Malformations" below; Medina, 2000) and is useful for pre-operative planning and assessing post-operative progress (Boyle & Rosenblum, 1997).

The sensitivity of CT scans approaches 100% when combined with physical examination and conventional 2D radiography. Danelson and associates (2009) investigated the benefits of using 3D models in pre-operative planning for craniosynostosis surgery, specifically spring-mediated cranioplasty and cranial vault reconstruction. They showed that the surgical procedure was less invasive using 3D models in planning surgery because less of the skull had to be exposed. Additionally, the force characteristics of the spring could be quantified better. The addition of this pre-surgical planning tool resulted in a less invasive approach and shorter procedure time.

Sagittal synostosis is the most common form of isolated craniosynostosis. It results in a dolicocephalic head shape, ridging over the sagittal suture, frontal bossing, and occipital protrusion due to compensatory growth along the coronal, metopic, and lambdoid sutures. 3D CT demonstrates focal or generalized suture absence with ridging over the sagittal suture (Figure 23.2A).

Coronal synostosis, the second most common isolated synostosis (18–29%), results in flattening of the ipsilateral parietal and frontal bones and compensatory bulging of the frontal and temporal regions on the opposite side of the deformity (Figure 23.2B). Metopic synostosis represents 10% of all craniosynostosis. It presents as narrowing of the anterior cranial fossa with a prominent mid-frontal ridge resulting in a pointed forehead (trigonocephaly; Figure 23.2C). Lambdoid synostosis (LS) is the least frequent type of craniosynostosis (<5%). It most often is unilateral, resulting in asymmetry, which is referred to as plagiocephaly. It is important to distinguish LS from positional plagiocephaly, which is a flattening of the back of the skull that develops when babies sleep on their backs. Importantly, as opposed to LS, the lambdoidal suture remains patent in positional plagiocephaly. The rates of positional plagiocephaly have increased since the National Institute of Child Health and Development initiated the Back-to-Sleep (BTS) program in 1994 in which parents are encouraged to monitor their baby's sleep position and to keep the baby on his or her back while asleep to reduce the risk of Sudden Infant Death Syndrome (SIDS; Willinger *et al.*, 1994). A 3D radiograph can distinguish the two conditions based on the patency of the lambdoidal sutures. Both right and left lambdoidal sutures are patent in babies with positional plagiocephaly, whereas one or both of these sutures are fused in LS. Also in LS patients, 3D CT shows a flattening of the skull on the side of suture fusion with an ipsilateral mastoid bulge (Figure 23.2D).

Craniosynostosis syndromes usually are associated with fusion of facial sutures as well as cranial sutures and present with underdevelopment of

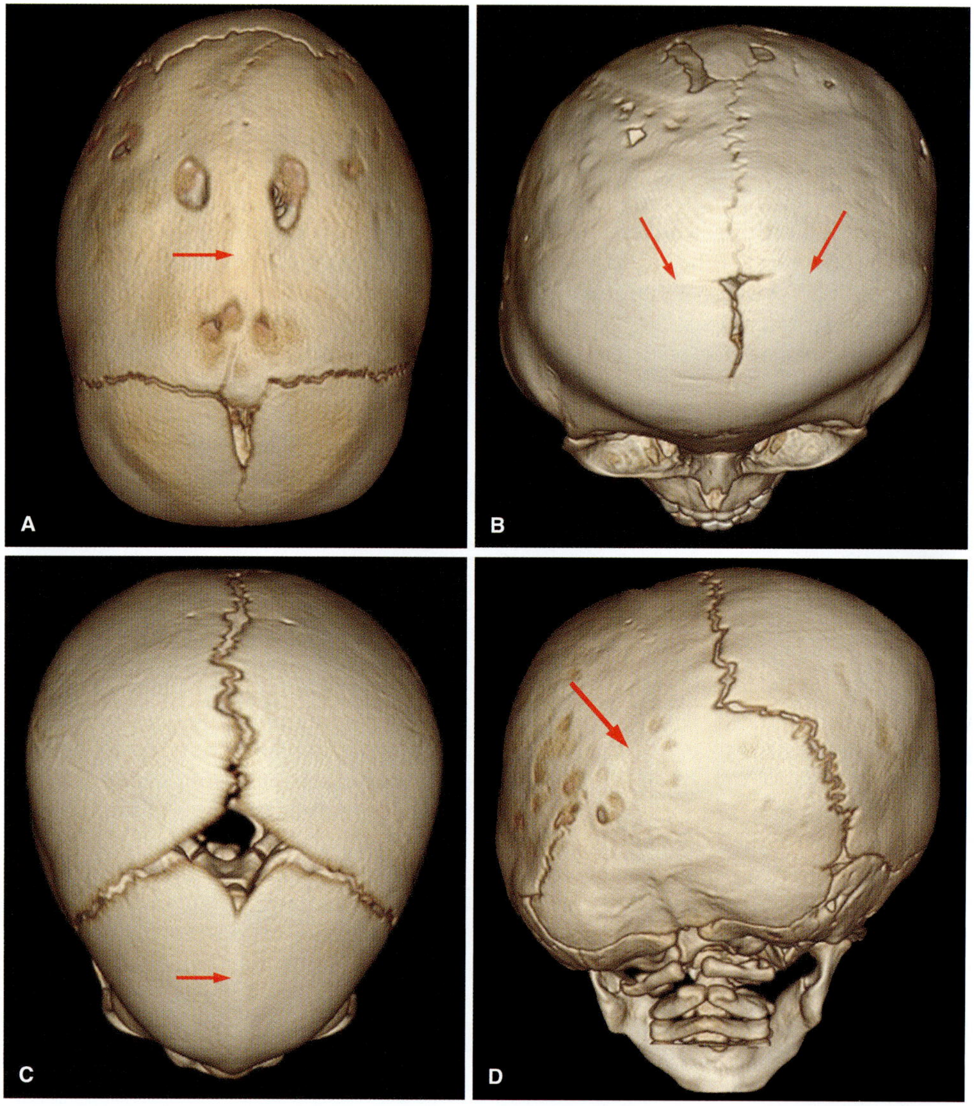

Figure 23.2 3D volumetric CT showing (*A*) sagittal synostosis with scaphocephaly where the fused sagittal suture (arrow) inhibits lateral expansion of the upper cranium, which produces a narrow, keel-shaped (scaphoid-shaped) skull to accommodate the growing brain; (*B*) bilateral coronal synostosis in which the fused coronal sutures (arrows) inhibit anterior expansion of the cranium, which produces a flattened and broadened forehead; (*C*) metopic synostosis where the fused metopic suture (arrow) produces a prominent vertical ridge and triangular shape to the forehead; and (*D*) lambdoid synostosis where the unilaterally fused lambdoidal suture produces a pronounced asymmetric flattening in the posterior skull.

the midface (Figure 23.3). The midface hypoplasia often compromises vital functions such as respiration and feeding. At some stage of development, surgical correction will become necessary in these patients. Functional, psychological, and esthetic factors play a role in determining the best time for the midface advancement (Vargervik *et al.*, 2012).

Management of craniosynostosis syndromes requires a team of experienced specialists and extends over the entire growth period from infancy to adulthood. Both the traditional Le Fort III and

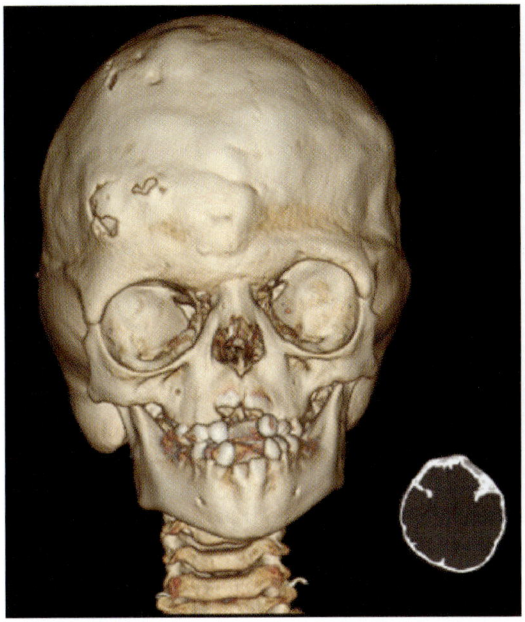

Figure 23.3 Surface-rendered CT of a child with Apert Syndrome. This image demonstrates the significant craniofacial dysmorphology in Apert Syndrome, one of the more common craniosynostoses. The lack of patent sutures and asymmetric skull are visible clearly in the 3D volume and the axial slice (lower right panel) of the skull. Clinically, 3D radiographs such as this are helpful for orthodontic and surgical treatment planning. Suture release, often needed more than once, and Le Fort advancement (see Figure 23.4) are planned more easily and accurately when detailed 3D digital images of the entire craniofacial complex are available.

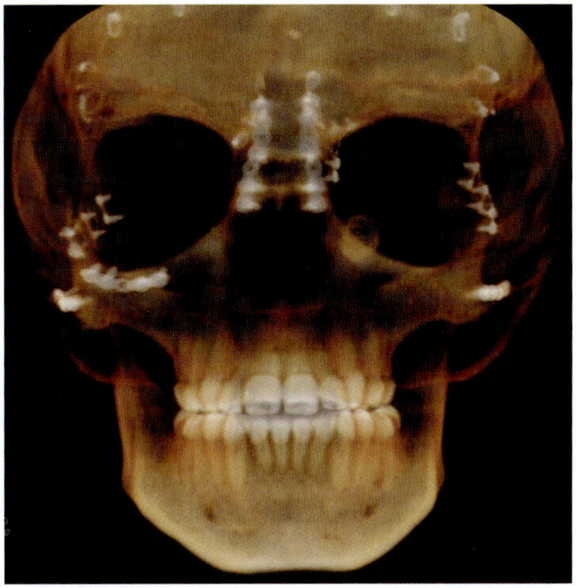

Figure 23.4 CBCT radiograph of an individual with Pfeiffer Syndrome after Le Fort III and Le Fort I advancement. Pfeiffer Syndrome is a craniosynostosis syndrome that results in a significant midface deficiency. As this image demonstrates, significant surgical correction along with orthodontics can provide these patients with a more normal facial appearance and occlusion.

distraction techniques are effective surgical techniques in correcting the midface hypoplasia (Oberoi *et al.*, 2012). Both CT and CBCT are used to assess malformations and functional impairments, to plan the surgical approach, and to perform long-term follow-up studies after major surgical interventions (Figure 23.4; Meazzini *et al.*, 2012; Ohtani *et al.*, 2012).

Cleft lip and palate (CL/P)

Assessment of the alveolar defect and planning for alveolar bone grafting

With relatively easy access to CBCT, this imaging approach has become standard for our CL/P patients at the start of Phase I orthodontic treatment. Maxillary expansion and protraction, if needed to correct crossbites in preparation for alveolar bone grafting, is a common treatment for individuals with complete CL/P. A successful alveolar bone graft results in continuity of the maxillary arch, facilitates eruption of permanent teeth, provides adequate bone support for erupting teeth, preserves periodontal health of teeth adjacent to the cleft, permits orthodontic tooth alignment, allows placement of osseointegrated implants, and improves alar base symmetry (Bergland *et al.*, 1986; Trindade *et al.*, 2005). Diagnostic imaging is essential before alveolar bone grafting to evaluate the size of the alveolar cleft defect, position and level of bone on adjacent teeth, and presence of supernumerary teeth. After bone grafting, radiographic evaluation helps to determine the outcome of the procedure by evaluating the bone fill of the defect, eruption status of the lateral incisor or canine adjacent to the cleft, and adequacy of bone for placement of endosseous implant (Figure 23.5).

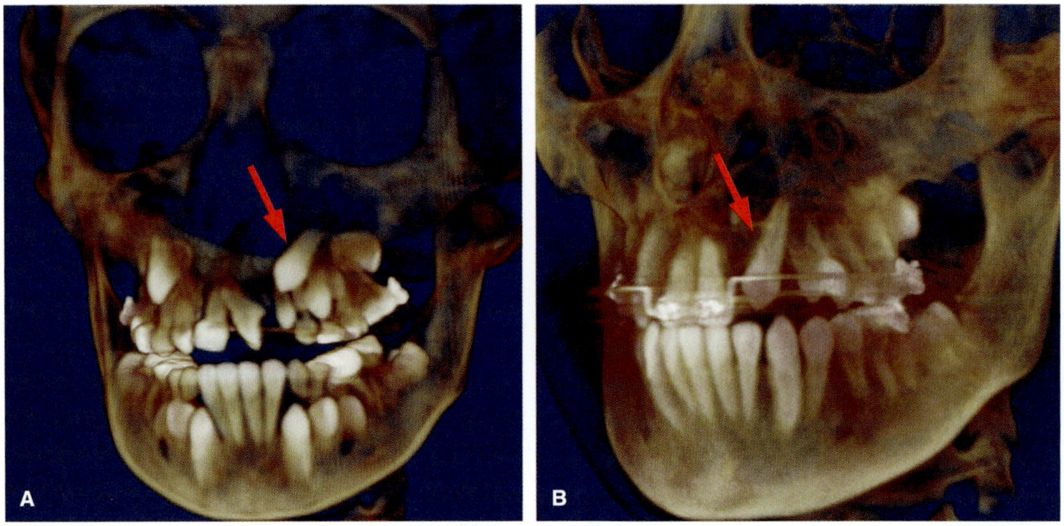

Figure 23.5 Volume rendering of CBCT scans of an individual with a unilateral CL/P (*A*) before and (*B*) after alveolar bone grafting. With CBCT imaging, assessing the morphology, locating the position, and determining the developmental stage of the unerupted maxillary left canine (arrow) permit the orthodontist and surgeon to time the placement of the alveolar graft ahead of canine eruption. Sufficient lead time allows the graft to mature and gives the orthodontist sufficient time for arch development to better support the canine as it erupts into the arch.

In our recent study to assess the radiographic outcome of alveolar bone grafting in 21 individuals with CL/P using CBCT, the average volume of the pre-operative alveolar cleft defect in unilateral CL/P was 0.61 cm^3, and the combined average volume of the right and left alveolar cleft defects in bilateral CL/P was 0.82 cm^3 (Oberoi *et al.*, 2009). The average percentage bone fill in both unilateral and bilateral CL/P was 84%. The CBCT also enabled the determination of the adequacy of bone height and width for placement of an implant to replace a missing lateral incisor. In a study to assess accuracy of CBCT measurements on bone height and thickness, buccal bone height and thickness were measured on CBCT scans and compared with direct measurements on human cadavers. The mean differences between CBCT and direct measurements were nearly zero (Timock *et al.*, 2011).

Assessment of individual teeth

CBCT is useful in assessing and treatment planning for teeth adjacent to the cleft as illustrated in a case in which the left maxillary permanent central incisor is impacted and erupting horizontally (Figure 23.6A). With the aid of the CBCT scans, exposure and bonding was carried out and the tooth was brought into the arch with appropriate force application (Figure 23.6B). CBCT studies to measure the length of the maxillary central incisor adjacent to the cleft have revealed that the cleft side incisor is shorter than the contralateral one (Zhou *et al.*, 2013). A pilot study on two individuals with van der Woude Syndrome using CBCT showed abnormal morphology of both crown and roots, which was not apparent on the standard panoramic radiograph. Further analyses using both the volumetric and linear measurements of the ratio of crown body to root were indicative of taurodontism in this patient (Figure 23.7; Nawa *et al.*, 2008).

Eruption status and eruption path of the maxillary canine in non-cleft and grafted cleft side

Several studies have found that the percentage of canines that erupt spontaneously through the

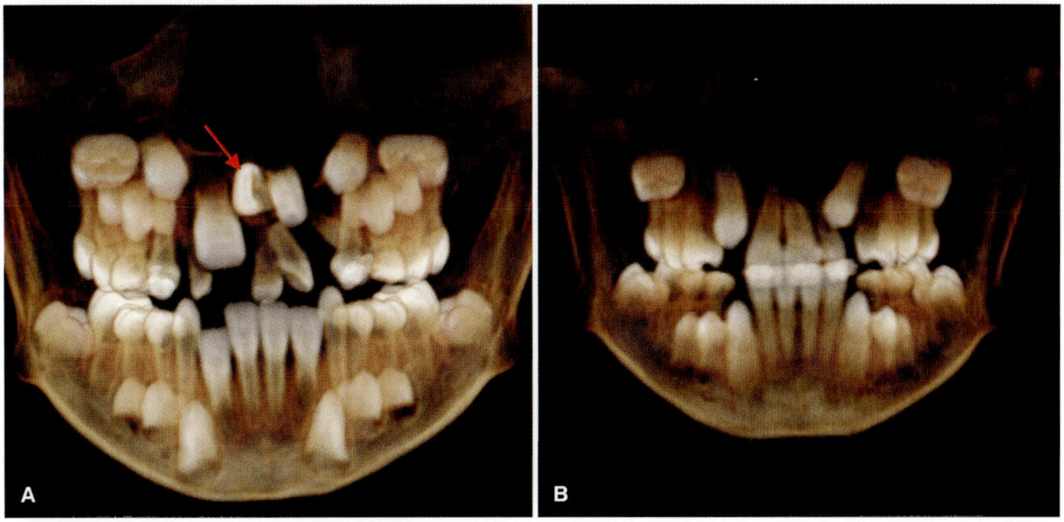

Figure 23.6 Volume rendering of CBCT scans of a CL/P patient showing impacted central incisor (*A*; red arrow) that was exposed, bonded, and orthodontically moved into the dental arch (*B*).

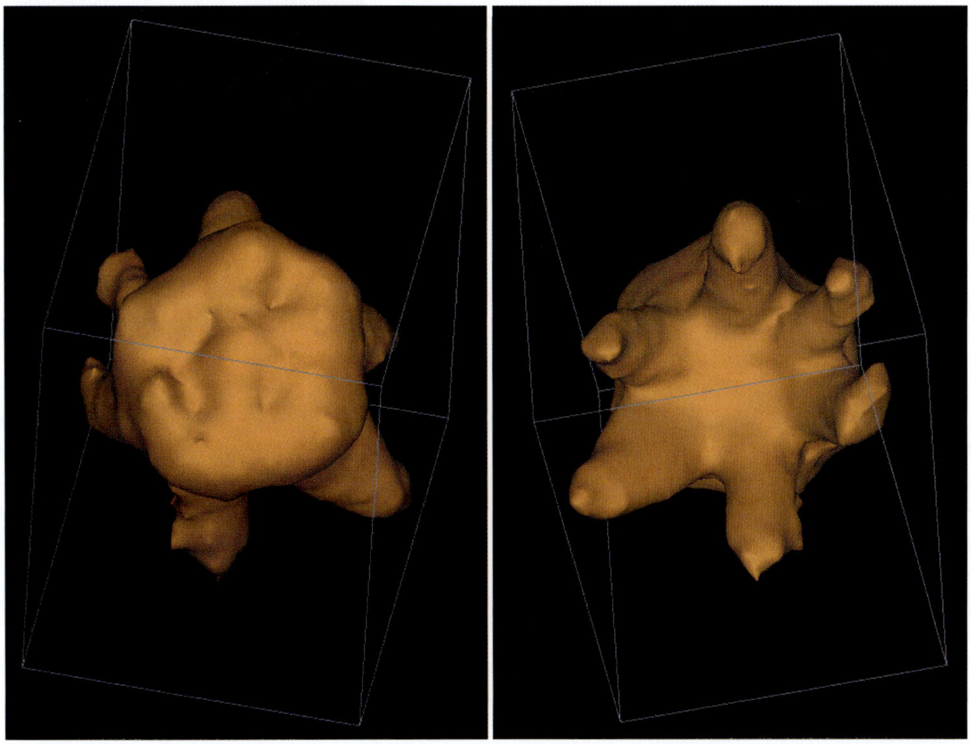

Figure 23.7 Volumetric CBCT segmentation of a taurodont in van der Woude Syndrome.

bone-grafted site can vary widely, from a low of 27% to a high of 97% (Turvey *et al.*, 1984; da Silva Filho *et al.*, 2000). A recent CBCT study on 21 consecutively treated unilateral CL/P patients showed that 12% of the canines did not erupt spontaneously (Oberoi *et al.*, 2010). Most canines on both the grafted cleft and non-cleft side moved incisally, facially, and mesially. Presence or absence of the lateral incisor did not affect the vertical eruption of the canine. The study showed that alveolar bone grafting after orthodontic expansion and before eruption of the permanent canine crown into the defect allows a normal path of eruption of the canine, predominantly without impaction, thereby enhancing alveolar bone development and facilitating orthodontic management.

Airway characteristics

Anatomical abnormalities associated with CL/P increase the risk of airway complications. Nasal abnormalities such as septal deviation, nostril atresia, turbinate hypertrophy, and maxillary constriction are frequent findings (Hairfield *et al.*, 1988). These abnormalities are attributed, in part, to the congenital defect itself and partly to the surgeries done to repair the orofacial defect. Collectively, the nasal abnormalities tend to reduce the dimensions of the nasal cavity and overall airway function.

Airway patency has been evaluated by 2D radiographic imaging, such as lateral and posteroanterior cephalometric films, and functional studies such as rhinomanometry and plethysmography (Smahel *et al.*, 1991; Drake *et al.*, 1993; Imamura *et al.*, 2002; Fukushiro & Trindade, 2005; see also Chapter 13). In contrast to 2D methods, MSCT or CBCT provide dimensional and volumetric airway data for accurate assessment of the airway in all three planes—coronal, sagittal, and axial (Figure 23.8). Due to the high radiation dose for standard MSCT scanning, however, CBCT is preferred for repeated longitudinal studies. Studies have shown that 3D imaging using CBCT is a simple and effective method to analyze the airway accurately (Abramson *et al.*, 2009; Iwasaki *et al.*, 2009; Olszewska *et al.*, 2009; Kim *et al.*, 2010; Hatcher, 2012; see also Chapter 13), and a systematic review of the literature indicates that 3D analysis of the upper airway using CBCT can provide accurate and reliable results (Guijarro-Martinez & Swennen, 2011). Nevertheless, important limitations including the impact of respiratory phase, influence of tongue position and mandibular morphology, and 3D CBCT definition of the anatomical boundaries of the upper airway must be taken into account for such an analysis.

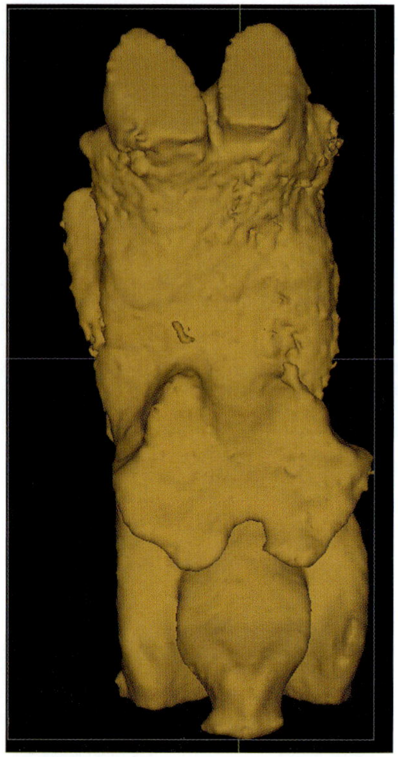

Figure 23.8 Segmented airway volume from a patient with unilateral CL/P.

In a recent study, we hypothesized that children with unilateral CL/P had smaller pharyngeal airways compared with non-CL/P controls. However, data showed that there were no significant differences in pharyngeal airway volume and smallest cross-sectional area and that the airway length was larger significantly in the CL/P group. The mean smallest cross-sectional area for CL/P individuals was 115.7 mm^2 (SD = 58.4 mm^2) and for controls 113.8 mm^2 (SD = 59.2 mm^2), with the large standard deviations signifying a wide range of values for airway cross-sectional area. This may be attributed to the age range of patients and the varying levels of growth for each patient (Oberoi *et al.*, 2011). An earlier CBCT study found differential growth in airway length in boys and girls during puberty, resulting in significantly longer airways in boys aged 14–19 (Ronen *et al.*, 2007). Future studies could compare the volume in different regions of the pharynx (naso-, oro-, and hypopharynx) to elucidate precisely where the airway is larger and also could explore airway length differences between CL/P individuals and controls.

Implant placement

The imaging technique of choice for implant placement is CBCT with curved and radial reconstructions, which enables the determination of bone height, width, and quality. CBCT also is valuable in the location or identification of several important anatomical structures or limitations. In the mandible, CBCT enables the visualization of inferior alveolar nerve canal, a structure of critical importance to avoid during implant placement. The depth of the submandibular fossa also can be assessed by CBCT such that if there is insufficient bone at this site, anterior implants can be placed mesial to the mental foramina, which can be used to support an overdenture. In the maxilla, CBCT can be used to assess the magnitude of proclination of the alveolar ridge and the relationship and size of the nasopalatine canal to the proposed implant site. In the posterior maxilla, CBCT allows the determination of bone width and height, typically revealing adequate bone width but reduced bone height, that would warrant the need for a sinus lift procedure (Boeddinghaus & Whyte, 2008).

CBCT increasingly has become valuable for implant placement to replace missing lateral incisors in CL/P individuals (Pena *et al.*, 2009). Virtual implant planning using CBCT data allows the clinicians to create and visualize the end result before initiating treatment. CBCT scans are accurate and cost-effective and can be used to improve communication and coordination of an interdisciplinary team to achieve the desired clinical outcome. The optimized virtual plan may be converted through modeling to create a surgical guide for clinical implementation (Worthington *et al.*, 2010; Benavides *et al.*, 2012).

Use of temporary anchorage devices (TADs) increasingly has become useful in orthodontic treatment planning (see also Chapter 18). CBCT to assess the quantity and quality of bone and location of adjacent structures can make placement of TADs easier and safer. For example, it has been shown that an ideal location for placement of palatal implants lies approximately 4 mm palatal to the incisive foramen (King *et al.*, 2007; Gracco *et al.*, 2008). Finally, a technique using CBCT scans and rapid prototyping to fabricate surgical guides has been used for placing TADs (Kim *et al.*, 2007).

Midface hypoplasia

The maxilla in cleft individuals often is deficient in all three planes of space. Maxillary deficiency is evident in the anterior-posterior (AP), vertical, and transverse dimensions. The causes of abnormal facial morphology in treated cleft individuals may result from one of two factors: intrinsic developmental deficiency or iatrogenic factors introduced by treatment.

When the degree of maxillary hypoplasia is severe, surgical correction with facial osteotomies is necessary. A Le Fort I maxillary osteotomy typically is used to correct this deformity. The literature indicates that the surgical correction is needed for 14–45%, with an average of 25% of such cases. Current advances in CBCT and CAD/CAM that allow clinicians to generate accurate diagnosis and treatment planning, surgical predictions, and surgical splints are making obsolete the traditional indirect planning techniques based on 2D cephalometry and articulated model surgery (Xia *et al.*, 2007; Orentlicher *et al.*, 2010; Bell, 2011; see also Chapters 4 and 20).

Hemifacial microsomia (HFM) and other asymmetries

CBCT can overcome many of the limitations of 2D radiography to aid clinicians in diagnosing and studying patients with asymmetries. The asymmetries often are discerned best in all planes of space in 3D by visualization of structures from all angles. In a recent study, CBCT and 2D postero-anterior cephalometric images were compared in

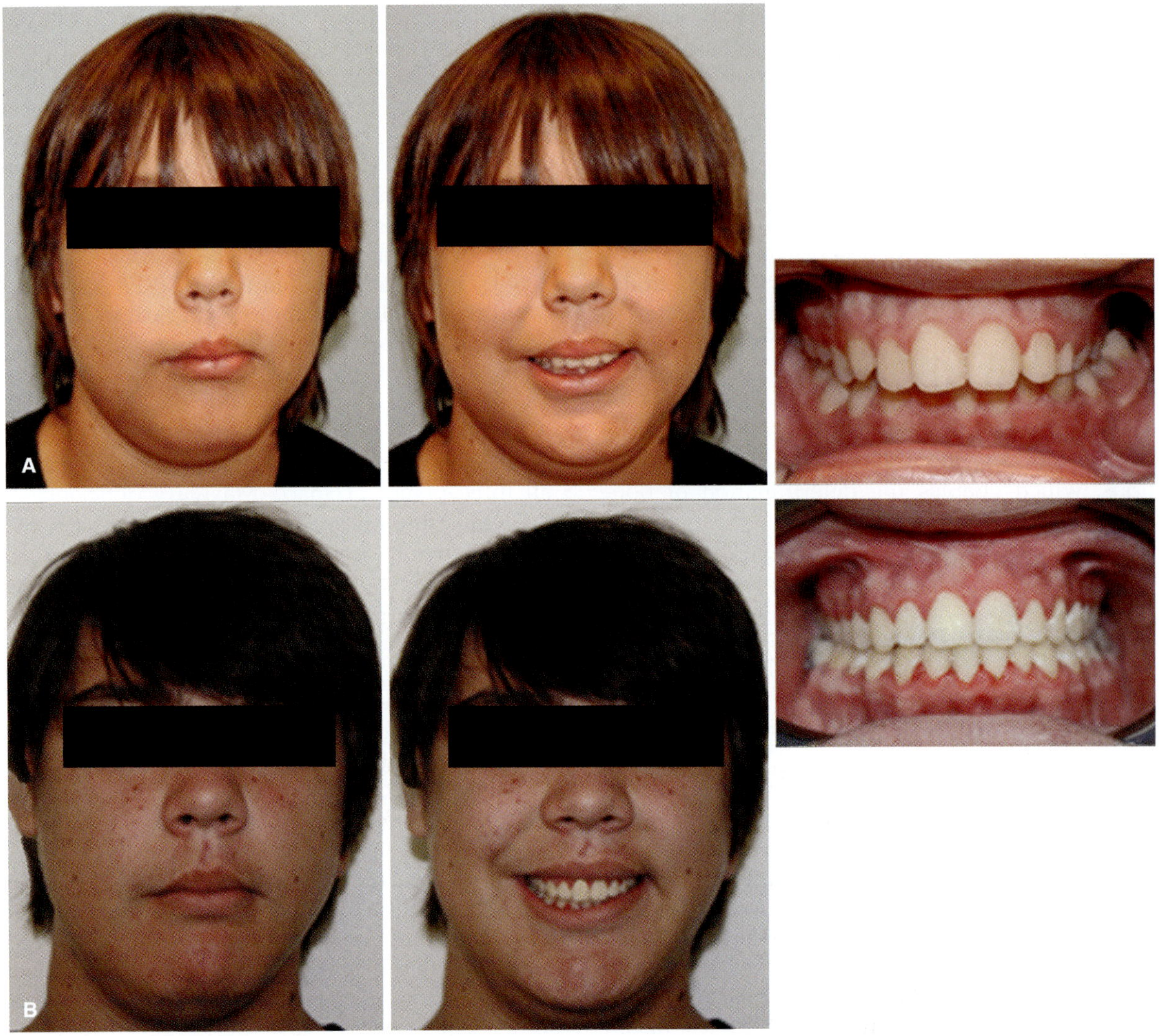

Figure 23.9 Photographs of a patient with hemifacial microsomia before (*A*) and after (*B*) orthognathic surgery and orthodontic treatment. (Reprinted with permission from Ohtani *et al.*, 2012.)

evaluating craniofacial asymmetry using 10 dry human skulls and radiopaque markers on 17 skeletal landmarks. The CBCT measurements and physical measurements were nearly identical, while the 2D postero-anterior radiograph gave less accurate values (de Moraes *et al.*, 2011).

Currently, CT with 3D reconstruction is used routinely to delineate clearly the asymmetries in patients with hemifacial microsomia (HFM; Marsh *et al.*, 1989; Ono *et al.*, 1992; Yune, 1993; Huisinga-Fischer *et al.*, 2001). These images not only demonstrate the asymmetry of the facial bones, but also allow assessment of tooth inclination, cranial base asymmetries, and soft tissue deficiencies (Figure 23.9 and Figure 23.10; Senggen *et al.*, 2011; Ohtani *et al.*, 2012). The main advantage of 3D CT is the accuracy in dimensional measurements, but it exposes the patient to a high radiation dose. In a study to compare the accuracy of 3D CT and panoramic radiography in the evaluation of

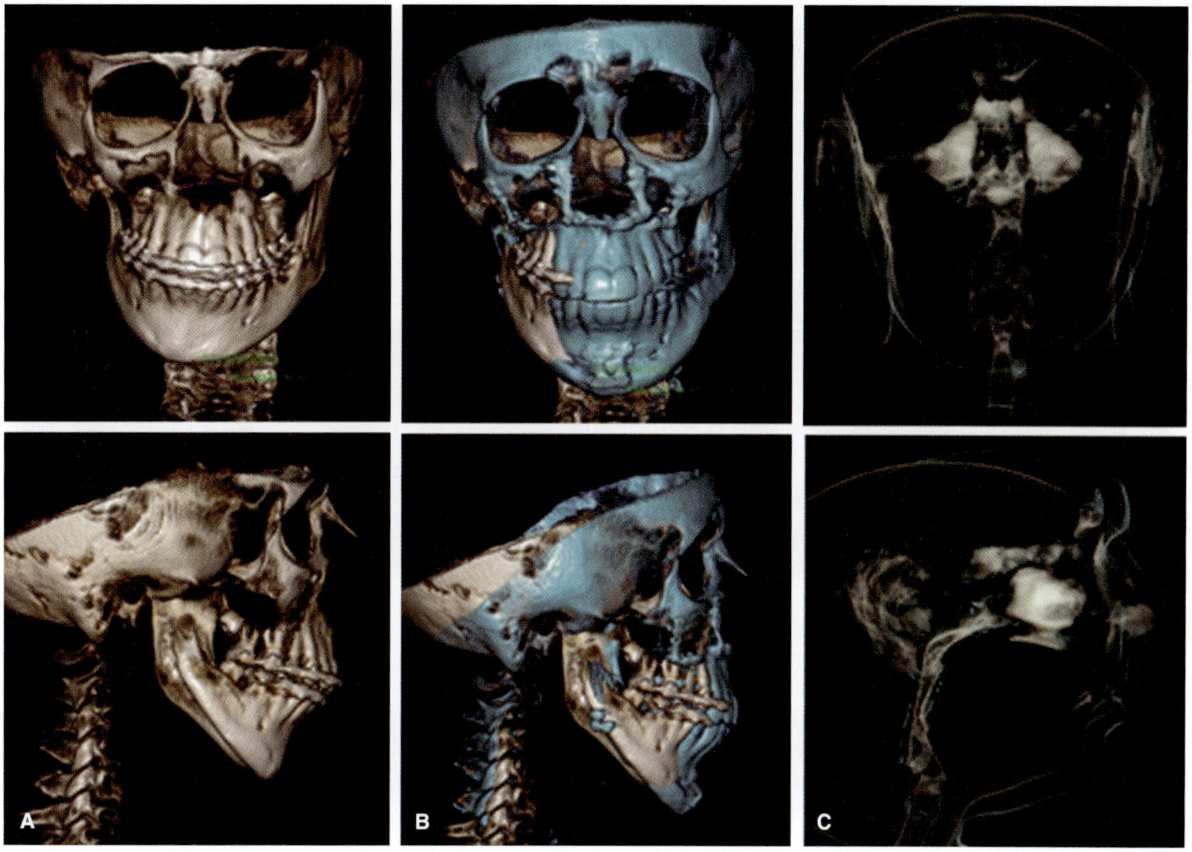

Figure 23.10 CBCT images. *A*: Before orthognathic surgery. *B*: Skeletal superimposition at 3 years 2 months after orthognathic surgery. *C*: Soft-tissue superimposition at 3 years 2 months after orthognathic surgery.

mandibular hypoplasia in individuals with HFM, 3D CT was found to be superior for Type II cases (Takahashi-Ichikawa *et al.*, 2013). In another study comparing two methods of quantifying mandibular asymmetry using CBCT image volumes, no differences were found between mirroring on the midsagittal plane versus registering on the cranial base (Cevidanes *et al.*, 2011). The advantages of CBCT in both the diagnosis and treatment of facial asymmetries are discussed in detail in Chapter 21.

22q11.2 Deletion Syndrome

3D imaging, particularly MRI and 3dMD cranial imaging systems, is being used widely to study 22q11.2 Deletion Syndrome, also known as Velocardiofacial Syndrome (VCFS). This genetic condition is associated with more than 180 clinical features and more than 25 dysmorphic craniofacial features (Oberoi *et al.*, 2011). Ruotolo and coworkers (2006) assessed one of these features, the abnormal velopharyngeal (VP) structure in individuals with 22q11.2 Deletion Syndrome by using 3D MRI analysis. This technique provides an accurate, reproducible, and quantifiable assessment of VP structures in 3D without having to expose the subject to ionizing radiation. By using 3D MRI analysis, Ruotolo and associates (2006) were able to demonstrate that individuals with the syndrome showed greater anterior and posterior cranial base and atlanto-dental angles. In addition, greater pharyngeal cavity volume and width and smaller tonsillar and adenoid volumes all contributed to VP dysfunction.

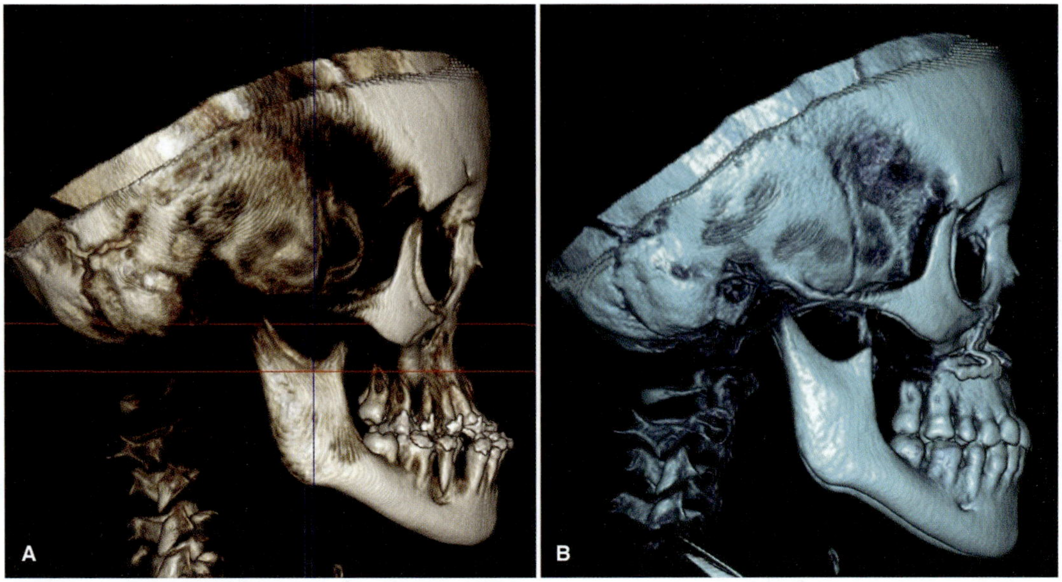

Figure 23.11 CBCT scans of a 17-year-old girl with Down Syndrome before (*A*) and after (*B*) a Le Fort I advancement. (Reprinted with permission from Ohtani *et al.*, 2012.)

The 3dMD cranial imaging system also has been developed to quantify facial dysmorphology in 22q11.2 Deletion Syndrome (Wilamowska *et al.*, 2012). This new methodology not only is useful in discriminating between 22q11.2 Deletion Syndrome individuals and the general population, but also can be used to study detailed characteristics in patients with any craniofacial condition.

Down Syndrome (DS)

The phenotypic expression of trisomy 21, or DS, produces variable, yet characteristic facial morphology. Although certain facial features have been documented quantitatively and qualitatively as characteristic of DS (e.g., epicanthic folds, macroglossia, and hypertelorism), all of these traits occur in other craniofacial conditions with an underlying genetic cause. Nonetheless, orthodontists and oromaxillofacial surgeons must contend with common dentoskeletal imbalances that contribute to malocclusion in DS patients. Maxillary hypoplasia (both sagittally and vertically), Class III malocclusion, and bilateral posterior crossbite are common in DS patients (Alio *et al.*, 2011). CBCT is useful in orthodontic and surgical treatment planning for these individuals. Figure 23.11 shows CBCT scans during pre-surgical orthodontic treatment and post-Le Fort I maxillary advancement in a DS patient.

While DS patients have a common set of phenotypic features, 3D imaging is being used to tease out subtle differences between DS patients to help us understand how trisomy 21 affects facial form. A recent study compared morphological integration patterns of immature DS faces with those of non-DS siblings, aged 6–12 years, using 3dMD facial images (Starbuck *et al.*, 2011). Facial features are affected differentially in DS, as evidenced by statistically significant differences in integration both within and between facial regions (Figure 23.12). These results suggest a differential effect of trisomy 21 on facial prominences during craniofacial development.

Cleidocranial dysplasia (CCD)

CCD presents with delayed exfoliation of primary teeth, delayed eruption or non-eruption of permanent teeth, presence of supernumerary teeth, and midface hypoplasia. The management of individu-

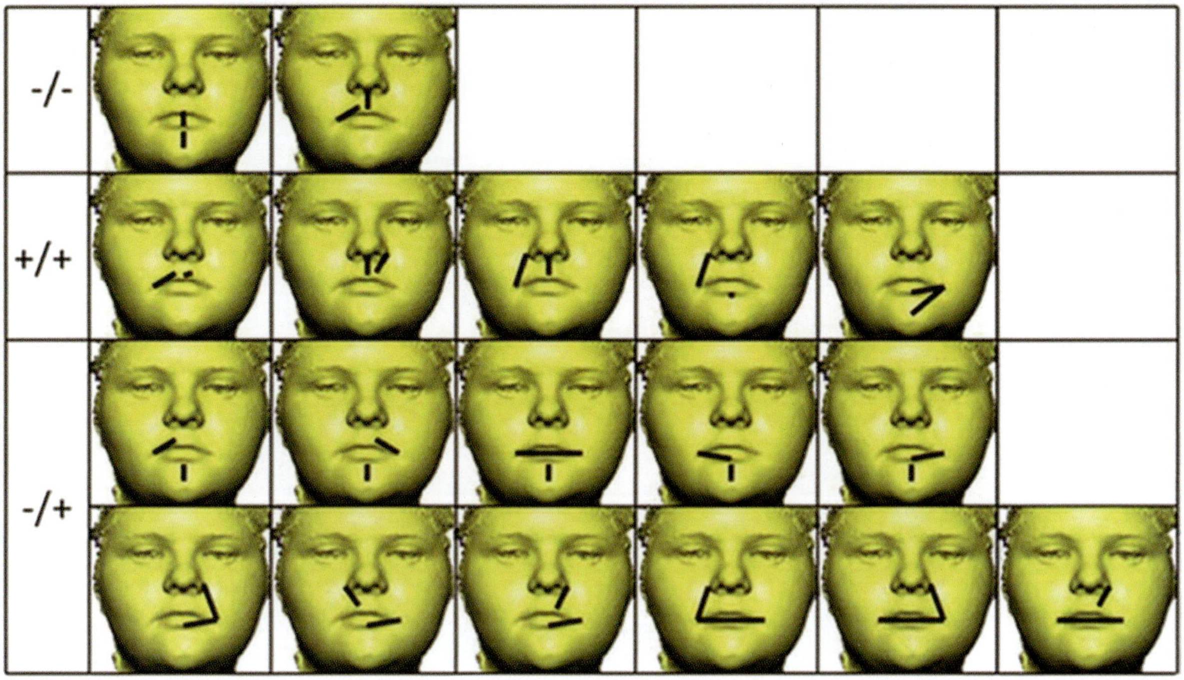

Figure 23.12 3D photography used to assess facial differences in children with Down Syndrome (DS) compared with their non-DS siblings. The findings demonstrated 18 lower face measurements (black lines) that were correlated either negatively in both DS and non-DS groups (−/−), positively in both DS and non-DS groups (+/+), or negatively in the DS group and positively in the non-DS group (−/+) when the DS is compared with the non-DS group. (Reprinted with permission from Starbuck *et al.*, 2011.)

als with CCD is challenging and requires comprehensive orthodontic and surgical treatment (Ishii *et al.*, 1998). In these and similar patients, CBCT is used routinely to provide a 3D image of the jaws and teeth, resulting in less guesswork and a more accurate anatomical location of the supernumerary and impacted teeth (Oberoi & Knueppel, 2012). 3D imaging provides precise location of a supernumerary tooth in relation to structures such as the cortex of the nasal floor, labial cortex of the nasal ridge, nasopalatine duct, or adjacent root apices (Figure 23.13). Accurate localization results in minimally invasive surgery and planning for the most effective orthodontic tooth movements (Dalessandri *et al.*, 2011). CT images allow visualization for best placement of TADs for orthodontic tooth movement that often is required in these patients due to multiple missing teeth (Kuroda *et al.*, 2007). All of the information derived from CBCT greatly improves the orthodontic and surgical treatment of CCD patients.

Ectodermal dysplasia (ED)

ED is characterized by poor development of ectodermal derivatives, including enamel, sweat glands, and hair. The need for comprehensive dental treatment to replace anomalous teeth in ED patients is a challenge for restorative dentists and orthodontists. Dental implants often are the treatment of choice for ED patients. CBCT imaging can provide valuable information for the placement of endosseous dental implants. As discussed previously, the evaluation of the quantity and quality of bone on CBCT scans helps in identifying optimal sites for the implant, thereby enhancing the chances of success. CBCT scans also can

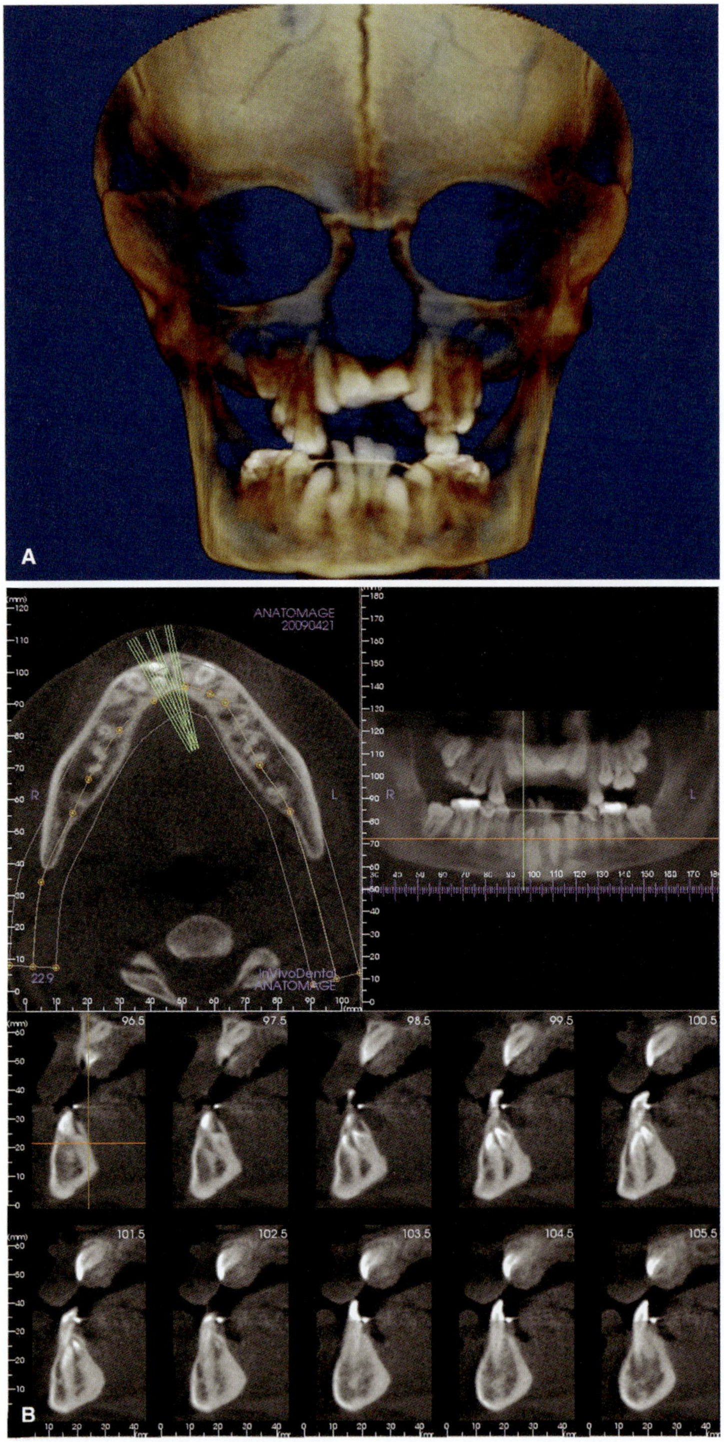

Figure 23.13 Volumetric (*A*) and segmental (*B*) CBCT images of a patient with cleidocranial dysplasia showing impacted and supernumerary teeth.

provide useful visualization of neighboring structures such as tooth roots, the mandibular canal, and maxillary sinus floor (Scarfe *et al.*, 2009). The indications for implant placement in the growing child have been described and the decision for implant placement is based not only on growth, but also on the number and location of the missing teeth (Sharma & Vargervik, 2006). A recent study identified detailed morphologic characteristics and growth and treatment changes by using a non-invasive 3D computerized digitizer on facial soft tissue (Dellavia *et al.*, 2010). During the first time point (8–11 years), the growth of all facial measurements was reduced in ED subjects compared with control subjects. During this interval, most of the ED children underwent a functional and/or prosthetic treatment. During adolescence, the width and height of the lower and upper facial thirds showed more increase in ED subjects than in control subjects, while all facial depths and all distances in the middle facial third remained deficient. These data demonstrate the important point that a disorder such as ED, with its well-known abnormalities in ectodermal derivatives, has much broader systemic effects of which the clinical team treating these patients must be aware. 3D imaging is proving to be an important tool to ensure that ED patients are diagnosed accurately and that appropriate treatment plans are made for orthodontic care.

RARE SYNDROMES

As access to and accuracy of genetic testing improve, rare syndromes may prove to be valuable for expanding our understanding of the genetic control of craniofacial development and growth. Combining 3D imaging with advanced genetic testing could prove to be a powerful combination for establishing a database of detailed phenotyping of known genotypes. This database then could be used to better understand the cause of mutations (random, environmental, or inherited) and lead to potential gene-targeted treatments. In this section, we will discuss briefly some rare syndromes for which 3D images are available.

Oculofacialcardiodental Syndrome (OFCD)

OFCD is an X-linked condition with characteristic ocular, cardiac, facial, and dental anomalies in affected females. It is lethal in males. The most typical dental abnormality is radiculomegaly. The roots of permanent teeth, particularly canines, can continue to grow until they reach the cortical plate of the orbit or the lower border of the mandible. Other findings include delayed tooth development and eruption, oligodontia, retained primary teeth, and variable root length (Figure 23.14; Oberoi *et al.*, 2005).

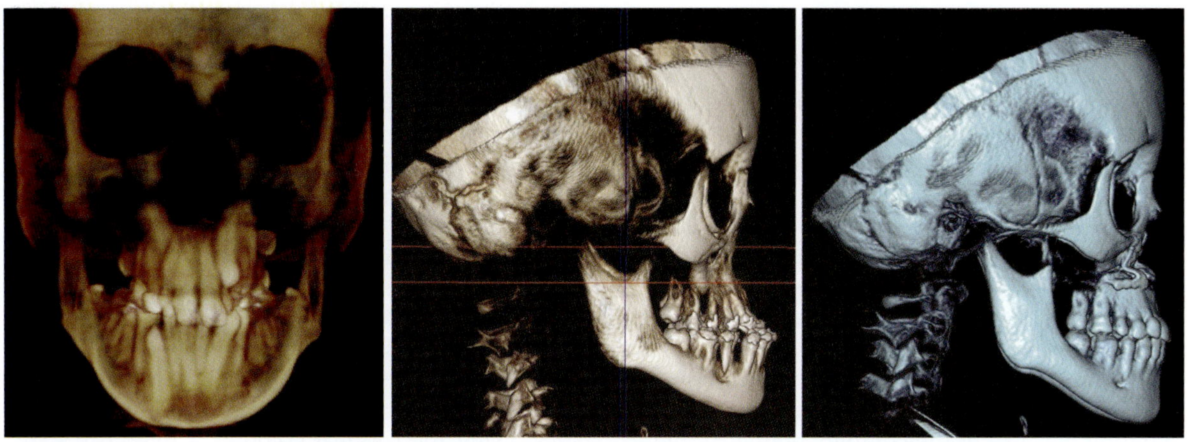

Figure 23.14 CBCT scan of a 16-year-old girl with OFCD Syndrome with radioculomegaly of the canines.

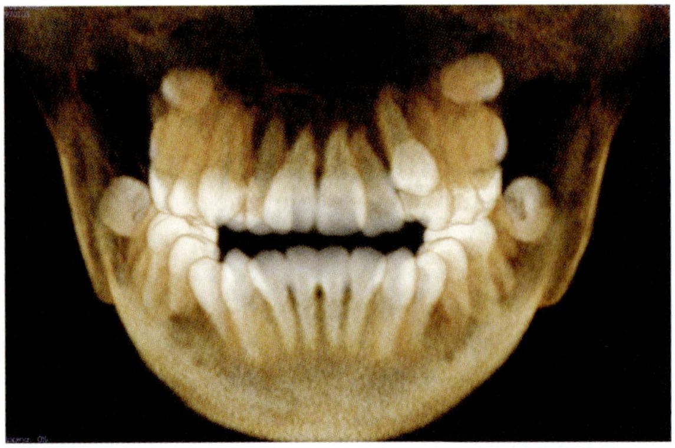

Figure 23.15 CBCT scan of a 14-year-old girl with Neonatal Onset Multisystem Inflammatory Disease Syndrome (NOMID). Children with this rare syndrome present with midface deficiency and frontal bossing. This scan demonstrates significant maxillary crowding and anterior open bite that are the challenges facing the orthodontist and surgeon who will treat this patient.

Neonatal Onset Multisystem Inflammatory Disease Syndrome (NOMID)

NOMID Syndrome is a rare congenital inflammatory disorder characterized by a triad of neonatal onset of cutaneous symptoms, chronic meningitis, and joint manifestations with recurrent fever and inflammation. Distinctive facies with characteristic frontal bossing and protruding eyes have been described. While midface hypoplasia has not been reported in these patients, Figure 23.15 shows CBCT image of a 14-year-old NOMID patient who has midface hypoplasia.

Incontinentia Pigmenti Syndrome (IP)

IP is a rare X-linked anomaly seen in females. As with OFCD, IP is lethal in males. In addition to skin manifestation, dental anomalies are found in 60% of IP patients. The most common findings are peg- or cone-shaped teeth. Late or incomplete eruption of teeth, oligodontia, dental agenesis, and mineralization defects are other dental anomalies. IP can affect both primary and permanent dentition, the latter more severely. CBCT is useful in treatment planning because of the complex dental problems with which IP patients often present. Figure 23.16 shows CBCT images of a 7-year-old girl with IP and multiple missing teeth.

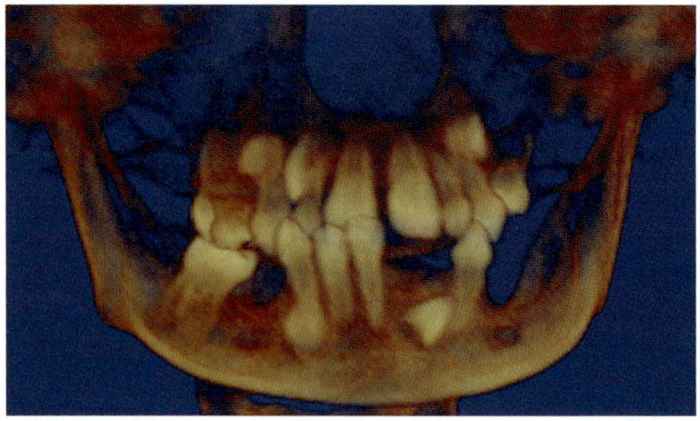

Figure 23.16 CBCT scan of a 7-year-old girl with Incontinentia Pigmenti Syndrome (IP). Another of the rare syndromes that have significant dental findings, IP is seen only in females because this X-linked mutation is lethal in males. Dental anomalies occur in 60% of IP patients. Peg- or cone-shaped teeth are seen most often, along with late or incomplete eruption of teeth. Oligodontia, dental agenesis, and mineralization defects are other dental anomalies. Many of these problems can be seen in this 3D volumetric image of a 8-year-old IP patient. With such a complex malocclusion, it is clear that the orthodontist, restorative dentist, and surgeon who will treat her will benefit from having the 3D images to map out their treatment strategy.

Cervical vertebral anomalies (CVA)

Orthodontists analyze the cervical vertebrae for several reasons. First, the cervical vertebrae are used to estimate skeletal age of individuals being considered for orthodontic treatment. The cervical spine previously was analyzed on the lateral cephalogram, sometimes in conjunction with hand–wrist radiographs and observations used to aid the orthodontist in the prediction of future growth, which is important in the orthodontic treatment plan. Second, cervical vertebrae anomalies (CVA) have been found to occur in individuals with CL/P, different dento-skeletal malocclusions, and craniofacial syndromes. Finally, an individual's natural head position commonly is assessed in orthodontics, using the cervical spine as a reference structure on the lateral cephalograms. The use of CBCT

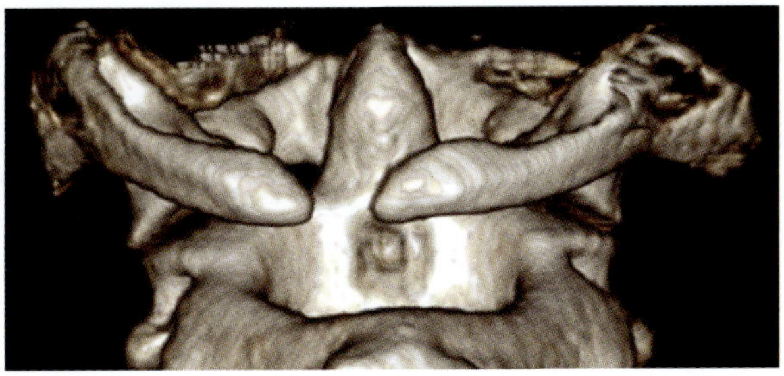

Figure 23.17 Surface rendering of a CBCT scan showing posterior arch deficiency of the first cervical vertebrae in a 10-year-old child with CL/P.

allows detailed analysis of structures, and programs can be developed to recognize and compare shape and size changes during growth (Miller, 2007). 3D imaging has increased diagnostic accuracy for CVA over conventional 2D and CBCT-generated cephalograms (Bebnowski *et al.*, 2012). In fact, there is a significant increase in false-positive CVA diagnosis on 2D radiographs, leading to an over-reported prevalence of CVA.

Several studies have described CVA in clefts and other craniofacial anomalies (Osborne *et al.*, 1971; Farman *et al.*, 1979; Shprintzen *et al.*, 1985; Lima *et al.*, 2009). The most common CVA is fusion, occurring most frequently between the second and third cervical vertebrae (C2-C3). The condition generally is asymptomatic, but increasing age or injury may precipitate symptoms (Yochum & Rowe, 2005). There is a high incidence of CVA, particularly fusions in hemifacial microsomia (Tsirikos & McMaster, 2006). A recent CBCT study found that 14% of individuals studied who had CL/P also had CVA (Figure 23.17; Maxfield *et al.*, 2012). Finally, an incidental finding on CBCT in an orthodontic patient showed cleft of the atlas vertebrae (Rogers *et al.*, 2011). Accurate diagnosis is important for these patients, who often undergo orthognathic surgery under general anesthesia with intubation, which exposes them to neck extension.

Vascular malformations

Vascular anomalies, particularly in the head and neck regions, often are difficult to treat due to complexities of diagnosis (Kramer *et al.*, 2011). They are subdivided into hemangiomas and vascular malformations. Vascular malformation is classified into high flow and low flow, with the latter accounting for more than 90% of all malformations. It is imperative that the imaging technology used for diagnosis is able to differentiate between the two for correct diagnosis (Flors *et al.*, 2011). MRI and ultrasound have been the imaging methods of choice, but over the past decade, magnetic resonance angiography (MRA) has been developed as an alternative imaging method to delineate size, location, and tissue involvement (Kramer *et al.*, 2011). Recently, 3D contrast-enhanced time-resolved MRA, which combines conventional MRI and high-radiation 3D CT angiography (CTA), uses parallel imaging to provide non-invasive comprehensive evaluation of vascular malformations by showing separation between arteries and veins, draining veins, and clear demarcation of the arterio-venous malformation (AVM; Oleaga *et al.*, 2010). The authors concluded that this imaging modality is a good alternative to more invasive digital subtraction catheter angiography (DSA), which is the standard technique for diagnosing and assessing intracranial AVM (Yilmaz *et al.*, 2011).

GROWTH AND TREATMENT CHANGES ASSESSED BY 3D TECHNIQUES

Current 3D imaging techniques can provide detailed measures of mandibular growth. Cevidanes and colleagues (2005) used high-resolution MRI scans to analyze the direction of growth and qualitative 3D growth visualizations positioned with skeletal landmarks. Medical software packages have allowed for the creation of 3D virtual models in the form of triangular mesh called stereolithograph (STL) from threshold segmented images. These 3D virtual models are powerful clinical tools for comparing 3D anatomic surfaces. STL files from successive years can be compared using software techniques for rapid prototyping and object verification. This method allows for production of a 3D deviation map between virtual models.

CBCT data also can be used to create a numerical growth map that illustrates the direction and magnitude of growth at different ages. Reynolds and coworkers (2011) evaluated 3D mandibular growth for an adolescent male patient using consecutive CBCT scans. 3D virtual models were created from the CBCT scans using medical software.

Surface scanning to study facial growth in 3D was used in the Cardiff 3D Facial Study (Kau & Richmond, 2008). This method will play an important role in the future in the study of growth, in diagnosis and treatment planning, and in the study of treatment outcomes. In the future, it is expected that 3D imaging will be used to establish population norms and, along with genome-wide association studies, will be utilized for establishing genotype–phenotype relationships.

CONCLUSIONS

Several ongoing technological advances in 3D imaging including CBCT are likely to continue its increased use in diagnosing and treatment planning of complex cases. For example, 3D imaging rapidly is replacing 2D imaging in diagnosis, treatment planning, and outcomes studies, particularly in patients with CFA. Its use in establishing population norms also likely will expand, so that together with genome-wide association studies, it will help in defining genotype–phenotype relationships. These technologies are likely to lead to increasing feasibility of facial animations for biometric identification and facial recognition. Virtual simulation for surgical planning and splint fabrication will become the standard of care. Recent advances in computer vision will automate image analyses and interpretation tasks, decreasing time of processing and human error. The future of 3D imaging in diagnosis and treatment planning of craniofacial anomalies will include "dynamic facial imaging" that will provide normative data for facial movements and post-surgical functional outcomes.

References

Abramson, Z., Susarla, S., Troulis, M., *et al.* (2009) Age-related changes of the upper airway assessed by 3-dimensional computed tomography. *Journal of Craniofacial Surgery*, 20 (Suppl 1), 657–663.

Alio, J., Lorenzo, J., Iglesias, M.C., *et al.* (2011) Longitudinal maxillary growth in Down syndrome patients. *The Angle Orthodontist*, 81 (2), 253–259.

Baumler, M., Faure, J.M., Bigorre, M., *et al.* (2011) Accuracy of prenatal three-dimensional ultrasound in the diagnosis of cleft hard palate when cleft lip is present. *Ultrasound in Obstetrics & Gynecology*, 38 (4), 440–444.

Bebnowski, D., Hanggi, M.P., Markic, G., *et al.* (2012) Cervical vertebrae anomalies in subjects with Class II malocclusion assessed by lateral cephalogram and cone beam computed tomography. *European Journal of Orthodontics*, 34 (2), 226–231.

Beegun, I., Dua, R., Connor, S., *et al.* (2012) Prenatal diagnosis and management of a craniofacial glioma detected at 20 weeks' gestation: case report and review of the literature. *International Journal of Oral and Maxillofacial Surgery*, 41 (2), 200–202.

Bell, R.B. (2011) Computer planning and intraoperative navigation in orthognathic surgery. *Journal of Oral and Maxillofacial Surgery*, 69 (3), 592–605.

Benavides, E., Rios, H.F., Ganz, S.D., *et al.* (2012) Use of cone beam computed tomography in implant dentistry: the International Congress of Oral Implantologists Consensus Report. *Implant Dentistry*, 21 (2), 78–86.

Bergland, O., Semb, G., & Abyholm, F.E. (1986) Elimination of the residual alveolar cleft by secondary bone grafting and subsequent orthodontic treatment. *Cleft Palate Journal*, 23 (3), 175–205.

Boeddinghaus, R. & Whyte, A. (2008) Current concepts in maxillofacial imaging. *European Journal of Radiology*, 66 (3), 396–418.

Boyle, C.M. & Rosenblum, J.D. (1997) Three-dimensional CT for pre- and post-surgical imaging of patients with craniosynostosis: correlation of operative procedure and radiologic imaging. *American Journal of Roentgenology*, 169 (4), 1173–1177.

Campbell, S., Lees, C., Moscosco, G., *et al.* (2005) Ultrasound antenatal diagnosis of cleft palate by a new technique: the 3D "reverse face" view. *Ultrasound in Obstetrics & Gynecology*, 25 (1), 12–18.

Cevidanes, L.H., Franco, A.A., Gerig, G., *et al.* (2005) Assessment of mandibular growth and response to orthopedic treatment with 3-dimensional magnetic resonance images. *American Journal of Orthodontics and Dentofacial Orthopedics*, 128 (1), 16–26.

Cevidanes, L.H., AlHadidi, A., Paniagua, B., *et al.* (2011) Three-dimensional quantification of mandibular asymmetry through cone-beam computerized tomography. *Oral Surgery, Oral Medicine, Oral Pathology, Oral Radiology, and Endodontology*, 111 (6), 757–770.

Chen, M.L., Chang, C.H., Yu, C.H., *et al.* (2001) Prenatal diagnosis of cleft palate by three-dimensional ultrasound. *Ultrasound in Medicine & Biology*, 27 (8), 1017–1023.

da Silva Filho, O.G., Teles, S.G., Ozawa, T.O., *et al.* (2000) Secondary bone graft and eruption of the permanent canine in patients with alveolar clefts: literature review and case report. *The Angle Orthodontist*, 70 (2), 174–178.

Dalessandri, D., LaFranchi, L., Tonni, I., *et al.* (2011) Advantages of cone beam computed tomography (CBCT) in the orthodontic treatment planning of cleidocranial dysplasia patients: a case report. *Head & Face Medicine*, 7, 6.

Danelson, K.A., Gordon, E.S., David, L.R., *et al.* (2009) Using a three dimensional model of the pediatric skull for pre-operative planning in the treatment of craniosynostosis: Biomed 2009. *Biomedical Sciences Instrumentation*, 45, 358–363.

de Moraes, M.E., Hollender, L.G., Chen, C.S., *et al.* (2011) Evaluating craniofacial asymmetry with digital cephalometric images and cone-beam computed tomography. *American Journal of Orthodontics and Dentofacial Orthopedics*, 139 (6), e523–e531.

Dellavia, C., Catti, F., Sforza, C., *et al.* (2010) Craniofacial growth in ectodermal dysplasia: an 8 year longitudinal evaluation of Italian subjects. *The Angle Orthodontist*, 80 (4), 733–739.

Donatsky, O., Bjorn-Jorgensen, J., Holmqvist-Larsen, M., *et al.* (1997) Computerized cephalometric evaluation of orthognathic surgical precision and stability in relation to maxillary superior repositioning combined with mandibular advancement or setback. *Journal of Oral and Maxillofacial Surgery*, 55 (10), 1071–1079.

Drake, A.F., Davis, J.U., & Warren, D.W. (1993) Nasal airway size in cleft and noncleft children. *The Laryngoscope*, 103 (8), 915–917.

Elia, D., Garel, C., Enjolras, O., *et al.* (2008) Prenatal imaging findings in rapidly involuting congenital hemangioma of the skull. *Ultrasound in Obstetrics & Gynecology*, 31 (5), 572–575.

Estroff, J.A. (2012) Imaging clues in the prenatal diagnosis of syndromes and aneuploidy. *Pediatric Radiology*, 42 (Suppl 1), 5–23.

Farman, A.G., Nortje, C.J., & Joubert, J.J. (1979) Radiographic profile of the first cervical vertebra. *Journal of Anatomy*, 128 (Pt 3), 595–600.

Flors, L., Leiva-Salinas, C., Maged, I.M., *et al.* (2011) MR imaging of soft-tissue vascular malformations: diagnosis, classification, and therapy follow-up. *Radiographics*, 31 (5), 1321–1340.

Fukushiro, A.P. & Trindade, I.E. (2005) Nasal airway dimensions of adults with cleft lip and palate: differences among cleft types. *Cleft Palate—Craniofacial Journal*, 42 (2), 396–402.

Gateno, J., Xia, J.J., Teichgraeber, J.F., *et al.* (2007) Clinical feasibility of computer-aided surgical simulation (CASS) in the treatment of complex cranio-maxillofacial deformities. *Journal of Oral and Maxillofacial Surgery*, 65 (4), 728–834.

Ginsberg, N.A., Cohen, L., Dungan, J.S., *et al.* (2011) 3-D ultrasound of the fetal ear and fetal autosomal trisomies: a pilot study of a new screening protocol. *Prenatal Diagnosis*, 31 (3), 311–314.

Gracco, A., Lombardo, L., Cozzani, M., *et al.* (2008) Quantitative cone-beam computed tomography evaluation of palatal bone thickness for orthodontic miniscrew placement. *American Journal of Orthodontics and Dentofacial Orthopedics*, 134 (3), 361–369.

Guijarro-Martinez, R. & Swennen, G.R. (2011) Cone-beam computerized tomography imaging and analysis of the upper airway: a systematic review of the literature. *International Journal of Oral Maxillofacial Surgery*, 40 (11), 1227–1237.

Hairfield, W.M., Warren, D.W., & Seaton, D.L. (1988) Prevalence of mouthbreathing in cleft lip and palate. *Cleft Palate Journal*, 25 (2), 135–138.

Hamada, Y., Kondoh, T., Nakaoka, K., *et al.* (2000) Magnetic resonance imaging findings and clinical symptoms in the temporomandibular joint in patients with mandibular continuity defects. *Journal of Oral Maxillofacial Surgery*, 58 (5), 487–493.

Hatcher, D.C. (2012) Cone beam computed tomography: craniofacial and airway analysis. *Dental Clinics of North America*, 56 (2), 343–357.

Huisinga-Fischer, C.E., Zonneveld, F.W., Vaandrager, J.M., *et al.* (2001) Relationship in hypoplasia between the masticatory muscles and the craniofacial skeleton in hemifacial microsomia, as determined by 3-D CT imaging. *Journal of Craniofacial Surgery*, 12 (1), 31–40.

Imamura, N., Ono, T., Hiyama, S., *et al.* (2002) Comparison of the sizes of adenoidal tissues and upper airways of subjects with and without cleft lip and palate. *American Journal of Orthodontics and Dentofacial Orthopedics*, 122 (2), 189–194.

Ishii, K., Nielsen, I.L., & Vargervik, K. (1998) Characteristics of jaw growth in cleidocranial dysplasia. *Cleft Palate–Craniofacial Journal*, 35 (2), 161–166.

Iwasaki, T., Hayasaki, H., Takemoto, Y., *et al.* (2009) Oropharyngeal airway in children with Class III malocclusion evaluated by cone-beam computed tomography. *American Journal of Orthodontics and Dentofacial Orthopedics*, 136 (3), 318.e1–e9.

Jayaratne, Y.S., Zwahlen, R.A., Lo, J., *et al.* (2010) Three-dimensional color maps: a novel tool for assessing craniofacial changes. *Surgical Innovation*, 17 (3), 198–205.

Kapila, S., Conley, R.S., & Harrell, W.E., Jr. (2011) The current status of cone beam computed tomography imaging in orthodontics. *Dentomaxillofacial Radiology*, 40 (1), 24–34.

Kau, C.H. & Richmond, S. (2008) Three-dimensional analysis of facial morphology surface changes in untreated children from 12 to 14 years of age. *American Journal of Orthodontics and Dentofacial Orthopedics*, 134 (6), 751–760.

Kim, S.H., Choi, Y.S., Hwang, E.H., *et al.* (2007) Surgical positioning of orthodontic mini-implants with guides fabricated on models replicated with cone-beam computed tomography. *American Journal of Orthodontics and Dentofacial Orthopedics*, 131 (Suppl 4), S82–S89.

Kim, Y.J., Hong, J.S., Hwang, Y.I., *et al.* (2010) Three-dimensional analysis of pharyngeal airway in preadolescent children with different anteroposterior skeletal patterns. *American Journal of Orthodontics and Dentofacial Orthopedics*, 137 (3), 306.e1–306.e11.

King, K.S., Lam, E.W., Faulkner, M.G., *et al.* (2007) Vertical bone volume in the paramedian palate of adolescents: a computed tomography study. *American Journal of Orthodontics and Dentofacial Orthopedics*, 132 (6), 783–788.

Krakow, D., Santulli, T., & Platt, L.D. (2001) Use of three-dimensional ultrasonography in differentiating craniosynostosis from severe fetal molding. *Journal of Ultrasound in Medicine*, 20 (4), 427–431.

Kramer, U., Ernemann, U., Fenchel, M., *et al.* (2011) Pretreatment evaluation of peripheral vascular malformations using low-dose contrast-enhanced time-resolved 3D MR angiography: initial results in 22 patients. *American Journal of Roentgenology*, 196 (3), 702–711.

Kuroda, S., Yanagita, T., Kyung, H.M., *et al.* (2007) Titanium screw anchorage for traction of many impacted teeth in a patient with cleidocranial dysplasia. *American Journal of Orthodontics and Dentofacial Orthopedics*, 131 (5), 666–669.

Lima, M.C., Franco, E.J., Janson, G., *et al.* (2009) Prevalence of upper cervical vertebrae anomalies in patients with cleft lip and/or palate and noncleft patients. *Cleft Palate–Craniofacial Journal*, 46, 481–486.

Lubbers, H.T., Medinger, L., Kruse, A., *et al.* (2010) Precision and accuracy of the 3dMD photogrammetric system in craniomaxillofacial application. *Journal of Craniofacial Surgery*, 21 (3), 763–767.

Luedders, D.W., Bohlmann, M.K., Germer, U., *et al.* (2011) Fetal micrognathia: objective assessment and associated anomalies on prenatal sonogram. *Prenatal Diagnosis*, 31 (2), 146–151.

Mailath-Pokorny, M., Worda, C., Krampl-Bettelheim, E., *et al.* (2010) What does magnetic resonance imaging add to the prenatal ultrasound diagnosis of facial clefts? *Ultrasound in Obstetrics & Gynecology*, 36 (4), 445–451.

Marsh, J.L., Baca, D., & Vannier, M.W. (1989) Facial musculoskeletal asymmetry in hemifacial microsomia. *Cleft Palate Journal*, 26, 292–302.

Maxfield, B., Doughlas, S., & Oberoi, S. (2012) Cervical spine abnormalities in individuals with craniofacial anomalies. University of California San Francisco Research Day poster presentation. *Informationen aus Orthodontie & Kieferorthopädie*. Submitted for publication.

Meazzini, M.C., Allevia, F., Mazzoleni, F., *et al.* (2012) Long-term follow-up of syndromic craniosynostosis after Le Fort III halo distraction: a cephalometric and CT evaluation. *Journal of Plastic Reconstronstructive and Aesthetic Surgery*, 65 (4), 464–472.

Medina, L.S. (2000) Three-dimensional CT maximum intensity projections of the calvaria: a new approach for diagnosis of craniosynostosis and fractures. *American Journal of Neuroradiology*, 21 (10), 1951–1954.

Merz, E. & Abramowicz, J.S. (2012) 3D/4D ultrasound in prenatal diagnosis: is it time for routine use? *Clinical Obstetrics and Gynecology*, 55 (1), 336–351.

Miller, G. (2007) Growth prediction based on a three-dimensional assessment of cervical vertebrae. Master's Thesis. University of California, San Francisco.

Munch, E.M., Cisek, L.J., Jr., & Roth, D.R. (2009) Magnetic resonance imaging for prenatal diagnosis of multisystem disease: megacystis microcolon intestinal hypoperistalsis syndrome. *Urology*, 74 (3), 592–594.

Nawa, H., Oberoi, S., & Vargervik, K. (2008) Taurodontism and Van der Woude syndrome: is there an association? *The Angle Orthodontist*, 78 (5), 832–837.

Nopoulos, P., Richman, L., Andreasen, N.C., *et al.* (2007) Abnormal brain structure in adults with Van der Woude syndrome. *Clinical Genetics*, 71 (6), 511–517.

Nopoulos, P., Boes, A.D., Jabines, A., *et al.* (2010) Hyperactivity, impulsivity, and inattention in boys with cleft lip and palate: relationship to ventromedial prefrontal cortex morphology. *Journal of Neurodevelopmental Disorders*, 2 (4), 235–242.

Oberoi, S. & Knueppel, S. (2012) Three-dimensional assessment of impacted canines and root resorption using cone beam computed tomography. *Oral Surgery, Oral Medicine, Oral Pathology, Oral Radiology, and Endodontology*, 113 (2), 260–267.

Oberoi, S., Winder, A.E., Johnston, J., *et al.* (2005) Case reports of oculofacio-cardiodental syndrome with unusual dental findings. *American Journal of Medical Genetics Part A*, 136 (3), 275–277.

Oberoi, S., Chigurupati, R., Gill, P., *et al.* (2009) Volumetric assessment of secondary alveolar bone grafting using cone beam computed tomography. *Cleft Palate–Craniofacial Journal*, 46 (5), 503–511.

Oberoi, S., Gill, P., Chigurupati, R., *et al.* (2010) Three-dimensional assessment of the eruption path of the canine in individuals with bone-grafted alveolar clefts using cone beam computed tomography. *Cleft Palate–Craniofacial Journal*, 47 (5), 507–512.

Oberoi, S., Huynh, L., & Vargervik, K. (2011) Velopharyngeal, speech and dental characteristics as diagnostic aids in 22q11.2 deletion syndrome. *Journal of the California Dental Association*, 39 (5), 327–332.

Oberoi, S., Hoffman, W.Y., & Vargervik, K. (2012) Craniofacial team management in Apert syndrome. *American Journal of Orthodontics and Dentofacial Orthopedics*, 141 (Suppl 4), S82–S87.

Ohtani, J., Hoffman, W.Y., Vargervik, K., *et al.* (2012) Team management and treatment outcomes for patients with hemifacial microsomia. *American Journal of Orthodontics and Dentofacial Orthopedics*, 141 (Suppl 4), S74–S81.

Oleaga, L., Dalal, S.S., Weigele, J.B., *et al.* (2010) The role of time-resolved 3D contrast-enhanced MR angiography in the assessment and grading of cerebral arteriovenous malformations. *European Journal of Radiology*, 74 (3), e117–e121.

Olszewska, E., Sieskiewicz, A., Rozycki, J., *et al.* (2009) A comparison of cephalometric analysis using radiographs and craniofacial computed tomography in patients with obstructive sleep apnea syndrome: preliminary report. *European Archives of Otorhinolaryngoly*, 266 (4), 535–542.

Ono, I., Ohura, T., Narumi, E., *et al.* (1992) Three-dimensional analysis of craniofacial bones using three-dimensional computer tomography. *Journal of Craniomaxillofacial Surgery*, 20 (2), 49–60.

Orentlicher, G., Goldsmith, D., & Horowitz, A. (2010) Applications of 3-dimensional virtual computerized tomography technology in oral and maxillofacial surgery: current therapy. *Journal of Oral Maxillofacial Surgery*, 68 (8), 1933–1959.

Osborne, G.S., Pruzansky, S., & Koepp-Baker, H. (1971) Upper cervical spine anomalies and osseous nasopharyngeal depth. *Journal of Speech and Hearing Research*, 14 (1), 14–22.

Parisi, M., Mehdizadeh, H.M., Hunter, J.C., *et al.* (1989) Evaluation of craniosynostosis with three-dimensional CT imaging. *Journal of Computer Assisted Tomography*, 13 (6), 1006–1012.

Pena, W.A., Vargervik, K., Sharma, A., *et al.* (2009) The role of endosseous implants in the management of alveolar clefts. *Pediatric Dentistry*, 31 (4), 329–333.

Plooij, J.M., Maal, T.J., Haers, P., *et al.* (2011) Digital three-dimensional image fusion processes for planning and evaluating orthodontics and orthognathic surgery: a systematic review. *International Journal of Oral Maxillofacial Surgery*, 40 (4), 341–352.

Proffit, W.R., White, R.P., & Sarver, D.M. (2003) *Contemporary Treatment of Dentofacial Deformity*. Mosby, St. Louis, MO.

Rathnayaka, K., Momot, K.I., Noser, H., *et al.* (2012) Quantification of the accuracy of MRI generated 3D models of long bones compared to CT generated 3D models. *Medical Engineering and Physics*, 34 (3), 357–363.

Rathnayaka, K., Cowin, G., Schuetz, M.A., *et al.* (2013) Correction of step artefact associated with MRI scanning of long bones. *Medical Engineering and Physics*, 35 (7), 988–993.

Reynolds, M., Adeeb, S., & El-Bialy, T. (2011) 3-D volumetric evaluation of human mandibular growth. *Open Biomedical Engineering Journal*, 5, 83–89.

Robson, C.D. & Barnewolt, C.E. (2004) MR imaging of fetal head and neck anomalies. *Neuroimaging Clinics of North America*, 14 (2), 273–291.

Rogers, S.A., Drage, N., & Durning, P. (2011) Incidental findings arising with cone beam computed tomography imaging of the orthodontic patient. *The Angle Orthodontist*, 81 (2), 350–355.

Ronen, O., Malhotra, A., & Pillar, G. (2007) Influence of gender and age on upper-airway length during development. *Pediatrics*, 120 (4), e1028–e1034.

Ruotolo, R.A., Veitia, N.A., Corbin, A., *et al.* (2006) Velopharyngeal anatomy in 22q11.2 deletion syndrome: a three-dimensional cephalometric analysis. *Cleft Palate–Craniofacial Journal*, 43 (4), 446–456.

Scarfe, W.C., Levin, M.D., Gane, D., *et al.* (2009) Use of cone beam computed tomography in endodontics. *International Journal of Dentistry*, 2009, 634567.

Senggen, E., Laswed, T., Meuwly, J.Y., *et al.* (2011) First and second branchial arch syndromes: multimodality approach. *Pediatric Radiology*, 41 (5), 549–561.

Sforza, C., De Menezes, M., Bresciani, E., *et al.* (2012) Evaluation of a 3D stereo-photogrammetric technique to measure the stone casts of patients with unilateral cleft lip and palate. *Cleft Palate–Craniofac Journal*, 49 (4), 477–483.

Sharma, A.B. & Vargervik, K. (2006) Using implants for the growing child. *Journal of the California Dental Association*, 34 (9), 719–724.

Shprintzen, R.J., Siegel-Sadewitz, V.L., Amato, J., *et al.* (1985) Anomalies associated with cleft lip, cleft palate, or both. *American Journal of Medical Genetics Part A*, 20 (4), 585–595.

Smahel, Z., Kasalova, P., & Skvarilova, B. (1991) Morphometric nasopharyngeal characteristics in facial clefts. *Journal of Craniofacial Genetics and Developmental Biology*, 11 (1), 24–32.

Starbuck, J., Reeves, R.H., & Richtsmeier, J. (2011) Morphological integration of soft-tissue facial morphology in Down Syndrome and siblings. *American Journal of Physical Anthropology*, 146 (4), 560–568.

Swennen, G.R., Mommaerts, M.Y., Abeloos, J., *et al.* (2009) A cone-beam CT based technique to augment the 3D virtual skull model with a detailed dental surface. *International Journal of Oral Maxillofacial Surgery*, 38 (1), 48–57.

Takahashi-Ichikawa, N., Susami, T., Nagahama, K., *et al.* (2013) Evaluation of mandibular hypoplasia in patients with hemifacial microsomia: a comparison between panoramic radiography and three-dimensional computed tomography. *Cleft Palate–Craniofacial Journal*, 50 (4), 381–387.

Timock, A.M., Cook, V., McDonald, T., *et al.* (2011) Accuracy and reliability of buccal bone height and thickness measurements from cone-beam computed tomography imaging. *American Journal of Orthodontics and Dentofacial Orthopedics*, 140 (5), 734–744.

Trindade, I.K., Mazzottini, R., Silva Filho, O.G., *et al.* (2005) Long-term radiographic assessment of secondary alveolar bone grafting outcomes in patients with alveolar clefts. *Oral Surgery, Oral Medicine, Oral Pathology, Oral Radiology, and Endodontology*, 100 (3), 271–277.

Trotman, C.A. (2011) Faces in 4 dimensions: why do we care, and why the fourth dimension? *American Journal of Orthodontics and Dentofacial Orthopedics*, 140 (6), 895–899.

Tsirikos, A.I. & McMaster, M.J. (2006) Goldenhar-associated conditions (hemifacial microsomia) and congenital deformities of the spine. *Spine*, 31 (13), e400–e407.

Turvey, T.A., Vig, K., Moriarty, J., *et al.* (1984) Delayed bone grafting in the cleft maxilla and palate: a retrospective multidisciplinary analysis. *American Journal of Orthodontics*, 86 (3), 244–256.

van Loon, B., Maal, T.J., Plooij, J.M., *et al.* (2010) 3D stereophotogrammetric assessment of pre- and post-operative volumetric changes in the cleft lip and palate nose. *International Journal of Oral Maxillofacial Surgery*, 39 (6), 534–540.

Vargervik, K., Rubin, M.S., Grayson, B.H., *et al.* (2012) Parameters of care for craniosynostosis: dental and orthodontic perspectives. *American Journal of Orthodontics and Dentofacial Orthopedics*, 141 (Suppl 4), S68–S73.

Wilamowska, K., Wu, J., Heike, C., *et al.* (2012) Shape-based classification of 3D facial data to support 22q11.2DS craniofacial research. *Journal of Digital Imaging*, 25 (3), 400–408.

Willinger, M., Hoffman, H.J., & Hartford, R.B. (1994) Infant sleep position and risk for sudden infant death syndrome: report of meeting held January 13 and 14, 1994, National Institutes of Health, Bethesda, MD. *Pediatrics*, 93 (5), 814–819.

Worthington, P., Rubenstein, J., & Harcher, D.C. (2010) The role of cone-beam computed tomography in the planning and placement of implants. *Journal of the American Dental Association*, 141 (Suppl 3), 19S–24S.

Xia, J.J., Gateno, J., Teichgraeber, J.F., *et al.* (2007) Accuracy of the computer-aided surgical simulation (CASS) system in the treatment of patients with complex craniomaxillofacial deformity: a pilot study. *Journal of Oral and Maxillofacial Surgery*, 65 (2), 248–254.

Yilmaz, K.B., Canter, H.I., Vargel, I., *et al.* (2011) Use of three-dimensional MRI-angiography in preoperative evaluation and postoperative management of hemangiomas of head and neck region. *Journal of Craniofacial Surgery*, 22 (5), 1814–1818.

Yochum, R.L. & Rowe, L.J. (2005) *Essentials of Skeletal Radiology*, 2nd ed. Lippincott/Williams & Wilkins, Philadelphia.

Yune, H.Y. (1993) Two-dimensional-three-dimensional reconstruction computed tomography techniques. *Dental Clinics of North America*, 37 (4), 613–626.

Zhou, W., Li, W., Lin, J., *et al.* (2013) Tooth lengths of the permanent upper incisors in patients with cleft lip and palate determined with cone beam computed tomography. *Cleft Palate–Craniofacial Journal*, 50 (1), 88–95.

Index

Note: Page numbers in *italics* represent figures; those in **bold**, tables.

Cone Beam Computed Tomography in Orthodontics: Indications, Insights, and Innovations, First Edition. Sunil D. Kapila.